THE COGNITIVE NE   ⌐NCE
OF MUSIC

THE COGNITIVE
NEUROSCIENCE OF
MUSIC

Edited by

ISABELLE PERETZ

Départment de Psychologie,
Université de Montréal, C.P. 6128,
Succ. Centre-Ville, Montréal,
Québec, H3C 3J7, Canada

and

ROBERT J. ZATORRE

Montreal Neurological Institute,
McGill University, Montreal,
Quebec, H3A 2B4, Canada

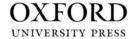

OXFORD
UNIVERSITY PRESS

OXFORD

UNIVERSITY PRESS

Great Clarendon Street, Oxford OX2 6DP

Oxford University Press is a department of the University of Oxford.
It furthers the University's objective of excellence in research, scholarship,
and education by publishing worldwide in

Oxford New York

Auckland Bangkok Buenos Aires Cape Town Chennai
Dar es Salaam Delhi Hong Kong Istanbul Karachi Kolkata
Kuala Lumpur Madrid Melbourne Mexico City Mumbai Nairobi
São Paulo Shanghai Taipei Tokyo Toronto

Oxford is a registered trade mark of Oxford University Press
in the UK and in certain other countries

Published in the United States
by Oxford University Press Inc., New York

A catalogue record for this title is available from the British Library

Library of Congress Cataloging in Publication Data

(Data available)

ISBN 0 19 852519 2 (Hbk)

0 19 852520 6 (Pbk)

10 9 8 7 6 5 4 3 2 1

Typeset by Newgen Imaging Systems (P) Ltd., Chennai, India
Printed in Great Britain
on acid-free paper by T.J. International Ltd, Padstow

PREFACE

Over the past decade there has been an explosion in research activities on music perception and performance, and their correlates in the human brain. This sudden increase in scientific work on music has been motivated in part by the idea that music offers a unique opportunity to better understand the organization of the human brain. The other major motivation for exploring the neural substrates of musical activities is that they may shed light on the functional origin and biological value of music. Like language, music exists in all human societies. Like language, music is a complex, rule-governed activity, and appears to be associated with a specific brain architecture. Moreover, sensitivity to musical structure develops early in life, without conscious effort, in the large majority of the population. Music also appears to be specific to humans, although some investigators have begun to examine its possible evolutionary origins in other species'.[1]

Unlike most other high-level functions of the human brain—and unlike language—only a minority of individuals become proficient performing musicians through explicit tutoring. This particularity in the distribution of acquired skills confers to music a privileged role in the study of brain plasticity. Another distinction from language is that a large variety of sensory-motor systems may be studied because of the many different ways of producing music. These variable modes of auditory expression enable interesting comparisons across systems.

Given both its similarities with language and its divergence from it, we believe that the relationship between music and the brain is of central importance for the domain of cognitive neuroscience. The fact that musical activities have generally been considered as an exquisite product of human culture, and as such are often assumed to be merely a cultural artifact, should not be taken as an impediment to achieving a scientific understanding of its underlying basis. In fact, we would argue that the cultural overlay associated with music confers upon it a key role for understanding the biology of human cognitive functions. Indeed, the ubiquity of music, its developmental features, and its brain substrates raise the question of the nature and the extent of its biological foundations, and how these interact with culture.

In this context, it is remarkable to note that the study of music as a major brain function has been relatively neglected. Neuropsychological questions related to musical abilities have been of occasional interest to neurologists and psychologists since the last century (e.g. Ref. 2 for pioneering work), but systematic, sustained investigations have been rare until recently. Several developments—both theoretical and technological—have created a profound change in the way in which music studies are perceived, thereby enabling us to present this volume as a beginning to the scientific study of the neurobiology of music. First, one should mention the development of cognitive psychology during the latter half of the twentieth century; cognitive psychologists were among the first to recognize the value of music as a means of studying perception, memory, attention, and performance (see Refs 2–5 for the three benchmark textbooks). Second, neuropsychology, which had always been based on knowledge from neurophysiology and neuroanatomy, began also to adopt experimental and cognitive paradigms, permitting advances in understanding lesion effects on musical functions. Third, developmental psychologists exploited new techniques that allowed them to probe the mind of even neonates. Finally, and most dramatically perhaps with the arrival on the scene of neuroimaging techniques such as fMRI and MEG, the stage was set for the explosion to which we alluded above, and which forms the core of the present volume.

The objective of the conference, from which most of the present texts are derived, was to demonstrate the dynamism and richness of the discipline. The conference was held in May 2000 in New York, and was initiated and sponsored by the *New York Academy of Science*. Major scientists from six different countries, working in a variety of interrelated disciplines and pursuing sustained research activities on music were invited to present their work. Most responded enthusiastically and addressed issues crucial to a better understanding of the neural substrates underlying musical functions. Their presentations first appeared in the *Annals of the New York Academy of Sciences*, volume 930, under the title 'The Biological Foundations of Music' in 2001. Given the success of this issue, Oxford University Press invited us to edit an updated version of it in their collection of books. We eagerly accepted and invited a few other major players in the field who originally presented a poster to publish a full chapter in the present volume. Therefore, you will find here an updated version of the 25 original chapters as well as three new chapters.

The contributions in the present volume will reveal how much progress has been made in the field over the last decade. Besides providing research overviews, many texts also delineate significant avenues for future research. Indeed, it is clear that this is a very young field still, and that much remains to be done. We hope that the material presented in this volume, coupled with an increase of interest for the biological foundations of music in the scientific and general community, represent the initial spark for building a solid and stimulating cognitive neuroscience of music.

I.P. and R.Z.

February 2003

References

1. **Wallin, N., B. Merker and S. Brown** (ed.) (2000) *The Origins of Music.* Cambridge, MA: MIT Press.
2. **Bouillaud, J.** (1865) Sur la faculté du langage articulé. *Bulletin de l'Académie de Médecine* 30, 752–68.
3. **Deutsch, D.** (ed.) (1982) *The Psychology of Music.* New York: Academic Press.
4. **Dowling, W. and D. Harwood** (1986) *Music Cognition.* Series in cognition and perception. New York. Academic Press.
5. **Sloboda, J.** (1985) *The Musical Mind: The Cognitive Psychology of Music.* London: Oxford University Press.

CONTENTS

Part IV Musical brain substrates

Part V Musical expertise/brain plasticity

Part VI Relation of music to other cognitive domains

LIST OF CONTRIBUTORS

Eckart O. Altenmüller Institut für Musikphysiologie und Musiker-Medizin der Hochschule für Musik und Theater Hannover, 30175 Hannover, Germany

Daisy Bertrand Laboratoire de Psychologie Expérimentale, CNRS UMR 8581, Université René Descartes, Institut de Psychologie, Centre Universitaire de Boulongne, 92774 Boulogne-Billancourt Cedex, France

Mireille Besson Language and Music Group, Institut de Neurosciences Physiologiques et Cognitives, CNRS, 31 ch. Joseph Aiguer, 13402 Marseille, Cedex 20, France

Jamshed J. Bharucha Language and Music Group, Institut de Neurosciences Physiologiques et Cognitives, CNRS, USA

Emmanuel Bigand Université de Bourgogne, LEAD-CNRS, Bd Gabriel, F-21000 Dijon, France

John C.M. Brust Department of Neurology, Harlem Hospital Center and Columbia University College of Physicians and Surgeons, New York, New York 10037, USA.

V. Candia Department of Psychology, University of Konstanz, Konstanz, Germany

Ian Cross Faculty of Music, University of Cambridge, West Road, Cambridge CB3 9DP, UK

Carolyn Drake Laboratoire de Psychologie Expérimentale, CNRS UMR 8581, Université René Descartes, Institut de Psychologie, Centre Universitaire de Boulogne, 92774 Boulogne-Billancourt Cedex, France

Nathalie Ehrlé Service de Neurologie, Hôpital Maison-Blanche, 45 Rue Cognacq-jay, 51092 Reims Cedex, France

T. Elbert Department of Psychology, University of Konstanz, Konstanz, Germany

A. Engelien Institute for Experimental Audiology, University of Münster, Münster, Germany

Timothy D. Griffiths Departments of Neurology and Physiological Sciences, Newcastle University Medical School, Newcastle-upon-Tyne NE2 4HH, United Kingdom

Andrea R. Halpern Psychology Department, Bucknell University, Lewisburg, Pennsylvania 17837, USA

David Huron School of Music, Ohio State University, Columbus, Ohio 43210, USA

Carol L. Krumhansl   Department of Psychology, Cornell University, Ithaca, New York 14853, USA

Fred Lerdahl   Department of Music, 602 Dodge Hall, University of Columbia, 2960 Broadway, New York NY 10027 6902, USA

Catherine Liégeois-Chauvel   INSERM EPI 9926, Laboratoire de Neurophysiologie et Neuropsychologie, Faculté de Medecine, 13005 Marseille, France

Daniel Matzkin   IRCAM-CNRS, 1 place Igor Stravinsky, F-75004 Paris, France

Stephen McAdams   IRCAM-CNRS, 1 place Igor Stravinsky, F-75004 Paris, France

Christo Pantev   Language and Music Group, Institut de Neurosciences Physiologiques et Cognitives, CNRS, Germany

Lawrence M. Parsons   University of Texas Health Science Center at San Antonio, San Antonio, Texas 78284-6240, USA

Alvaro Pascual-Leone   Behavioral Neurology Unit, Beth Israel Deaconess Medical Center, Harvard Medical School, Boston, Massachusetts 02215, USA

Aniruddh D. Patel   The Neurosciences Institute, 10640 John Jay Hopkins Drive, San Diego, CA 92121, USA

Isabelle Peretz   Département de Psychologie, Université de Montréal, C.P. 6128, succ. Centre-Ville, Montréal (Qué), H3C 3J7, Canada

Josef P. Rauschecker   Department of Physiology and Biophysics, Georgetown Institute for Cognitive and Computational Sciences, Georgetown University School of Medicine, Washington, DC 20057-1460, USA

Jenny R. Saffran   Department of Psychology, University of Wisconsin-Madison, Madison, WI 53706, USA

Séverine Samson   Laboratoire URECA, UFR de Psychologie, Universite Charles de Gaulle Lille-III, BP 149-59653 Villeneuve d'Ascq Cedex, France

E. Glenn Schellenberg   Department of Psychology, University of Toronto at Mississauga, Mississauga, ON L5L 1C6, Canada

Gottfried Schlaug   Beth Israel Deaconess Medical Center and Harvard Medical School, 330 Brookline Ave., Boston, MA 02215, USA

Louis Schmidt   Department of Psychology, McMaster University, Hamilton, ON L8S 4B2, Canada

Daniele Schön   Language and Music Group, Institut de Neurosciences Physiologiques et Cognitives, CNRS, 31 ch. Joseph Aiguer, 13402 Marseille, Cedex 20, France

Mari Tervaniemi   Cognitive Brain Research Unit, Department of Psychology, P.O. Box 13, FIN-00014 University of Helsinki, Finland

Barbara Tillmann   Université Claude Bernard Lyon 1, Laboratoire Neurosciences et Systèmes Sensoriels, CNRS-UMR 5020, 50 Avenue Tony Garnier, F-69366 Lyon Cedex 07, France

Petri Toiviainen   Department of Music, University of Jyväskylä, Jyväskylä, Finland

Laurel J. Trainor   Department of Psychology, McMaster University, Hamilton, ON, L8S 4B2 Canada

Mark Jude Tramo   Department of Neurology, Harvard Medical School and Massachusetts General Hospital, Boston, Massachusetts 02114-2696, USA

Sandra E. Trehub   Department of Psychology, University of Toronto at Mississauga, Mississauga, ON L5L 1C6, Canada

Robert J. Zatorre   Montreal Neurological Institute, McGill University, Montreal, Quebec, H3A 2B4, Canada

PART I

THE ORIGINS OF MUSIC

CHAPTER 1

MUSICAL PREDISPOSITIONS IN INFANCY: AN UPDATE

SANDRA E. TREHUB

For contributors to this volume on the cognitive neuroscience of music, the consideration of musical predispositions seems reasonable. By contrast, the larger scientific community is highly skeptical about links between music and biology. For example, Pinker,[1] who popularized the notion of a *language instinct*, dismisses music as 'auditory cheesecake'—a pleasant but superfluous confection. 'As far as biological cause and effect are concerned, music is useless. It shows no signs of design for attaining a goal such as long life, grandchildren, or accurate perception and prediction of the world. Compared with language, vision, social reasoning, and physical know-how, music could vanish from our species and the rest of our lifestyle would be virtually unchanged' (p. 528).[2]

Pinker's[2] thinking in this regard is flawed. He makes no distinction between musical *competence* and *performance*, or between underlying knowledge and demonstrable skill, as he does for language. He notes that while *all* normal children speak and comprehend language without explicit instruction, many adults are unmusical, as evidenced by their inability to sing in tune. Although developmental disorders of language occur in the absence of other disabilities,[3] developmental disorders of music are rare[4] even though music perception requires finer pitch resolution than does speech perception.

Pinker[2] emphasizes the training and practice required for mastering a musical instrument while de-emphasizing the daily language (speaking and listening) practice that all children experience. Caregivers, peers, and others function as language mentors, modelling target behaviours in age-appropriate ways. Similarly, informal musical mentoring is much more common than formal musical training in much of the world. Admittedly, individuals without certain kinds of mentoring or training may be limited in their explicit musical knowledge, but their implicit knowledge is similar, in many respects, to that of trained individuals.[5] Pinker also contrasts the wide variations in musical ability (i.e. tuneless singing to expert performance) with the presumed uniformity in language ability (i.e. the basic ability to speak and listen). In so doing, he applies a magnifying lens to music, which exaggerates individual differences, and a minifying lens to language, which reduces or eliminates individual differences. There is no evidence, however, of anything other than a normal distribution of language and musical abilities. Finally, Pinker's vision of life without music betrays considerable ethnocentrism—music as material for concerts, dance halls, and movie soundtracks rather than something entwined in the fabric of life. It ignores the historical and cross-cultural importance of music in ritual ceremonies,[6–9] work,[10,11] and child care[12] as well as the inextricable links between music and movement.[13]

Miller,[14] by contrast, considers music to exemplify many of the classic criteria for a complex human adaptation: (1) No culture in any period of recorded history has been without music (i.e. universality). (2) The development of musical abilities is orderly.[15] (3) The ability is widespread in the sense that almost every normal adult can appreciate music and carry a tune (i.e. basic perceptual and performing skills). (4) Adults can recognize thousands of melodies, implying specialized memory. (5) Special-purpose cortical mechanisms are involved.[16] (6) There are analogues in the signals of other species such as songbirds,[17] gibbons,[18] and whales,[19] raising the possibility of convergent evolution. (7) Finally, music can evoke strong emotions,[20–23] which implies receptive as well as productive adaptations.

If music is a complex biological adaptation rather than a by-product of other evolutionary processes, it must have conferred survival or reproductive benefits through the cumulative effect, over generations, of natural selection or sexual selection.[14,24,25] The costs of music production—energy expenditure—must be balanced by benefits. Because no survival benefits are obvious, Miller[14] argues for the evolution of music on the basis of its reproductive benefits. In other words, he makes a case for music as sexual courtship. He argues that although music is typically performed *in* groups, it is not *for* groups (but see Ref. 26; Huron, Chapter 4, this volume). In the context of the tribal group, dancing (i.e. vigorous movement to music) could have provided a means for young women to assess the strength, endurance, and motor coordination of potential mates. The relative stability of ancestral social groups would have allowed women to scrutinize prospective partners over an extended period. Miller[14] acknowledges, however, that aesthetic preferences would have been equally effective as a basis for sexual selection.

Sexual (or natural) selection of this nature would lead to the replication of genes related to receptive and productive musical potential. In fact, genetic correlates of musical pitch processing have been identified.[27] Musical processing predispositions or biases might be evident in infancy, well before they have obvious utility. As Cross[28] argues, it may be possible to observe the impact of evolutionary processes in infancy before any musical culture has left its indelible impression.

Uncovering musical predispositions

Accessing the music processing skills of preverbal listeners is no easy matter. Nevertheless, researchers have made considerable headway by means of conditioning procedures,[29] habituation procedures,[30,31] and preference procedures.[32,33] The most common conditioning procedure involves the presentation of a repeating melody or tone sequence from a laterally displaced loudspeaker while infants watch a puppet show. Periodically, the repeating pattern changes in some way, which prompts infants to turn towards the loudspeaker. Correct responses (i.e. turns) immediately following the change are rewarded by the presentation of a colourful mechanical toy (e.g. dancing bear, acrobatic monkey). Failure to turn at such times and turns at other times have no consequences. Such response-contingent rewards motivate attentive listening for 10–15 min, or 20–30 test trials. Aside from the bears, monkeys, puppets, and other paraphernalia that facilitate communication with nonverbal participants, the task is similar to adult same–different tasks. Infants turn to the loudspeaker when they consider the comparison pattern to be different from the standard pattern (i.e. response of *different*). They continue watching the puppet show (i.e. no turning response) when they fail to notice the change or if they consider the change unimportant (i.e. response of *same*). Significantly more responses (turns) to trials with changes than to those without changes indicate that infants can detect the target change. Successful detection of such changes also sheds light on infants' encoding of the standard melody. For example, infants' detection of a pitch change in the comparison melody implies that they noticed the specific pitches or pitch patterning of the original melody.

Relational processing of pitch and duration

Infants' perception of frequency,[34,35] timing,[36,37] and timbre[38,39] is finer than that required for musical purposes. Moreover, perceptual grouping principles that are relevant to music[40,41] are operative in infancy. Like adults, infants group isochronous tone sequences on the basis of similarities in pitch, loudness, and timbre.[42,43]

Infants go well beyond these minimal criteria for music perception. They recognize a melody in transposition, that is, when its pitch level is shifted upward or downward so long as the relations between tones are preserved.[30,44] An analogous situation prevails with respect to timing. Infants recognize a tone sequence when the tempo is altered so long as the relative durations remain unchanged.[45] In other words, they can focus on relational attributes of a melody, transforming a potentially unmanageable feat—encoding the exact pitches and durations—into a manageable task. Saffran[33,46] contends that infants preferentially attend to absolute rather than relative pitch cues in music, but support for her claim is lacking.[47] In principle, infants could retain absolute information along with relational information. In fact, infants and adults differentiate instrumental performances heard previously from subtly different performances of the same melody.[48] On balance, however, relational information seems to dominate melodic processing in infancy as in adulthood.[49,50]

One relational feature, melodic contour, is especially potent. For example, infants notice contour similarities and differences when the standard and comparison melodies are separated by a full 15 s[30] or when distractor tones are inserted between standard and comparison sequences.[29] Indeed, there are indications that pitch contour is the most salient musical feature for infant listeners.[50,51] Pitch contour may also be the most salient feature of mothers' speech to prelinguistic infants.[52–55] In the case of adult listeners, contour processing seems to be fundamental and relatively impervious to musical experience.[15] During contour-processing tasks, for example, the amplitude and latency of event-related potentials do not differ for musicians and nonmusicians, in contrast to interval-processing tasks, where experience-dependent differences are apparent.[56]

Interval processing

For adults, the extraction of pitch information is not limited to melodic contour, except for novel, unconventional melodies.[57,58] When adults hear unfamiliar but conventional melodies (i.e. those that conform to familiar musical conventions), they remember more detailed pitch information than they would otherwise.[59–61] In the case of highly familiar melodies, adults are thought to encode and retain precise pitch distances between tones (i.e. intervals) but not the absolute pitches.[62] There are indications, however, that even untrained adults retain the pitch level of familiar music, as reflected in their reproduction of familiar pop songs within two semitones of the original recordings.[63] More compelling evidence of the encoding of absolute pitch cues comes from adults' ability to distinguish the original pitch level of television soundtracks from versions that are pitch shifted by as little as a semitone.[64]

Despite infants' contour processing bias,[29] they can extract detailed interval information from patterns that elicit enhanced pitch processing in adults. For example, infants detect interval changes in brief melodies that conform to the conventions of their culture-to-be, but they fail to do so for melodies that violate those conventions.[65–68] It is highly unlikely that 6-month-old infants have acquired such musical knowledge. Indeed, the available evidence indicates that 6- to 10-month-old infants lack implicit knowledge of Western musical conventions.[61,69,70] The mistaken impression that they are sensitive to these conventions arises from commonalities in musical structure across cultures.[49,50]

In studies of infant melody perception, the presence of a prominent seven-semitone interval, or *perfect fifth*, has been associated with success in interval discrimination, and its absence with failure.[65–68,71] The *perfect fifth* is not alone in enhancing infants' perception of pitch relations.[72] Rather, infants, children, and adults detect interval changes more easily in the context of small-integer ratios—the octave (2 : 1), *perfect fifth* (3 : 2), and *perfect fourth* (4 : 3)—than in the context of large-integer ratios such as the *tritone* (45 : 32 ratio).[72–74] For example, Schellenberg and Trehub[72] had 6-month-old infants listen to a repeating tone sequence consisting of alternating tones separated by a *perfect fifth* (seven semitones), *perfect fourth* (five semitones), or *tritone* (six semitones). Their task was to respond (i.e. by turning) whenever a semitone change occurred. As can be seen in Figure 1.1, they succeeded when the standard pattern was consonant (i.e. *perfect fourth* or *fifth*) but not when it was dissonant (i.e. *tritone*). The implication is that *perfect fifths* and *fourths* are

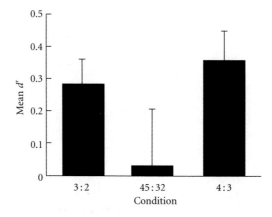

Figure 1.1 Infant discrimination (d') scores as a function of the frequency ratios of tones in melodic (sequential) intervals. Figure reprinted from Schellenberg and Trehub[72] with permission. Error bars indicate standard errors.

inherently easier to encode than are tritones. No doubt, the inherent ease of processing consonant intervals has contributed to their prominence in most musical systems.[50,75,76] Historical and cross-cultural records document the inequality of intervals, with numerous references to the beauty of octaves, *perfect fifths*, and *perfect fourths*[77,78] and the ugliness of the *tritone*—'the devil in music' in medieval times.[79]

Not only do consonant intervals promote ease of processing, they also influence infant attention and affect. For example, infants are more attentive and exhibit more positive affect when listening to consonant music than to music with many dissonant intervals.[80–82] In principle, these preferences could arise from the predominance of consonant intervals in the infant's environment (e.g. speech, music, environmental sounds). In the absence of such environmental input, as is the case for newborn infants whose deaf parents communicate by means of sign language, a similar pattern of preferences is evident.[83]

Processing of scale structure

Scales across cultures are diverse, but they exhibit some common features. For example, the octave is typically divided into five to seven discrete pitches, a design feature that is often attributed to cognitive constraints.[84] Another similarity is the ubiquitous *perfect fifth*, which is associated with enhanced processing in listeners of all ages.[72,74,85] Scales, for the most part, have unequal steps[86]—for example, one- and two-semitone steps in diatonic scales—a feature that is thought to confer processing advantages.[87,88]

To evaluate potential processing advantages of equal steps in scales, Trehub *et al.*[70] presented 9-month-old infants and adults with one of three ascending–descending scales: (1) the major scale, which is highly familiar to adults and potentially familiar to infants, (2) an artificial analogue of the major scale that was created by dividing the octave into 11 equal units, and selecting a seven-tone subset (featuring 1- and 2-unit steps), and (3) an artificial equal-step scale that was created by dividing the octave into seven equal steps.[89,90] These scales are depicted in Figure 1.2. Infants and adults were required to detect a mistuned tone (0.75- and 0.5-semitone change for infants and adults, respectively) in the comparison pattern. Adults' performance was highly accurate on the familiar major scale and equally poor on the two unfamiliar scales. By contrast, scales with unequal steps, major or artificial, enhanced infant performance relative to their performance on the equal-step scale (see Figure 1.3). Thus, unequal-step scales, which are universal or near-universal, facilitate musical pitch processing in infancy.

Infants' performance cannot be attributed to familiarity. It is possible, although highly unlikely, that infants heard adults or siblings practising the major scale, but they could not have heard the invented unequal-step scale that generated similar performance. By extension, other instances of enhanced processing—small-integer ratios, for example—are unlikely to stem from exposure. Adults' performance is informative in revealing how culture-specific experience, such as long-term exposure to the major scale, can override inherent processing biases (e.g. advantages of unequal-step scales in general).

There are other examples of culture-specific exposure attenuating or eliminating initial processing biases. For example, pitch processing in infancy is enhanced when the standard and comparison patterns are presented in related keys—specifically, keys standing in a 3 : 2 ratio—rather than unrelated keys.[66] For adults, such enhancement is limited to melodies that

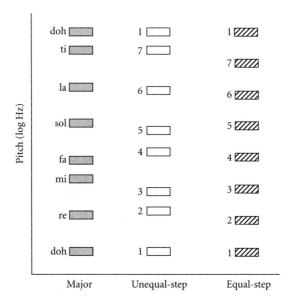

Figure 1.2 Schematic depiction of the major, artificial unequal-step, and equal-step scales. Figure reprinted from Trehub *et al.*[70] with permission.

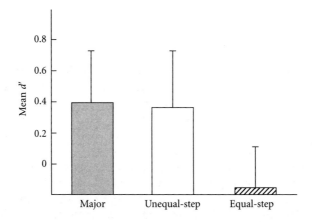

Figure 1.3 Infant discrimination (d') scores on the ascending-descending major scale, artificial, unequal-step scale, and equal-step scale. Error bars indicate standard errors. Figure reprinted from Trehub *et al.*[70] with permission.

are structured in a conventional manner.[66] Similarly, melodic redundancy enhances infants' retention of conventional and unconventional melodies, but comparable redundancy enhances adult performance for conventional melodies only.[61] In general, musics of the world capitalize on human processing predispositions (e.g. the preference for consonance and unequal scale steps), which means that musical experience tends to intensify the initial biases or predispositions.

Temporal processing

Similar adult–infant parallels are observable in the temporal domain (see Drake and Bertrand, Chapter 2, this volume). For example, infants differentiate tone sequences with identical pitches but contrasting rhythmic arrangements.[31,45,91] They also impose rhythmic groupings on isochronous tone sequences on the basis of pitch or timbre similarities.[42,43] The temporal organization of a sequence also has implications for infants' processing of pitch and timing details.[92] For example, melodic processing is enhanced when tone durations are related by binary ratios,[93,94] as is the case for children and adults.[95–97] Temporal processing predispositions (Drake and Bertand, Chapter 2, this volume) may account for the fact that adults' preferred rhythmic arrangements of melodies generate better infant performance than do non-preferred arrangements.[94] They may also account for superior infant performance on patterns with regular rather than syncopated rhythms.[93]

Hemispheric specialization

Well before infants understand language, they show a right-ear (i.e. left hemisphere) advantage for speech and a left-ear (i.e. right hemisphere) advantage for music.[98,99] Moreover, 8-month-old infants exhibit a left-ear superiority for contour processing and a right-ear superiority for interval processing.[100] Such laterality effects parallel those reported for adults[101,102] (but see Zatorre, Chapter 16, this volume).

Maternal music

The relevance of these processing predispositions to the daily lives of infants is unclear. Typical laboratory studies use musical stimuli (e.g. sequences of pure tones) that differ dramatically from the music that infants experience. Caregivers across cultures produce distinctive, solo performances of songs for infant listeners.[12,103–105] They also speak to infants in a sing-song manner that incorporates a number of musical features.[52,106,107] For example, mothers' speech differs from women's usual speech (e.g. pitch level, pitch contours, tempo, rhythm) in ways that reflect its greater emotional expressiveness.[52,55,108] Infants prefer this maternal speaking style to the usual adult style.[109–111]

When caregivers sing to infants, they generally use a special-purpose repertoire consisting of lullabies and play songs.[12,104] To the naïve adult listener, the tunes of unfamiliar lullabies, including those from foreign musical cultures, sound much like those of familiar lullabies. In fact, adults successfully identify unfamiliar lullabies from pairs of novel lullabies and nonlullabies matched on culture of origin and tempo.[112] Adults also perceive foreign lullabies as simpler and more repetitive than nonlullabies.[113]

Among the performance alterations that distinguish singing to infants from other singing are raised pitch level, decreased tempo, and an emotive voice quality.[114–116] In addition, mothers' song renditions are tailored to the age and needs of the listener. For example, maternal singing is approximately one-semitone higher in pitch level for infant than for preschool audiences, and the articulation of lyrics is more slurred for infants than for preschoolers.[117] Expressive features of the 'maternal' style are also evident when fathers sing to their infant offspring[116,118,119] and when preschoolers sing to their infant siblings.[120]

There are parallels between maternal speech and singing to infants,[12,51,104] but there are differences as well. In general, women's singing is higher pitched than their speech, but maternal speech to infants is higher pitched than maternal singing.[121] This situation results from a three- to four-semitone increase in pitch level when mothers speak to infants,[122] in contrast to an increase of approximately one-semitone when they sing to infants.[114,116]

Despite considerable variation across mothers, there is dramatic intra-individual consistency. When mothers sing the same song to infants on different occasions separated by a week or more, their pitch level and tempo (see Table 1.1) are virtually identical.[121] Variations in mothers' pitch and tempo are smaller than those observed in adults' repeated renditions of pop or folk songs.[63,123,124] By contrast, mothers' repeated utterances to infants exhibit large variations in pitch and tempo (see Table 1.1) but relatively stable rhythms. If singing to infants affects maternal mood or state, it could contribute to the stability of pitch and tempo over extended periods—a possible consequence of mood-dependent memory.[125] Frequent singing to infants may also implicate motor memory. In any event, mothers' sung performances seem to become ritualized, which could promote infants' recognition of mother's voice and the songs she sings.

Responsiveness to maternal music

How do infants respond to these maternal singing rituals? In the newborn period and beyond, infants listen significantly longer to audio recordings of infant-directed singing than to typical informal singing.[126,127] They also exhibit greater attention to higher- than to lower-pitched versions of the same song.[128] These preferences indicate the potency of the maternal style of singing, even in the absence of the familiar voice and expressive gestures that typically accompany maternal performances.

Table 1.1   Absolute pitch and tempo differences for mothers' infant-directed speech and singing across weeks

Mother	Pitch (semitones)		Tempo (beats per minute)	
	Speech	Singing	Speech	Singing
1	4.0	1.0	16	0
2	6.0	0.0	32	4
3	5.0	1.0	6	0
4	3.0	2.0	32	6
5	4.0	0.0	88	0
6	4.5	0.0	0	0
7	5.5	0.0	4	12
8	16.0	0.0	16	0
9	6.5	3.0	18	18
10	0.0	0.0	8	0
11	0.0	1.0	31	0

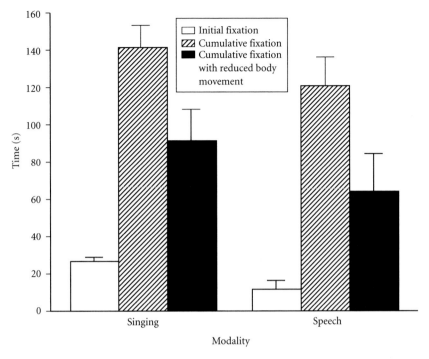

Figure 1.4   Initial fixation, cumulative fixation, and cumulative fixation with minimal body movement as a function of maternal speech and singing. Error bars indicate standard errors.

When 6-month-old infants view (and hear) videotaped speech and singing by their own mother, they exhibit longer visual fixations and greater reductions in body movement during singing than during speaking episodes (see Figure 1.4).[129,130] These sung performances have a hypnotic effect on infants, who remain glued to their mother's image. Maternal speaking is also engaging but not nearly as engaging as maternal singing.

There has been much discussion of maternal speech and singing as modulators of infant arousal,[12,52,108] but the available research has focused largely on attention rather than arousal. To explore the arousal consequences of maternal speech and singing, Shenfield, Trehub, and Nakata[131] took saliva samples from 6-month-old infants before the onset of maternal speech and singing (on different days) as well as 20 and 25 min later. As can be seen in Figure 1.5, cortisol levels decreased systematically across the three sampling periods of the singing condition. There was a similar decrease in cortisol levels 20 min after speaking onset, but this decrease was not sustained at the 25-minute period (see Figure 1.5). Maternal music as a means of optimizing infant mood or arousal parallels adolescents' and adults' use of music for self-regulation.[132,133] It appears that some forms of music, maternal singing in particular, modulate arousal level in healthy, nondistressed infants, as they do for distressed newborns in intensive care units.[134] There are indications, moreover, that maternal singing is a more effective regulator of arousal than is maternal speech.

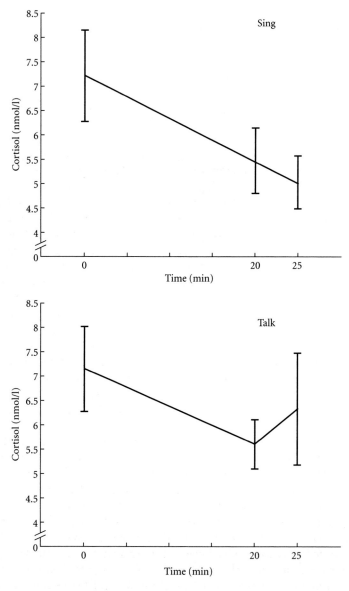

Figure 1.5 Baseline cortisol levels and cortisol levels at 20 and 25 min after the onset of singing (upper panel) and speaking (lower panel). Error bars indicate standard errors.

Biological significance of singing to infants

The ubiquity of maternal singing and the impact of such singing on infant attention and arousal raise the possibility that maternal singing could have enhanced infant survival in difficult (e.g. ancestral) conditions. To the extent that maternal singing optimizes infant mood, it could contribute to infant growth and development by facilitating feeding, sleeping, and even learning. Children's extended period of helplessness creates intense selection pressures for parental commitment and for infant behaviours to reward such commitment. Falling asleep to lullabies or entering trance-like states to performances of other songs might be suitable rewards for maternal effort. In general, favourable consequences of maternal singing on infant arousal, whether through cry reduction, sleep induction, or positive affect, would contribute to infant well-being while sustaining such maternal behavior. Presumably, the healthy and contented offspring of singing mothers would be more likely to pass on their genes than would the offspring of non-singing mothers.

Maternal singing may also be self-soothing, providing a safe outlet for negative as well as positive feelings.[12] There are numerous examples of lullabies across cultures that combine laments on life with sleep-inducing singing.[12,135] Maternal singing is likely to strengthen the emotional ties between mother and infant[106,119] just as singing in other contexts reduces the psychological distance between singer and listener.[136,137] Indeed, maternal singing may set the stage for the subsequent role of music in group bonding.[26,138] In any case, singing to infants seems to enhance maternal as well as infant well-being.

If women's expressive singing captures the attention and hearts of infant listeners, it may have been equally captivating to young adult males in the distant past. In some avian species, females sing to attract mates, and they lead duets with their male partner.[17,139] There is speculation, moreover, that such duetting fosters long-term pair bonding.[140] These notions are inconsistent with Miller's[14] view of music as male sexual courtship. To evaluate his hypothesis, Miller compared the recorded output of prominent jazz, rock, and classical musicians. Male musicians produced 10 times as much music as female musicians, their output reaching its peak near the age of peak mating effort. This led Miller[14] to conclude that music continues to function as a courtship display to attract females. To date, however, there is no evidence of sexual dimorphism in musical ability or achievement that cannot be accounted for by sociocultural factors.

Tooby and Cosmides[141] offer a radically different evolutionary account of the universal attraction to the imaginative arts (e.g. fiction, visual art, music). Unlike human activities that have fitness-enhancing consequences in the external world (e.g. sex) or on the body (e.g. eating), aesthetic activities promote fitness-enhancing activities in the human brain. According to Tooby and Cosmides,[140] readying the brain for its mature role is one of the most critical and most exacting developmental tasks. They contend that artistic or imaginative actions (or action tendencies) play a key role in mental development. In line with their view, infants' attraction to music may reflect motivational guidance systems designed to develop and fine-tune the brain mechanisms that subserve cognitive and social competence. Part of what may make music so important in this regard is its lack of immediate consequences (Cross, this volume)—the very factor that leads others[2] to dispute its biological basis.

Conclusion

It is clear that infants do not begin life with a blank musical slate. Instead, they are predisposed to attend to the melodic contour and rhythmic patterning of sound sequences, whether music or speech. They are tuned to consonant patterns, melodic as well as harmonic, and to metric rhythms. Surely these predispositions are consistent with a biological basis for music, specifically, for the core abilities that underlie adult musical skill in all cultures. As Cross[28] notes, evolution acts on the mind by shaping infant predispositions, and culture shapes the expression of those predispositions. In effect, music is part of our nature as well as being part of our culture.

Mothers cater to infants' musical inclinations by singing regularly in the course of caregiving and by adapting their singing style in ways that are congenial to infant listeners. These ritualized vocal interactions may reflect caregivers' predisposition to share affect and forge emotional ties by means of temporal synchrony.[142] Perhaps it is not surprising that infants are predisposed to attend to and appreciate the species-typical vocalizations of their primary caregiver. Is it surprising that they are also predisposed to attend to specific structural features of music? Only if music is viewed in a narrow sense, as fully developed musical systems of particular cultures. Viewed broadly, music embraces what all musical systems have in common. In that sense, infants begin life as musical beings, being responsive to the primitives or universals that are the foundation of music everywhere.

Acknowledgements

The preparation of this paper was assisted by grants from the Natural Sciences and Engineering Research Council and the Social Sciences and Humanities Research Council of Canada.

References

1. **Pinker, S.** (1994) *The Language Instinct: How the Mind Creates Language.* New York: William Morrow.

2. **Pinker, S.** (1997) *How the Mind Works.* New York: Norton, p. 528.

3. **Fletcher, P.** (1999) Specific language impairment. In M. Barrett (ed.) *The Development of Language.* Hove, East Sussex, UK: Psychology Press, pp. 349–71.

4. **Peretz, I., J. Ayotte, R. Zatorre, J. Mehler, P. Ahad, V. Penhune**, and **B. Jutras** (2002) Congenital amusia: a disorder of fine-grained pitch discrimination. *Neuron* 33, 185–91.

5. **Smith, J. D., D. G. Kemler Nelson, L. A. Grohskopf**, and **T. Appleton** (1994) What child is this? What interval was that? Familiar tunes and music perception in novice listeners. *Cognition* 52, 23–54.

6. **Basso, E.** (1985) *A Musical View of the Universe: Kalapalo Rhythmic and Ritual Performance.* Philadelphia: University of Pennsylvania Press.

7. **Dissanayake, E.** (1992) *Homo Aestheticus: Where Art Comes From and Why.* New York: Free Press.

8. **Merriam, A. P.** (1964) *The Anthropology of Music.* Evanston, Ill: Northwestern University Press.

9. **Sarno, L.** (1993) *Song from the Forest: My Life among the Ba-Benjelle Pygmies.* Boston: Houghton Mifflin.

10. **Deng, F. M.** (1973) *The Dinka and their Songs.* London: Oxford University Press.

11. **Firth, R.** (1961) *Elements of Social Organization.* London: Watts.

12. **Trehub, S. E.** and **L. J. Trainor** (1998) Singing to infants: lullabies and play songs. *Advances in Infancy Res.* 12, 43–77.

13. Blacking, J. (1995) *Music, Culture, and Experience.* London: University of Chicago Press.

14. Miller, G. (2000) Evolution of human music through sexual selection. In N. L. Wallin, B. Merker, and S. Brown (eds) *The Origins of Music.* Cambridge, MA: MIT Press, pp. 329–60.

15. Dowling, W. J. (1999) The development of music perception and cognition. In D. Deutsch (ed.) *The Psychology of Music.* San Diego, CA: Academic Press, pp. 603–25.

16. Peretz, I. and J. Morais (1993) Specificity for music. In F. Boller and J. Grafman (eds) *Handbook of Neuropsychology,* vol. 8. Amsterdam: Elsevier, pp. 373–90.

17. Slater, J. B. (2000) Birdsong repertoires: their origins and use. In N. L. Wallin, B. Merker, and S. Brown (eds) *The Origins of Music.* Cambridge, MA: MIT Press, pp. 49–63.

18. Geissmann, T. (2000) Gibbon songs and human music from an evolutionary perspective. In N. L. Wallin, B. Merker, and S. Brown (eds) *The Origins of Music.* Cambridge, MA: MIT Press, pp. 103–23.

19. Payne, K. (2000) The progressively changing songs of humpback whales: a window on the creative process in a wild animal. In N. L. Wallin, B. Merker, and S. Brown (eds) *The Origins of Music.* Cambridge, MA: MIT Press, pp. 135–50.

20. Blood, A. J. and R. J. Zatorre (2001) Intensely pleasurable responses to music correlate with activity in brain regions implicated in reward and emotion. *Proc. Nat. Acad. Sci.* 98, 11818–23.

21. Gabrielsson, A. (2001) Emotions in strong experiences with music. In P. N. Juslin and F. A. Sloboda (eds) *Music and Emotion: Theory and Research.* Oxford: Oxford University Press, pp. 431–49.

22. Peretz, I. (2001) Listen to the brain: a biological perspective on musical emotions. In P. N. Juslin and J. A. Sloboda (eds) *Music and Emotion: Theory and Research.* Oxford: Oxford University Press, pp. 105–34.

23. Sloboda, J. A. (1992) Empirical studies of emotional response to music. In M. R. Jones and S. Holleran (eds) *Cognitive Bases of Musical Communication.* Washington, DC: American Psychological Association, pp. 33–50.

24. Dawkins, R. (1996) *Climbing Mount Improbable.* London: Penguin Books.

25. Williams, G. C. (1966) *The Selfish Gene. Adaptation and Natural Selection.* Princeton, NJ: Princeton University Press.

26. Brown, S. (2000) Evolutionary models of music: from sexual selection to group selection. In F. Tonneau and N. S. Thompson (eds) *Perspectives in Ethology, vol. 13: Evolution, Culture, and Behavior.* New York: Kluwer Academic, pp. 231–81.

27. Drayna, D., A. Manichaikul, M. de Lange, H. Sneider, and T. Spector (2001) Genetic correlates of musical pitch recognition in humans. *Science* 291, 1969–72.

28. Cross, I. (2001) Music, mind, and evolution. *Psychol. Music* 29, 95–102.

29. Trehub, S. E., D. Bull, and L. A. Thorpe (1984) Infants' perception of melodies: the role of melodic contour. *Child Dev.* 55, 821–30.

30. Chang, H. W. and S. E. Trehub (1977) Auditory processing of relational information by young infants. *J. Exp. Child Psychol.* 24, 324–31.

31. Chang, H. W. and S. E. Trehub (1977) Infants' perception of temporal grouping in auditory patterns. *Child Dev.* 48, 1666–70.

32. Krumhansl, C. L. and P. W. Jusczyk (1990) Infant's perception of phrase structure in music. *Psychol. Sci.* 1, 70–3.

33. Saffran, J. R. and G. J. Griepentrog (2001) Absolute pitch in infant auditory learning: evidence for developmental reorganization. *Developmental Psychol.* 37, 74–85.

34. Olsho, L. W., C. Schoon, R. Sakai, R. Turpin, and V. C. Sperduto (1982) Preliminary data on frequency discrimination in infancy. *J. Acoust. Soc. Am.* 71, 509–11.

35. Werner, L. A. (1992) Interpreting developmental psychoacoustics. In L. A. Werner and E. W. Rubel (eds) Developmental Psychoacoustics. Washington, DC: American Psychological Association, pp. 47–88.

36. Trehub, S. E., B. A. Schneider, and J. L. Henderson (1995) Gap detection in infants, children, and adults. *J. Acoust. Soc. Am.* 98, 2532–41.

37. Werner, L. A, G. C. Marean, C. F. Halpin, N. B. Spetner, and J. M. Gillenwater (1992) Infant auditory temporal acuity: gap detection. *Child Dev.* 63, 260–72.

38. Clarkson, M. G. and R. K. Clifton (1995) Infants' pitch perception: inharmonic tonal complexes. *J. Acoust. Soc. Am.* 98, 1372–9.

39. Trehub, S. E., M. Endman, and L. A. Thorpe (1990) Infants' perception of timbre: Classification of complex tones by spectral structure. *J. Exp. Child Psychol.* 49, 300–13.

40. Bregman, A. S. (1990) *Auditory Scene Analysis.* Cambridge, MA: MIT Press.

41. Deutsch, D. (1999) Grouping mechanisms in music. In D. Deutsch (ed.) *The Psychology of Music.* San Diego, CA: Academic Press, pp. 299–348.

42. Thorpe, L. A. and S. E. Trehub (1989) Duration illusion and auditory grouping in infancy. *Developmental Psychol.* 25, 122–7.

43. Thorpe, L. A., S. E. Trehub, B. A. Morrongiello, and D. Bull (1988) Perceptual grouping by infants and preschool children. *Developmental Psychol.* 24, 484–91.

44. Trehub, S. E., L. A. Thorpe, and B. A. Morrongiello (1987) Organizational processes in infants' perception of auditory patterns. *Child Dev.* 58, 741–9.

45. Trehub, S. E. and L. A. Thorpe (1989) Infants' perception of rhythm. Categorization of auditory sequences by temporal structure. *Canadian J. Psychol.* 43, 217–29

46. Saffran, J. R. (2003) Absolute pitch in infancy and adulthood: the role of tonal structure. *Developmental Science* 6, 37–45.

47. Trehub, S. E. (2003) Absolute and relative pitch processing in tone learning tasks. *Developmental Science* 6, 46–7.

48. Palmer, C., M. K. Jungers, and P. W. Jusczyk (2001) Episodic memory for musical prosody. *J. Mem. Lang.* 45, 526–45.

49. Trehub, S. E. (2000) Human processing predispositions and musical universals. In N. L. Wallin, B. Merker, and S. Brown (eds) *The Origins of Music.* Cambridge, MA: MIT Press, pp. 427–48.

50. Trehub, S., E. G. Schellenberg, and D. Hill (1997) The origins of music perception and cognition: a developmental perspective. In I. Deliège and J. Sloboda (eds) *Perception and Cognition of Music.* Hove, UK: Psychology Press, pp.103–28.

51. Trehub, S. E., L. J. Trainor, and A. M. Unyk (1993) Music and speech processing in the first year of life. *Advances Child Dev. Behav.* 24, 1–35.

52. Fernald, A. (1991) Prosody in speech to children: prelinguistic and linguistic functions. *Annals Child Dev.* 8, 43–80.

53. Fernald, A. and P. K. Kuhl (1987) Acoustic determinants of infant preference for motherese. *Infant Behav. Dev.* 10, 279–93.

54. Lewis, M. M. (1951) *Infant Speech.* London: Routledge and Kegan Paul.

55. **Papoušek, M.** (1992) Early ontogeny of vocal communication in parent–infant interactions. In H. Papoušek, U. Jürgens, and M. Papoušek (eds) *Nonverbal Vocal Communication: Comparative and Developmental Approaches.* Cambridge: Cambridge University Press, pp. 230–61.

56. **Trainor, L. J., R. N. Desjardins**, and **C. Rockel** (1999) A comparison of contour and interval processing in musicians and nonmusicians using event-related potentials. *Australian J. Psychol.* 51, 147–53.

57. **Bartlett, J. C.** and **W. J. Dowling** (1980) Recognition of transposed melodies: a key-distance effect in developmental perspective. *J. Exp. Psychol.: Hum. Percept. Perform.* 6, 501–15.

58. **Dowling, W. J.** (1978) Scale and contour: two components of a theory of memory for melodies. *Psychological Rev.* 85, 341–54.

59. **Cuddy, L. L., A. J. Cohen**, and **D. J. K. Mewhort** (1981) Perception of structure in short melodic sequences. *J. Exp. Psychol.: Hum. Percept. Perform.* 7, 869–83.

60. **Krumhansl, C. L., J. J. Bharucha** and **E. J. Kessler** (1982) Perceived harmonic structure of chords in three related keys. *J. Exp. Psychol.: Hum. Percept. Perform.* 8, 24–36.

61. **Schellenberg, E. G.** and **S. E. Trehub** (1999) Culture-general and culture-specific factors in the discrimination of melodies. *J. Exp. Child Psychol.* 74, 107–27.

62. **Dowling, W. J.** and **D. Fujitani** (1971) Contour, interval, and pitch recognition in memory for melodies. *J. Acoust. Soc. Am.* 49, 524–31.

63. **Levitin, D. J.** (1994) Absolute memory for musical pitch: evidence from the production of learned melodies. *Percept. Psychophys.* 56, 414–23.

64. **Schellenberg, E. G.** and **S. E. Trehub** (2003). Good pitch memory is widespread. *Psychol. Sci.* 14, 262–6.

65. **Cohen, A. J., L. A. Thorpe**, and **S. E. Trehub** (1987) Infants' perception of musical relations in short transposed tone sequences. *Canadian J. Psychol.* 41, 33–47.

66. **Trainor, L. J.** and **S. E. Trehub** (1993) Musical context effects in infants and adults: key distance. *J. Exp Psychol.: Hum. Percept. Perform.* 19, 615–26.

67. **Trainor, L. J.** and **S. E. Trehub** (1993) What mediates infants' and adults' superior processing of the major over the augmented triad? *Music Percept.* 11, 185–96.

68. **Trehub, S. E., L. A. Thorpe**, and **L. J. Trainor** (1990) Infants' perception of *good* and *bad* melodies. *Psychomusicology* 9, 5–19.

69. **Trainor, L. J.** and **S. E. Trehub** (1992) A comparison of infants' and adults' sensitivity to Western musical structure. *J. Exp. Psychol.: Hum. Percept. Perform.* 18, 394–402.

70. **Trehub, S. E., E. G. Schellenberg**, and **S. B. Kamenetsky** (1999) Infants' and adults' perception of scale structure. *J. Exp. Psychol.: Hum. Percept. Perform.* 25, 965–75.

71. **Lynch, M. P., R. E. Eilers, D. K. Oller**, and **R. C. Urbano** (1990) Innateness, experience, and music perception. *Psychol. Sci.* 1, 272–6.

72. **Schellenberg, E. G.** and **S. E. Trehub** (1996) Natural musical intervals: evidence from infant listeners. *Psychol. Sci.* 7, 272–7.

73. **Schellenberg, E. G.** and **S. E. Trehub** (1994) Frequency ratios and the discrimination of pure tone sequences. *Percept. Psychophys.* 56, 472–8.

74. **Schellenberg, E. G.** and **S. E. Trehub** (1996) Children's discrimination of melodic intervals. *Developmental Psychol.* 32, 1039–50.

75. **Meyer, L. B.** (1956) *Emotion and Meaning in Music.* Chicago: University of Chicago Press.

76. **Sachs, C.** (1943) *The Rise of Music in the Ancient World: East and West.* New York: Norton.

77. **Bower, C.** (1980) Boethius, Anicius, Manlius Severinus. In S. Sadie (ed.) *The New Grove Dictionary of Music and Musicians,* vol. 2. London: Macmillan, p. 844.

78. **Hill, C. C.** (1986) Consonance and dissonance. In D. M. Randel (ed.) *The New Harvard Dictionary of Music.* Cambridge, MA: Belknap Press, pp. 197–9.

79. **Kennedy, M.** (1994) Song. *The Oxford Dictionary of Music,* 2nd edn. Oxford: Oxford University Press.

80. **Trainor, L. J.** and **B. M. Heinmiller** (1998) Infants prefer to listen to consonance over dissonance. *Infant Behav. Dev.* 21, 77–88.

81. **Zentner, M. R.** and **J. Kagan** (1996) Perception of music by infants. *Nature* 383, 29.

82. **Zentner, M. R.** and **J. Kagan** (1998) Infants' perception of consonance and dissonance in music. *Infant Behav. Dev.* 21, 483–92.

83. **Masataka, N.** (1999) Personal communication.

84. *Burns,* E. M. (1999) Intervals, scales, and tuning. In D. Deutch (ed.) *The Psychology of Music,* 2nd edn. San Diego, CA: Academic Press, pp. 215–64.

85. **Schellenberg, E. G.** and **S. E. Trehub** (1994) Frequency ratios and the perception of tone patterns. *Psychonomic Bulletin and Rev.* 1, 191–201.

86. **Sloboda, J. A.** (1985) *The Musical Mind: The Cognitive Psychology of Music.* Oxford: Clarendon Press.

87. **Butler, D.** (1989) Describing the perception of tonality in music: a critique of the tonal hierarchy theory and proposal for a theory of intervallic rivalry. *Music Percept.* 6, 219–42.

88. **Shepard, R. N.** (1982) Geometrical approximations to the structure of musical pitch. *Psychological Rev.* 89, 305–33.

89. **Jordan, D. S.** and **R. N. Shepard** (1987) Tonal schemas: evidence obtained by probing distorted scales. *Percept. Psychophys.* 41, 489–504.

90. **Shepard, R. N.** and **D. C. Jordan** (1984) Auditory illusions demonstrating that tones are assimilated to an internalized scale. *Science* 226, 1333–4.

91. **Demany, L., B. McKenzie,** and **E. Vurpillot** (1977) Rhythm perception in early infancy. *Nature* 266, 718–19.

92. **Trainor, L. J.** and **B. Adams** (2000) Infants' and adults' use of duration and intensity cues in the segmentation of tone patterns. *Percept. Psychophys.* 62, 333–40.

93. **Bergeson, T. R.** (2002) *Perspectives on Music and Music Listening in Infancy.* Unpublished doctoral dissertation, University of Toronto.

94. **Trehub S. E., D. S. Hill,** and **S. B. Kamenetsky** (1997) *Infants' Perception of Melodies with "Good" or "Bad" Rhythms.* Presented at the biennial meeting of the Society for Research in Child Development. Washington, DC.

95. **Drake, C.** (1993) Reproduction of musical rhythms by children. *Percept. Psychophys.* 53, 25–33.

96. **Drake, C.** (1998) Psychological processes involved in the temporal organization of complex auditory sequences: universal and acquired processes. *Music Percept.* 16, 11–26.

97. **Parncutt, R.** (1994) A perceptual model of pulse salience and metrical accent in musical rhythms. *Music Percept.* 11, 409–64.

98. **Bertoncini, J., J. Morais, R. Bijeljac-Babic, S. McAdams, I. Peretz,** and **J. Mehler** (1989) Dichotic perception and laterality in neonates. *Brain Lang.* 37, 591–605.

99. **Best, C. T., H. Hoffman,** and **B. B. Glanville** (1982) Development of infant ear asymmetries for speech and music. *Percept. Psychophys.* 31, 75–85.

100. Balaban, M. T., L. M. Anderson, and A. B. Wisniewski (1998) Lateral asymmetries in infant melody perception. *Developmental Psychol.* 34, 39–48.

101. Peretz, I. (1987) Shifting ear differences in melody comparison through transposition. *Cortex* 23, 317–23.

102. Peretz, I. and M. Babaï (1992) The role of contour and intervals in the recognition of melody parts: Evidence from cerebral asymmetries in musicians. *Neuropsychologia*, 30, 277–92.

103. Brakeley, T. C. (1950) Lullaby. In M. Leach and J. Fried (eds), *Standard Dictionary of Folklore, Mythology, and Legend*. New York: Funk and Wagnalls, pp. 653–4.

104. Trehub, S. E. and E. G. Schellenberg (1995) Music: its relevance to infants. *Annals Child Dev.* 11, 1–24.

105. Tucker, N. (1984) Lullabies. *History Today* 34, 40–6.

106. Dissanayake, E. (2000) Antecedents of the temporal arts in early mother–infant interaction. In N. L. Wallin, B. Merker, and S. Brown (eds) *The Origins of Music*. Cambridge, MA: MIT Press, pp. 389–410.

107. Fernald, A. (1992) Meaningful melodies in mothers' speech to infants. In H. Papoušek, U. Jurgens, and M. Papoušek (eds) *Nonverbal Vocal Communication: Comparative and Developmental Approaches*. Cambridge, UK: Cambridge University Press, pp. 262–82.

108. Trainor, L. J., C. M. Austin, and R. N. Desjardins (2000) Is infant-directed speech prosody a result of the vocal expression of emotion? *Psychol. Sci.* 11, 188–95.

109. Cooper, R. P. and R. N. Aslin (1990) Preference for infant-directed speech in the first month after birth. *Child Dev.* 61, 1584–95.

110. Fernald, A. (1985) Four-month-old infants prefer to listen to motherese. *Infant Behav. Dev.* 8, 181–95.

111. Werker, J. F. and P. J. McLeod (1989) Infant preference for both male and female infant-directed talk: a developmental study of attentional and affective responsiveness. *Canadian J. Psychol.* 43, 230–46.

112. Trehub, S. E., A. M. Unyk, and L. J. Trainor (1993) Adults identify infant-directed music across cultures. *Infant Behav. Dev.* 16, 193–211.

113. Unyk, A. M., S. E. Trehub, L. J. Trainor, and E. G. Schellenberg (1992) Lullabies and simplicity: a cross-cultural perspective. *Psychol. Music* 20, 15–28.

114. Trainor, L. J., E. D. Clark, A. Huntley and B. Adams (1997) The acoustic basis of infant preferences for infant-directed singing. *Infant Behav. Dev.* 20, 383–96.

115. Trehub, S. E., A. M. Unyk, and L. J. Trainor (1993) Maternal singing in cross-cultural perspective. *Infant Behav. Dev.* 16, 285–95.

116. Trehub, S. E., A. M. Unyk, S. B. Kamenetsky, D. S. Hill, L. J. Trainor, J. L. Henderson and M. Saraza (1997) Mothers' and fathers' singing to infants. *Developmental Psychol.* 33, 500–7.

117. Bergeson, T. R. and S. E. Trehub (1999) Mothers' singing to infants and preschool children. *Infant Behav. Dev.* 22, 51–64.

118. O'Neill, C., L. J. Trainor, and S. E. Trehub (2001) Infants' responsiveness to fathers' singing. *Music Percept.* 18, 409–25.

119. Trehub, S. E., D. S. Hill, and S. B. Kamenetsky (1997) Parents' sung performances for infants. *Canadian J. Exp. Psychol.* 51, 385–96.

120. Trehub, S. E., A. M. Unyk, and J. L. Henderson (1994) Children's songs to infant siblings: parallels with speech. *J. Child Lang.* 21, 735–44.

121. **Bergeson, T. R.** and **S. E. Trehub** (2002) Absolute pitch and tempo in mothers' songs to infants. *Psychol. Sci.* 13, 71–4.

122. **Fernald, A.** and **T. Simon** (1984) Expanded intonation contours in mothers' speech to newborns. *Developmental Psychol.* 20, 104–13.

123. **Halpern, A. R.** (1989) Memory for the absolute pitch of familiar songs. *Memory and Cognition* 17, 572–81.

124. **Levitin, D. J.** and **P. R. Cook** (1996) Memory for musical tempo: additional evidence that auditory memory is absolute. *Percept. Psychophys.* 58, 927–35.

125. **Eich, E.** and **D. Macaulay** (2000) Are real moods required to reveal mood-congruent and mood-dependent memory? *Psychol. Sci.* 11, 244–8.

126. **Masataka, N.** (1999) Preference for infant-directed singing in 2-day-old hearing infants of deaf parents. *Developmental Psychol.* 35, 1001–5.

127. **Trainor, L. J.** (1996) Infant preferences for infant-directed versus noninfant-directed playsongs and lullabies. *Infant Behav. Dev.* 19, 83–92.

128. **Trainor, L. J.** and **C. A. Zacharias** (1998) Infants prefer higher-pitched singing. *Infant Behav. Dev.* 21, 799–805.

129. **Nakata, T.** and **S. E. Trehub** (2000) *Maternal Speech and Singing to Infants.* Presented at the Society for Music Perception and Cognition. Toronto, ON.

130. **Trehub, S. E.** and **T. Nakata** (2001–2002) Emotion and music in infancy. *Musicae Scientiae,* Special Issue, 37–61.

131. **Shenfield, T., S. E. Trehub,** and **T. Nakata** (2002) *Salivary Cortisol Responses to Maternal Speech and Singing.* Presented at the International Conference on Infant Studies, Toronto, ON.

132. **Sloboda, J. A.** and **S. A. O'Neill** (2001) Emotions in everyday listening to music. In P. N. Juslin and J. A. Sloboda (eds) *Music and Emotion: Theory and Research. Series in Affective Science.* London, UK: Oxford University Press, pp. 415–29.

133. **Zillman, D.** (1988) Mood management: using entertainment to full advantage. In L. Donohew, H. E. Syhper, and E. T. Higgens (eds) *Communication, Social Cognition, and Affect.* Hillsdale, NJ: Erlbaum, pp. 147–71.

134. **Standley, J. M.** and **R. S. Moore** (1995) Therapeutic effects of music and mother's voice on premature infants. *Pediatric Nursing* 21, 509–12.

135. **Masuyama, E. E.** (1989) Desire and discontent in Japanese lullabies. *Western Folklore* 48, 144–8.

136. **Lomax, A.** (1968) *Folk Song Style and Culture.* Washington, DC: American Association for the Advancement of Science.

137. **Pantaleoni, H.** (1985) *On the Nature of Music.* Oneonta, NY: Welkin Books.

138. **Kogan, N.** (1997) Reflections on aesthetics and evolution. *Critical Rev.* 11, 193–210.

139. **Levin, R. N.** (1996) Song behaviour and reproductive strategies in a duetting wren, Thryothorus Nigricapillus: II playback experiments. *Animal Behavior* 52, 1107–17.

140. **Hooker, T.** and **B. I. Hooker** (1969) Duetting. In R. A. Hinde (ed.) *Bird Vocalizations.* Cambridge: Cambridge University Press, pp. 185–205.

141. **Tooby, J.** and **L. Cosmides** (2001) Does beauty build adapted minds? Toward an evolutionary theory of aesthetics, fiction and the arts. *SubStance* 30, 6–27.

142. **Dissanayake, E.** (2001) Becoming homo aestheticus: sources of aesthetic imagination in mother-infant interactions. *SubStance* 30, 85–103.

CHAPTER 2

THE QUEST FOR UNIVERSALS IN TEMPORAL PROCESSING IN MUSIC

CAROLYN DRAKE AND DAISY BERTRAND

> One would ultimately hope to specify these cognitive principles or "universals" that underlie all musical listening, regardless of musical style or acculturation. To what extent is it learned, and to what extent is it due to an innate musical capacity or general cognitive capacity?
>
> Lehrdal & Jackendoff[1]

Abstract

Music perception and performance rely heavily on temporal processing: for instance, each event must be situated in time in relation to surrounding events, and events must be grouped together in order to overcome memory constraints. The temporal structure of music varies considerably from one culture to another, and so it has often been supposed that the specific implementation of perceptual and cognitive temporal processes will differ as a function of an individual's cultural exposure and experience. In this paper we examine the alternative position that some temporal processes may be universal, in the sense that they function in a similar manner irrespective of an individual's cultural exposure and experience. We first review rhythm perception and production studies carried out with adult musicians, adult nonmusicians, children, and infants in order to identify temporal processes that appear to function in a similar fashion irrespective of age, acculturation, and musical training. This review leads to the identification of five temporal processes that we submit as candidates for the status of 'temporal universals'. For each process, we select the simplest and most representative experimental paradigm that has been used to date. This leads to a research proposal for future intercultural studies that could test the universal nature of these processes.

Keywords: Temporal processing; Rhythm perception; Segmentation; Grouping; Regularity; Duration ratios

Towards intercultural research in temporal processing

We plead guilty to the charge of cultural egocentricity. In previous research, we have proceeded as if the musical environment the world over is identical to that in France, Belgium, England, and the United States (the countries in which we have carried out our experiments). The musical environment in these countries is relatively homogenous in the sense that it is dominated by a Western tonal tradition (although we acknowledge significant differences even between these environments). From a rhythmic point of view, both our 'classical' and 'popular' musics are dominated by relatively simple rhythmic structures, organized around a regular beat, with binary or ternary multiplications and subdivisions of this beat.[1,2] By focusing on the auditory world around us, we have identified some of the psychological rhythmic processes that appear to function in our particular instance when listening to or producing 'our' type of music. Following the results of this developmental prospective, we have even made the claim that some of these processes function the same way whatever the musical environment in which a listener is immersed.[3] Despite this previous highly focused position, we are fully aware that our assumptions concerning the generalizability of these processes to other cultures are only that—assumptions. This paper is an attempt to make amends for our previous cultural egocentricity by suggesting how our psychological developmental prospective could be adapted to an intercultural one, into which existing knowledge from the field of ethnomusicology and future cross-cultural studies could be incorporated.

Our previous research has focused on how people hear musical and nonmusical rhythms in order to identify the underlying psychological processes that make the perception of music such a fulfilling and satisfying activity. Music is typical of all forms of sustained activity over time, in that it can be successfully perceived or performed only if the individual events from which it is composed are perceptually integrated into larger units spread over time. Indeed, music has been defined as the art of organizing events in time. As such, it provides an ideal opportunity to investigate the perceptual and cognitive temporal processes that make such activity possible.

In the past we have adopted the experimental principle of comparing performances on both perceptual and motor rhythmic tasks by people varying in levels of rhythmic skill, be it by age (as children get older there is a gradual increase in their exposure to, and experience with, the rhythmic structures around them) or musical training (the musical training common to our culture is particularly characterized by the development of explicit knowledge about musical structure). Such an experimental principle allows us to tease apart the processes that appear to be 'innate' or 'hard-wired' (functioning at birth, determined by genes, independent of environmental influence, and experience) and those that develop with maturation, acculturation (learning by immersion in the auditory world around us), or explicit training. The principle has been that if young infants, children, and nonmusician and musician adults display similar functioning modes on a particular task, then we conclude that this process may be 'innate' or at least 'functional' at an early age. Alternatively, if differences are observed between these populations, we then conclude that this type of functioning is acquired, either through acculturation or explicit learning.

We have, in the past avoided the word *innate* due to strong theoretical and philosophical connotations, referring rather to processes that may be universal—that is, that function in the same way in everyone. However, as has been pointed out to us, this wording is ambiguous. If we claim that a process is universal, we must demonstrate that it occurs the world over, irrespective of the cultural environment in which the individual lives and grew up. The present paper proposes such a research project. Whereas we have the know-how about both the psychological processes involved and appropriate paradigms to demonstrate the functioning of these processes, we are quite ignorant of the enormously exciting field of ethnomusicology, and our attempts at contact have so far been limited. Such a project cannot be accomplished on our own, or even with just one or two colleagues, but requires numerous sites the world over with researchers collaborating within a network.

Temporal processing is limited by memory space and processing time

If a computer programmer wanted to make a computer reproduce a musical rhythm, the program would probably record the precise duration (in milliseconds or computer clicks) of each interval in the sequence, put them in a lookup table, and then recall these values to produce the rhythm. The result would be that the reproduced rhythmic structure would be identical to that of the model. Is this a good model for the functioning of the human perceptual system? Probably not. Whereas human beings are able to reproduce musical rhythms so that they sound satisfactorily similar to the model, previous research suggests that our perceptual system does not function in the same way as the computer. The main difference in the way computers and humans function concerns memory limitations: computer memory is usually not a problem, while human memory is severely limited. As psychologists, our task is thus to describe the way in which our perceptual system analyses incoming temporal information and how it overcomes the main enemies: memory space and processing time.

Sound events usually do not occur in isolation, but rather are surrounded by other events, with each sound embedded within a sequence. Each event takes its existence from its relation with these surrounding events, rather than from its own specific characteristics. The task of situating each event in relation to surrounding events is quite simple when the sequence is short in duration and when it contains a limited number of events (i.e. three or four intervals). However, as the sequence becomes longer we very quickly run into problems of memory space and processing time. Imagine the number of intervals that would need to be stored and accessed when listening to a Beethoven sonata!

The idea is that all events would be stored in a memory buffer lasting several seconds (psychological present, probably corresponding to echoic or working memory), allowing the system to extract all relevant information (interval duration). One can imagine a temporal window gliding gradually through time, with new events arriving at one end and old events disappearing at the other due to decay. Thus only events occurring within a span of a few seconds would be accessible for processing at any one time, and only events occurring within this limited time window can be situated in relation to each other by the coding of relevant relational information. However, when the sequence becomes more complicated (longer and/or more events), the number of events that must be processed quickly goes beyond the limits of this buffer. Consequently, simple concatenation models that propose the maintenance in memory of the characteristics of each event are not able to account for the perception of long sequences because of problems of memory overload.

In this chapter, we present a set of five temporal processes that overcome these constraints, at least partially. These processes have been selected because previous research in the field of rhythmic perception suggests that they function in a similar fashion in all the populations examined so far. They are therefore candidates for the status of 'temporal universal'. This is not an exhaustive list, and other candidates could certainly be added as the project advances. As mentioned above, this list emerges from previous developmental and comparative studies. In each case we select key paradigms that we have used successfully in the past to demonstrate the lack of difference between populations differing in age and musical experience. An essential characteristic of developmental research is that the tasks used must be conceptually simple; must not require reading, writing, or any other specific knowledge such as musical notation; must be short (usually not more than 20 min of experimenting time); and must be technically transportable (into schools). As such, the paradigms we have used for children should be easily adaptable for intercultural research, which faces similar constraints. Taken together, this set of experimental paradigms could be used as a basis for answering the question of the true 'universal' nature of these psychological processes.

Candidate 1: segmentation and grouping

We tend to group into perceptual units events that have similar physical characteristics or that occur close in time.

One way to overcome processing limitations and to allow events to be processed together is to group the events into small perceptual units. These units result from a comparison process that compares incoming events with events that are already present in memory. If a new event is similar to those that are already present, it will be assimilated. If the new event differs too much (by its acoustical and/or temporal characteristics), the sequence will be segmented. This segmentation leads to the closure of one unit and the opening of the next. Elements grouped together will be processed together within a single perceptual unit and thus can be situated in relation to each other.

Several studies support these ideas. Listeners usually segment sequences as a function of the surface characteristics (timbre, pitch, intensity, event duration, pauses, etc.), following the principles laid down by the Gestalt psychologists: a change in any sound parameter leads to the perception of a break in the sequence and thus to the creation of groups separated by the changes (see Ref. 5 for a summary). For instance, the occurrence of a longer temporal gap or a major change in pitch leads to the segmentation of the sequence at that point, with the termination of one perceptual unit and the beginning of the next.

Paradigm 1: online segmentation

Many variations on a simple segmentation paradigm have been used. Usually participants listen to a musical excerpt and are asked to indicate, by pressing a button or drawing a line on a musical score, whenever they hear a 'break' in the sequence, so that events that belong together go together. The sequences are constructed in such a way as to establish whether each type of segmentation is used, as well as to indicate the relative importance of each segmentation principle.

Arguments in favour of universal status

Comparisons across musical skill levels.   Grouping appears unaffected by musical training, as similar segmentation principles are observed for adult musicians and nonmusicians, although musicians are more systematic in their responses.[6–8]

Infants.   Grouping also appears to function from an early age. For instance, studies using a gap detection paradigm suggest that six- to eight-month-old infants segment in a similar fashion to adults, at least for timbre and pitch, although a much greater pitch change was necessary for infants compared with adults.[9,10]

Comparisons across ages.   Findings are even less clear in children. Among the few previous studies on rhythmic development, we often find suggestions that this sort of grouping process is functioning in relatively young (five- to seven-year-old) children. However, these studies employ extremely indirect methodologies, and the conclusions are tentative.[10–15] With this criticism in mind, a major research project has been undertaken to examine the principles governing segmentation in 4- to 12-year-old musician and nonmusician children.[16] The children's task was to listen to short musical sequences composed of nine tones and to indicate, during a second listening, the point at which they would break the sequence into two (group boundary). Each sequence contained two changes in either pitch, intensity, tone duration, or pause duration. The question was whether or not their perceived boundaries were induced by the physical changes in the sequence, as observed previously in adults. The results provide a clear answer to this question: segmentations were well above chance level for all four segmentation principles, even for the youngest children (four years). On average, more than three-quarters of the segmentations corresponded to the physical change; this effect was equally strong for the four indices (pitch, intensity, tone duration, and pause duration). There was a slight improvement with age and musical experience, probably due to improved task-related skills.

Comparisons across cultures.   The online segmentation paradigm can easily be adapted for intercultural research, as the stimuli are nonculture-specific, and the task does not require any specific learned skill. If these basic processes of segmentation and grouping are unaffected by experience with a particular type of sequence, then the same types of segmentation should be observed in all cultures.

Candidate 2: predisposition towards regularity

Processing is better for regular than irregular sequences. We tend to hear as regular sequences that are not really regular.

As mentioned above, rather than coding the precise duration of each interval, our perceptual system compares each newly arriving interval with preceding ones. If the new interval is similar in duration to preceding intervals (within an acceptable temporal window, the 'tolerance window'), it will be categorized as 'same'; if it is significantly longer or shorter than the preceding intervals (beyond the tolerance window), it will be categorized as 'different'. There may be an additional coding of 'longer' or 'shorter'. Thus, our system may code two or three categories of durations (same/different, or same/longer/shorter); but note that this is a relative, rather than absolute, coding system.

One consequence of this type of processing is that if a sequence is irregular (each interval has a different duration) but all the intervals remain within the tolerance window, then we will perceive this sequence as the succession of 'same' intervals and so perceive a regular sequence. Such a tolerance in our perceptual system is quite understandable when we examine the temporal microstructure of performed music: local lengthenings and shortenings of more than 10 per cent are quite common[17,18] and are not necessarily picked out by listeners as irregularities.[19]

Paradigm 2: tempo discrimination for regular and irregular sequences

This predisposition towards regularity has been investigated using a tempo discrimination paradigm. Listeners hear two sequences that differ slightly in tempo, and they must say which is the fastest. The degree of regularity of the sequences is varied from completely regular (isochronous) to extremely irregular (based on the standard deviation of the interval durations).[20] Results show that up to a certain degree of irregularity, irregular sequences are processed as well as the regular sequences: they are 'assimilated' towards regularity. However, above a certain degree of irregularity, discrimination performance drops considerably. This cut-off point corresponds to the tolerance window mentioned above.

Arguments in favour of universal status

Comparisons across musical skill levels. The tolerance window appears to function in a similar fashion for both musicians and nonmusicians, with slightly irregular sequences being assimilated to regular sequences, although temporal thresholds are lower in musicians than nonmusicians.[20]

Comparison across ages. To our knowledge, nothing is known about children's ability to process irregular sequences. We do know, however, that from the age of four years, children are able to detect a small change in tempo of an isochronous sequence.[21] Another way of demonstrating the importance of temporal regularity in processing sequences involves rhythm reproduction tasks. For instance, when five- and seven-year-old children reproduced both regular and irregular rhythms, performance was much better for the regular ones.[22]

Infants. We also know little about infants' ability to process irregular sequences. We do know, however, that the capacity to detect a small change in tempo of an isochronous sequence is already functional at two months in infants.[23] They are able to habituate to a particular tempo, and there is a reaction to novelty if the tempo changes.

Comparison across cultures. This tempo discrimination task for regular and irregular sequences is easily adaptable to people from other cultures. If this process is universal, we should observe the same low tempo discrimination thresholds for regular and slightly irregular sequences, with considerably higher thresholds for very irregular sequences.

Candidate 3: active search for regularity

We spontaneously search for temporal regularities and organize events around this perceived regularity.

Coding events in terms of temporal regularity is thus an economical processing principle, and it has implications. If an incoming sequence can be coded in such a fashion, the needed processing resources are reduced, thus making it easier to process such a sequence. Indeed, we can say that the perceptual system exploits this predisposition, by actively 'looking for' temporal regularities in all types of sequences. We therefore suggest that when listening to a piece of music, we are predisposed to finding a regular pulse, that which is emphasised by tapping our foot in time with the music (*tactus* in musical terms). Once this underlying pulse has been identified, it is used as an organizational framework around which other events are situated.

Paradigm 3: synchronization with musical sequences

A simple way of investigating this process is to ask people to listen to a musical sequence, and then to tap in time with the music in a regular fashion at the rate that they think 'goes best' with the music. Synchronization is considered to be accomplished if successive taps coincide with tones within the music (at a particular hierarchical level) within a 10 per cent window. This is quite a strict criteria when you take into consideration the considerable temporal variations observed in performed music. In order to accomplish this task, listeners must abstract an underlying regularity, even if the performance variations tend to mask 'pure' temporal regularity.

Arguments in favour of universal status

Comparison across musical skill levels.   Synchronization success rates for both musicians and nonmusicians are very high (more than 90 per cent) when they are asked to tap in synchrony with music, even if the music contains many temporal and other performance microvariations.[24]

Comparison across ages.   All 20 four-year-olds (as well as the older children aged 6–10 years) examined in our study were able to successfully synchronize with the beginning of Ravel's *Boléro*.[21]

Infants.   Infants are able to adapt their spontaneous sucking rate to the rate of an auditory sequence,[25] at least under certain circumstances.

Comparison across cultures.   In order to adapt this paradigm to intercultural research, musical excerpts must be selected to include both music that respects the temporal structure with which the participants are familiar (their own musical idiom) and music that does not.

Candidate 4: temporal zone of optimal processing

We process information best if it arrives at an intermediate rate.

A fourth processing principle concerns the rate of temporal sequences. People spontaneously 'listen for' important events occurring at equally spaced moments in time, and the rate at which they 'search for' important information is specific to each individual.[26,27] Thus, the search for temporal regularities described above occurs at a particular rate. A zone of optimal processing has been demonstrated with numerous paradigms and types of sequences. The results are concordant: sensitivity to change is highest if events occur about every 600 ms, with a range stretching between about 300 and 800 ms interonset interval (IOI).

Paradigm 4: irregularity detection in complex sequences

How can we demonstrate that people focus spontaneously on events occurring at intermediate rates? A first method is simply to compare tempo discrimination thresholds of different rates,[20] as mentioned above. However, a more ecologically valid paradigm is currently being developed that would be ideal for the present requirements. When participants listen to complex sequences composed of two cooccurring isochronous subsequences, they should focus on the subsequence closest in rate to the optimal processing zone (300–800 ms IOI). We therefore introduce a temporal irregularity into one of the subsequences, which listeners should be able to detect only if they are focusing on that particular subsequence. The overall rate of the complex sequence is varied from very fast to very slow. Our results indicate that, as expected, detection was better for the slowest subsequence when the complex sequence was fast, and better for the fastest subsequence when the complex sequence was slow.[28] This promising paradigm has been applied only to nonmusician adults.

Arguments in favour of universal status

Comparison across musical skill levels.   Although musicians demonstrate a wider range of optimal tempi than nonmusicians, this optimal zone is still centred around the same value of 600 ms IOI.[20]

Comparison across ages.   Children between the ages of 4 and 10 years also demonstrate the same zone of optimal tempi, although the range increases with age.[21]

Infants.   Two-month-old infants demonstrate a reaction to novelty only for sequences at 600 ms IOI, demonstrating the same optimal zone from a very young age.[23]

Comparison across cultures.   This paradigm can be easily adapted to people of other cultures.

Candidate 5: predisposition towards simple duration ratios

We tend to hear a time interval as twice as long or short as previous intervals.

A fifth principle concerns the perceptual status of the 'longer' and 'shorter' durations: longer time intervals tend to be perceived and produced twice as long as the 'same' intervals, and shorter intervals tend to be perceived and produced twice as short as the same intervals.[29–31] The implication is that a categorization process is involved here, with clear-cut passages from one category to another.[30,32] Such an organization principle results in the dominance of binary, rather than ternary or more complex ratios between the three categories of intervals.

Paradigm 5: rhythm reproduction

One consequence of this process is that people are better able to reproduce rhythms containing only 1:2 ratios than rhythms containing 1:3 ratios[33] or even more complicated ratios.[34] Also, when people reproduce complex musical rhythms, the duration of some intervals undergoes a distortion towards one of the categories—that is, the rhythm is simplified so that the produced intervals respect a 1:2 ratio.[29]

Arguments in favour of universal status

Comparison across musical skill levels.   The same pattern of perceptual and motor distortions are observed in musicians and nonmusicians.[34]

Comparison across ages. From the age of 5 years, children are able to reproduce short rhythms based on binary (1:2), but not ternary (1:3) ratios.[33] When five- and seven-year-old children reproduce complex rhythms, their reproductions undergo simplification towards simple ratios.[22] Their incorrect reproductions contain only two durations, in a 2:1 ratio.[22]

Infants. To our knowledge, no data exists concerning the functioning of this duration categorization process in infants.

Comparison across cultures. A rhythm reproduction task can be adapted for intercultural research. Participants can be asked to reproduce rhythms varying in the number of different durations they contain. Reproductions should be best when they contain only two different durations in a ratio of 1:2. Ratios of 1:3 should be harder, and more complex ratios (which are perceived as irregular—see Candidate 2) even harder. The reproductions of complex rhythms should demonstrate simplification towards simple ratios.

Conclusion

We have thus proposed a series of five experimental paradigms, designed and tested to demonstrate the functioning of five temporal processes. If our hypotheses are correct concerning the universal nature of these processes, then whatever the culture or origin of the people being tested, we should observe the same results. This list of potential candidates for the status of temporal universals is probably far from complete, but it provides a starting point. Further suggestions are welcome.

References

1. **Lerdahl, F.** and **R. Jackendoff** (1983) *A Generative Theory of Tonal Music.* Cambridge, MA: MIT Press.
2. **Cooper, G.** and **L. G. Meyer** (1960) *The Rhythmic Structure of Music.* Chicago: University of Chicago Press.
3. **Yeston, M.** (1976) *The Stratification of Musical Rhythm.* New Haven, CT: Yale University Press.
4. **Drake, C.** (1998) Psychological processes involved in the temporal organization of complex auditory sequences: universal and acquired processes. *Music Percept.* 16, 11–26.
5. **Handel, S.** (1989) *Listening. An Introduction to the Perception of Auditory Events.* Cambridge, MA: MIT Press.
6. **Deliège, I.** (1987) Grouping conditions in listening to music: an approach to Lerdahl and Jackendoff's grouping preference rules. *Music Percept.* 4, 325–60.
7. **Fitzgibbons, P. J., A. Pollatsek,** and **I. B. Thomas** (1974) Detection of temporal gaps within and between perceptual tonal groups. *Percept. Psychophys.* 16, 522–8.
8. **Peretz, I.** and **J. Morais** (1989) Music and modularity. *Contemp. Music Rev.* 4, 279–93.
9. **Krumhansl, C. L.** and **P. W. Jusczyk** (1990) Infants perception of phrase structure in music. *Psychol. Sci.* 1, 70–3.

10. **Thorpe, L. A.** and **S. E. Trehub** (1989) Duration illusion and auditory grouping in infancy. *Dev. Psychol.* 25, 122–7.

11. **Drake, C.** (1993) Influence of age and experience on timing and intensity variations in the reproduction of short musical rhythms. *Psychol. Belg.* 33, 217–28.

12. **Drake, C.** (1993) Perceptual and performed accents in musical sequences. *Bull. Psychon. Soc.* 31, 107–10.

13. **Drake, C., J. Dowling,** and **C. Palmer** (1991) Accent structures in the reproduction of simple tunes by children and adult pianists. *Music Percept.* 8, 313–32.

14. **Gérard, C.** and **C. Drake** (1990) The inability of young children to reproduce intensity differences in musical rhythms. *Percept. Psychophys.* 48, 91–101.

15. **Bamberger, J.** (1980) Cognitive structuring in the apprehension and description of simple rhythms. *Arch. Psychol.* 48, 177–99.

16. **Bertrand, D.** (1999) Groupement rythmique et representation mentale de mélodies chez l'enfant. Ph.D. Thesis. Belgium: Liège University.

17. **Penel, A.** and **C. Drake** (1997) Perceptual and cognitive sources of timing variations in music performance: a psychological segmentation model. *Psychol. Res.* 61, 12–32.

18. **Repp, B. H.** (1992) Diversity and commonality in music performance: an analysis of timing microstructure in Schumann's Träumerei. *J. Acoust. Soc. Am.* 92, 2546–68.

19. **Repp, B. H.** (1992) Probing the cognitive representaion of musical time: structural constraints on the perception of timing perturbations. *Cognition* 44, 241–81.

20. **Drake, C.** and **M. C. Botte** (1993) Tempo sensitivity in auditory sequences: evidence for a multiple-look model. *Percept. Psychophys.* 54, 277–86.

21. **Drake, C., M. R. Jones,** and **C. Baruch** (2000) The development of rhythmic attending in auditory sequences: attunement, reference period, focal attending. *Cognition* 77, 251–88.

22. **Drake, C.** and **C. Gérard** (1989) A psychological pulse train: how young children use this cognitive framework to structure simple rhythms. *Psychol. Res.* 51, 16–22.

23. **Baruch, C.** and **C. Drake** (1997) Tempo discrimination in infants. *Infant Behav. Dev.* 20, 573–7.

24. **Drake, C., A. Penel,** and **E. Bigand** (2000) Tapping in time with mechanically and expressively performed music. *Music Percept.* 18(1), 1–24.

25. **Pouthas, V.** (1995) The development of the perception of time and temporal regulation of action in infants and children. In I. Deliège and J. A. Sloboda (Eds) *Musical Beginnings: The Origins and Development of Musical Competence.* New York: Oxford University Press, pp. 115–41.

26. **Jones, M. R.** (1976) Time, our last dimension: toward a new theory of perception, attention, and memory. *Psychol. Rev.* 83, 323–55.

27. **Jones, M. R.** and **M. Boltz** (1989) Dynamic attending and responses to time. *Psychol. Rev.* 96, 459–91.

28. **Brochard, R.** (1997) Role of attention in the perceptual organisation of complex auditory sequences. Ph.D. Thesis, University of Paris.

29. **Fraisse, P.** (1956) Les structures rythmiques. Publications Universitaires de Louvain. Louvain.

30. **Clarke, E. F.** (1987) Categorical rhythm perception: an ecological perspective. In A. Gabrielsson (ed.) *Action and Perception in Rhythm and Musica.* Stockholm: Royal Swedish Academy of Music, pp. 19–34.

31. **Parncutt, R.** (1994) A perceptual model of pulse salience and metrical accent in musical rhythms. *Music Percept.* 11, 409–64.

32. **Schulze, H. H.** (1989) Categorical perception of rhythmic patterns. *Psychol. Res.* 51, 10–15.

33. **Drake, C.** (1993) Reproduction of musical rhythms by children, adult musicians, and adult nonmusicians. *Percept. Psychophys.* 53, 25–33.

34. **Sternberg, S., R. L. Knoll,** and **P. Zukofsky** (1982) Timing by skilled musicians. In D. Deutsch (ed.) *The Psychology of Music.* New York: Academic Press, pp. 182–237.

CHAPTER 3

MECHANISMS OF MUSICAL MEMORY IN INFANCY

JENNY R. SAFFRAN

Abstract

How do infants learn about their auditory world, and what do they remember? In this chapter, we review recent findings suggesting that as previously observed in the language domain, infants possess powerful memory abilities that allow them to represent myriad aspects of their musical environments. These memories provide a corpus of musical experiences from which infants can begin to acquire the structures that characterize their native musical systems.

Introduction

From the perspective of an infant just beginning to make sense of the world, music is an extremely complex and attractive stimulus. Not only is music itself of great interest to the youngest listeners, but it is also the case that the musical aspects of language—the pitch and rhythmic patterns that constitute native language prosodic structure—are the most likely to capture infants' attention, and are the first components of language that infants learn (e.g. Refs 1–3). Moreover, infant-directed music may be more speech-like, with more communicative value, than adult-directed music, suggesting that the input to infant listeners may be particularly similar in these two domains (e.g. Ref. 4 and Chapter 1). Linguistic and musical input both present a vast array of information to listeners—including many levels of structure that are simultaneously available—that must be acquired by infants on the road to becoming native listeners. How does this process unfold, and what are the mechanisms that allow infants to learn from their musical experiences?

While we will focus primarily on music in this chapter, we will use the literature on infant speech and language perception to suggest avenues of overlap and difference, and as a source of potentially fruitful areas for future study. Before doing so, however, it is necessary to step back and consider the hypothesized relationships between these two systems. In particular, the connection between linguistic and musical processes in infancy is currently unknown. Language and music are clearly not isomorphic in the adult brain, and are dissociable in many important ways (for recent reviews, see Chapters 12 and 13). Despite these differences in the mature state, it is possible that some of the same mechanisms are engaged in learning in both domains. It is important to note that any observed modularity in the adult brain does not necessarily mean that the learning mechanisms which initially supported learning during infancy are themselves modular. While there is some evidence that some specifically musical processes are subject to congenital impairments,[8] it is also the case that some learning mechanisms have been shown to operate equivalently for both speech-like and music-like stimuli in both infancy and adulthood.[9] Similarly, related patterns of adult brain electrical activity occur in response to some aspects of music and language, but not to others (for review, see Chapter 18). The level of plasticity evident for both types of auditory learning, particularly during childhood, suggests that at least some of the underlying processes for music and language may overlap developmentally.

Consider a specific example of the possible relationship between representations of auditory information in memory with respect to speech and music. The relevance of pitch for music perception is obvious; what is less obvious but also important is the role played by pitch in language learning. The most easily observed use of linguistic pitch lies in the melodic contours which signal sentence meaning, such as the rising contour that is indicative of question prosody. There are also many languages which use pitch and/or pitch contour contrastively with respect to word meaning; these tonal languages, such as Mandarin, Thai, and Vietnamese, are acquired readily by infants and young children. For this learning to occur, all infants—regardless of their native language-to-be—must possess the capacity to attend to pitch cues as a possible component of lexical items. At the same time, many aspects of pitch in linguistic stimuli must be ignored by infants engaged in learning their native language. As in music perception, the absolute pitches with which words are spoken are not informative as to their meaning. Even deeper relationships between the use of pitch in speech and music processing have been hypothesized; for example, processing speech may lead the auditory system to acquire the specific pitch relationships between harmonics in speech sounds, which become the intervals in music.[11] It is thus likely that the learning mechanisms that subserve the acquisition both speech and music are related to one another in some fashion, despite the eventual deep differences in the knowledge acquired; however, the nature of this relationship is currently unknown.

Infant music perception and possible relationships with speech perception

The task of learning about how music works appears to be partially solved for the infant quite early in life, either via biological predispositions or through extremely rapid learning. Infants show early preferences for consonant musical intervals such as octaves and perfect fifths, are highly attuned to rhythm, can represent both relational and absolute pitch information under different circumstances, and are sensitive to cues correlated with musical phrase boundaries (for a recent review, see Chapter 1). These early emerging capacities provide support for the infant's initial representations of musical structure and events.

Despite this early head-start, there remains a tremendous amount of information for infants to learn. Just as in language, where learners must acquire knowledge of the systematic structure in their native language (e.g. phonological and grammatical generalizations) as well as specific knowledge about individual experiences (e.g. individual phonemes, lexical items, and voices), infants must learn the structure of the musical system present in their environment (e.g. tonality, conventional structures) as well as specific pieces of music. Infants must therefore possess abilities which allow them to represent musical experiences, and to learn from those experiences.

Of particular interest is the question of which aspects of music are represented in infants' memories. Any given musical experience contains information which is relevant for discerning the deep structure of the piece, including its melodic structure, harmonic structure, and rhythm. There is also myriad information which is less important musically, such as the specific key of the piece, the exact tempo of the performance, and the instruments upon which it is played. Despite the seeming irrelevance of these highly specific aspects of particular musical experiences, adult listeners' representations of highly familiar pieces include information about absolute pitch,[12] absolute tempo,[13] and timbre.[14] It appears that at least for adult listeners, 'memory representations for complex auditory stimuli contain information about the absolute properties of the stimuli, in addition to more meaningful information abstracted from the relations between stimulus components'[14] (p. 646). This model of auditory memory also captures what is currently known about adult representations of linguistic auditory events, which include seemingly irrelevant specific information such as talker-specific cues as well as linguistically meaningful information; for example, adult listeners appear to include speaker voice and rate (though not amplitude) in their representations of spoken words.[15]

Which aspects of auditory experiences are represented by infant listeners in memory? Research focused on infant speech perception suggests that infants as young as 7.5 months of age can reliably remember new words after just a few exposures embedded in fluent speech, and that these representations are specific enough that infants exposed to 'cup' do not incorrectly recognize 'tup' (e.g. Ref. 16). Moreover, infants at this age can remember words heard multiple times in stories over multi-week delays.[17] Even younger infants can recognize their names and other words that are heard frequently in their environments (e.g. Refs 18 and 19). The literature also provides some indications that like adults, infants represent multiple levels of auditory stimuli, including both those that are linguistically relevant and those that are not. For example, 7.5-month-old infants include talker-specific cues in their representations of spoken words.[20] However, infants are able to ignore talker-specific properties under other circumstances—in particular, infants readily exhibit vowel normalization, categorizing individual exemplars according to vowel identity despite differences in speaker sex (e.g. Refs 21 and 22). Infants thus appear to process linguistic auditory events at multiple levels of detail simultaneously.

These findings from the domain of speech suggest potential avenues of study for infant musical learning and memory. Is infant memory for musical experiences as powerful and as detailed as memory for language? It is possible that infants' representations of music are even more specific than their representations of speech; mothers' songs to infants are remarkably consistent over time with respect to their pitch and tempo, providing a highly reliable set of musical cues to infant listeners, whereas their infant-directed-speech is less consistent in pitch and tempo.[23]

To learn about music, infants must acquire knowledge both about musical structure in general and about specific pieces of music. The literature suggests that the former process— learning one's native musical system—is quite extended developmentally. Indeed, while there are some indications that infants acquire rudimentary knowledge about how tonal systems work during their first year of life (e.g. Ref. 24), most of this knowledge is not fully acquired until childhood (e.g. Refs 25–27). For example, Schellenberg and Trehub[28] demonstrated that the degree to which novel melodies adhere to Western tonal conventions affected the performance of 5-year-old children, but not 9-month-old infants. These findings diverge from the literature on infant speech perception, which suggests that infants have acquired the bulk of their native language's sound structure by the time they are a year of age (for extensive review, see Ref. 29). It is possible that the acquisition of Western tonal structure is more akin to the acquisition of syntax and morphology than to the acquisition of phonology, as the grammatical aspects of language are acquired slightly later (primarily in the second and third postnatal year). Alternatively, the fact that infants presumably receive more exposure to speech than to music (although this has never been quantified) may account for the relative rapidity with which knowledge of the native language emerges relative to knowledge of the native musical system.

Infants' memory capacity for specific musical experiences—individual pieces of music present in the infant's environment—has received far less attention in the literature. In the remainder of this chapter, we will review recent evidence suggesting that infants possess the capacity to remember individual pieces of music over multiweek delays. These accumulated memory representations presumably provide a corpus of musical knowledge from which infants can learn about the structure of their native musical system, analogous to the specific linguistic experiences from which infants begin to glean phonological and grammatical generalizations. As described above with reference to adult musical memory and infant linguistic memory, infants appear to attend to many levels of musical structure which are manifest in their memory representations, suggesting interesting parallels in memory both across age (infants vs adults) and domain (music vs language).

Long-term memory for music in infancy

To what extent do young infants maintain specific musical experiences in long-term memory? Recent findings in the language domain suggest that 8-month-old infants can remember words from stories over time delays of two weeks.[17] Because music, along with language, is among the most complex auditory learning tasks facing infants, it is possible that infant memory for musical stimuli is equally powerful. Little research, however, has addressed the question of whether infants remember particular musical pieces heard during passive listening experiences.

To ask whether infants possess long-term memory for musical materials, we adapted the experimental procedures used by Jusczyk and Hohne[17] to assess the maintenance of linguistic materials over multiweek delays.[30] We exposed a group of 7-month-old infants to a 10 min. recording of two Mozart piano sonata movements: KV 281 in B-flat major, Andante, and KV 282 in E-flat major, Adagio. Each infant listened to the music once a day, at home, for 14 consecutive days. Following a two week retention interval, during which the infants did not hear these pieces, we assessed the infants' long-term memory for the Mozart sonatas in the laboratory. To do so, we measured listening preferences using the head-turn preference procedure (e.g. Ref. 31), a standard computer-automated method used in studies of infant auditory perception.

We hypothesized that if infants remembered the music with which they were familiarized at home, they would show recognition by listening longer to passages of familiar music

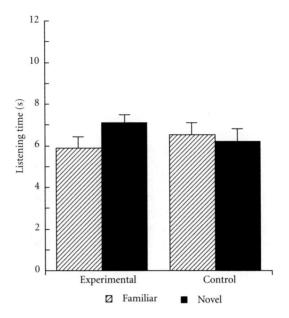

Figure 3.1 Experiment 1: listening times for familiar and novel test passages for infants from the experimental (prior exposure) and control (no prior exposure) groups.[30]

than to novel passages (as observed in Ref. 17 research on infant linguistic long-term memory). The test consisted of two familiar and two novel passages, all 20 s in duration. The familiar test passages were drawn from the middle of each of the two familiarized sonata movements. The novel test stimuli were drawn from two other Mozart sonatas (taken from the same CD recording and also composed during late 1774-early 1775: KV 280 in F-major, Adagio, and KV 283 in G-major, Andante). To ensure that arbitrary properties of the test stimuli could not account for the infants' performance, we also tested a control group of 8-month-old infants who received no prior exposure to any of these pieces.

Mean listening times for the familiar and novel musical passages were calculated for each infant (see Figure 3.1). Consistent with the hypothesis that infants maintain musical experiences in long-term memory, there was a significant difference in listening times for the familiar and novel passages for infants in the experimental group. However, the direction of the preference was contrary to our hypothesis; the infants preferred the novel passages over the familiar passages. To ensure that this pattern of results was not due to biased test materials, we also examined the performance of the infants in the control group. These infants did not show a significant preference for either type of test passage, suggesting that the preferences which emerged for the experimental group reflected long-term memory for the familiar passages.

Why did the infants prefer the novel passages in the first experiment? This direction of preference is the opposite of the results from Jusczyk and Hohne's linguistic study,[17] in which infants preferred familiar stimuli after a two week delay. There are (at least) two possible explanations: (1) Mastery: If infants mastered the familiarized music, they might now

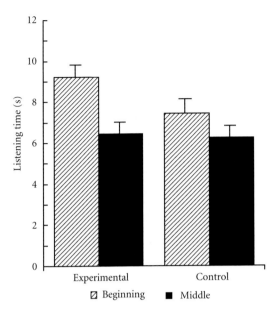

Figure 3.2   Experiment 2: listening times for passages from the beginnings and middles of the familiar music for infants from the experimental (prior exposure) and control (no prior exposure) groups.[30]

prefer to hear something new, despite the two week retention period during which they did not hear the familiarized music. (2) Musical context: The familiar test passages were taken from the middles of the familiar sonata movements. Thus, when they were played during testing, they were removed from the musical context within which they were originally learned. Because infants typically prefer to listen to stimuli that are maximally natural, in both the linguistic and musical domains (e.g. Refs 32 and 33), passages removed from context may have been dispreferred.

The second experiment was designed to test these two hypotheses. A second group of 7-month-old infants was familiarized with the same two sonata movements, following procedures identical to Experiment 1. Following a two week retention interval, the infants were tested in the laboratory on two different types of *familiar* passages: passages taken from the middles of the sonatas (which were the familiar passages used in Experiment 1), and the beginning passages from the two familiarized sonatas. If the results of Experiment 1 reflected mastery as evidenced by relative disinterest in the familiar music, then the infants should now prefer the *middle* passages, as the beginnings are presumably more memorable than the middle passages. However, on the musical context hypothesis, infants should prefer the familiar passages taken from the *beginnings* of the sonatas. Even in the context of the full sonata movements, the beginning passages were always preceded by silence. Thus, unlike the passages taken from the middles of the sonatas, the beginning test passages were not removed from their musical context when played in isolation.

As in Experiment 1, there was a significant difference in listening times (see Figure 3.2). The direction of the preference was consistent with the musical context hypothesis: the infants preferred the passages from the beginnings rather than the middles of the familiarized sonatas. Again, we tested a separate control group to ensure that biased test passages could not account for the experimental group's performance; these infants did not show a significant preference for either type of test passage. Along with Experiment 1, the results of Experiment 2 strongly suggest that infants do remember the music that they hear; the existence of a preference for passages drawn from the beginnings, rather than the middles, of the familiar music indicates that the infants remembered the pieces last heard at home two weeks before. Moreover, the infants preferred music that was not taken out of context. The control infants showed no such bias; even out of context, these passages sounded coherent to listeners who were not familiar with the pieces from which they were drawn.

These results suggest that infants are sophisticated musical listeners. Their representations of music in long-term memory are not undifferentiated sequences of notes. Instead, passages are linked together to form coherent musical events. Other recent studies investigating infant long-term memory for music similarly suggest that infants' representations are quite nuanced. For example, infants can represent far more complex pieces of music (such as Ravel) in long-term memory.[34] Moreover, the content of infants' memories includes some extremely specific aspects of musical performances. For example, 10-month-olds represent acoustic patterns specific to the particular performances with which they were previously familiarized.[35] Six-month-old infants remember the specific tempo and timbre of music with which they are familiarized, failing to recognize pieces when they are played at new tempos or with new timbres.[36] It thus appears that infant representations are extremely specific, without the flexibility to generalize to include changes in tempo or timbre. This level of specificity must change with age, as either a function of experience or development, else listeners would not be able to recognize familiar music played on different instruments or at different rates. Indeed, preschool children can recognize familiar tunes across many different types of transformations, suggesting that children are in the process of developing more flexible musical representations.[37]

Interestingly, infants can recognize previously familiarized melodies when they are played in a new key,[36] suggesting that for highly familiar pieces, infants represent the relative pitches of melodies. Such interval-level information is the appropriate level of specificity for generalizing memories from one experience to another, and is the preferential level of processing for most adult listeners. These results reinforce the suggestion that task demands determine the level of processing of pitch cues in musical materials: infants represent pitch contour and/or relative pitches more readily given familiar pieces, or given familiarization with repeating brief tunes (for review, see Ref. 38), but appear to rely on absolute pitches given unsegmented stretches of previously unfamiliar tone sequences.[24,39] Infants have access to multiple levels of pitch representations, much like adults (e.g. Refs 40 and 12); the structure of the task and the familiarity of the stimulus domain may influence which levels of representation are prioritized. For example, when absolute pitch cues are rendered uninformative in a task which previously elicited the use of absolute pitch information, infants shift to rely on relative pitch cues (Saffran, Reeck, Niebuhr, and Wilson, in prep.). These results mirror data from an avian species—starlings—who can switch from relying on absolute pitch cues to using relative pitch cues when necessitated by the structure of the task.[41]

Conclusion

We thus see a surprising level of similarity in infant memory representations for music and for language. In both cases, infants readily represent the input at multiple levels of analysis, from highly specific surface-level cues to the structural information that eventually conveys meaning. Moreover, these processes of learning and memory proceed without instruction or any reinforcement other than the pleasure of listening and the instinct to learn. These findings lend further support to an emerging picture of infants as remarkably adept at implicitly learning and remembering the structured information that characterizes the environment in which they develop. From the infant's perspective, music and language may not be nearly as different as they are for the adult listener, at least when considering what is to be gleaned from a listening experience. Just how distinct these processes are remains to be seen. Might the eventual differences in how the adult brain represents music and language be due to predetermined differences in the brain, or to differences in the structure of the input drawn from these two domains, or both? Regardless, it is evident that even the youngest listeners are already accomplished musicians in their own right.

Acknowledgements

The preparation of this chapter was made possible by a grant from the International Foundation for Music Research. Thanks to the many students and research assistants who have collaborated on the conduct of this research, and to Erik Thiessen for helpful comments on a previous draft.

References

1. **Cooper, R. P.** and **R. N. Aslin** (1990) Preference for infant-directed speech in the first month after birth. *Child Dev.* 61, 1584–95.
2. **Fernald, A.** (1989) Intonation and communicative intent in mothers' speech to infants: is the melody the message? *Child Dev.* 60, 1497–510.
3. **Mehler, J., P. W. Jusczyk, G. Lambertz, N. Halsted, J. Bertoncini,** and **C. Amiel-Tison** (1988) A precursor of language acquisition in young infants. *Cognit.* 29, 144–78.
4. **Trehub, S. E.** and **L. J. Trainor** (1998) Singing to infants: lullabies and play songs. In C. Rovee-Collier, L. Lipsitt, and H. Hayne (eds) *Advances in Infancy Research.* Stamford, CT: Ablex, pp. 43–77.
5. **Ayotte, J., I. Peretz,** and **K. Hyde** (2002) Congenital amusia: a group study of adults afflicted with a music-specific disorder. *Brain*, 125, 238–51.
6. **Saffran, J. R., E. K. Johnson, R. N. Aslin,** and **E. L. Newport** (1999) Statistical learning of tone sequences by human infants and adults. *Cognit.* 70, 27–52.
7. **Terhardt, E.** (1974) Pitch, consonance, and harmony. *J. Acoust. Soc. Am.* 55, 1061–9.
8. **Levitin, D.** (1994) Absolute memory for musical pitch: evidence from the production of learned melodies. *Percept. Psychophy.* 56, 414–23.
9. **Levitin, D.** and **P. R. Cook** (1996) Memory for musical tempo: additional evidence that auditory memory is absolute. *Percept. Psychophy.* 58, 927–35.

10. Schellenberg, E. G., P. Iverson, and M. C. McKinnon (1999) Name that tune: identifying popular recordings from brief excerpts. *Psychonomic Bulletin Rev.* 6, 641–6.

11. Bradlow, A. R., L. C. Nygaard, and D. B. Pisoni (1999) Effects of talker, rate, and amplitude variation on recognition memory for spoken words. *Percept. Psychophy.* 61, 206–19.

12. Jusczyk, P. W. and R. N. Aslin (1995) Infants' detection of the sound patterns of words in fluent speech. *Cognit. Psychol.* 29, 1–23.

13. Jusczyk, P. W. and E. A. Hohne (1997) Infants' memory for spoken words. *Sci.* 277, 1984–86.

14. Mandel D. R., P. W. Jusczyk, and D. B. Pisoni (1995) Infants' recognition of the sound patterns of their own names. *Psychological Sci.* 6, 314–17.

15. Tincoff, R. and P. W. Jusczyk (1999) Some beginnings of word comprehension in 6-month-olds. *Psychological Sci.* 10, 172–5.

16. Houston, D. M. and P. W. Jusczyk (2000). The role of talker-specific information in word segmentation by infants. *J. Exp. Psychol.: Hum. Percept. Perform.* 26, 1570–82.

17. Kuhl, P. K. (1979) Speech perception in early infancy: perceptual constancy for spectrally dissimilar vowel categories. *J. Acoust. Soc. Am.* 66, 1668–79.

18. Kuhl, P. K. (1983) Perception of auditory equivalence classes for speech in early infancy. *Infant Behav. Dev.* 6, 263–85.

19. Bergeson, T. R. and S. E. Trehub (2002) Absolute pitch and tempo in mothers' songs to infants. *Psychological Sci.* 13, 72–5.

20. Saffran, J. R. (2003) Absolute pitch in infancy and adulthood: the role of tonal structure. *Dev. Sci.* 6, 37–49.

21. Krumhansl, C. L. and F. C. Keil (1982) Acquisition of the hierarchy of tonal functions in music. *Mem. Cognit.* 10, 243–51.

22. Lynch, M. P. and R. E. Eilers (1992) A study of perceptual development for musical tuning. *Percept. Psychophy.* 52, 599–608.

23. Trainor, L. J. and S. E. Trehub (1992) A comparison of infants' and adults' sensitivity to Western musical structure. *J. Exp. Psychol.: Hum. Percept. Perform.* 18, 394–402.

24. Schellenberg, E. G. and S. E. Trehub (1999) Culture-general and culture-specific factors in the discrimination of melodies. *J. Exp. Child Psychol.* 74, 107–27.

25. Jusczyk, P. W. (1997) *The Discovery of Spoken Language*. Cambridge: MIT Press.

26. Saffran, J. R., M. M. Loman, and R. R. W. Robertson (2000) Infant memory for musical experiences. *Cognit.* 77, 15–23.

27. Kemler Nelson, D. G., P. W. Jusczyk, D. R. Mandel, J. Myers, A. Turk, and L. A. Gerken (1995) The head-turn preference procedure for testing auditory perception. *Infant Behav. Dev.* 18, 111–16.

28. Krumhansl, C. L. and P. W. Jusczyk (1990) Infants' perception of phrase structure in music. *Psychological Sci.* 1, 70–3.

29. Hirsh-Pasek, K., D. G. Kemler Nelson, P. W. Jusczyk, K. Wright Cassidy, B. Druss, and L. Kennedy (1987) Clauses are perceptual units for young infants. *Cognit.* 26, 269–86.

30. Ilari, B. and L. Polka (2002) Memory for music in infancy: the role of style and complexity. Poster presented at the International Conference on Infant Studies, Toronto, April, 2002.

31. Palmer, C., M. K. Jungers, and P. W. Jusczyk (2001) Episodic memory for musical prosody. *J. Mem. Language* 45, 536–45.

32. **Trainor, L. J., L. Wu, C. D. Tsang**, and **J. Plantinga** (2002) Long-term memory for music in infancy. Poster presented at the International Conference on Infant Studies, Toronto, April, 2002.

33. **Schellenberg, E. G.** and **S. E. Trehub** (2000) Children's memory for familiar music. Paper presented at the meeting of the Psychonomic Society, New Orleans.

34. **Trehub, S. E., E. G. Schellenberg**, and **D. Hill** (1997) The origins of music perception and cognition: a developmental perspective. In I. Deliège and J. Sloboda (eds) *Perception and Cognition of Music*. East Sussex, UK: Psychology Press, pp. 103–28.

35. **Saffran, J. R.** and **G. J. Griepentrog** (2001) Absolute pitch in infant auditory learning: evidence for developmental reorganization. *Dev. Psychol.* 37, 74–85.

36. **Halpern, A. R.** (1989) Memory for the absolute pitch of familiar songs. *Mem. Cognit.* 17, 572–81.

37. **MacDougall-Shackleton, S. A.** and **S. H. Hulse** (1996) Concurrent absolute and relative pitch processing by European starlings. *J. Comparative Psychol.* 110, 139–46.

38. **Jusczyk, P. W.** and **C. L. Krumhansl** (1993) Pitch and rhythmic patterns affecting infants' sensitivity to musical phrase structure. *J. Exp. Psychol.: Hum. Percept. Perfor.* 19, 627–40.

39. **Schellenberg, E. G.** and **S. E. Trehub** (1996) Natural musical intervals: evidence from infant listeners. *Psychological Sci.* 7, 272–7.

CHAPTER 4

MUSIC, COGNITION, CULTURE, AND EVOLUTION

IAN CROSS

Abstract

We seem able to define the biological foundations for our musicality within a clear and unitary framework, yet music itself does not appear so clearly definable. Music is different things and does different things in different cultures; the bundles of elements and functions which are music for any given culture may overlap minimally with those of another culture, even for those cultures where 'music' constitutes a discrete and identifiable category of human activity in its own right. The dynamics of culture, of music as cultural praxis, are neither necessarily reducible, nor easily relatable, to the dynamics of our biologies. Yet music appears to be a universal human competence. Recent evolutionary theory, however, affords a means for exploring things biological and cultural within a framework within in which they are at least commensurable. The adoption of this perspective shifts the focus of the search for the foundations of music away from the mature and particular expression of music within a specific culture or situation and on to the human capacity for musicality. This paper will survey recent research that examines that capacity and its evolutionary origins in the light of a definition of music that embraces music's multifariousness. It will be suggested that 'music', like speech, is a product of both our biologies and our social interactions: that 'music' is a necessary and integral dimension of human development: and that 'music' may have played a central role in the evolution of the modern human mind.

We can express our understanding of biology within a framework that enables us to relate it, if not reduce it, to our understanding of the world in physical and material terms. Biological and physical understandings of the world are *commensurable*, in at least one of the senses that Lakoff[1] (p. 322) proposes. An understanding of ourselves as biological beings appears to be an understanding of 'natural kinds'.[a] But is music a 'natural kind', comprehensible within the generalized framework that is science?

---

[a] This is not to endorse the idea that there are 'natural kinds', that science provides an account of the essences of things in the world. The term 'natural kind' is used here simply as a concise way of referring to the objects of scientific discourse. As Rose[2] (p. 42) points out, even a concept as seemingly 'natural' and unambiguous as a 'protein' is susceptible to multiple and differing levels of definition that are dependent on 'the purposes for which we need to make the definition'. There is an incontestably societal dimension to the make-up of what is taken to constitute science at any time. But the notion that scientific procedures and understandings are simply varieties of social practice definable by their particular vocabularies[3] or by their poverty and abstraction[4] is insufficient to account for the instrumentality of those procedures and for the commensurability of the understandings that they afford.

Many argue that music is not a natural kind. Indeed, following a conventional dictionary definition of music—'The art of combining sounds of voices or instruments to achieve beauty of form and expression of emotion'—it would be difficult to do so. The consensual view from within the humanities appears to be that music is cultural rather than natural; music is viewed as constituted of practices, concepts, and perceptions that are grounded in particular social interactions and constructions. Molino[5] (p. 169), in questioning the status of music as a natural kind, proposes that 'Nothing guarantees that all the forms of human music contain a nucleus of common properties that would be invariant since the origination of music'.

As Geertz[6] (p. 5) put it, in promoting a semiotic and interpretive approach to culture, 'man is an animal suspended in webs of significance he himself has spun', and within Geertz's humano-centric web of culture there is little room for the 'natural'. For Treitler[7] (p. 203), 'Meaning in music is a function of the engagement of codes or orders by the note complexes of which the musical event is comprised', and musical phenomena are thus 'intelligible only in the light of an interpretation which intuits the purpose or intention that they embody'. Tomlinson, inciting musicologists to embrace Geertz's concept of culture, makes explicit the idea that scientific generalization is incompatible with musicological method; he asserts[8] (p. 352) that the essence of cultural—and hence musicological—explanation is 'not to codify abstract regularities but to make thick description possible, not to generalize across cases but to generalize within them'. Indeed, Abbate[9] has suggested (p. xv) that 'There is nothing immanent in a musical work (beyond the material reality of its written and sonic traces) and our perceptions of forms, configurations, meanings, gestures, and symbols are always mediated by verbal formulas, as on a broader scale by ideology and culture'. And Garnett[10] proposes that 'there is...no extra-cultural locus from which to observe music, nor extra-cultural meaning to observe'. 'Music' is seen as the expression of discrete, contingent, and socially conditioned factors in respect of which a generalizable—and hence scientific— account is neither relevant nor possible.

Such an approach to understanding music appears justified in view of the heterogeneity of forms that music can take. What 'nucleus of common properties' other, perhaps, than the very concept of the musical work (see Ref. 11) underlies such diverse products of western culture (or, as Slobin[12] has put it, musical microcultures) as (i) a performance of a Machaut motet; (ii) the autograph score of a Beethoven string quartet; (iii) the concept of Alvin Lucier's 'I am sitting in a room...'; (iv) a live broadcast of Brian Ferneyhough's 'Transit'; (v) the grooves in the vinyl that constitute the recording of the Holy Modal Rounders' track 'Half a mind to have a mind'; (vi) and the samples that make up part of the mastering materials of a Dr Dre CD? And indeed this last example undermines the very concept of the musical work itself. It might be suggested that 'the art of combining sounds of voices or instruments...' provides such a common property (though the issue of 'the achievement of beauty...' seems moot). But if we look beyond what Tomlinson[8] refers to as a 'presentist'[b] view of our own culture, that common property evanesces.

---

[b] Tomlinson[8] (p. 358): 'The presentist view of art works as transcendent entities fully comprehensible without reference to the conditions of their creation sacrifices Geertz's expansion of human discourse for a solipsistic and ultimately narcissistic aestheticism'.

Indeed, when we look to other cultures, the notion of music *per se* is called into question. For example, Malm[13] (p. 5) questions whether or not the sound of the bull roarer used in some Arnhem Land aboriginal ceremonies constitutes 'music', as 'its sounds in secret rituals are not considered as independent sonic events but rather are thought to be the sounds of the supernatural itself'. And a culture may be constituted such that it does not distinguish a discrete category of practices that map onto those that would comprise music from a western perspective. Gourlay[14] notes that some cultures employ terms far more inclusive than the western notion of music; for the Igbo of Nigeria, *nkwa* denotes 'singing, playing instruments, and dancing'. Thus the anthropologist approaching Igbo culture with a view to examining its 'music' is confronted by a dilemma; as Gourlay[14] puts it (p. 35) 'By forcing the Igbo concept into the Procrustean bed of western conceptualization, she is in fact surrendering to the dominance of western ideas—or at least to the dominance of the English language. How different things would be if the Igbo tongue had achieved the same 'universality' as English! We should then have been seeking for universals in *nkwa*, and regarding the whole process of western "serious" music as an aberration because it excluded dance'. If the very concept of 'music' is so variable and inextricable from its cultural context how can we expect to seek, far less find, its biological foundations?

Perhaps some space for the 'natural' in conceptions of music might be found through recourse to cognitive anthropology rather than to anthropology *per se*, using the notion of mind to connect culture with biology. As D'Andrade[15] notes, the tacit notion of culture even within the anthropological consensus is that it is *in the mind*. He suggests (p. 146) that 'Since the 1950s most anthropologists have defined culture as a purely *mental* phenomenon'. Hence if culture is a mental phenomenon 'The structures that exist in the physical world as objects or events...are all thought to be...more or less a reflection of these mental cultural structures'. And given the success of cognitive science in instating mind in the material, it seems reasonable to expect that notions of mind might furnish terms that could connect the discourses of anthropology and of the natural sciences.

But cognitive anthropology, or from another perspective, cultural psychology (see Ref. 16) offers little comfort. For there is little consensus about the depth to which culture permeates the grain of our experience. The question of whether we should conceive of some psychic unity upon which culture forms an overlay, or a psychic diversity that is principally constructed by culture, remains unresolved. D'Andrade[15], for example, leaves space for the notion of a primitive and perceptual psychic unity when he suggests (p. 217) that 'culture seems to have its greatest effect...on semantic memory and complex reasoning'. But he undermines that notion by suggesting (p. 184) that 'In general, naive perception can be influenced by cultural schemas'. A practical musical example might uphold the second suggestion by showing that culture indeed appears to determine the grain of our unreflective perceptions.

One factor that appears to apply to almost all the world's musics is that there is a level of temporal organization that is regular and periodic, sometimes called the tactus. It is taken to correspond to the regular points in the music where one would tap one's foot or clap along. In listening to a piece in a familiar idiom, all listeners are capable of tapping along without thinking (even if it is frowned upon in the concert hall). And even when encountering previously unheard music from an unknown culture, a listener can still 'keep a beat'. Most western listeners confronted by this particular piece from Northern Potosí in Bolivia (recorded by my friend and colleague Henry Stobart, an ethnomusicologist specializing in Andean music) are likely to clap or tap along with the regularly spaced longer and louder notes:

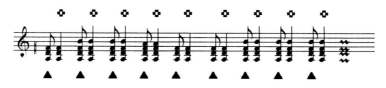

❖ = Clapping of western listeners

▲ = performers' footfalls

An example of a recording of this piece can be heard on the Internet by accessing http://www.mus.cam.ac.uk/~cross/BJE/ and selecting Example III(a). At the end of the recording something occurs that gives the game away; for the first time the regular footfalls that accompany—that are part of—the performance can be heard. And they coincide not with the longer and louder notes, but with the short, sometimes almost inaudible notes that alternate with the long notes. For the people of the culture from which this music comes, these appear to be the appropriate places to tap the feet—that is, the point at which the tactus occurs. For western listeners, while one can *learn* to clap or tap at those points in the piece, it does not appear to *feel*—and I speak from long experience—as though one is tapping on the beat. It always feels as though one is tapping on an offbeat.

While certain features of this music's organization can be accounted for by invoking the operation of perceptual processes underpinning the experience of time that appear genuinely universal, the fact that longer, more intense, notes do not mark out the tactus cannot be explained in this way. In fact it seems likely that prosodic features of the language of Northern Potosí, Quechua, relate to the way in which tactus is organized, projected, and experienced in that culture's music (see Ref. 17).

That even such an apparently unreflective act as regularly tapping the foot in time to a piece of music is so susceptible to cultural differentiation appears to suggest either that tapping one's foot in time to music has a semantic component (if D'Andrade's proposal that culture impacts cognition primarily at the conceptual level is accepted) or that human cognitive capacities are so grounded in culture that any elementary commonalities are over-ridden, and that minds are only susceptible to explanation in terms specific to the particular cultures in which those specific minds are rooted—a return to the position of Geertz. In other words, culture is in the bones and science has no place in its understanding.

We appear to have reached an impasse; it seems that music is cultural, variable and particular, and not susceptible to explanation in general and scientific terms. Yet there are those who argue that music is, nevertheless, a human universal. Blacking[18] (p. 224) states that 'every known human society has what trained musicologists would recognize as "music", while Merriam[19] (p. 227) bluntly asserts that music 'is a universal behavior'. How can these claims be squared with music's cultural particularity?

As a first step we must enquire what Blacking and Merriam mean by 'music' in this universal manifestation. For both, music is not just sound. Indeed, the musical example given above is not 'the music'; it was a recording of the sound of a musical activity in a particular cultural context. To experience 'the music', you might have to undergo what has been called[20] the 'Total Turing Test' of lifelong immersion in the culture; at the least you would have get the feel of the instrument and of the movements involved. The 'music' would involve embodied action as much as disembodied sound. Even in our own culture it is only in the last hundred years, with music becoming an increasingly commodified aural consumable, that the self-evident ties between musical sound and human movement have been rendered obscure. For John Blacking, the claim that music is a human universal explicitly involves acknowledgement of the embodied nature of music, the *indivisibility* of movement and sound in characterizing music across times and cultures; he claims[18] (p. 241) that '"Music" as a human capability is a cognitive, and hence affective, activity of the body'. For the greater number of cultures in the world, and for the greater part of the historical existence of our culture, 'music' appears to have involved and to involve *movement* just as much as sound.

But music in its universal guise not only involves sound and movement, but also it involves multiplicity of reference and meaning; for Blacking and Merriam music is intrinsically polysemic. For example, music can function as a means of communication with the dead for the Kaluli of Papua New Guinea, binding birds, souls, places, and people at a time of transformation; or music can function in the restructuring of social relations, as in the *domba* initiation of the Venda.[21] In each of these two very different ceremonies, music is central, its meaning rarely if ever explicit but its fugitive significances essential. Blacking[18] notes (p. 237) 'the "same" sound patterns…can…have different meanings within the same society because of different social contexts'. And as Merriam[19] (p. 221) suggests, a defining characteristic of the musical utterance is its property of being 'unrepudiable in form but repudiable as to content'. In other words, music has the capacity to *lack* consensual reference; it can be *about* something, but its *aboutness* can vary from context to context and even within context.

Not only may music's significance vary according to social context, but the significances of a singular musical activity can vary from individual to individual. We know this from our experience of music in our own cultures and we can see it in others; for example, in the *gisalo* ceremonies of the Kaluli, some performers seek to dominate and direct while the performances of others appear to emerge from performer-audience interaction[22] and in any particular performance some participants weep while others do not.[23]

And finally, music in general has a further, peculiarly negative, feature; it appears to have no immediate and evident efficacy. Music neither ploughs, sows, weaves nor feeds; in itself, if it can be considered to exist outwith its context of use, it does not seem to be capable of being a material cause of anything other than a transient hedonic encounter. It is inefficacious.

From these considerations of the 'universal' characteristics of music we can return to the original question of whether music can be construed as a natural kind. We now appear to have a basis for proposing an operational definition of music that might afford the commonalities that would allow an instatement of the natural in the musical. It seems that a generalizable definition of music would refer to music's two roots in sound and movement, to music's heterogeneity of meaning, to its grounding in social interaction yet personalized significance, and to its inefficacy. Putting these four premises together yields the following operational definition:

> Musics can be defined as those temporally patterned human activities, individual and social, that involve the production and perception of sound and have no evident and immediate efficacy or fixed consensual reference.

When applied to the mature expressions of music in particular cultures, this definition does no more than provide a conceptual umbrella for otherwise potentially heterogeneous ethnographies; in that context it is descriptive rather than explanatory. It constitutes a general proposition that applies to the universal presence of something like 'music' in all human cultures. However, in claiming that music is universal Blacking goes further than this; he suggests that music is ubiquitous not only across human societies but across all members of those societies. As he states[18] (p. 236) '...the almost universal distribution of musical competence in African societies suggested that musical ability [is] a general characteristic of the human species rather than a rare talent'. This suggestion squares with recent research into the precursors of musical ability in a western context, notwithstanding those such as Barrow[24] (p. 194) who asserts that 'musical ability is...limited in its distribution'. While it is self-evidently true that the production of 'music' in contemporary western society is in the hands of a specialized class of performers and composers (and lawyers), musical ability cannot be defined solely in terms of productive competence; (almost) every member even of our own, highly specialized, society is capable of listening to and hence of *understanding* music. Indeed, recent research[25] can be interpreted as suggesting that musical productive abilities in a western context, rather than being rare capacities that are evidence of some inborn 'talent', are better explained in terms of the effects of motivation and of practice. In other words, music is not just universal across cultures; it appears that everyone has the capacity to be musical, though this capacity is likely to be realized to different degrees and in different ways in different cultural and social environments.

It is within this broader notion of music as a universal human attribute that the operational definition of music given above might be informative, as applied to the human *capacity* for musicality; if borne in mind in the exploration of the propensities for, and the functionalities of, music for infants and children, it might yield an understanding of the commonalities that appear necessary in order to relate music to our biologies. And as Sandra Trehub notes in this volume, investigations of infant and childhood musical capacities do appear to reveal cross-cultural invariants.

Sandra Trehub and her collaborators have shown that even young infants possess the capacities to perceive significant structural and affective features of musical sounds.[26] The real-world context in which such capacities are most evident is the typically affect-laden interaction of the infant with a care-giver (and it is notable that, irrespective of culture, even adults appear sensitive to features of infant directed song[27].) Other researchers such as the Papouseks and, more recently Colwyn Trevarthen and his collaborators have focused closely on the musicality of such interactions.

The Papouseks have been particularly concerned with infant vocal capacities and interactions. Hanus Papousek[28] (p. 43) has noted that 'musical elements participate in the process of communicative development very early', suggesting that 'they pave the way to linguistic capacities earlier than phonetic elements'. He sees (pp. 46–47) infant and early childhood musical behaviours as forms of play involving higher level integrative processes that act to nurture 'exploratory competence' (a notion that seems to rely on the idea of musical signification as transposable); these exploratory competences entail the participation of emotions and constitute precursors of artistic or scientific competencies.

Mechthild Papousek focuses on the musicality of infant-caregiver interactions, stressing the indivisibility in these of music and movement and the fact that they appear to involve patterns of infant *and* caregiver behaviour that are singularly invariant across cultures. She notes[29] (p. 100) that 'parents' multimodal stimulation is tailored to infants' early competence for perceiving information through different senses as coordinated wholes', and that 'regular synchronization of vocal and kinaesthetic patterns provides the infant with multimodal sensory information including tactile, kinaesthetic, and visual information'.

The work of Trevarthen and his colleagues has centred on these temporal characteristics of infant-caregiver interaction. Trevarthen[30] states that, from birth, central to our neuronal anatomy is a 'body-imaging core system' that comes to act so as to integrate attention, learning, and self-regulating physiology with actions of expression and execution; this he terms the Intrinsic Motive Formation (IMF). In operation, the IMF incorporates periodic timing mechanisms that give rise to a 'hierarchy of motor rhythms'; these, governing movement and binding affect in rhythmic time, he calls the Intrinsic Motive Pulse. For Trevarthen[30] (p. 160) 'Musicality…is the aurally appreciated expression of the IMF with the Intrinsic Motive Pulse as its agent'. From these premises, Trevarthen develops a conceptual framework to explore the expression and development of communication—of intersubjectivity, in his terms—through empirical observations and analyses of infant-caregiver interaction.

The rhythmicity of caregiver-infant interaction, in terms of the capacity of the infant to follow and respond in kind to temporal regularities in vocalization and in movement, and in time to initiate temporally regular sets of vocalizations and movements, is seen here as central to the development of human significative and communicative capacities; its embodied nature enables the sharing of patterned time with others and facilitates harmonicity of affective state and interaction. For Trevarthen, that rhythmicity is also a manifestation of a fundamental musical competence. As he frames it[30] (p. 194), 'Musicality is part of a natural drive in human socio-cultural learning which begins in infancy'.

There is, thus, an increasing amount of evidence that musicality is in our birthright; the capacity for music is an integral component of the infant mind. However, the notion of music as innate that emerges from the research just cited does not sit easily with current general theories of the infant mind. While these theories are increasingly nativist in suggesting that the infant mind, rather than being domain general, is endowed with either modular or domain-specific competences, they tend to account for the existence of these competences on the basis of their adaptive value in evolution and most theorists see no adaptive role for human musicality in evolution. The present consensus (see, e.g. Ref. 31) suggests that the infant mind is primed for the rapid emergence of competence in (at the least) interpreting social relations, physical and mechanical interactions, and the behaviour of biological systems. This view is supported by a substantial quantity of empirical research, in particular by recent work[32] that supports the cross-cultural generality of some of these domains.

There have been some suggestions that musicality might constitute one of these 'native domains'. Gelman and Brenneman[33] propose that a domain-specific competence in music is evidenced by the results of Trehub and others, suggesting that sensitivities to harmonicity of tonal relations and to melodic contoural formations constitute evidence of a music-specific competence. However, their conclusions are rather undermined by their focus on perceptual capacities of which the existence might equally well be accounted for by their utility in other cognitive domains; the tendency to link sounds that are perceived as harmonically related, and to differentiate between sequences of sounds that differ in their contour, appears more likely to derive from a general capacity for auditory scene analysis[34] than to testify to the existence of an early and specifically musical competence. In other words, the suite of perceptual capacities that Gelman and Brenneman identify as making up the domain of musical competence might be epiphenomenal; each capacity might be more securely considered as being proper to other domains that are more self-evidently and immediately functional than is music.

Indeed when music has been viewed from an evolutionary perspective it has often been viewed as contingent, at best exaptive, a view most clearly exemplified by Steven Pinker[35] and endorsed by others such as Barrow[24] and Sperber.[36] For Pinker, music is famously 'auditory cheesecake'; while music in his view is bound to the domains of language, auditory scene analysis, habitat selection, emotion, and motor control, it does no more than exploit the capacities that have evolved to subserve each of these areas. Music is thus 'exaptive', an evolutionary by-product of the emergence of other capacities that have direct adaptive value. Barrow[24] similarly suggests that human musicality has had no role in our survival as a species, suggesting that it derives from an 'optimal instinctive sensitivity for certain sound patterns' that itself arose because it proved adaptive. Sperber[36] goes furthest in condemning music as an evolutionary 'parasite', though he explicitly disavows serious intent in formulating that view. Nevertheless, he does suggest that music is a human activity that arose to exploit parasitically the operation of a cognitive capacity to 'process complex sound patterns discriminable by pitch variation and rhythm' that was originally functional in primitive human communication but that fell into disuse with the emergence of the modern vocal tract and the finer shades of differentiation in sound pattern that it afforded. For Pinker, Sperber and Barrow, music exists simply because of the pleasure that it affords; its basis is purely hedonic, and, as Pinker puts it 'Compared with language, vision, social reasoning, and physical know-how, music could vanish from our species and the rest of our lifestyle would be virtually unchanged'.

These three views appear to constitute the beginnings of a consensus that would relegate music to the status of evolutionary footnote and would seem to vitiate the idea that its bio-logical foundations deserve any attention. However, all three theories suffer from an attrib-ute that disqualifies their conclusions from serious consideration, that of ethnocentricity. Theirs is a 'culture-lite' view of music. They take no account in their conclusions of the *indivisibility* of movement and sound in music,[c] focusing on only one dimension of music as defined above, that of music's inefficacy in any domain other than the individually hedonistic. Despite lip-service paid to the notion that music might take other forms in other cultures, music appears in these theories largely as disembodied sound oriented

---

[c] Although Pinker explicitly addresses the link between music and movement he treats this simply in terms of music 'tapping in' to systems of motor control.

towards individual hedonism, a notion quite untenable before the advent of recording technology. Indeed, over the last 100 years, recording technology together with the reification of intellectual property and the globalization of its law has sanctioned the subsumption of music into the capitalist economy as a tradable and consumable commodity. It might well be that Pinker's view of music is an accurate reflection of what music is now for some within western culture, but that culture-specific 'music' is scarcely representative of the complex and embodied set of activities and interpretations that are evident in most nonwestern 'musics'. To put it another way, what music is for some at present is not what music is for others, was for our predecessors or could be for our children.

Even when music has been viewed as adaptive in human evolution, the problem of ethnocentricity can remain. Miller,[37] in promoting the notion that 'Machiavellian intelligence' played and still plays a significant role as an agent in processes of sexual selection, suggests that musicality constitutes a marker for possession of such intelligence; musical performance constitutes a display of protean behaviours and functions so as to advertise to prospective mates the possession of the 'protean' capacity to be 'unpredictable', a capacity that he suggests is of value in social interaction. The putative link between music and sex certainly motivates many adolescents in our society to engage in 'musical' behaviours, but most will realise only too quickly that mere presence onstage is no guarantee of successful subsequent sexual interaction. If it could be demonstrated from a comprehensive cross-cultural survey that music's primary function is as a vehicle for the display of 'protean behaviours', it would be reasonable to infer that this was music's *raison d'être*. However, the available evidence does not sustain this view; music is and has been employed for many different ends by different societies, and in most the role of music in courtship is positively subsidiary to its value in activities of healing, praying, mourning, or instructing. Miller's view of music seems as bound to the peculiarities of current western practice as does that of Pinker.

For Pinker, Barrow, Sperber, and Miller, the effects of music are at the level of the individual, whether in terms of affording hedonic experience or exhibiting protean attributes. It's notable that much of the research into infant musicality (particularly that of Trevarthen) suggests a different locus for music's functionality (if any), that of human interaction. Several recent theories of music as adaptive in human evolution have located its functionality at the level of the group, including the writings of Kogan and of Brown. Kogan[38] (p. 197) notes that current evolutionary theory suggests that 'natural selection operates not only within groups but also between them'. He follows McNeill's[39] notion of 'muscular bonding' in proposing that the communal experience of affect elicited by moving together rhythmically in music and dance could have enhanced cooperative survival strategies for early humans, for example, in hunting or in inter-group conflict. This efficacy of rhythmic synchronicity in promoting group identity can be related back to the 'time-sharing' capacities exhibited in infant-caregiver interaction, though here it seems limited to its impact on affect, ignoring any broader functionality.

For Brown,[40] the adaptive features of music for the group go beyond those on which Kogan relies. Brown adduces the notion of music as reinforcing 'groupishness', which he defines as a 'suite of traits that favour the formation of coalitions, promote cooperative behaviour towards group members and create the potential for hostility towards those outside the group'. Music supports these traits through the opportunities that it offers for the formation and maintenance of *group identity*, for the conduct of *collective thinking* (as in the transmission of group history and planning for action), for *group synchronization*—the sharing of time—between members of a group, and for *group catharsis*, the collective expression and experience of emotion. Ultimately, Brown sees music as having become instantiated in human cultures through its role as 'ritual's reward system'; music, for him, is a type of 'modulatory system acting at the group level to convey the reinforcement value of these activities... for survival'. And if Brown is correct in his portrayal of music's role in promoting 'groupishness', music is likely to have been a major contributor to what Smith and Szathmáry[41] hold to have constituted one of the major transitions in evolution: the very emergence of human culture.

Dissanayake[42] see the mature expression of music in human culture as intimately linked to the characteristics of mother–infant interaction. She views music (p. 390) as 'multimodal or multimedia activity of temporally patterned movements' that has 'the capacity to coordinate the emotions of participants and thus promote conjoinment'. She suggests that features of the musicality of mother–infant interaction might lay the foundations for a 'grammar of the emotions' that can be expressed in mature musical (and other artistic) activities. For the developing child, the musical characteristics of mother-infant interaction are of critical importance in the acquisition of capacities for 'social regulation and emotional bonding'; these characteristics also provide the elements in the 'musical play' of later childhood that will equip the adult with the predisposition and capacity to engage in the structured interactions of ceremony and ritual as well as in specifically musical behaviours. However, other significant and functional roles have been proposed for music in individual development and in the development of capacities for social interaction; music can be both a consequence free means of exploring social interaction and a 'play space' for rehearsing processes that may be necessary to achieve cognitive flexibility.[43]

Music is consequence free in that it is not *directly* functional; it is noneffacacious. It is specifically suited to testing out aspects of social interaction by virtue of both its noneffi-caciousness and its polysemic nature, its multiple potential meanings. For each child in a group ostensibly involved in a cooperative musical activity, that musical activity can mean something different yet the singularity of the collective musical activity is not threatened by the existence of multiple simultaneous and potentially conflicting meanings. Music provides for a child a medium for the gestation of a capacity for social interaction, a risk-free space for the exploration of social behaviour that can sustain otherwise potentially risky action and transaction.

Just as one can posit a role for music in the socialization of the child, one can also postulate a role for music in the development of the child's individual cognitive capacities that is quite distinct from its efficacy in the child's acculturation. Again, this role is motivated by the intrinsically polysemic nature of music, the fact that its significances can modulate from situation to situation and can even be simultaneously multiple. If music is *about* anything, it exhibits a deictic intentionality, a 'transposable aboutness'. And it is conceivable that music's 'transposable aboutness' is exploited in infancy and childhood as a means of forming connections and interrelations between different domains of infant and childhood competence such as the social, biological, and mechanical. To give a crude example; the arc of a ball thrown through the air, the prosodic contour of a comforting utterance, the trajectory of a swallow as it hawks an insect, the pendular ballistics of a limb swung in purposive movement, might, for a child, each underlie the significances of a single musical phrase or proto-musical behaviour on different occasions. Indeed, these heterogeneous incidents may be bound together simultaneously in the significance of that phrase or behaviour, the music thus exhibiting what I have called elsewhere a 'floating intentionality'. The 'floating intentionality' of the music can provide for the child a space within which she can explore the possible bindings of these multidomain representations. Hence one and the same musical activity might, at one and the same time, be about the trajectory of a body in space, the dynamic emergence or signification of an affective state, the achievement of a goal and the unfolding of an embodied perspective. All these 'aboutnesses' exist not in respect of objects but events, ongoing structures in time, and music or proto-musical behaviours afford the opportunity to explore the cross-domain mappings that the representation of temporal sequences of object states as events makes available.

From this perspective one can advance a second definition of music, one that rests on the idea that what 'music' is for any given culture may vary immensely but will derive from the same general human propensities:

> Musics are cultural particularisations of the human capacity to form multiply-intentional representations through integrating information across different functional domains of temporally extended or sequenced human experience and behaviour, generally expressed in sound.

In this view, music, or proto-musical behaviours, subserve a *metaphorical* domain or perhaps more appropriately, underpin a metaphorical stance, acting to create and to maintain the cognitive flexibility that marks off humans from all other species. And it could be that the emergence of proto-musical behaviours and their cultural realization as music (and, for the matter, dance) might themselves have been crucial in precipitating the emergence of the cognitive flexibility that marks the appearance of *Homo sapiens*. For if Smith and Szathmáry[41] are correct in maintaining that human culture constitutes one of the major transitions in evolution, and Mithen[44] is correct in claiming that the appearance of *Homo sapiens sapiens*, ourselves, is marked by the emergence of a flexible cross-domain cognitive capacity, then music is uniquely fitted to have played a significant role in facilitating the acquisition and maintenance of the skill of being a member of a culture—of interacting socially with others—as well as providing a vehicle for integrating our domain-specific competences so as to endow us with the multipurpose and adaptive cognitive capacities that make us human.

Of course, what music, or more appropriately proto music, is for infants and children and what it might have been in evolution, is not necessarily what music is for a mature culture or society. Culture shapes and particularizes proto-musical behaviours and propensities into specific forms for specific functions, and those, as noted at the outset of this paper, can be so divergent that they do not appear to be mutually reducible—they do not appear to exhibit a 'nucleus of common properties' (after Molino[5]). However, it is noteworthy that for most cultures, music—and here one might almost prefer to use the Igbo term *nkwa*, as it seems to capture the interlinking of sound and action that characterizes music for most cultures—the functions that music fulfils, the contexts in which it appears most efficacious, often lie in the realm of ritual and of psychic healing. That is, music often functions in individual and group encounters with the numinous and in the modulation of affective state.

The affective functionality of music can certainly be referred to its embodiment in action and to the contexts within which proto-musical activities occur for infants and children,[42] as well as to a broad range of different circumstances in specific cultures.[45] But it seems that music's ubiquity and efficacy in encounters with the numinous are best accounted for by reference to proto-music's polysemy, its 'floating intentionality'. This property of proto-musical activities may facilitate the mature use of music in those cultural contexts that deal with what Sperber has called 'relevant mysteries'. Sperber applies this term to situations where beliefs or mental representations arise which are contradictory but are each separately related to (and hence relevant in respect of) other mental representations and beliefs. When simultaneously foregrounded by actions or circumstances, these contradictory beliefs then become 'mysteries' and 'achieve relevance because of their paradoxical character—that is because of the rich background of everyday empirical knowledge from which they systematically depart'[36] (p. 72). Within the framework of Sperber's theory, religious ideas are distinguished from everyday beliefs by their paradoxicality and their relevance, by their broad applicability and their ambiguity; and the view of music's functionality outlined above would suggest that music is also distinguished by just such a broad applicability and ambiguity. By virtue of these attributes music may thus be particularly appropriate as a means of amplifying, exemplifying or reinforcing in the course of ongoing experience just these attributes of belief that are interpretable as religious; music's indeterminacy may suit it for use as a means of pursuing and perhaps even parsing the numinous.

But the factors that endow music with its efficacy for individual cognitive development and socialization in infancy and childhood cannot by themselves determine the multiplicitous forms and functions that music takes and that music serves in mature cultural contexts. The meaning of a musical activity for a mature individual will necessarily depend at any given moment on that person's own history and narratives, and on the situational significances that culture's 'shared system of meanings' confer on that activity. The polysemic potential that characterises proto-musical activity is likely to underpin the social functionality of music and to contribute to, but not determine, music's meaning. The functionalities and functions of music or proto-musical behaviours for the individual, whether in their own cognitive development or in their socialization, must be set in the context of the functionalities and functions of music as a cultural phenomenon. Music, like language, cannot be wholly private; it is a property of communities, not individuals. And these different levels at which music may be efficacious must be integrated in any understanding of its foundations. Music's very existence is best evidenced in interaction. If music is of importance in human development, evolution and life, then an attempt to render commensurable our understanding of music as interaction with our understanding of music's biological foundations is crucial in coming to terms with what Henry Plotkin[46] (p. 222) calls 'the most complicated thing in the universe—the collective of human brains and their psychological processes that make up human culture'.

To return to the beginning; what are the implications for this view of music as something more than patterned sound, for an understanding of its biological foundations? We would expect its neurophysiology to be complex, reaching beyond the auditory pathways to the limbic system and to centres of motor behaviour. We would expect that the cultural context of music—the forces that shape music for any given culture—should condition its neurophysiological correlates. And we might expect music and language to share many, but not all, neurophysiological correlates.[47] While music and language might meet somewhere near poetry, music can never attain the unambiguous referentiality of language (which Deacon[48] holds to be language's primary defining characteristic), nor language the absolute ambiguity of music.

But at the limit, while music may be in our biologies, our culture is in our music. If the roots of human musicality are to be found in infancy, particularly in infant-caregiver interaction, its potency might be tied to the support provided by society for those interactions. In an intriguing study Maya Gratier[49] investigated the coherence of interactions between caregivers and infants in three different contexts: French mothers in France, Southern Indian mothers in South India, and Southern Indian mothers who were recent immigrants to France. She found a difference between the coherence of the immigrant mother-infant interactions and those of the other two culturally embedded groups; interaction between the immigrant mothers and their infants was significantly less coherent than was interaction in the other two groups. She suggests that the cultural dislocation of the immigrant mothers had impacted directly on their capacities to interact 'musically' with their infants. Something as individual and putatively innate as the capacity of a mother to interact coherently in time with her child seems to be dependent on the mother's rootedness in her cultural environment. In other words, if music is in our birthright, its inheritance appears to be a fragile gift that rests on the humaneness and sympathy of the culture that surrounds us.

References

1. Lakoff, G. (1987) *Women, Fire and Dangerous Things.* Chicago: University of Chicago Press.
2. Rose, S. (1996) *Lifelines: Biology, Freedom, Determinism.* London: Allen Lane.
3. Rorty, R. (2000) Being that can be understood is language. *London Rev. Books* 126, 23–5.
4. Feyerabend, P. (1981) *Problems of Empiricism,* vol. 2. Cambridge: Cambridge University Press.
5. Molino, J. (2000) Towards an evolutionary theory of music and language. In N. Wallin, B. Merker, and S. Brown (eds) *The Origins of Music.* Cambridge, MA: MIT Press, pp. 165–76.
6. Geertz, C. (1973) *The Interpretation of Cultures: Selected Essays.* New York: Basic Books.
7. Treitler, L. (1980) History, criticism and Beethoven's ninth symphony. *Nineteenth Century Music* 3, 193–210.
8. Tomlinson, G. (1984) The web of culture. *Nineteenth Century Music* 7, 350–62.
9. Abbate, C. (1991) *Unsung Voices: Opera and Musical Narrative in the Nineteenth Century.* Oxford: Princeton University Press.
10. Garnett, L. (1998) Musical meaning revisited: thoughts on an 'epic' critical musicology. *Critical Musicology.* http://www.leeds.ac.uk/music/Info/CMJ/Articles/(1998)/01/01.html.
11. Goehr, L. (1992) *The Imaginary Museum of Musical Works.* Oxford: Clarendon Press.

12. **Slobin, M.** (1993) *Subcultural Sounds: Micromusics of the West.* Hanover: Weslyan University Press.

13. **Malm, M.** (1977) *Music Cultures of the Pacific, the Near East and Asia.* Englewood Cliffs, NJ: Prentice-Hall.

14. **Gourlay, K. A.** (1984) The non-universality of music and the universality of non-music. *World Music* **26**, 25–36.

15. **D'Andrade, R.** (1996) *The Development of Cognitive Anthropology.* Cambridge: Cambridge University Press.

16. **Cole, M.** (1996) *Cultural Psychology.* London: Belknap Press of Harvard University Press.

17. **Stobart, H. F.** and **I. Cross** (2000) The Andean Anacrusis? rhythmic structure and perception in Easter songs of Northern Potosí, Bolivia. *Br. J. Ethnomusicol.* 9(2), 63–94.

18. **Blacking, J.** (1995) *Music, Culture and Experience.* London: University of Chicago Press.

19. **Merriam, A. P.** (1964) *The Anthropology of Music.* Chicago: Northwestern University Press.

20. **Harnad, S.** (1992) There is only one mind/body problem. *Intl. J. of Psychol.* 27, 521.

21. **Blacking, J.** (1976) *How Musical is Man?* London: Faber.

22. **Scheifflin, E. L.** (1993) Performance and the cultural construction of reality: a New Guinea example. In R. Rosaldo, S. Lavie, and K. Narayan (eds) *Creativity/Anthropology.* London: Cornell University Press, pp. 270–295.

23. **Feld, S.** (1982) *Sound and Sentiment: Birds, Weeping, Poetics and Song in Kaluli Expression.* Philadelphia: University of Pennsylvania Press.

24. **Barrow, J. D.** (1995) *The Artful Universe.* Oxford: Clarendon Press.

25. **Sloboda, J. A., J. W. Davidson, M. J. A. Howe,** and **D. G. Moore** (1996) The role of practice in the development of performing musicians. *Br. J. Psychol.* 87, 287–309.

26. **Trehub, S. E., G. Schellenberg,** and **D. Hill** (1997) The origins of music perception and cognition: a developmental perspective. In I. Deliège and J. Sloboda (eds) *Perception and Cognition of Music.* Hove: The Psychology Press, pp. 103–28.

27. **Trehub, S. E., A. M. Unyk,** and **L. J. Trainor** (1993) Adults identify infant-directed music across cultures. *Infant Behavior Development* 16, 193–211.

28. **Papousek, H.** (1996) Musicality in infancy research: biological and cultural origins of early musicality. In I. Deliège and J. Sloboda (eds) *Musical Beginnings.* Oxford: Oxford University Press, pp. 37–55.

29. **Papousek, M.** (1996) Intuitive parenting: a hidden source of musical stimulation in infancy. In I. Deliège and J. Sloboda (eds) *Musical Beginnings.* Oxford: Oxford University Press, pp. 88–112.

30. **Trevarthen, C.** (1999) Musicalty and the intrinsic motive pulse: evidence from human psycho-biology and infant communication. *Musicae Scientiae* (Special Issue), 155–215.

31. **Spelke, E.** (1999) Infant cognition. In R. A. Wilson and F. C. Keil (eds) The MIT Encyclopedia of Cognitive Sciences. Cambridge, MA: MIT Press, pp. 402–4.

32. **Medin, D.** and **S. Atran** (1999) *Folk Biologies.* Cambridge, MA: MIT Press.

33. **Gelman, R.** and **K. Brenneman** (1994) First principles can support both universal and culture-specific learning about number and music. In L. A. Hirschfeld and S. A. Gelman (eds) *Mapping the Mind: Domain Specificity in Cognition and Culture.* Cambridge: Cambridge University Press, p. 396.

34. **Bregman, A.** (1990) *Auditory Scene Analysis.* Cambridge, MA: MIT Press.

35. **Pinker, S.** (1997) *How the Mind Works.* London: Allen Lane.

36. **Sperber, D.** (1996) *Explaining Culture.* Oxford: Blackwell.

37. **Miller, G. F.** (1997) Protean primates: the evolution of adaptive unpredictability in competition and courtship. In A. Whiten and R. W. Byrne (eds) *Machiavellian Intelligence II: Extensions and Evaluations.* Cambridge: Cambridge University Press, pp. 312–40.

38. **Kogan, N.** (1997) Reflections on aesthetics and evolution. *Critical Rev.* 11, 193–210.

39. **McNeill, W. H.** (1995) *Keeping Together in Time.* London: Harvard University Press.

40. **Brown, S.** (2000) Evolutionary models of music: from sexual selection to group selection. In F. Tonneau and N. S. Thompson (eds) *Perspectives in Ethology. 13: Behavior, Evolution and Culture.* New York: Plenum Publishers, pp. 231–81.

41. **Smith, J. M.** and **E. Szathmáry** (1995) *The Major Transitions in Evolution.* Oxford: Oxford University Press.

42. **Dissanayake, E.** (2000) Antecedents of the temporal arts in early mother-infant interactions. In N. Wallin, B. Merker, and S. Brown (eds) *The Origins of Music.* Cambridge, MA: MIT Press, pp. 389–407.

43. **Cross, I.** (1999) Is music the most important thing we ever did ? Music, development and evolution. In Suk Won Yi (ed.) *Music, Mind and Science.* Seoul: Seoul National University Press, pp. 10–39.

44. **Mithen, S.** (1996) *The Prehistory of the Mind.* London: Thames and Hudson.

45. **Sloboda, J. A.** and **P. Juslin** (eds) (2001) *Music and Emotion: Theory and Research.* Oxford: Oxford University Press.

46. **Plotkin, H.** (1997) *Evolution in Mind.* London: Allen Lane.

47. **Peretz, I., S. Belleville,** and **S. Fontaine** (1997) Dissociation between music and language following cerebral hemorrhage – another instance of amusia without aphasia. *Canadian J. Exp. Psychol.* 51, 354–68.

48. **Deacon, T.** (1996) *The Symbolic Species: The Co-evolution of Language and the Human Brain.* London: Allen Lane.

49. **Gratier, M.** (1999) Expressions of belonging: the effect of acculturation on the rhythm and harmony of mother-infant interaction. *Musicae Scientiae,* (Special Issue), 93–122.

CHAPTER 5

IS MUSIC AN EVOLUTIONARY ADAPTATION?

DAVID HURON

Abstract

In contemplating the function and origin of music, a number of scholars have considered whether music might be an evolutionary adaptation. This article reviews the basic arguments related to evolutionary claims for music. Although evolutionary theories about music remain wholly speculative, musical behaviours satisfy a number of basic conditions, which suggest that there is indeed merit in pursuing possible evolutionary accounts.

Keywords: Evolutionary theories of music; Music industry; Evolutionary origin of language; Music and social bonding; Oxytocin; Mood regulation

Addressing the question of music's origins has a long history and is patently speculative. Although several cultures have provided colourful stories describing how people acquired the capacity for music, most contemporary scholars have focused on possible psychological, social, and cultural beginnings. In this chapter, I propose to offer a social account of music's origins that is explicitly linked to one of the most successful theories yet devised: the theory of evolution by natural selection.

Evolution is often thought of in purely physiological rather than psychological terms.[1-5] It is not simply that evolution has shaped immune systems, digestive tracts, and knee caps. Evolution has also shaped our attitudes, dispositions, emotions, perceptions, and cognitive functions. Some of our deepest convictions can be traced to plausible evolutionary origins: we love life, we fear death, and we nurture our children because these dispositions better ensure the propagation of our genes.

The theory of evolution by natural selection is a distal theory. It is not a theory that explains specific behaviours, such as why you chose to cook ravioli for dinner last night, or why you parked in a particular parking spot this morning. Similarly, if music is an evolutionary adaptation, this will not allow us to account for particular musical acts, such as Mendelssohn's writing of the *Scottish Symphony*. Evolution proceeds by selecting traits that are adaptive to an organism's environment. For example, evolution did not 'originate' or 'create' the phenomenon of altruism. Instead, given a certain environment, natural selection favoured individuals who exhibited certain altruistic traits. Evolution does not dictate our behaviour: it selects which behaviours are likely to be passed on to subsequent generations—and it selects only those behaviours that have a genetic component. So in discussing possible evolutionary origins for musical behaviours, the question is not, What caused people to make music? but rather, How might music-making behaviours have escaped the hatchet of natural selection? or more precisely, What advantage is conferred on those individuals who exhibit musical behaviours over those who do not?

Does music have survival value?

Many knowledgeable people have concluded that music has no survival value. Indeed, a number of esthetic philosophers have argued that an essential, defining characteristic of the arts is that they serve no practical function.[6] Accordingly, any music that is created for biological (or even economic) reasons cannot be considered art. Even among evolutionary psychologists such as Steven Pinker, it has been common to suppose that music is not adaptive.[7]

Many linguists—Pinker included—believe that language is likely an evolutionary adaptation.[8] However, the evidence in support of language as an adaptation is not notably stronger than comparable evidence for music. Where pertinent evidence is available, music exhibits the essential properties of all adaptations. My goal in this chapter is not to attempt to prove that music is adaptive. (Like others, I am not at all convinced that music has evolutionary origins.) Rather, my goal here is to convince you that the question of music's origins remains open and warrants further investigation (see also several articles in Ref. 9).[10]

Of course there are a number of dangers attending evolutionary speculation.[11,12] Popper (1935/1959) pointed out that no scientist has yet formulated the theory of evolution by natural selection in such a way that a set of observations could, in principle, be used to falsify it.[13] Gould and Lewontin[14] have noted that evolutionary reasoning is plagued by *post hoc* reasoning. Evolutionary theory has been used to defend all sorts of nefarious ideologies, from racism to sexism. Philosophers note that evolutionary arguments often lead to the naturalist fallacy where what is is confused with what ought to be. In the case of music, there is an undistinguished history of polemical writing where certain kinds of music have been condemned for being 'unnatural'. Finally, by focusing on biological issues, one can leave the false impression that the effects of culture on music are minimal.

If music is an evolutionary adaptation, then it is likely to have a complex genesis. Any musical adaptation is likely to be built on several other adaptations that might be described as premusical or protomusical. Moreover, the nebulous rubric *music* may represent several adaptations, and these adaptations may involve complex coevolutionary patterns with culture (see Ref. 15). In biological matters, things are rarely straightforward.

Given these possible dangers, why bother attempting to formulate an evolutionary theory of music? Isn't it premature? First, as noted above, my goal here is not to convince you that music is adaptive; my goal is only to convince you that this is a worthwhile question. Understanding the possible origins of music might help inform us about some of the reasons we tend to respond in certain ways. Second, in the spirit of Popper, I will aim to tell an evolutionary story that is able to generate testable hypotheses. Like other evolutionary accounts, my own theory will draw on existing knowledge, and so be *post hoc* in character. As long as this account remains *post hoc*, Gould and Lewontin's criticisms raise justified and paramount difficulties. However, it is my hope that the theory can be developed to the point where testable hypotheses might be derived.

Before entertaining some possible evolutionary views of music's origins, let us first consider two pertinent complicating points of views. One view is that music is a form of nonadaptive pleasure seeking (NAPS). A second view is that music is an evolutionary vestige.

NAPS theory of music

Most pleasurable activities, such as eating and sex, have clear links to survival. Such activities ultimately stimulate brain mechanisms that are specifically evolved to reward and encourage adaptive behaviours. Note that once brain mechanisms are in place that permit the experience of pleasure, it may be possible to stimulate those mechanisms in ways that do not confer a survival advantage. We can call these behaviours NAPS. An example of NAPS behaviour is found in the human taste for sugars and fats. In premodern times, sugars and fats were rare in human diets, but highly nutritious in the amounts available. There are good reasons why human tastes would evolve to reward the ingestion of foods with high fat or sugar content. However, centuries of human ingenuity have succeeded in generating a modern diet that contains unnaturally high levels of fats and sugars—levels so high as to cause health problems such as diabetes and heart disease. Although such tastes originally conferred an increased chance of survival, in the modern environment, these behaviours have become less adaptive.

Another example of NAPS behaviour is found in drug use, such as heroin or cocaine. These drugs can directly activate the brain's pleasure centers, simply by injecting or imbibing a substance. Although the channel for pleasure exists for good evolutionary reasons, it may be possible to exploit the channel without any concomitant survival-enhancing result.

As in the case of drugs, it is possible that musical behaviours are forms of nonadaptive pleasure seeking. That is, music itself may not enhance human survival; music may merely exploit one or more existing pleasure channels that evolved to reinforce some other adaptive behaviour(s). We might call this view the 'NAPS theory of music'.

One way to determine whether some pleasure-seeking behaviour is adaptive or nonadaptive is to consider how long the behaviour has been around. In the long span of evolutionary history, nonadaptive pleasure-seeking behaviours tend to be short-lived. For example, heroin users tend to neglect their health and are known to have high mortality rates. Furthermore, heroin users make poor parents; they tend to neglect their offspring. Poor health and neglect of offspring are infallible ways of reducing the probability that one's genes will be present in a future gene pool. After many generations, natural selection will tend to militate against heroin use. Those individuals who are not disposed (for whatever reason) to use heroin, are much more likely to procreate and so pass along their aversion to the use of such drugs, provided that the aversive behaviour is somehow linked to a gene or genes.

The use of alcohol already suggests how NAPS behaviours can transform a gene pool. Although no gene has been identified, either for alcohol susceptibility or for alcohol tolerance, the responses of different human populations to alcohol show a suggestive pattern. Large quantities of alcohol became possible only with the advent of agriculture. Modern European and Asian descendents of early agrarian cultures (such as originated in Mesopotamia) manage to deal with alcohol better than descendents of traditional hunter-gatherer societies, such as indigenous peoples in the Americas and in the arctic regions of Europe. Of course there are certain to be nongenetic factors influencing alcohol tolerance and abuse. However, alcohol researchers suspect that genetic factors are at work. Those people who have descended from traditional agricultural societies have a clear statistical advantage in dealing with the nonadaptive consequences of alcohol, and this would be expected if alcohol had been prevalent in these societies for thousands of years.

If music itself has no survival value (and merely exploits an existing pleasure channel), then any disposition towards musical behaviours would tend to worsen one's survival. Spending inordinate amounts of resources (such as time and money) on music would be expected to place music lovers at an evolutionary disadvantage. In other words, if the NAPS theory of music is true, then we would expect music appreciation to be correlated with marginal existence: as in the case of alcohol, music lovers would be disproportionally more likely to end up on 'skid row'.

In addition, if music is nonadaptive, then it must be the case that music is historically recent; otherwise music lovers would have become extinct some time ago. As we will see, the archaeological evidence indicates that music is very old—much older than agriculture—and this great antiquity is inconsistent with music originating as a nonadaptive pleasure-seeking behaviour. In short, there is little evidence that musical behaviours have been selected against. All of these suggest that there is little support for the NAPS theory of music.

Music as an evolutionary vestige

Another possibility is that, although music at one time did indeed confer some survival values, it is now merely vestigial. Like the human appendix, at one time this 'organ' may have contributed directly to human survival, but now it is largely irrelevant—a piece of evolutionary litter. If this view is true, then we would have to ask What advantage did music once confer? and How have things changed so that music is no longer adaptive?

Measuring the adaptive value of music

The adaptive value of some function is often evident in the individual survival costs arising from that function. For example, the larynx of newborn infants is anatomically arranged so that breathing and swallowing can happen at the same time. When the larynx enlarges, our physiological capacity for speech is purchased at the price of the danger of choking. In effect, one measure of the evolutionary advantage of speech is the mortality rate due to choking.

Similarly, an estimate of the evolutionary advantage conferred by music is to measure the amount of time people spend in musical behaviours. In the Atlas mountains of Morocco, full-time Jujuka mountain musicians are supported by the local villagers. That is, there is an entire caste of people whose principal productive activity is music making. A ready index of the importance of music in such a society may be the ratio of the number of musicians to the number of farmers and herders.

Some evolutionary theories of music

Of the various proposals concerning a possible evolutionary origin for music, eight broad theories can be identified:

Mate selection. In the same way that some animals find colourful or ostentatious mates attractive, music making may have arisen as a courtship behaviour. For example, the ability to sing well might imply that the individual is in good health.

Social cohesion. Music might create or maintain social cohesion. It may contribute to group solidarity, promote altruism, and so increase the effectiveness of collective actions such as defending against a predator or attacking a rival clan.

Group effort. More narrowly, music might contribute to the coordination of group work, such as pulling a heavy object.

Perceptual development. Listening to music might provide a sort of 'exercise' for hearing. Music might somehow teach people to be more perceptive.

Motor skill development. Singing and other music-making activities might provide (or have provided) opportunities for refining motor skills. For example, singing might have been a necessary precursor to the development of speech.

Conflict reduction. In comparison with speech, music might reduce interpersonal conflict. Campfire talk may well lead to arguments and possible fights. Campfire singing might provide a safer social activity.

Safe time passing. In the same way that sleep can keep an animal out of harm's way, music might provide a benign form of time passing. Evolutionary biologists have noted, for example, that the amount of sleep an animal requires is proportional to the effectiveness of food gathering. Efficient hunters (such as lions) spend a great deal of time sleeping, whereas inefficient feeders (such as grazing animals) sleep relatively little. Sleep is thought to help keep an animal out of trouble. A lion is more apt to injure itself if it is engaged in unnecessary activities. As early humans became more effective at gathering food, music might have arisen as a harmless pastime. (Note, e.g. that humans sleep more than other primates.)

Transgenerational communication. Given the ubiquity of folk ballads and epics, music might have originated as a useful mnemonic conveyance for useful information. Music might have provided a comparatively good channel of communication over long periods of time.

Sexual selection

Before continuing, we should take a moment to discuss a variant of the mate selection theory. Charles Darwin identified a form of natural selection known as sexual selection. The classic example of sexual selection is the peacock's tail. The function of the tail is not to promote the survival of the peacock; rather, the function is to promote the survival of the peacock's genes. Sexual selection arises once a particular genetic preference is established by the opposite sex—in this case, the preference of the peahen for flashy tails. Even if one peahen is not particularly impressed by Las Vegas-style tails, it remains to the female's benefit to mate with the most colourful male if her offspring are more likely to be desired by other females who are fond of colourful tails.

Darwin himself suggested that music might have arisen due to sexual selection in mating calls.[16] Like the peacock's tail, the preferences of hominid women could create an escalating competition for ever more elaborate and beautiful melodies. Miller[17] has suggested that sexual selection accounts for why musical interests appear to peak in adolescence. However, the members of the all-male Vienna Philharmonic notwithstanding, there is nothing to indicate that one sex is more musical than the other, and so there is no evidence of the dimorphism commonly symptomatic of sexual selection. Women may be impressed by men who serenade them outside their balcony windows, but unlike female songbirds, female humans are perfectly capable of serenading men. Currently, there is no other known example of sexual selection that does not exhibit high sexual dimorphism—although one should note that biology is full of surprises.

Types of evidence

In presenting a case for the evolutionary origins of music, we can consider four types of evidence:

Genetic evidence. The best evidence of an evolutionary origin would be the identification of genes whose expression leads to the behaviour in question. Unfortunately, it is rare for scientists to be able to link particular behaviours to specific genes. Although behaviour-linked genes have been discovered in other animals (such as fruit flies), no behaviour-linked gene has yet been conclusively established in humans. As in so many other areas, music has attracted a kind of folklore related to heritability. In some cultures, it is common for people to assume or believe that musical talent is partly inherited. More recently, work at the University of California, San Francisco by Baharloo *et al.*[18] appears to suggest a genetic component for absolute pitch.

Neurological evidence. The existence of specialized brain structures is neither a sufficient nor a necessary condition for music to be an evolutionary adaptation. Nevertheless, if stable anatomical brain structures exist for music, then this is consistent with music arising from innate development rather than being due solely to a generalized learning.

Ethological evidence. Are musical behaviours consistent with survival and the propagation of genes? In order for music to be an evolutionary adaptation, music-related behaviours must somehow increase the likelihood that the musical person's genes will be propagated.

Archaeological evidence. Since complex evolutionary adaptations arise over many thousands of generations, we must ask how widespread music is in biological history? If music originated in the past few thousand years, then it is highly unlikely to be an evolutionary adaptation. Evolution does not work that fast.

As noted, there is currently no evidence that links music to any gene. Let us consider the other areas of evidence in more detail.

Archaeological evidence

Let us begin by considering some of the archaeological facts. The archaeological record shows a continuous record of music making in human settlements. Wherever you find evidence of human settlement, you find evidence of musical activities.

In 1995, paleontologist Ivan Turk discovered a bone flute while excavating an ancient burial mound in Divje Babe, Slovenia.[19,20] This flute has been determined to be between

43,000 and 82,000 years old, using electron spin dating. The instrument was fashioned from the femur of the now-extinct European bear.

Of course, finding this flute does not mean we have found the earliest musical instrument; this is just the earliest found instrument. As musical instruments go, flutes are rather complicated devices. If we look at contemporary hunter-gatherer societies, the most common instruments are rattles, shakers, and drums. For example, prior to the arrival of Europeans, by far the most common instruments in native American cultures were rattles and drums. The same pattern of preferred instruments is evident in African and Polynesian cultures. If we assume that rattles and drums typically predated the use of flutes, then the ancient music makers of Slovenia might well have been creating instrumental music somewhat earlier than 100,000 years ago.

What sort of music making, however, might have existed prior to the fashioning of musical instruments? It is not unreasonable to assume that singing preceded the making of musical instruments by some length of time. If we suppose that singing predated instrument making by 50 per cent of the intervening time, then music making might have existed 150,000 years ago—roughly twice the age of the older estimate for the Divje Babe flute. Even this figure might be a conservative estimate, and the actual origin of music might be twice as old, say around 250,000 years ago.

On the other hand, the Divje Babe flute might truly be an early specimen, and singing might have developed about the same time. Using the most recent estimate for the Divje Babe flute would therefore place the origins of music making about 50,000 years ago.

In summary, the archaeological record implies that music making likely originated between 50,000 years ago and a quarter of a million years ago. Although Wurlitzer organs, American Bandstand, and MTV are relatively recent phenomena, music making, in general, is really quite old. The evidence pointing to the great antiquity of music satisfies the most basic requirement for any evolutionary argument. Evolution proceeds at a very slow pace, so nearly all adaptations must be extremely old. Music making satisfies this condition.

Incidentally, the antiquity of music raises problems for those who would wish to use evolutionary arguments in esthetic debates by claiming that one music is 'more natural' than another. Whatever the origins of music, the vast majority of people have long ceased to live in Pleistocene conditions. In deciding whether Twisted Sister is better or worse than the Grateful Dead, appealing to the sounds of neolithic caves is unlikely to help.

Anthropological evidence

Turning to contemporary anthropology, we can ask, What does the plethora of existing human cultures tell us about music? Without taking time to review the evidence, there is one overwhelming conclusion from the modern anthropological record. There is no human culture known in modern times that did not, or does not, engage in recognizably musical activities.

Not only is music making very old, it is ubiquitous; it is found wherever humans are found.[21] Moreover, I neglected earlier to mention one important fact about the bone flute at Divje Babe: the flute was found in a Neanderthal burial site. The Divje Babe flute isn't even a human artifact. In short, it may be that music making is not just ubiquitous among *Homo sapiens*; music making may possibly be characteristic of the entire genus *Homo*.

The evidence pointing to the ubiquity of music satisfies another important basic requirement for any evolutionary argument. Relatively few adaptations are not found throughout the entire population of the affected species. For example, if eyelashes confer an evolutionary advantage, then just about everyone should have eyelashes. There are some exceptions to this principle, some of which are very important. For example, humans divide into female and male versions, so there are some genes that are not shared by everyone. Another more subtle example is the gene that codes for sickle-cell—a gene that protects against malaria, but that can also cause anemia. In general, however, adaptive genes are typically ubiquitous throughout a gene pool.

Ethological evidence

When studying a particular animal, ethologists often begin by making an inventory of observed behaviours. What does the animal do, and how often does it do it? Activities that require a great deal of time and large expenditures of energy are understandably considered important. Ethologists assume that behaviours are likely to be optimized. Even behaviours that seem unimportant (such as infant play or sleeping) often have a serious or critical purpose.

Primates, for example, spend an extraordinary amount of time grooming each other. Ethologists feel obliged to formulate theories that account for the various proportions of resources dedicated by an animal to different activities.

Let us apply the ethological approach to the behaviours we call musical. For the purposes of illustration, we will consider two case descriptions. The first case is that of the Mekranoti Indians of the Brazilian Amazon, and the second case is that of contemporary society in the United States.

The Mekranoti Indians

The Mekranoti Indians are primarily hunter-gatherers who live in the Amazon rain forest of Brazil. In Mekranoti culture, singing plays a prominent role in daily life. For several months of the year, every morning and evening the women lay banana leaves on the ground where they sit and sing for between one and two hours. The men sing early every morning, starting typically around 4:30, but sometimes as early as 1:30 AM. The men sing for roughly two hours each day, and often they will also sing for a half hour or so before sunset.

When singing, the Mekranoti men hold their arms in a sort of cradling position and swing their arms vigorously. The men endeavour to sing in their deepest bass voices and heavily accent the first beats of a pervasive quadruple meter with glottal stops that make their stomachs convulse in rhythm. Anthropologist Dennis Werner[22] describes their singing as a 'masculine roar'. When gathering in the middle of the night, the men are obviously sleepy, and some men will linger in their lean-tos well after the singing has started. These malingerers are often taunted with shouted insults.

Werner reports that 'Hounding the men still in their lean-tos [is] one of the favourite diversions of the singers. "Get out of bed! The Kreen Akrore Indians have already attacked and you're still sleeping", they [shout] as loudly as they [can] . . . . Sometimes the harassment [is] personal as the singers [yell] out insults at specific men who rarely [show] up'.[23]

What is extraordinary about the Mekranoti singing is the amount of time involved—roughly two hours per day. (Remember, this is a subsistence society.) For the evolutionary ethologist, the important question arising from the Mekranoti Indians is why music making would attract so much of the tribe's resources. We will return to this question later.

Modern United States of America

By way of comparison, consider now the prevalence of music in a modern industrialized society like the United States. For the ethologist looking at modern human behaviours, a crude though ready index of the amount of resources we dedicate to a particular activity can be found by measuring economic activity.

There is a widespread misconception that the foremost export sector in the US economy is 'high technology'. In fact, the preeminent export sector in the US economy is entertainment. Of the various component areas—films, sports, television, toys, and games—it is music that ranks foremost.

How big is the music industry? The music industry is comparable in size to the pharmaceutical industry. People spend more money on music than on prescription drugs. We purchase recordings, go to concerts, buy sheet music, take our children to music lessons, listen to commercial radio, watch film accompanied by music, and encounter Muzak in the local shopping mall. The most active concert venues in the world are freeways: a major preoccupation for millions of drivers is listening to music.

Of course financial measures are crude indicators of behavioural significance. The ethological point is simple. In both a hunter-gatherer society and a modern industrial society, we find humans dedicating a notable proportion of the available resources to music making and listening. Music may not be more important than sex; but it is arguably more expensive, and it is certainly more time consuming.

In order to put these behaviours in perspective, suppose you were a Martian anthropologist visiting Earth. There are many aspects of human behaviour that would have recognizable value. You would see people engaged in growing and preparing food, in raising and educating children, people involved in transportation, health, and governance; but even if Martian anthropologists had ears, I suspect they would be stumped by music.

If you are still not convinced that music attracts a peculiarly excessive proportion of human resources, consider another comparison. Think of how important food is to human well-being, of how tasty and enjoyable food is and can be. Now how many universities have departments of cuisine or nutrition, or departments of food sciences, or even departments of home economics? Now consider how many universities have departments of music. Why would music figure more prominently than food? To a visiting tourist from Mars, music sticks out; it is a remarkable and bizarre activity that earthlings do.

Of course, we must be careful in drawing any conclusions about adaptations based on observations of modern behaviours. If music making is an adaptive behaviour, then it must have arisen long ago in the environment of evolutionary adaptedness—namely, the Pleistocene period, when the vast majority of human evolution occurred.

Ethology and evolution

Just because an animal spends a lot of time on certain activities does not mean that the activity represents an evolutionary adaptation. Ethologists must connect the behaviour to an explicit evolutionary account. That is, there must exist a plausible explanation of how the behaviour would be adaptive.

Before considering such a theory for music, let us examine a nonmusical example—an example that has a richer theoretical literature about its origins. Specifically, we will consider some of the evolutionary arguments that have been advanced to account for the origins of language.

On the evolutionary origin of language

As in the case of music, views concerning the origins of language are necessarily speculative. Nevertheless, we can learn a great deal by considering some of the theories that have been advanced concerning its origin. Until recently, the principal view of language was that it facilitated complex collaborative activities such as coordinating actions during hunting. This account seems unlikely, first, because talking is a bad idea when tracking prey, and second, because men as a group display inferior language skills compared with women.

A number of anthropological psychologists have suggested that language (and even music) evolved as surrogates for social bonding.

The grooming and gossip theory of language origins

The most empirically grounded of the recent theories of language origins is what might be called the 'grooming and gossip hypothesis'. Its principal advocate is Robin Dunbar.[24] The theory proposes the following logic.

Animals often live in groups for mutual protection against predators. In general, larger groups are more effective in detecting and warding off predators than smaller groups, but there are costs associated with maintaining a large group. One cost is that feeding must be much more intensive in a given area and so a larger group must travel greater distances in search of food. A second cost is that as group size increases, threats are more likely to arise from internal conflict within the group rather than from external predators. That is, there is a point where group size effectively minimizes predation, but at the cost of threats from members of the group itself. Nowhere is this more evident than in primates. As a consequence of internal threats, animals within the group begin to form alliances with one another. These alliances reduce the likelihood of conflict due to the threat of group retaliation.

In primates, the principal means by which alliances are formed and bonds maintained is through grooming. Grooming accounts for between 10 and 20 per cent of an individual's daytime activities.

There is good evidence to suggest that the principal purpose of grooming is to form alliances between individuals. First, grooming partners are much more likely to come to the defence of one another when threatened by another member of the group. Even more important evidence comes from relating the amount of time spent grooming to the size of the group. Different primate species have different typical group sizes. Gorillas, macaques, chimpanzees, and bonobos, among other groups, tend to form groups that have different average sizes. Primatologists have measured the different amounts of time each species engages in grooming.[25]

A major discovery has been that there is a consistent relationship between group size and the amount of time spent grooming. As the group size increases, the average grooming time also increases. This is an unusual finding: there is no reason to suppose that animals in larger groups tend to get dirtier than animals in smaller groups, so the increase in grooming is unlikely to be related to cleanliness. Primatologists widely agree that the increase in grooming time for larger groups arises from the need to form more extensive networks of alliances. In a large group, an individual fares better by having a wider circle of friends, and the way to build primate friendships is through mutual grooming.

In the case of humans, the common 'group size' has been estimated at roughly 150 people. This is approximately the size of most rural villages in the world. This means that human groups are especially large when compared with other primates. As Dunbar has pointed out, 'If modern humans tried to use grooming as the sole means of reinforcing their social bonds, as other primates do, then the equation for monkeys and apes suggests we would have to devote around 40 per cent of our day in mutual mauling'.[26]

Dunbar has suggested that language evolved as an alternative to physical grooming. In effect, physical grooming was replaced by 'vocal grooming', whose purpose remains the formation and maintenance of friendships or alliances. Such vocal grooming has a distinct advantage over physical grooming: we can talk to several people simultaneously. This increases the number of people we can bond with at the same time.

Note, however, that even language has significant limitations for multiple concurrent social interaction. Dunbar[27] has noted that 'there appears to be a decisive upper limit of about four on the number of individuals who can be involved in a conversation'. When a fifth or sixth person joins a conversation there is a marked tendency for the group to subdivide into two or more concurrent conversations. It is only in hierarchical situations (such as in a formal lecture) where a single conversation can be maintained in a larger group.

All of this suggests that language is most useful in close interpersonal interactions, such as grooming, gossiping, courting, and conspiring. Note, however, that there are other activities that are of value to members of a social group that involve the entire group (or at least large segments) rather than groups of twos or threes. Chief among these group activities is defence. When under threat, uniform group action is indeed a mighty force, much more powerful than smaller groups of twos and threes.

Music and social bonding

At this point, we might speculate how music might fit into this account. Let us assume, for the moment, that the hypothesis that language evolved as a surrogate for physical grooming is true, and that language thereby allowed humans to live in larger groups with their attendant complex social relations. We could certainly conceive of a similar function for music. In some ways, music provides several advantages over language. Singing is much louder than speaking, so singing may facilitate group interactions involving more than the four individuals posited as the upper limit for conversation.

This view of the possible origins for music was essentially proposed by Juan Roederer in 1984: '... the role of music in superstitious or sexual rites, religion, ideological proselytism, and military arousal clearly demonstrates the value of music as a means of establishing behavioural coherency in masses of people. In the distant past this could indeed have had an important survival value, as an increasingly complex human environment demanded coherent, collective actions on the part of groups of human society'.[28]

In light of later work by primatologists such as Dunbar, there appears to be merit in Roederer's hypothesis. Music might have originated as an adaptation for social bonding—more particularly, as a way of synchronizing the mood of many individuals in a larger group. That is, music helps to prepare the group to act in unison.

Perhaps a helpful image is to imagine the cackling of geese prior to their taking off. How is it that individual geese manage to synchronize their actions so that the entire flock takes flight more or less simultaneously? For anyone who has watched geese take off, there is a clear increase in the volume of cackling: more and more geese start honking. The general hubbub of honking geese is apt to raise the arousal levels of all geese in the vicinity. This increased arousal (which includes increased heart rate) would prepare the geese for a significant collective expenditure of energy.

Music and social bonding—further evidence

It is this theory of music and social bonding that I believe holds the greatest promise as a plausible evolutionary origin for music. For the remainder of this article, I would like to review further phenomena that provide support for this hypothesis. The evidence is going to come from the following five sources: various mental disorders imply a strong link between sociability and musicality; child development implies a social role for music; brain structures related to music are linked to social and interpersonal functions; the most popular musical works imply social functioning; music modifies hormone production in groups of people.

Complementary disorders: Williams syndrome and Asperger autism

Consider two mental disorders: Williams syndrome and Asperger-type autism. The principal feature of Williams syndrome is mental retardation. Williams syndrome is unique in that sufferers display three additional characteristics. One characteristic is high verbal abilities. Individuals suffering from Williams syndrome take a great interest in words. Their speech is fluent and peppered with a remarkably sophisticated vocabulary. In fact, when first encountering someone with Williams syndrome, the language fluency tends to mask the mental handicap.

In addition to high verbal abilities, Williams syndrome individuals also exhibit high sociability. They are gregarious and sociable. Coupled with the high verbal abilities, this makes Williams syndrome children a delight to work with. Finally, Williams syndrome children exhibit high musicality.

Daniel Levitin and Ursula Bellugi[29] have described the musical activities of Williams syndrome children at a summer camp in New York State. The children are remarkable. The entire camp is alive with music. Although the children have been shown to have no greater musical aptitude than normals, they clearly relish both the musical activities and the social environment in which their musical enthusiasms can flower.

Now consider the case of Asperger-type autism. Autism is a general diagnosis that is applied to individuals who exhibit a diverse range of symptoms. For example, some autistics are hyper-musical whereas others exhibit complete amusia. Autism is characterized by a strong aversion to social interaction. Although most autism is associated with reduced mental functioning, mental retardation is not always evident. There are autistic individuals with normal and above-average intelligence as well. Autism is related to an emotional deficit—notably the failure to develop the so-called secondary or social emotions, including shame, pride, guilt, love, and empathy. For normal children, these secondary emotions typically appear by the age of about four.

Temple Grandin is a high functioning Asperger-type autistic who has become well known through her writings about her own condition. Concerning love, Grandin talks about her confusion in high school when reading Shakespeare's *Romeo and Juliet*. 'I never figured out what it was all about', said Grandin. In a trip through the Rocky Mountains with Oliver Sacks, Grandin remarked, 'The mountains are pretty, . . . but they don't give me a special feeling, the feeling you seem to enjoy'. 'You get such joy out of the sunset', she said. 'I wish I did, too. I know it's beautiful, but I don't "get" it'.[30] Grandin's experience of music is similar. Although Grandin has perfect pitch and what she describes as a tenacious and accurate auditory memory, she finds music leaves her cold. She finds the sounds 'pretty', but in general, she just doesn't get it.[31] All the fuss about music leaves her mystified.

Grandin's own explanation is that not all of the 'emotional circuits' are connected. Sacks interprets the phenomenon as follows: 'An autistic person can have violent passions, intensely charged fixations and fascinations, or, like Temple [Grandin], an almost overwhelming tenderness and concern in certain areas. In autism, it is not affect in general that is faulty but affect in relation to complex human experiences, social ones predominantly, but perhaps allied ones—esthetic, poetic, symbolic, etc. No one, indeed, brings this out more clearly than Temple herself . . . She feels that there is something mechanical about her mind, and she often compares it to a computer ... She feels that there are usually genetic determinants in autism; she suspects that her own father, who was remote, pedantic, and socially inept, had Asperger's—or, at least, autistic traits—and that such traits occur with significant frequency in the parents and grandparents of autistic children'.[32]

The contrast between Asperger-type autism and Williams syndrome is striking. On the one hand we have a group of people whose symptoms include high sociability linked with high musicality. On the other hand we have a group of people whose symptoms include low sociability often linked with low musicality. Together, these mental conditions are consistent with a relationship between sociability and musicality—and this link is the principal assumption of a group-oriented evolutionary account.

Music and social function

Consider the following question: What is the most successful piece of music in modern history? Of course the answer to this question depends on how we define success—and this is far from clear, as esthetic philosophers have shown. Nevertheless, I want to use a straightforward criterion: let us assume that the most successful musical work is the one that is most performed and most heard. Using this criterion, you might be surprised by the answer. The most successful musical work was composed by Mildred and Patti Hill in 1893, and revised in the 1930s.[33] The piece in question is, of course, 'Happy Birthday'. 'Happy Birthday' has been translated into innumerable languages and is performed on the order of a million times a day. It remained under copyright protection until the middle of the twentieth century. For many people, the singing of 'Happy Birthday' is the only time they sing in public. For other people, the singing of 'Happy Birthday' constitutes the only time they sing.

In some ways, 'Happy Birthday' is the quintessential feminist work. Its composers remain unknown and uncelebrated; the work was created by the collaboration of two women rather than as an egotistic expression of one man. It is a thoroughly domestic work: 'Happy Birthday' is performed in the kitchen or lunch room rather than in the concert hall. No other musical work has evoked so much spontaneous music making. The work is domestic, amateur, and relationally oriented. Despite its extraordinary success, it remains undervalued as a musical creation.

'Happy Birthday' plays a role in our evolutionary story because I suspect that for the vast majority of human history, music making was of this ilk. In Western culture, it is surely the camp songs sung by Girl Scouts or the songs sung by British soccer fans that come closest to what might be imagined in Pleistocene *Homo sapiens*. In all these cases, the music serves an obvious social role and in helping to define a sense of identity and common purpose.

In light of our evolutionary hypothesis, let us return and reconsider the singing of the Mekranoti Indians. Recall some of the characteristic features—especially the singing done by the men: the men's singing is done late at night and in the early morning, and their singing is associated with a high degree of machismo. Like most native societies, the greatest danger facing the Mekranoti Indians is the possibility of being attacked by another human group. The best strategic time to attack is in the very early morning while people are asleep. Recall the insult shouted at men who continued to sleep in their lean-tos: 'Get out of bed! The Kreen Akrore Indians have already attacked and you're still sleeping'. The implication is obvious. It appears that the nightly singing by the men constitutes a defensive vigil. The singing maintains arousal levels and keeps the men awake.

Of course music making is also associated with stirring a war party. North American Indians famously sang and danced prior to initiating an attack on another tribe. One might suppose that engaging in an activity that publicly announces a hostile intention would be counterproductive. War dances might possibly warn an enemy of an impending attack. However, the music making seems to serve a more important role: that of raising arousal and synchronizing individual moods to serve the larger goal of the group.

Social bonding and hormones

Apart from arousing individuals, music can also pacify. Experimental work by Fukui has shown that listening to music can reduce testosterone levels. Fukui himself was quick to point out the possible social and evolutionary significance of this finding. In human social groups, lower levels of testosterone are likely to result in less aggression, less conflict, less sexual confrontation or sexual competition, and consequently more group cohesiveness.

A problem with Fukui's experiment is that he did not manipulate the type of music heard by his listeners. Listeners simply listened to their favourite music. Depending on his sample of listeners, we might expect whole genres of music were not represented. We might suppose, for example, that heavy metal, hard rock, or thrash music might well have increased rather than decreased testosterone levels. Further research is necessary to document the specific hormonal changes associated with different types of musical experiences. However, Fukui's work at least shows that music can have marked effects on hormone levels—specifically, hormones that relate especially strongly to sociability.

Oxytocin and the biology of social bonding

An important question to ask is how precisely music might bring about social bonding. Neurophysiologist Walter Freeman[34] has proposed a pertinent theory related to the hormone oxytocin.

Oxytocin is most commonly associated with the 'let-down' response in new mothers—that is, the response that enables the flow of breast milk following childbirth. The presence of oxytocin also has dramatic effects on the brain. For example, when a ewe gives birth to a lamb, the olfactory bulb in the ewe's brain is bathed in oxytocin. Following the birth of the new lamb, a ewe will imprint on the smell of the new lamb, but will subsequently fail to recognize the smell of her former offspring. The result is that the ewe will suckle only the newborn lamb.

Neurophysiological research has shown that oxytocin acts as a sort of 'eraser' that wipes away previous memories and simultaneously facilitates the storage of new memories. When linked with significant life events, oxytocin is the cement that binds new memories. The amnesic properties of oxytocin are evident in all kinds of learning episodes. However, their strongest effects occur during major limbic activations, such as those resulting from trauma or from ecstasy. Pavlov discovered this phenomenon when serious spring flooding affected his lab and nearly drowned his caged dogs. Following their rescue it was discovered that the dogs had to be retrained from scratch.[35]

In his book, *Societies of Brains*, Freeman chronicles a number of circumstances where oxytocin release occurs and the effects of these releases on neural organization. As we have noted, oxytocin releases are associated with trauma and ecstasy. In addition to childbirth, oxytocin is released in males and females following sexual orgasm. Freeman also suggests that oxytocin is released during trance and while listening to music.

In many cases, the presence of oxytocin is correlated with human and animal bonding circumstances. For example, in the case of sexual orgasm, oxytocin may significantly facilitate pair bonding in the same way that oxytocin following childbirth facilitates mother–child bonding. Freeman's suggestion that music causes oxytocin to be released has important repercussions for instances of peer-group bonding and social identity. If Freeman is correct, there would be good neurophysiological reasons for lovers to enjoy music while courting, for union members to sing while on the picket line, for religious groups to engage in collective music making, for colleges to promote alma mater songs, and for warriors to sing and dance prior to fighting.

Mood regulation

Thayer and his colleagues have carried out a number of studies concerning how people regulate their moods. One study attempted to determine what people do to try to get out of a bad mood. Of 29 categories of activities, the foremost activity was calling or talking to a friend. The second most frequently reported activity was trying to think positive thoughts—to give oneself a sort of 'pep talk'. The third most frequently reported activity—ahead of a wide variety of behaviours—was listening to music. Forty-seven per cent of respondents reported that they used music to temper or eliminate a bad mood.[36]

Thayer *et al.*[37] carried out a similar study to determine what people do to raise their alertness or energy level. Listening to music was reported by 41 per cent of respondents, following activities such as sleeping, taking a shower, getting some fresh air, and drinking coffee. Finally, in a third study investigating what people do to reduce nervousness, tension, or anxiety, listening to music ranked third at 53 per cent, following after only calling or talking to someone, and trying to calm down by thinking about a situation.

There are two points to highlight from these studies. The first is that the foremost category of behaviour for mood regulation is being with or conversing with a friend. That is to say, our first tendency is to seek mood regulation through social interaction. Moods are contagious, and we rely to some extent on each other to modulate, reinforce, or temper our moods. Although we know that moods are highly influenced by the individual's physiological state—notably through food, exercise, or rest—behaviours such as eating, exercise, and rest are less frequently used for mood regulation than music.

The second point to highlight is the obvious point that music appears to figure prominently as a method for mood regulation. Although in contemporary society music tends to be experienced in a personalized or individualized listening context, we already know that this context is historically unprecedented. Most music making in hunter-gatherer societies occurs in a social or group context. Until the invention of the phonograph, the vast majority of music in Western culture was also experienced in social or group contexts. In short, music is not out of place in the list of socialized behaviours used for mood regulation.

Conclusion

By way of conclusion, first let me reiterate that I do not think the evidence in support of music as an evolutionary adaptation is strong. The purpose of this article has been to show that there are no obvious or fatal impediments that rule out a possible evolutionary origin.

We might summarize the basic evidence as follows:

1. Complex evolutionary adaptations arise only over many millennia. Accordingly, in order for a behaviour to be adaptive, it must be very old. As we have seen, music making does indeed conform to the criterion of great antiquity.

2. Behavioural specializations are often expected to be associated with specific anatomical or functional brain structures. Lesions and other neurological assaults can leave an individual with impaired musical functioning. There are double-dissociations between

various amusias and virtually every other kind of functional mental loss. This does not prove that music is not acquired by general learning, but the neurological evidence is at least consistent with the possibility that there are specialized music-related brain structures.

3. In order for a behaviour to be adaptive, the behaviour itself must enhance the propagation of the individual's genes. As we have seen, musical behaviours are consistent with mood modification and group mood synchronization—and these synchronous states are at times clearly associated with situations where group efforts are adaptive—such as in the case of defence against other human groups. In addition, high musical involvement is not associated with dereliction or poor survival (such as the case for alcohol); this raises problems for the view that music is a form of nonadaptive pleasure seeking.

The evidence we have for mood regulation and synchronization is suggestive:

1. We have noted contrasting disorders in Williams syndrome and Asperger-type autism. In one case, we see a group of individuals who are highly sociable and also highly musical. In the other case, we see some individuals who display extremely low sociability and also low musical understanding or affinity.

2. Although we did not review this literature, the emergence of the secondary or socialized emotions in child development is strongly associated with musical empathy, understanding, and sophistication. The pertinent research on child development implies a social role for music.

3. We noted that the most popular musical works often imply some sort of social function. 'Happy Birthday' is only one example. Group identity is often expressed through, for example, folk songs, Girl Scouts' camp songs, sports, and war dances.

4. Although we did not review the literature, it is also known that the emergence of musical tastes relates to postpubescent socializing and group identity.

5. Finally, we discussed how music modifies hormone production in groups of people.

As noted at the beginning of this essay, there is a long history of abuse of genetic claims serving ulterior and often nefarious motives. Even if we assume that musicality has some adaptive function, the repercussions for modern music making and modern musical enjoyment are likely to be minimal. Music is now deeply embedded in a cultural/historical context where human musical memories span centuries, and the fashion cycle is a significant engine of change. Music is now part of a Lamarckian system where acquired characteristics are transmitted in Dawkinsean 'meme pool' rather than in Mendelian 'gene pool'.[38] Like language, the details of musical culture and tastes are largely a product of enculturation.

Nevertheless, it remains worthwhile to attempt to understand where music comes from and why it has achieved such a ubiquitous presence in human lives. Evolutionary theorizing about music may well remain in the realm of *Just-So* stories. There is always the possibility, however, of a testable hypothesis emerging, and if so, we will all wait with interest to see the results.

Acknowledgements

I would like to extend my thanks to Dr Kristin Precoda for drawing my attention to the work of Werner regarding the Mekranoti Indians, and to Dr David Wessel for drawing my attention to Freeman's work concerning oxytocin. This lecture was originally presented at the Department of Music, University of California, Santa Barbara, 6 March 1998. A shortened version was presented at the Society for Music Perception and Cognition Conference, Evanston, Illinois, 16 August 1999.

References

1. **Barkow, J., L. Cosmides**, and **J. Tooby** (eds) (1992) *The Adapted Mind: Evolutionary Psychology and the Generation of Culture*. Oxford: Oxford University Press.

2. **Tooby, J.** and **L. Cosmides** (1992) The psychological foundations of culture. In J. Barkow, L. Cosmides, and J. Tooby (eds). *The Adapted Mind: Evolutionary Psychology and the Generation of Culture*. Oxford: Oxford University Press, pp. 19–136.

3. **Baron-Cohen, S.** (ed.) (1997) *The Maladapted Mind: Classic Readings in Evolutionary Psychopathology*. East Sussex, UK: Psychology Press.

4. **Shepard, R. N.** (1992) The perceptual organization of colors: an adaptation to regularities of the terrestrial world? In J. Barkow, L. Cosmides, and J. Tooby, (eds) *The Adapted Mind: Evolutionary Psychology and the Generation of Culture*. Oxford: Oxford University Press, pp. 495–532.

5. **Wright, R.** (1994) *The Moral Animal: The New Science of Evolutionary Psychology*. New York: Vintage Books.

6. **Dissanayake, E.** (1988) *What Is Art For?* Seattle: University of Washington Press.

7. **Pinker, S.** (1997) *How the Mind Works*. New York: W.W. Norton.

8. **Pinker, S.** (1994) *The Language Instinct*. New York: Morrow.

9. **Wallin, N. L., B. Merker**, and **S. Brown** (2000) *The Origins of Music*. Cambridge, MA: MIT Press.

10. **Williams, L.** (1980) *The Dancing Chimpanzee: A Study of the Origin of Music in Relation to the Vocalising and Rhythmic Action of Apes*. Revised edition London: Allison and Busby.

11. **Lewontin, R. C.** (1991) *Biology as Ideology; The Doctrine of DNA*. Concord, Ontario: House of Anansi Press.

12. **Symons, D.** (1992) On the use and misuse of Darwinism in the study of human behaviour. In J. Barkow, L. Cosmides, and J. Tooby (eds) *The Adapted Mind: Evolutionary Psychology and the Generation of Culture*. Oxford: Oxford University Press, pp. 137–59.

13. **Popper, K.** (1935/1959) *Logik der Forschung*. Vienna, 1935. Translated as The Logic of Scientific Discovery. New York: Basic Books.

14. **Gould, S. J.** and **R. C. Lewontin** (1979) The spandrels of San Marco and the Panglossian program: a critique of the adaptationist programme. *Proc. R. Soc. Lond.* 250, 281–8.

15. **Durham, W.** (1991) *Coevolution: Genes, Culture, and Human Diversity*. Stanford, CA: Stanford University Press.

16. **Darwin, C.** (1872) *The Expression of Emotion in Man and Animals*. London: Murray.

17. **Miller, G.** (2000) Evolution of human music through sexual selection. In N. L. Wallin, B. Merker, and S. Brown (eds) *The Origins of Music*. Cambridge, MA: MIT Press, pp. 329–60.

18. Baharloo, S., P. A. Johnston, S. K. Service, *et al.* (1998) Absolute pitch: an approach for identification of genetic and nongenetic components. *Am. J. Hum. Genet.* 62, 224–31.

19. Anon (1997) Neanderthal notes: did ancient humans play modern scales? *Sci. Am.* 277, 28–30.

20. Turk, I. (ed.) (1997) *Mousterian "Bone Flute" and Other Finds from Divje Babe I Cave Site in Slovenia.* Ljubljana: Zalozba ZRC.

21. Brown, D. (1991) *Human Universals.* New York: McGraw-Hill.

22. Werner, D. (1984) *Amazon Journey; An Anthropologist's Year among Brazil's Mekranoti Indians.* New York: Simon and Schuster.

23. Werner, D. (1984) *Amazon Journey; An Anthropologist's Year among Brazil's Mekranoti Indians.* New York: Simon and Schuster, pp. 245–47.

24. Dunbar, R. (1997) *Grooming, Gossip and the Evolution of Language.* New York: Faber & Faber.

25. Aiello, L. and R. I. M. Dunbar (1993) Neocortex size, group size and the evolution of language. *Curr. Anthropol.* 34, 184–93.

26. Dunbar, R. (1997) *Grooming, Gossip and the Evolution of Language.* New York: Faber & Faber, p. 78.

27. Dunbar, R. (1997) *Grooming, Gossip and the Evolution of Language.* New York: Faber & Faber, p. 121.

28. Roederer, J. (1984) The search for a survival value of music. *Music Percept.* 1, 350–6.

29. Levitin, D. L. and U. Bellugi (1997) *Musical abilities in individuals with Williams Syndrome.* Paper presented at the 1997 Society for Music Perception and Cognition. Cambridge, MA: Massachusetts Institute of Technology.

30. Sacks, O. (1996) *An Anthropologist on Mars.* New York: Random House, p. 124.

31. Sacks, O. (1996) *An Anthropologist on Mars.* New York: Random House, p. 122.

32. Sacks, O. (1996) *An Anthropologist on Mars.* New York: Random House, p. 123.

33. Fuld, J. J. (1995) *The Book of World-famous Music; Classical, Popular and Folk,* 4th edn. New York: Dover.

34. Freeman, W. J. (1995) *Societies of Brains: A Study in the Neuroscience of Love and Hate.* Hillsdale, NJ: Lawrence Erlbaum Associates.

35. Pavlov, I. P. (1955) *Selected Works.* Translated by S. Belsky, edited by J. Gibbons. Moscow: Foreign Languages Publishing House.

36. Thayer, R. E. (1996) *The Origins of Everyday Moods.* New York: Oxford University Press.

37. Thayer, R. E., J. R. Newman, and T. M. McLain (1994) The self-regulation of mood: strategies for changing a bad mood, raising energy, and reducing tension. *J. Pers. Soc. Psychol.* 67, 910–25.

38. Dawkins, R. (1976) *The Selfish Gene.* Oxford: Oxford University Press.

PART II

THE MUSICAL MIND

CHAPTER 6

THE ROOTS OF MUSICAL VARIATION IN PERCEPTUAL SIMILARITY AND INVARIANCE

STEPHEN McADAMS AND DANIEL MATZKIN

Abstract

Perceptual similarity underlies a number of important psychological properties of musical materials including perceptual invariance under transformation, categorization, recognition, and the sense of familiarity. Mental processes involved in the perception of musical similarity may be an integral part of the functional logic of music composition and thus underly important aspects of musical experience. How much and in what ways can musical materials be varied and still be considered as perceptually related or as belonging to the same category? The notions of musical material, musical variation, perceptual similarity and invariance, and form-bearing dimensions are considered in this light. Recent work on similarity perception has demonstrated that the transformation space for a given musical material is limited by several factors ranging from degree of match of the values of auditory attributes of the events composing the sequences, to their relations at various levels of abstraction, and to the degree that the transformation respects the grammar of the musical system within which the material was composed. These notions and results are considered in the light of future directions of research, particularly concerning the role of similarity and invariance in the understanding of musical form during listening.

Keywords: Similarity in music; Invariance in music; Musical variation; Perception of music

Introduction

Perceptual similarity underlies a number of important psychological properties of musical materials including perceptual invariance under transformation, categorization, recognition, and the sense of familiarity. Mental processes involved in the perception of musical similarity may be an integral part of the functional logic of music composition and may thus underly important aspects of musical experience. We are interested in the perception of musical materials and of their musical transformations, that is, 'themes' and 'variations' but in a much larger sense than is usually attached to this specific form in Western tonal music.

A longer term goal of this approach is to understand the role of the perception of similarity and invariance, as well as that of the change produced by variations of the original materials in the experience of musical form. We hesitate to say 'perception' of musical form since most musical forms are too long to be 'perceived' as such. By understanding the mental processing underlying similarity perception, it may be possible to explain in part how listeners form hierarchical and associative relations among features of a musical piece belonging to a given musical system and thereby explain in some musical situations how they manage or fail to establish these relations. How much and in what ways can musical materials be varied and still be considered as perceptually related or as belonging to the same category? Can there be a repertoire of possible transformational rules that the cognitive system can decipher, allowing listeners to perceive a relation between a variation and a theme and perhaps even the nature of the transformation process itself?

We will first of all consider in a general way the notions of musical material, musical variation, perceptual similarity, and perceptual invariance, and then what these all suggest for the development of the notion of form-bearing dimensions in music as originally proposed in McAdams.[1] Subsequently, preliminary experiments on musical similarity that we have conducted[2,3] will be summarized. In this work, pitch and duration variations are studied for both tonal/metric and nontonal/nonmetric musical systems. A number of theoretical issues will finally be developed in the hopes of stimulating and orienting further work in this area, notably concerning: (1) the nature of the representation of musical materials and transformation processes, (2) modularity and dimensional interactions within the realm of music cognition, (3) parallelism and associative structures in music, and (4) the notion of musical development and musical process.

Musical materials

We take the notion of musical material in a very broad way. Materials may be more conventionally considered as simple figures or themes such as the opening 5-note figure of Anton Webern's *Sechs Stücke für großes Orchester*, op. 6 (1909) (only slightly more complex than Beethoven's famous ta-ta-ta-tum, although not as explicitly developed) or slightly more lengthy themes such as a Bach fugue subject. They may also be more fully developed musical ideas such as the thematic materials used by Roger Reynolds in pieces such as *Archipelago* for chamber orchestra and computer-processed sound (1982–3) or *The Behavior of Mirrors* for guitar (1986). He calls these materials core elements.[4] They may vary in duration anywhere from several seconds to several tens of seconds and any given piece will have several of them, each designed to have distinctive characteristics in terms of pitch materials, durational proportions, textures, and gestural movements. Musical materials can also be complex textures: the dense blocks of sound used emblematically by Krzysztof Penderecki in *Threnody for the Victims of Hiroshima* for 52 strings (1960), the architectonic gestures often used by Iannis Xenakis in his orchestral works such as *Pithoprakta* (1956), or the rich micromelodic tapestries in early orchestral and choral works by György Ligeti such as *Atmosphères* (1961) and *Lux Æterna* (1966). And finally, we should not leave out the realm of electroacoustic music in which spectral and temporal sound structures can be imagined from scratch and become the basis for compositional development or in which recorded sounds can become musical materials in their own right as the composer delves into and transforms the inner structure of the sound itself. Notable examples of the latter class are the deep church bell tone and the boy soprano's voice that are the two concrete sound sources from which the computer-generated piece *Mortuos Plango, Vivos Voco* (1980) was composed by Jonathan Harvey or the interpolations between unlikely partners such as a horse's whinny and a baby's cry in *Vox 5* (1986) by Trevor Wishart.

Musical variation

Given the variety of types of musical materials, there is obviously an infinity of ways that even simple ones can be varied in order to generate new material to fill the needs of musical discourse, all the while maintaining (most often) some kind of perceptual link to the original material so that the listener not only recognizes the relation (implicitly or explicitly), but also senses the kind of variation that has been applied. This trajectory of change is one of the perceptual components of musical development, and our intuition is that it contributes to the sense of larger-scale movement and cohesion in a work. In the simplest (operational) terms, musical variation or transformation may be taken to be simply the change along one or more musical dimensions of a given musical material.

In most musics, the principal dimensions targeted for transformation of materials are pitch and duration, although space and timbre have also become the focus of musical structuring in the twentieth century. A complete catalogue of transformation devices is of course impossible, so only a few clearly definable types will be mentioned below. The simplest kind of (non)variation is the repetition of the same material at a different point in time. In this case there is absolute identity in a physical sense and the perception of similarity and the recognition of the return of the material depend only on the listener and the intervening materials.

Another version would keep the pitch and rhythmic values constant and change the timbre through orchestration. A blatantly clear example of this approach is the piece *Boléro* for symphonic orchestra (1928) by Maurice Ravel in which two themes are alternated AABB four times and then AB at the end. However each time, the A and B melodies and their accompaniment are orchestrated differently. The similarity and sense of repetition are strong and it is the pattern of change in orchestration, dynamics, and articulation that create the expressive trajectory of the work. Similarly, in *The Angel of Death* for solo piano, chamber orchestra and computer-processed sound (2001) by Roger Reynolds, the five thematic elements are composed both for solo piano and for the 16-instrument chamber orchestra.[5] The piece is organized in two halves, in both of which the central 'core identities' of the five themes appear. However, if one core appears in the piano in one half, it returns in nearly identical form as concerns pitch and rhythm in the other half, but in the orchestra. Other core elements have the reverse relationship. Bigand *et al.*[6] have shown that for these contemporary musical materials musicians are more perturbed in a recognition task by the instrumentation change than are nonmusicians, although both groups perform in equivalent manner for tonal materials. Further, for materials from the piece by Reynolds, the similarity relations among excerpts are affected by changes in orchestration for some materials and are not affected for others,[7] demonstrating the complexity of perception and memory processes implicated in orchestration practice.

A more complex approach would be to change the timbre on each note, a true *Klangfarbenmelodie* as proposed by Schoenberg[8] and then have different timbral compositions for each new return of the theme. The danger in this case, as will be discussed below is that the melody may become fragmented perceptually if the timbre change is too drastic, bringing about the assignment of different subsets of notes to different auditory streams and thus compromising the psychological coherence of the melody as a whole.[9]

Transposition of pitch and change of tempo are the simplest kinds of transformations and testify to the fact that the representation of relations between events (exact intervals or number of scale steps related to a given scale) are prominent in musical memory. The perception of similarity of transposed melodies is indicative of the influence of internalized musical systems on recognition and similarity perception. An exactly transposed melody (one that maintains the same pitch intervals between successive notes) will in many cases be perceived as a change in key. A melody that is transposed, keeping the same number of scale steps between successive notes, but with pitches that remain within the current key is often perceived as more similar as suggested by recognition studies, although this ability depends on musical training, musical context, and task instructions.[10] At any rate, what seems to be the important aspect of the perceptual representation underlying melodic and rhythmic similarity here is the relations among notes, that is, the relative distance in terms of intervals or scale-steps. Note that the slight interval changes generally preserve the contour (pattern of ups and downs), a component of melody representation that has been shown to be particularly cogent for the similarity of unfamiliar melodies as measured by false recognitions.[11]

Some studies have shown that the perception of timbral intervals is also possible.[12,13] This work was based on the notion of timbre space in which the perceptual relations among sounds equated for pitch, duration, and loudness are represented mathematically as a multidimensional space. Timbral intervals are defined as oriented vectors in the space and timbral contours could be defined by the relative patterns of up and down along the various dimensions. A transformation of a timbre melody such as transposition would simply be the translation of the timbre vectors in the space, keeping their lengths and orientations constant. Although the precise reproduction of timbral intervals is problematic with instrumental music, such musical structures are quite possible with synthesized sounds.

A variant on the simple translation operation is the inversion operation in which the sign of the intervals and contour directions are changed. This technique is used in mirror canon writing and is also quite prominent in serial music in the twentieth century.

Another class of transformations involves temporal rearrangement of the musical material. For example, playing a melody backward is called retrogradation and is often found in music of the Common Practice, romantic, and contemporary periods of Western music. Mirror and cancrizans canons use this technique and it also became a prominent operation in serial music. A particularly intriguing compositional problem-solving task involves creating a melody that can be played forwards and backwards (the cancrizans or 'crab' canon). Often the material that is retrograded may not reproduce the exact interval structure for reasons related to the musical syntax. In such cases, certain prominent intervals or the inverted melodic contour may preserve the sense of similiarity. Take, for example, the opening five-note figure of Anton Webern's *Sechs Stücke*, op. 6 mentioned above in which the flute plays C#4-E4-F4-G4 followed by a D5 on the muted trumpet. Subsequently the sustained trumpet tone becomes the first note of the retrograded pattern D5 (trumpet), Bb4-Eb4-Db4 (flute), B3 (French horn). Although the intervals are slightly different, the pitch contour (small skip, two steps, large skip) is inverted, as is a timbral contour, moving from the low register flute to a bright muted trumpet in one direction and the flute to a lower darker French horn in the other. The mirror image is quite convincing perceptually. Various other techniques of recombination have been used as well, often involving the choice of particularly salient figures from the theme and their subsequent development, a practice quite prominent in Beethoven piano sonatas, for example.

All of the preceding examples are based on rearrangements of symbolically notated events. However, in electroacoustic music, where the material is a continuous sound wave-form, the operations need not be limited to predefined events. Granular synthesis, for example, takes bits of recorded sound from different parts of the original sample, applies a smoothing envelope to them and then recombines them in ingenious ways to create rich sound textures.[14] The larger the grains, the more the original sound quality 'comes through' in the recombination. Roger Reynolds has used a technique involving segmentation and rearrangement in several pieces, applied either to sound samples (as in *Archipelago*, 1982–3) or to note lists representing symbolic events (as in *Variation* for piano, 1988).[4] He has developed two classes of algorithms (SPLITZ and SPIRLZ) that transform the original samples within a space of variation constrained by the variables of the algorithm. The first one segments the sound sequence into units of different durations and then plays the odd ones in one order and the even ones in reverse order. The spacing and timing of the segmented unfolding can be controlled, as can the amplitude envelopes applied to the seg-ments (usually different for even and odd ones). This gives a kind of alternation between the front and back ends of the sound sequence that move towards the centre and then back to the extremities. The technique is obvious when applied to musical gestures with a clear trajectory, but can give stunning results in other cases even though the listener may not be able to follow explicitly the algorithm's logic. As for granular synthesis, the transformed sequences may have a more or less strong similarity to the original material depending on the size and ordering of the segments. When applied within a piece to several different themes, it may be that the transformation device itself takes on an identity across mater-ials that is stronger than the relations between the original and transformed materials in some cases. The perception of these kinds of materials is currently under study in our laboratory in collaboration with the composer, particularly as concerns interactions in memory between original and transformed materials.[15]

Staying within the realm of electroacoustic music, there are a plethora of digital techniques now that allow an extremely fine-grained analysis of a sound's spectral and temporal structure, and then either a direct modification of certain of these parameters, or even a modelling of their behaviour and a subsequent resynthesis with changes in the model para-meters. This kind of sonic elaboration is a class of transformation that remains quite close to the timbre and sound source identity of the materials to be transformed. Compelling examples of this approach can be found in Trevor Wishart's *Vox 5* (1986), Jean-Claude Risset's *Sud* (1985), and Jonathan Harvey's *Ritual Melodies* (1990). In particular, in the Harvey piece, models of various kinds of non-Western instruments and vocal styles are used to create interpolations between the sound universes of each, including not only the sound qualities themselves, but also the styles of playing (forms of vibrato, tremolo, portamento, etc.).[16] Harvey found that without the expressive performance gestures, many of the musical phrases for a given simulated instrument or voice were unconvincing, and the zone in which the heard sound source was between the two originals was musically untenable.

By far the most widely used type of variation involves change in the surface level structure while some invariant is retained at a higher hierarchical level. This kind of technique is quite common in theme-and-variations forms in music of the Common Practice period. The notions of elaboration and reduction have been formalized to a large extent by Lerdahl and Jackendoff,[17] although their applicability to contemporary music as proposed by Lerdahl[18] has been questioned. Indeed Dibben[19] suggests that since structurally important events that 'stand for' sets of subordinate events in tonal music, do not have the same kind of representation in atonal music, it may be necessary to consider more associational structures to explain formal coherence in this latter kind of music as will be discussed at the end of this chapter. Evidence for similarity among musical materials related by a common reduced structure in tonal/metric music is clear, for example,[20–22] and will not be belaboured here. However, notions of elaboration also exist in contemporary music, although it is not clear to what extent commonalities of mental processing exist between the different musical systems.

Some of the psychological questions that arise from this brief and extremely schematic consideration of the possibilities of musical variation may include the following: How far can one transform an original musical material before it becomes completely new, and perceptually unrelated, material, that is, what are the bounds of perceptual similarity? What does the answer to this question tell us about the representations of musical materials and the nature of the psychologically realistic processes of transformation that can operate on them?

Similarity and invariance

At the crux of the issue of musical variation are the notions of perceptual similarity and invariance, provided of course that the varied material appears to have at least some relation to the original material. What we actually mean by 'similarity' is not that easy to pin down operationally. Let us just assume that it is some degree of perceptual match between the properties and features of two materials. The experimental question is thus to understand what properties contribute to perceived similarity and how the degree of match between these (to-be-determined) properties affects its strength. We will speculate on the nature of various kinds of properties and levels of abstraction that might contribute to musical similarity as judged directly by listeners.

Properties that contribute to similarity may be of various levels of abstraction, moving from the most concrete (specific values of attributes of individual events in the sequence, such as melodic and rhythmic configurations) to the most abstract (higher-level reductions of the hierarchical event structure, if such exists for the material being heard, or harmonic contours that provide a kind of skeleton for a tonal work).

Concerning surface values, the surface content of a material and of its transformation (specific pitches, durations, loudnesses, timbres, etc.) may have more or less events in common along the different auditory dimensions. Also the temporal order of these events may be the same or may be transformed to a greater or lesser extent. Exact repetition would of course have the highest similarity and completely different values would have no similarity. However, under some situations the exact same number of events with specific attributes in completely different orders (a random rearrangement of the events, e.g.), may still be experienced as similar due to identical statistical distributions of material properties. Krumhansl[23] has shown, for example, that listeners are sensitive to the combinations of pitch and duration in Olivier Messiaen's *Modes de Valeurs et d'Intensités* for piano (1950). After having heard half of the piece, they were asked to rate new material according to the degree with which it corresponded to that already heard. The specific melodic and rhythmic structures were different, but the tight melodic-rhythmic correspondence was either identical to that of the first half (it was indeed drawn from the second half) or this correspondence was perturbed to a greater or lesser extent in a series of systematic modifications of the score materials. Listeners gave the highest ratings to the repetition of (already heard) excerpts from the first half, followed by excerpts from the second half and then the various modified versions that changed the correspondences between chroma, register, and duration.

As mentioned above, however, musical material can also be represented in terms of relations among attributes in a more or less precise way: exact intervals, relations within a musical system such as a scale, contours, and so on. The perception of similarity would thus be based on a match between relations abstracted from the material attributes rather than directly on the values of the attributes themselves. A melodic contour in Béla Bartók's *Music for Strings, Percussion and Celesta* (1936), for example, might undergo an expansive transformation in which all of the intervals are increased, and yet the whole stays within a certain pitch system and the pitch contour is preserved. Since the rhythmic material is relatively similar between the versions, listeners may hear a strong link between this variation and the original.

Finally, as also mentioned previously, research[20,21] has shown that materials that are quite different in surface structure (affecting specific surface values and the relations between adjacent events) may still be perceived as similar if they share an underlying structure such as the reduced structure proposed by Lerdahl and Jackendoff[17] and Schenker[24] before them. In these cases, it is necessary to postulate that the representation of the event structure of the material is organized to some extent in a hierarchical fashion and that it is some level of this hierarchy that is compared between versions. The experimental question here concerns the depth of the hierarchical representation that can be used to derive a sense of similarity between materials that differ drastically in surface structure. It would seem that it is this kind of structural abstraction that would be one of the main bases of the musical invariance underlying theme and variations forms. Bigand,[20] for example, has demonstrated that listeners group together musical excerpts that have the same underlying reduced structure although they may vary considerably at the surface level.

From these various considerations, we propose that there are (at least) three types of similarity that should be taken into consideration, all the while understanding that they are overlapping and not mutually exclusive categories. The first is relatively abstract and concerns similarity of the statistical distribution of surface values and their derivatives as well as of surface relations of first and higher orders, including perhaps even transitional probabilities from one value or relation to another (cf. Ref. 25 for implicit learning of transitional probabilities for pitch and Ref. 26 for those for timbre). This kind of similarity would seem to be involved in the perception of similar textures, where it is not the exact values that count but the probability of occurrence and of transition that define the texture. The second kind concerns figural similarity, specific patterns of attributes (perhaps associated intimately across auditory dimensions), that give perceptual landmarks within an extended material that allow its recognition when a transformed version still contains the same identifying pattern, or something very similar to it. This notion of figural similarity is akin to the notion of imprint proposed by Deliège.[27] The third kind of similarity is structural and relies on the abstraction of structural invariants related to the event hierarchy, often defined by underlying harmonic and metric templates that are maintained constant in cases of elaborative or reductive transformations of thematic materials.

Form-bearing dimensions

A framework concerning the psychological constraints on form-bearing dimensions in music has been developed.[1] Among these psychological constraints, some seem particularly cogent for the present concerns. Form-bearing dimensions are those along which invariant relations can be configured. For them to be useful in musical discourse these relations must be easily discriminable. Further in evaluating the degree of similarity between thematic materials and their transformations, time has necessarily passed between the two, often several tens of seconds in real music. The configurations must thus be memorizable to some degree of precision either in their absolute form or in some abstracted relative form.

In real music, several dimensions may be varied for a given material. For example, transposing a melody in pitch that is played by the same instrument maintains the same rhythmic structure, and while globally the timbre may change slightly, it remains roughly constant. One psychological constraint on form-bearing dimensions that merits extensive consideration is the resistance of perceived invariance on one dimension to independent variation on other dimensions. In other words, to what extent are the dimensions processed independently or do they interact? This raises the modularity question that has been addressed in both theoretical and experimental terms.[28–30] Both the psychological and the musical issues are extremely complex here since it becomes clear that one may have varying degrees of identity and difference on different dimensions, and the question would be to know how strong the sense of similarity was under certain conditions, or even whether similarity could be maintained. The perception of such transformations would depend on several factors. At the level of the stimulus, it would depend on the way the composer used variation across dimensions and on the types of interactions between dimensions, which may indeed by asymmetric. For example, in Olivier Messiaen's *Mode de Valeurs et d'Intensités* for piano (1950), many dimensions are used: pitch, dynamics, articulation, duration. However, as mentioned above, there is a coupling between the values of one and those of the others. Krumhansl[23] has shown that listeners pick up on these interdimensional correlations and can judge that new material fits or does not fit with the rules developed by the composer. In integral serialism on the other hand, the composer may have series of pitches, dynamics, articulations, and durations, each series having a different number of elements, and they thus become uncorrelated with one another as in Pierre Boulez' *Structures* for two pianos (1952). It would be interesting to repeat Krumhansl's experiment on such material. However, she and her colleagues[31] have shown that many listeners do hear different transformations of row forms (retrograde, inversion, and retrograde inversion) as being related to the original prime series in twelve-tone rows drawn from Schoenberg's *Wind Quintet* (1924) and *Fourth String Quartet* (1936).

A psychological factor that needs to be considered is the resistance of perceived invariance/similarity to perturbation by intervening material. We often presume as score gazers that recognition of the return of a theme is unaffected by new intervening material. However, work in auditory short-term memory has shown that relations of attribute similarity between the to-be-remembered information and the intervening material can degrade recognition and discrimination performance. This kind of auditory memory does seem to be somewhat modular however in that intervening material that is different on the criterial dimension but similar on other dimensions does not necessarily degrade performance, at least when the attributes of single tones are to be remembered.[11,31–40] At a more complex level and for longer term effects in the memory of musical materials varying along several auditory dimensions, it is unclear at present what kinds of contextual effects may exist that would render some intervening material more or less perturbing of the memory trace of the original material and thus hinder its recognition. If such were the case then the 'success' of a given theme in contributing to a sense of coherence in a musical form would certainly be compromised.

Given that materials can vary on different dimensions and that there have been strong tendencies in many cultures to focus primarily on pitch and duration, another psychological question that comes to the fore is the extent to which listeners can learn to focus on changes along a dimension not usually used in one's past experience as a structuring dimension in musical discourse, such as timbre or space, for example. That listeners do not have experience in listening for such structures would probably show up in psychological testing, but we could not conclude from such results that the use of these dimensions was impossible or doomed to failure from the outset. And so the question of perceptual learning will need to be addressed within the framework of contemporary musical experience.

Finally, one of the crucial problems of the perception of musical transformations in relation to their original material concerns perceptual coherence. Variations that affect stream formation or change the availability of properties of the material in working memory may indeed render what is perceived unsimilar to the original material since relations among perceptual attributes would appear to be computed on events belonging to the same auditory stream.[9,41]

Experiments on musical similarity

Having drawn with broad strokes a rough and largely intuitive account of what musical similarity might be and what it's role in music might be, let us examine a few studies that have specifically addressed this question, focusing in particular on recent work from our laboratory that takes a few small steps towards the answer. Several experiments have studied the implication of musical training, musical memory, pitch hierarchy, and musical context in the perception of tonal and nontonal transformations and their similarity ratings.[11,31,37-40] For example, similarity perception is not a symmetrical phenomenon: the similarity perceived between a melody A and a melody B does not automatically predict the similarity perceived between B and A.[37] Finally, although participants show an ability to recognize the type of transformations applied to a nontonal material presented isochronously, this ability tends to decline when transformations are multidimensional, that is when both pitch and rhythm dimensions vary simultaneously.[11,31,38] All these facts however do not explore or explain the computational basis of melodic similarity perception. In fact, is it plausible to imagine that melodic similarity perception could rely on general mental processes that are common to all listeners, independently from the melody's morphology (i.e. number of pitches, rhythmic figures, metronomical speed, etc.) and the listener's musical aptitude?

In recent work, we asked the following questions: What is the nature of musical transformation space and how is it constrained by the type of musical material and musical training (Ref. 2, exp. 1)? To what extent do pitch and duration components of musical materials contribute independently to global similarity judgements and discrimination focussed on each (Ref. 2, exp. 2)?

Musical transformation space: limits of similarity

Three tonal melodies were used as reference material (Ref. 2, exp. 1). Following Serafine et al.[21] a lure melody was constructed for each one such that the surface characteristics were very similar, while the underlying reduced structure was different. For each melody, 16 transformations were composed that differed from the original in terms of pitch content, rhythmic content or both. The transformations could be either elaborations or reductions of the original material, reduction being taken in the sense of a simplified abstract representation of a musical structure that keeps structural information such as important notes in the tonal and metric hierarchies.[17] Further, the pitch and rhythmic transformations either respected tonal/metric syntax (reasonable variations within the scale and meter) or departed from it (unlikely chromatic and unmetrical variations). Corresponding structural transformations were applied to the lure melodies as well. The melodies were verified with respect to the desired properties by a practising composer (Joshua Fineberg) working at IRCAM.

Musician and nonmusician listeners heard one of the three reference melodies followed by a test melody. The test melodies could be the reference or its corresponding lure or any of their transformations. The listeners made a similarity rating on a scale of 1–9 with the high end corresponding to maximum similarity.

The experiment was designed to test several hypotheses:

1. Musicians should be able to hear similarity to greater degrees of transformation if the transformations respect the syntactical rules.

2. If listeners are sensitive to commonalities at certain levels of hierarchical reduction, transformations that respect the reduction should be more similar than those that violate it (including the lure transformations).

3. Drastic transformations in both pitch and rhythm should render the variation as dissimilar to the reference as unrelated material, represented by the lure transformations.

4. The same types of transformation should have similar effects on the three reference melodies, although local morphological differences may prevail due to figural properties of the melodies.

The data revealed no systematic differences between the two populations of listeners. This last finding is concordant with previous studies that have specifically examined effects of musical training on musically realistic tasks.[42–46] Transformations that respected the reduced structure were judged significantly more similar to the reference than those that did not. The dissimilarity was particularly strong for chromatic transformations and for combined chromatic and nonmetric transformations, many of which were judged as dissimilar from the original as were the lure melody and its transformations. This latter result, when combined with the fact that the large majority of lure transformations were judged quite dissimilar to the original, indicates that some transformations of the original were perceived as completely unrelated. And finally, the three reference melodies were different concerning the perceived effects of the transformation types, demonstrating the importance of local surface features in the perception of melodic similarity and the fact that a transformational algorithm must necessarily interact complexly with the to-be-transformed material. However, rank correlations between reference melodies were very high indicating similar qualitative effects of the set of transformations applied to all three melodies.

Modularity of pitch and rhythm in perceived similarity

The answer to one question that cannot be easily gleaned from the results of the first study is the degree to which pitch and rhythmic materials interact in the perception of similarity. Another experiment (Ref. 2, exp. 2) was designed to address this problem more explictly. We therefore introduced a simple computational model based on a modular hypothesis that could represent the basis of the mental processing underlying melodic similarity perception. If the computational model turns out to be reliable for tonal melodies, can it also predict similarity perception of nontonal melodies and thus indicate general processing mechanisms independently of the musical system? One may wonder whether a modular approach is relevant or not to the study of music perception in general and of similarity perception in particular. Examples taken from vision, language, audition, and neuropsychology lead us to consider the modular hypothesis in order to clarify the specificities of similarity perception. Interestingly, aside from modular considerations in music theory,[30] the only consequential empirical research done within an explicitly modular perspective comes from the neuropsychological work of Peretz and collaborators.[29,47,48]

Based on previous findings, which argue in favour of independent pitch and duration processing structures,[40,49] the main hypothesis posited here is that a similarity judgement made between a reference melody and a transformation of that melody can be understood as an additive integration of two similarity coefficients computed by the two hypothetical pitch and duration modules. While such an additive approach is certainly a simplistic way to consider the relations between the two modules, such a general principle should be applicable to any musical system without regard to the nature of the underlying musical grammar, the tonal and twelve-tone systems in our case.

To test this independence, a paradigm similar to that of Garner and Morton[50] was used in which discriminations of changes on one dimension were made in the presence or absence of changes along another dimension, and vice versa, by different groups of listeners. A third group was required to make both discriminations. We coupled this discrimination task with a similarity judgement task. This paradigm was used in order to investigate whether the listeners could recognize a pitch or duration pattern independently from the values taken by the other dimension. Note that since the judgement is focused on a single dimension, at times in the face of variation on the other dimension, perfect discrimination performance across all conditions indicates an ability to ignore the other dimension, implying perceptual independence.

Four reference melodies were composed: one major, one minor, and two twelve-tone melodies. In addition to the original pitch or rhythm patterns, three variations of each dimension were created. These variations were designed to be progressively less similar to the reference pattern. The pitch and rhythm patterns were crossed giving 15 transformations of each reference. The melodies were all composed to achieve the desired properties by a practising composer (Jacopo Baboni-Schilingi) working at IRCAM. The transformations could thus differ only in pitch, only in rhythm or in both. Listeners were divided into three groups: pitch discrimination, rhythm discrimination or both. They first made discrimination judgements on the pitch and/or temporal dimension and then judged globally on a 10-point scale the strength of similarity for each type of transformation in relation to the reference melody.

The discrimination results globally corroborate the modularity hypothesis, although complete perceptual independence was not observed. In particular, the pitch and duration modules do not exhibit the same processing properties since duration processing seems to be less permeable to pitch information than pitch is to duration (at least for tonal melodies). This is reflected when comparing participants' discrimination performance on the two musical dimensions for the two musical systems. For all melodies, duration configurations were better discriminated than pitch configurations and in particular identical pitch patterns were judged as being progressively different when the rhythm pattern was indeed more and more removed from the reference, even though the pitch pattern was identical. By deduction this finding is coherent with existing empirical data in melodic similarity perception where it has been shown that the duration dimension was the major one used by participants for establishing similarity judgements.[51] The pitch permeability to duration configuration was limited to tonal melodies suggesting a functional interaction between the two in that musical system which is decoupled in the twelve-tone system.

Variations among listeners' similarity judgements showed that tonal and nontonal transformations were globally perceived in different ways. While the tonal transformations were hierarchically distinguished, this was not the case for the perception of the nontonal transformations where the pitch and duration modalities were not hierarchically differentiated. Further, whereas the perception of tonal transformations appeared to be perceived in a systematic way over repetitions and for the two reference melodies, this was not the case for the nontonal transformations where the range of variation of listeners' judgements was found to be much greater. Consequently, it seems reasonable to infer that similarity perception of tonal and nontonal melodies depended at least partly on different mental processing mechanisms.

Under the perceptual independence hypothesis, we claimed that similarity perception could be approximated by an elementary additive model. The model decomposes the listeners' similarity ratings into two numerical values: basic pitch and duration values (averaged across listeners) for each level of transformation of that dimension without change on the other dimension. The mean of the basic values for pitch and duration gives the model prediction. For three of the four reference melodies (including both tonal melodies and the first nontonal melody), listeners' mean similarity judgements for the nine two-dimensional transformations were highly correlated with model predictions. So although some differences between the tonal and nontonal melodies exist, they also seem to have certain commonalities as concerns processing in terms of rhythmic and pitch similarity. There are nonetheless deviations of the data from model predictions for each transformation, and these will need to be examined in detail to determine their cause, particularly for the second nontonal melody. There are perhaps salient surface or structural features not taken into account by this simplistic model that played a role in the perceived similarity.

Conclusions/questions

From the data, it is clear that the space of possible variation of thematic material that still maintains a link of perceptual similarity to the original is limited. Although conditions of direct comparison are different from those in real music where intervening material or competing material would often be present, a number of factors can be targeted in provisory fashion for more contextually realistic work in the future. A transformation that maintains a majority of exact values or relations among values in the correct temporal order will be more strongly similar than one that changes all values and all relations. Although this has not been explicitly tested, it may be that maintaining the same distribution of values or relations could still elicit a sense of similarity if compared with material that had dramatically different distribution of attribute values. Further relations of similarity can exist at more abstract levels of a hierarchical reduction, indicating something about the hierarchical nature of the mental representation of musical material in both tonal and nontonal music. From examining the similarity judgements on elaborative and reductive transformations, it would seem that these kinds of transformations retain similarity to the extent that the transformations do not violate the 'grammaticality' of the musical system within which the material has been conceived, suggesting a close link between comprehension of the musical system and the categorization processes that one may hypothesize to operate in the recognition of variations of an original theme.

Another issue of major import for the notion of musical similarity and invariance is the notion of perceptual independence between patterns on different musical dimensions. While there seems to be some degree of independence between pitch and duration structures at a global level, there are also asymmetrical interactions in which duration changes more strongly affect the perceived similarity of identical pitch patterns than is the case for the reverse. More refined experimentation will be necessary to probe the nature of the interaction between the dimensions that gives rise to such asymmetries. Also future research should clearly study more thoroughly different musical systems, including those of other cultures, in an attempt to distinguish the more general cognitive processes from those that are specific to a particular musical grammar.

And finally future research should examine the role that the perception of musical similarity plays in the apprehension or experience of musical form. The process of similarity perception necessarily involves comparison across time of different manifestations of musical material and thus memory processes. One might imagine that the recognition of similarity could thus establish some kind of associative link between different points in the piece and thus contribute in some way to a sense of formal cohesion over longer time spans. Further, one not only recognizes the link between two manifestations but can also appreciate the difference between the two, which perhaps contributes to a perception of the kind of change or the trajectory of change that has taken place. This trajectory may contribute in itself to a sense of musical development over longer time spans and also reinforce the integration of materials at different points in time into a greater whole. There are numerous theoretical and methodological obstacles to be overcome in the design of appropriate experiments to test these contributions in ongoing music listening.

Acknowledgements

This work has benefitted from fruitful discussions with several composers (Jacopo Baboni-Schilingi, Benjamin Carson, Joshua Fineberg, and Roger Reynolds), a musicologist (François Madurell), and two fellow psychologists (Emmanuel Bigand and Sandrine Vieillard), to whom we express our gratitude.

References

1. **McAdams, S.** (1989) Psychological constraints on form-bearing dimensions in music. *Contemporary Music Rev.* 4(1), 181–98.
2. **Matzkin, D.** (2001) Perception de similarité de mélodies tonales et non tonales: Etude pluridisciplinaire. Unpublished PhD thesis, Ecole des Hautes Etudes en Sciences Sociales, Paris.
3. **Matzkin, D.** and **S. McAdams** (2000) Similarity perception of variations of tonal and twelve-tone melodies. In *Proceedings of the 6th International Conference on Music Perception and Cognition.* Keele.
4. **Reynolds, R.** (2002) *Form and Method: Composing Music* (The Rothschild Essays). New York: Routledge.
5. **Reynolds, R.** (2002) Compositional strategies in The Angel of Death for piano, chamber orchestra and computer-processed sound. In C. Stevens, D. Burnham, G. McPherson, E. Schubert, and J. Renwick (eds) *Proceedings of the 7th International Conference on Music Perception and Cognition.* Sydney, Adelaide: Causal Productions.
6. **Bigand, E., S. Vieillard, F. Madurell, S. McAdams,** and **B. Poulin** (2002) Effects of instrumentation on the memorization of musical materials. In C. Stevens, D. Burnham, G. McPherson, E. Schubert,

and J. Renwick (eds) *Proceedings of the 7th International Conference on Music Perception and Cognition.* Sydney, Adelaide: Causal Productions.

7. **Vieillard, S., S. McAdams, O. Houix,** and **R. Reynolds** (2002) Perceptual and cognitive criteria used in the categorization of thematic excerpts from a contemporary musical piece. In C. Stevens, D. Burnham, G. McPherson, E. Schubert, and J. Renwick (eds) *Proceedings of the 7th International Conference on Music Perception and Cognition.* Sydney, Adelaide: Causal Productions.

8. **Schoenberg, A.** (1978) *Theory of Harmony.* Berkeley, CA: University of California Press.

9. **McAdams, S.** and **A. S. Bregman** (1979) Hearing musical streams. *Computer Music J.* 3(4), 26–43.

10. **Dowling, W. J.** (1986) Context effects on melody recognition: scale-step versus interval representations. *Music Percept.* 3, 281–96.

11. **Dowling, W. J.** (1972) Recognition of melodic transformations: inversion, retrograde, and retrograde inversion. *Percep. and Psychophysics* 12, 417–21.

12. **Ehresman, D.** and **D. L. Wessel** (1978) Perception of timbral analogies. IRCAM Report no. 13, IRCAM, Paris.

13. **McAdams, S.** and **J. C. Cunibile** (1992) Perception of timbral analogies. *Philosophical Transactions of the Royal Society, London, Series B* 336, 383–9.

14. **Roads, C.** (1985) Granular synthesis of sound. In C. Roads and J. Strawn (eds) *Foundations of Computer Music.* Cambridge, MA: MIT Press, pp. 145–59.

15. **Vieillard, S., E. Bigand, F. Madurell, S. McAdams,** and **R. Reynolds** (2002) Can listening to excerpts of original versions of contemporary musical materials facilitate recognition of their transformed versions? In C. Stevens, D. Burnham, G. McPherson, E. Schubert, and J. Renwick (eds) *Proceedings of the 7th International Conference on Music Perception and Cognition.* Sydney, Adelaide: Causal Productions.

16. **Vandenheede, J.** (1992) Jonathan Harvey's Ritual Melodies. *Interface* 21(2), 149–83.

17. **Lerdahl, F.** and **R. Jackendoff** (1983) *The Generative Theory of Tonal Music.* Cambridge, MA: MIT Press.

18. **Lerdahl, F.** (1989) Atonal prolongational structure. *Contemporary Music Rev.* 4, 65–87.

19. **Dibben, N.** (1994) The cognitive reality of hiearchical structure in tonal and atonal music. *Music Percept.* 12, 1–25.

20. **Bigand, E.** (1990) Abstraction of two forms of underlying structures in a tonal melody. *Psychol. of Music,* 18, 45–60.

21. **Serafine, M. L., N. Glassman,** and **C. Overbeek** (1989) The cognitive reality of hierarchic structure in music. *Music Percept.,* 6, 397–430.

22. **Stoffer, T. S.** (1985) Representation of phrase structure in the perception of music. *Music Percept.* 3, 191–220.

23. **Krumhansl, C. L.** (1991) Memory for musical surface. *Memory and Cognit.* 19, 401–11.

24. **Schenker, H.** (1935/1979) *Free Composition.* New York: Longman.

25. **Saffran, J. R., E. K. Johnson, R. N. Aslin,** and **E. L. Newport** (1999) Statistical learning of tone sequences by human infants and adults. *Cognition,* 70, 27–52.

26. **Bigand, E., P. Perruchet,** and **M. Boyer** (1998) Implicit learning of artificial grammar of musical timbres. *Current Psychol. of Cognit.* 17, 577–600.

27. **Deliège, I.** (1989) A perceptual approach to contemporary musical forms. *Contemporary Music Rev.* 4, 213–30.

28. **Fodor, J.** (1983) *The Modularity of Mind.* Cambridge, Mass: MIT Press.

29. Peretz, I. and J. Morais (1989) Music and modularity. *Contemporary Music Rev.* 2(1), 279–94.

30. Temperley, D. (1995) Motivic perception and modularity. *Music Percept.* 13, 141–70.

31. Krumhansl, C. L., G. J. Sandell, and D. C. Sergeant (1987) The perception of tone hierarchies and mirror forms in twelve tone serial music. *Music Percept.* 5, 31–78.

32. Deutsch, D. (1970) Tones and numbers: specificity of interference in immediate memory. *Science* 168, 1604–5.

33. Deutsch, D. (1972) Mapping of interactions in the pitch memory store. *Science* 175, 1020–2.

34. Semal, C. and L. Demany (1991) Dissociation of pitch from timbre in auditory short-term memory. *J. Acoust. Soc. of Am.* 89, 2404–10.

35. Semal, C. and L. Demany (1993) Further evidence for an autonomous processing of pitch in auditory short-term memory. *J. Acoust. Soc. Am.* 94, 1315–22.

36. Starr, G. and M. Pitt (1997) Interference effects in short-term memory for timbre. *J. Acoust. Soc. Am.* 102, 486–94.

37. Bartlett, J. C. and W. J. Dowling (1988) Scale structure and similarity of melodies. *Music Percept.* 5, 286–313.

38. Francès, R. (1972) *La perception de la musique.* Paris: Vrin.

39. Halpern, A. R., J. C. Bartlett, and W. J. Dowling (1998) Perception of mode, rhythm, and contour in unfamiliar melodies. Effect of age and experience. *Music Percept.* 15, 335–55.

40. Pitt, M. A. and C. B. Monahan (1987) The perceived similarity of auditory polyrhythms. *Percept. Psychophys.* 41, 534–46.

41. Bregman, A. S. (1990) *Auditory Scene Analysis: The Perceptual Organization of Sound.* Cambridge, MA: MIT Press.

42. Bigand, E. (1993) The influence of implicit harmony, rhythm, an musical training on the abstraction of tension-relaxation schemas in tonal musical phrases. *Contemporary Music Rev.* 9, 123–37.

43. Bigand, E. (1997) Perceiving musical stability: the effect of tonal structure, rhythm and musical expertise. *J. Exp. Psychol., Hum. Percep. Perform.* 23, 808–18.

44. Bigand, E. and M. Pineau (1996) Context effects on melody recognition: a dynamic interpretation. *Curr. Psychol. of Cognit.* 15, 121–34.

45. Bigand, E., B. Poulin, B. Tillmann, F. Madurell, and D. D'Adamo. Sensory versus cognitive components in harmonic priming. *J. Exp. Psychol.: Hum. Percept. Perform.*, in press.

46. Bigand, E., B. Tillmann, B. Poulin, D. D'Adamo, and F. Madurell (2001) The effect of harmonic context on phoneme monitoring in vocal music. *Cognition,* 81, 11–20.

47. Peretz, I. (1993) Auditory agnosia: a functional analysis. In S. McAdams and E. Bigand (eds) *Thinking in Sound: The Cognitive Psychology of Human Audition.* Oxford: Oxford University Press, pp. 199–230.

48. Peretz, I. and R. Kolinsky (1993) Boundaries of separability between melody and rhythm in music discrimination: a neuropsychological perspective. *Quarterly J. Exp. Psychol.* 46A, 301–25.

49. Palmer, C. and C. L. Krumhansl (1987) Independent temporal and pitch structures in the determination of musical phrases. *J. Exp. Psychol: Hum. Percept. Perform.* 13, 116–26.

50. Garner, W. R. and J. Morton (1969) Perceptual independence: definition, models, and experimental paradigms. *Psychol. Bulletin* 72, 233–59.

51. Monahan, C. B. and E. C. Carterette (1985) Pitch and duration as determinants of musical space. *Music Percept.* 1, 1–32.

CHAPTER 7

TONAL COGNITION

CAROL L. KRUMHANSL AND PETRI TOIVIAINEN

Abstract

This chapter presents a self-organizing map (SOM) neural network model of tonality based on experimentally quantified tonal hierarchies. A toroidal representation of key distances is recovered in which keys are located near their neighbours on the circle of fifths, and both parallel and relative major/minor key pairs are proximal. The map is used to represent dynamic changes in the sense of key as cues to key become more or less clear and modulations occur. Two models, one using tone distributions and the other using tone transitions, are proposed for key-finding. The tone transition model takes both pitch and temporal distance between tones into account. Both models produce results highly comparable to those of musically trained listeners, who performed a probe tone task for ten nine-chord sequences. A distributed mapping of tonality is used to visualize activation patterns that change over time. The location and spread of this activation pattern is similar for experimental results and the key-finding model.

Keywords: Music; Tonality; Cognition; Probe tone

Introduction

Tonality induction refers to the process through which the listener develops a sense of the key of a piece of music. The concept of tonality is central to Western music, but eludes definition. From the point of view of musical structure, tonality is related to a cluster of features, including musical scale (usually major or minor), chords, the conventional use of sequences of chords in cadences, and the tendencies for certain tones and chords to suggest or be 'resolved' to others. From the point of view of experimental research on music cognition, tonality has implications for establishing hierarchies of tones and chords, and for inducing certain expectations in listeners about how melodic and harmonic sequences will continue. One method for studying the perception of tonality is the probe tone method, which quantifies the tonal hierarchy. When applied to unambiguous key-defining contexts, it provides a standard for determining key strengths when more ambiguous and complex musical materials are presented. In addition to experimental studies, considerable effort has been spent developing computational models. This effort has produced various symbolic and neural network models, including a number that take musical input and return a key identification, sometimes called key-finding models.

Probe tone methodology

An experimental method introduced to study tonality is sometimes referred to as the probe tone method.[1] It is best illustrated with a concrete example. Suppose you hear the tones of the ascending C major scale: C D E F G A B. There is a strong expectation that the next tone will be the tonic, C, first, because it is the next logical tone in the series and, second, because it is the tonic of the key. In the experiment, the incomplete scale context was followed by the tone C (the probe tone), and listeners were asked to judge how well it completed the scale on a numerical scale (1 = very bad, 7 = very good). As expected, the C received the maximal rating. Other probe tones, however, also received fairly high ratings, and they were not necessarily those that are close to the tonic C in pitch. For example, the most musically trained listeners also gave high ratings to the dominant, G, and the mediant, E. In general, the tones of the scale received higher ratings than the nonscale tones, C♯ D♯ F♯ G♯ A♯. This suggested that it is possible to get quantitative judgements of the degree to which different tones are perceived as stable, final tones in tonal contexts.

A subsequent study[2] used this method with a variety of musical contexts at the beginning of the trials. They were chosen because they are clear indicators of a key. They included the scale, the tonic triad chord, and chord cadences in both major and minor keys. These were followed by all possible probe tones in the chromatic scale, which musically trained listeners were instructed to judge in terms of how well they fit with the preceding context in a musical sense. Different major keys were used, as were different minor keys. The results for contexts of the same mode were similar when transposed to a common tonic. Also, the results were similar independent of which particular type of context was used. Consequently, the data were averaged over these factors. We call the resulting values the K-K profiles, which can be expressed as vectors. The vector for major keys is: K-K major profile = $\langle 6.35, 2.23, 3.48, 2.33, 4.38, 4.09, 2.52, 5.19, 2.39, 3.66, 2.29, 2.88 \rangle$. The vector for minor keys is: K-K minor profile = $\langle 6.33, 2.68, 3.52, 5.38, 2.60, 3.53, 2.54, 4.75, 3.98, 2.69, 3.34, 3.17 \rangle$.

We can generate K-K profiles for 12 major keys and 12 minor keys from these. If we adopt the convention that the first entry in the vector corresponds to the tone C, the second to C♯/D♭, the third to D, and so on, then the vector for C major is: $\langle 6.35, 2.23, 3.48, 2.33, 4.38, 4.09, 2.52, 5.19, 2.39, 3.66, 2.29, 2.88 \rangle$, the vector for D♭ major is: $\langle 2.88, 6.35, 2.23, 3.48, 2.33, 4.38, 4.09, 2.52, 5.19, 2.39, 3.66, 2.29 \rangle$, and so on. The vectors for the different keys result from shifting the entries the appropriate number of places to the tonic of the key.

Tracing the developing and changing sense of key

The probe tone method was then used to study how the sense of key develops and changes over time.[2] Ten nine-chord sequences were constructed, some of which contained modulations between keys. Musically trained listeners did the probe tone task after the first chord, then after the first two chords, then after the first three chords, and continued until the full sequence was heard. This meant that 12 (probe tones) × 9 (chord positions) × 10 (sequences) = 1080 judgements were made by each listener. Each of the 90 sets of probe tone ratings was compared with the ratings made for the unambiguous key-defining contexts. That is, each set of probe tone ratings was correlated with the K-K profiles for the 24 major and minor keys. For some of the sets of probe tone ratings (some probe positions in some of the chord sequences), a high correlation was found, indicating a strong sense of key. For other sets of probe tone ratings, no key was highly correlated, which was interpreted as an ambiguous or sense of key.

As should be obvious from the above, the probe tone task requires an intensive empirical effort to trace how the sense of key develops and changes, even for short sequences. In addition, the sequence needs to be interrupted, and the judgement is made after the sequence has been interrupted. For these reasons, the judgements may not faithfully mirror the experience of music in time. Hence, we[3] have tested an alternative form of the probe tone methodology. In this method, which we call the concurrent probe tone task, the probe tone is presented continuously while the music is played. The complete passage is sounded together with a probe tone. Then the passage is sounded again, this time with another probe tone. This process is continued until all probe tones have been sounded. Preliminary results suggest this methodology produces interpretable results, at least for musically trained participants. Our focus here, however, is on how the sense of key can be represented, whether the input to the representation is from a probe tone task or from a model of key-finding as described later.

A geometric map of key distances from the tonal hierarchies

The K-K profiles generated a highly regular and interpretable geometric representation of musical keys.[2] The basic assumption underlying this approach was that two keys are closely related to each other if they have similar tonal hierarchies. That is, keys were assumed to be closely related if tones that are stable in one key are also relatively stable in the other key. To measure the similarity of the profiles, a product–moment correlation was used. It was computed for all possible pairs of major and minor keys, giving a 24×24 matrix of correlations showing how similar the tonal hierarchy of each key was to every other key. To give some examples, C major correlated relatively strongly with A minor (0.651), with G major and F major (both 0.591), and with C minor (0.511). C minor correlated relatively strongly with Eb major (0.651), with C major (0.511), with Ab major (0.536), and less strongly with F minor and G minor (both 0.339).

A technique called multidimensional scaling was then used to create a geometric representation of the key similarities. The algorithm locates 24 points (corresponding to the 24 major and minor keys) in a spatial representation to best represent their similarities. It searches for an arrangement such that points that are close correspond to keys with similar K-K profiles (as measured by the correlations). In particular, non-metric multidimensional scaling seeks a solution such that distances between points are (inversely) related by a monotonic function to the correlations. A measure (called 'stress') measures the amount of deviation from the best-fitting monotonic function. The algorithm can search for a solution in any specified number of dimensions. In this case, a good fit to the data was found in four dimensions.

The four-dimensional solution located the 24 keys on the surface of a torus (generated by one circle in dimensions 1 and 2, and another circle in dimensions 3 and 4). Because of this, any key can be specified by two values: its angle on the first circle and its angle on the second circle. Thus, the result can be depicted in two dimensions as a rectangle where it is understood that the left edge is connected to the right edge, and the bottom edge is connected to the top edge. The locations of the 24 keys were interpretable in terms of music theory. There was one circle of fifths for major keys (...F#/Gb, Db, Ab, Eb, Bb, F, C,

G, D, A, E, B, F♯/G♭ ...) and one circle of fifths for minor keys (... f♯, c♯, g♯, d♯/e♭, b♭, f, c, g, d, a, e, b, f♯ ...). These wrap diagonally around the torus such that each major key is located near both its relative minor (e.g. C major and A minor) and its parallel minor (e.g. C major and C minor). (See Figures 7.1 and 7.2.)

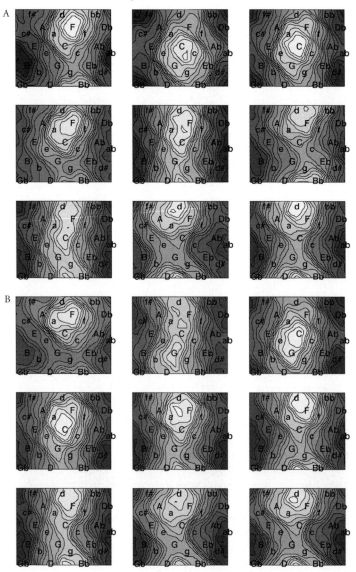

Figure 7.1 (A) Distributed mapping of tonality on the SOM for probe tone judgements for the nine-chord sequence modulating from C major to D minor. The *top row* shows the results for chords 1, 2, and 3 (*left to right*), the *second row* for 4, 5, and 6 (*left to right*), and the *bottom row* for chords 7, 8, and 9 (*left to right*). (B) Distributed mapping of model 1 for the same sequence.

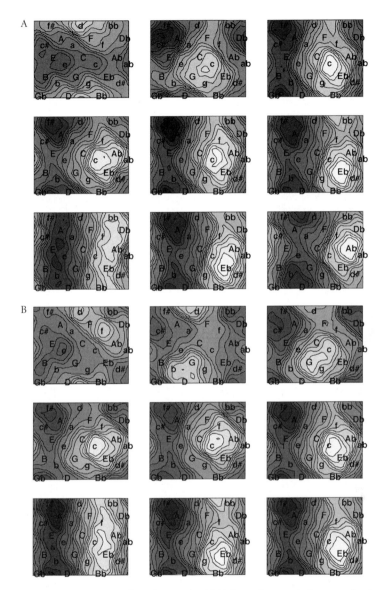

Figure 7.2 (A) Distributed mapping of tonality on the SOM for probe tone judgements for the nine-chord sequence modulating from C minor to Ab minor. Distributing mapping of model 1 for the same sequence.

Representing the sense of key on the torus

The continuous spatial medium containing the 24 major and minor keys affords representing the sense of key in a graphical form,[2] using a technique called multidimensional unfolding. It is a method that is closely related to multidimensional scaling.

Multidimensional unfolding begins with a multidimensional scaling solution, in this case the torus representation of the 24 major and minor keys. This solution is considered fixed. The algorithm then finds a point in the multidimensional scaling solution to best represent the sense of key at each point in time. Let P_1 be the probe tone ratings after the first chord in a sequence; it is a 12-dimensional vector of ratings for each tone of the chromatic scale. This vector was correlated with each of the 24 K-K vectors, giving a 24-dimensional vector of correlations. The unfolding algorithm finds a point to best represent these correlations. Suppose P_1 correlates highly with the K-K profile for F major and fairly highly with the K-K profile for D minor. Then the unfolding algorithm will produce a point near these keys and far from the keys with low correlations. Then the vector of correlations was computed for P_2, giving a second point. This process continues until the end of the sequence.

In this manner, each of the ten nine-chord sequences[2] generated a series of nine points on the torus representation of keys. For nonmodulating sequences, the points remained in the neighbourhood of the intended key. For the modulating sequences, the first points were near the initial intended key, then shifted to the region of the second intended key. Modulations to closely related keys appeared to be assimilated more rapidly than those to distantly related keys. That is, the points shifted to the region of the new key earlier in sequences containing close modulations than in sequences containing distant modulations.

Measurement assumptions of the multidimensional scaling and unfolding methods

The above methods make a number of assumptions about measurement, only some of which will be noted here. The torus representation is based on the assumption that correlations between the K-K profiles are appropriate measures of interkey distance. It further assumes that these distances can be represented in a relatively low-dimensional space (four dimensions). This latter assumption was supported by the low stress value (high goodness-of-fit value) of the multidimensional scaling solution. It was further supported by a subsidiary Fourier analysis of the K-K major and minor profiles, which found two relatively strong harmonics.[4] In fact, plotting the phases of the two Fourier components for the 24 key profiles was virtually identical to the multidimensional scaling solution. This supports the torus representation, which consists of two orthogonal circular components. Nonetheless, it would seem desirable to see whether an alternative method with completely different assumptions recovers the same toroidal representation of key distances.

The unfolding method also adopts correlation as a measure of distances from keys, this time using the ratings for each probe position in the chord sequences and the K-K vectors for the 24 major and minor keys. The unfolding technique finds the best-fitting point in the four-dimensional space containing the torus. It does not provide a way of representing cases in which no key is strongly heard, because it cannot generate points outside the space containing the torus. Thus, an important limitation of the unfolding method is that it does not provide a representation of the strength of the key or keys heard at each point in time. For this reason, we sought a method that is able to represent both the region of the key or keys that are heard, together with their strengths.

In addition, the unfolding approach assumes that spatial locations between the 24 points for major and minor keys are meaningful. An intermediate position would result from a blend of tonal hierarchies of nearby keys. However, other sets of probe tone ratings might also map to the same position. Thus, the identification of points between keys is not necessarily unique. This motivated an alternative model which explicitly specifies the meaning of positions between keys.

The self-organizing map (SOM) of keys

The self-organizing map (SOM)[5] is an artificial neural network that simulates the formation of ordered feature maps. The SOM consists of a two-dimensional grid of units, each of which is associated with a reference vector. Through repeated exposure to a set of input vectors, the SOM settles into a configuration in which the reference vectors approximate the set of input vectors according to some similarity measure; the most commonly used similarity measures are the Euclidean distance and the direction cosine. The direction cosine between an input vector $\mathbf{x}$ and a reference vector $\mathbf{m}$ is defined by

$$\cos \theta = \frac{\sum_i x_i m_i}{\sqrt{\sum_i x_i^2} \sqrt{\sum_i m_i^2}} = \frac{\mathbf{x} \cdot \mathbf{m}}{\| \mathbf{x} \| \| \mathbf{m} \|}. \tag{1}$$

Another important feature of the SOM is that its configuration is organized in the sense that neighbouring units have similar reference vectors. For a trained SOM, a mapping from the input space onto the two-dimensional grid of units can be defined by associating any given input vector with the unit whose reference vector is most similar to it. Because of the organization of the reference vectors, this mapping is smooth in the sense that similar vectors are mapped onto adjacent regions. Conceptually, the mapping can be thought of as a projection onto a nonlinear surface determined by the reference vectors.

We trained the SOM with the 24 K-K profiles. The SOM was specified in advance to have a toroidal configuration, that is, the left and the right edges of the map were connected to each other as were the top and the bottom edges. Euclidean distance and direction cosine, when used as similarity measures in training the SOM, yielded identical maps. (The resulting map is displayed in Figures 7.1 and 7.2.) The map shows the units with reference vectors that correspond to the K-K profiles. The SOM configuration is highly similar to the multidimensional scaling solution[2] and the Fourier-analysis-based projection[4] obtained with the same set of vectors. Unlike those maps, however, all locations in the map are explicitly associated with a reference vector so that they are uniquely identified.

Representing the sense of key on the SOM

A distributed mapping of tonality can be defined by associating each unit with an activation value. For each unit, this activation value depends on the similarity between the input vector and the reference vector of the unit. Specifically, the units whose reference vectors are highly similar to the input vector have a high activation, and vice versa. The activation value of each unit can be calculated, for instance, using the direction cosine of Equation 1. Dynamically changing data from either probe tone experiments or key-finding models can be visualized as an activation pattern that changes over time. The location and spread of this activation pattern provides information about the perceived key and its strength. More specifically, a focused activation pattern implies a strong sense of key and vice versa.

Key-finding models

A variety of key-finding algorithms have been proposed. The objective of these models is to assign a key to an input sample of music (such as the fugue subjects of J. S. Bach's *Well-Tempered Clavier*). Symbolic models, reviewed elsewhere,[4] have taken into consideration a number of factors in assigning key, including scales that contain the tones of the sample, and the presence of such cues to key as the tonic-fifth, tonic-third, and tonic—leading-tone intervals, characteristic tone sequences, and cadences. Some effort has been made to take phrasing, melodic accent, and rhythm into account. More recently proposed symbolic models[6,7] have made advances in both computational and music-analytic sophistication.

Concurrently, neural network models have provided an alternative subsymbolic approach.[8,9] In these, the input sample typically gives rise to activation levels of units associated with different keys. Thus, these models return graded measures of key strength. The problem of representing these in a way that takes into account the distances between keys, however, remains unsolved. In addition, little has been done to compare the output of key-finding algorithms to perceptual judgements, which may change over time as the cues to key become more or less clear and as the music may modulate to other keys. For the most part, the model's output has been compared with the composer's key signature.

Both these issues were addressed by a key-finding algorithm developed using the K-K profiles.[4] The input to this algorithm was a 12-dimensional vector specifying the total durations of the twelve chromatic scale tones in the musical selection to which the key was to be assigned. One application was to Bach's *C Minor Prelude* from Book II of the *Well-Tempered Clavier*. It was treated on a measure-by-measure basis. Each input vector was projected onto the toroidal map of keys using the phases of the two strong Fourier components. Two musical experts gave quantitative judgements of key strength in each measure of the piece, which were also projected onto the map. The key-finding algorithm followed the same pattern of modulations found by the experts, suggesting the approach lends itself to tracing dynamic changes in key as modulations occur. One obvious limitation of this approach is that it ignores the order of the tones in the input sample. This potentially important cue for key led to the development of the tone transition model described below.

Tone transitions and key-finding

The order in which tones are played may provide additional information that is useful for key-finding. This is supported by studies on both tone transition probabilities[10,11] and perceived stability of tone pairs in tonal contexts.[4,13] In samples of compositions by Bach,

Beethoven, and Webern, only a small fraction of all the possible tone transitions were actually used (the fractions were 23, 16, and 24 per cent, respectively).[10] Furthermore, in a sample of 20 songs by Schubert, Mendelssohn, and Schumann, there was an asymmetry in the transition frequencies in the sense that certain tone transitions were used more often than the same tones in the reverse temporal order.[11] For instance, the transition B-C was used 93 times, whereas the transition C-B was used only 66 times. A similar asymmetry was found in studies on perceived stability of tone pairs in a tonal context.[4,13] After the presentation of a tonal context, tone pairs that ended with a tone that was high in the tonal hierarchy were given higher ratings than the reverse temporal orders. For instance, in the context of C major, the ratings for the transitions B-C and C-B were 6.42 and 3.67, respectively.

Determining tone transitions in a piece of polyphonic music is not a trivial task, especially if one aims at a representation that corresponds to perceptual reality. Even in a monophonic piece, the transitions can be ambiguous in the sense that their perceived strengths may depend on the tempo. Consider, for example, the tone sequence C4-G3-D4-G3-E4, where all the tones have equal durations. When played slowly, this sequence is heard as a succession of tones oscillating up and down in pitch. With increasing tempi, however, the subsequence C4-D4-E4 becomes increasingly prominent. This is because these tones segregate into one stream due to the temporal and pitch proximity of its members, separate from G3-G3. With polyphonic music, the ambiguity of tone transitions becomes even more obvious. Consider, for instance, the sequence consisting of a C major chord followed by a D major chord, where the tones of each chord are played simultaneously. In principle, this passage contains nine different tone transitions. Some of these transitions are, however, perceived as stronger than others. For instance, the transition G–A is, due to pitch proximity, perceived as stronger than the transition G–D.

It seems, thus, that the analysis of tone transitions in polyphonic music should take into account principles of auditory stream segregation.[14] Furthermore, it may be necessary to code the presence of transitions on a continuous instead of a discrete scale. In other words, each transition should be associated with a strength value instead of just coding whether that particular transition is present or not. Below, a dynamic system that embraces these principles is described. In regard to the evaluation of transition strength, the system bears a resemblance to a proposed model applying the concept of apparent motion to music.[15]

Tone transition model

Let the piece of music under examination be represented as a sequence of tones, where each tone is associated with pitch, onset time, and duration. The main idea of the model is the following: given any tone in the sequence, there is a transition from that tone to all the tones following that particular tone. The strength of each transition depends on three factors: pitch proximity, temporal proximity, and the duration of the tones. More specifically, a transition between two tones has the highest strength when the tones are proximal in both pitch and time and have long durations. These three factors are included in the following dynamic model.

Representation of input

The pitches of the chromatic scale are numbered consecutively. The onset times of tones having pitch k are denoted by t_{ki}^n, $i = 1, \ldots, n_k$, and the offset times by, t_{ki}^f, $i = 1, \ldots, n_k$, where n_k is the total number of times the kth pitch occurs.

Pitch vector $p(t) = (p_k(t))_k$

Each component of the pitch vector has nonzero value whenever a tone with the respective pitch is sounding. It has the value of 1 at each onset at the respective pitch, decays exponentially after that, and is set to zero at the tone offset. The time evolution of $\mathbf{p}$ is governed by the equation

$$\dot{p}_k = -p_k \tau_p + \sum_{i=1}^{n_k} \delta\left(t - t_{ki}^n\right) - p_k \sum_{i=1}^{n_k} \delta\left(t - t_{ki}^f\right), \tag{2}$$

where $\dot{p}_k$ denotes the time derivative of p_k and $\delta(\cdot)$ the Dirac delta function (unit impulse function). The time constant τ_p has the value of $\tau_p = 0.5$ s. With this value, the integral of p_k saturates at about 1 s after tone onset, thus approximating the durational accent as a function of tone duration.[16]

Pitch memory vector $m(t) = (m_k(t))_k$

The pitch memory vector provides a measure of both the perceived durational accent and the recency of notes played at each pitch. In other words, a high value of m_k indicates that a tone with pitch k and a long duration has been played recently. The dynamics of $\mathbf{m}$ are governed by the equation

$$\dot{\mathbf{m}} = \mathbf{p} - \mathbf{m}/\tau_m, \tag{3}$$

The time constant τ_m determines the dependence of transition strength on the temporal distance between the tones. In the simulations, the value of $\tau_m = 3$ s has been used, corresponding to typical estimates of the length of the auditory sensory input.[17–19]

Transition strength matrix $S(t) = (s_{kl}(t))_{kl}$

The transition strength matrix provides a measure of the instantaneous strengths of transitions between all pitch pairs. More specifically, a high value of s_{kl} indicates that a long tone with pitch k has been played recently and a tone with pitch l is currently sounding. The temporal evolution of S is governed by the equation

$$s_{kl} = m_k \frac{1 + \text{sgn}(p_i - p_k)}{2} p_l e^{-(k-l)^2/\alpha^2}, \tag{4}$$

In this equation, the nonlinear term $(1 + \text{sgn}(p_l - p_k))/2$ is used for distinguishing between simultaneously and sequentially sounding pitches. This term is nonzero only when $p_l > p_k$, that is, when the most recent onset of pitch l has occurred more recently than that of pitch k.

The term $e^{-(k-l)2/\alpha 2}$ weights the transitions according to the interval size. For the parameter α, the value $\alpha = 6$ has been used. With this value a perfect fifth gets a weight of about 0.37 times the weight of a minor second.

Dynamic tone transition matrix $N(t) = (n_{kl}(t))_{kl}$

The dynamic tone transition matrix is obtained by temporal integration of the transition strength matrix. At a given point of time, it provides a measure of the strength and recency of each possible tone transition. The time evolution of N is governed by the equation

$$\dot{N} = S - N/\tau_N, \tag{5}$$

where the time constant τ_N is equal to τ_m, that is, $\tau_N = 3$ s.

To examine the role of tone transitions in key-finding, we developed two key-finding models. Model 1 is based on pitch class distributions. Model 2 is based on tone transition distributions. Below, a brief description of the models is given.

Key-finding model 1

Model 1 is based on pitch class distributions only. Like the earlier algorithm based on the K-K profiles,[4] it does not take tone transitions into account. However, it has a dynamic character in that both the pitch vector and the pitch memory vector depend on time. It uses a pitch class vector $p_c(t)$, which is similar to the pitch vector $p(t)$ used in the dynamic tone transition matrix, except that it ignores octave information. Consequently, the vector has 12 components that represent the pitch classes. The pitch class memory vector $m_c(t)$ is obtained by temporal integration of the pitch class vector according to the equation

$$\dot{m}_c = p_c - m_c/\tau_d. \tag{6}$$

is correlated with the K-K profiles for each key. Alternatively, or in addition, the vectors $m_c(t)$ can be projected onto the toroidal key representation using activation values as described earlier. Both approaches will be taken here.

Key-finding model 2

Model 2 is based on tone transitions. Using the dynamic transition matrix N, it calculates the octave-equivalent transition matrix $N' = (n'_{ij})_{ij}$ according to

$$n_{ij}'(t) = \sum_{\substack{i = p \bmod 12 \\ j = p \bmod 12}} n_{pq}(t). \tag{7}$$

In other words, transitions whose first and second tones have identical pitch classes are considered equivalent, and their strengths are added. Consequently, the melodic direction of the tone transition is not taken into account. To obtain estimates for the key, the pitch class transition matrix is correlated with the matrices representing the perceived stability of two-tone transitions for each key.[4]

Application of models 1 and 2 to the chord sequence data

The probe tone data for the ten chord sequences described earlier[2] were compared with the results of models 1 and 2 applied to those sequences. An interchord onset time of one second was used. The perceptual judgements were correlated with the K-K profiles, and these were compared with the key correlations of the two models. Model 1 results correlated highly ($r(2158) = 0.87$, $p < 0.0001$) with the experimental data. Model 2 also correlated highly ($r(1918) = 0.86$, $p < 0.0001$). (Model 2 produces an output only after the first two chords.) Model 2 contributed additional precision when combined with model 1, as shown by a multiple regression predicting the experimental data from both models ($R(2, 1917) = 0.89$, $p < 0.0001$, with both models contributing significantly at $p < 0.0001$; the standard coefficient was 0.50 for model 1 and 0.43 for model 2). Thus, the two models generally matched well the experimental results, and modelled slightly different aspects of the listeners' responses.

Figures 7.1 and 7.2 show the distributed mapping of tonality on the SOM for the listeners (Figures 7.1A and 7.2A) and model 1 (Figures 7.1B and 7.2B) for two illustrative chord sequences. (Because of issues about how best to visualize the results of model 2, we show only model 1 here.) In these representations, a single contour outlines correlations 0.70 or above, double contours outline correlations 0.80 or above, triple contours outline correlations 0.90 or above, and quadruple contours outline correlations 0.95 or above.

The sequence depicted in Figure 7.1 consists of the chords F G C F d B♭ e° A d, containing a relatively distant modulation from C major to D minor. After the first chord, F, appeared, the listeners and the model had a clear focus on the key of F major in which the chord is I. When the second chord, G, was sounded, listeners apparently interpreted this as a IV–V progression in C major, resulting in a focus near that key. The model, however, did not find this focus until the tonic triad, C, in the third position. For the fourth and fifth chords, F and d, the focus of both listeners and model remained in the region of C major but was shifted somewhat towards F major and D minor. The sixth chord, B♭, which is contained in D minor but not C major, shifted the focus farther towards D minor. The seventh chord, e° , greatly weakened the sense of key for both listeners and model; a diffuse elongated region of weak activation was found. With the last two chords, A and d, the final focus on D minor (in which these are V–I) was arrived at.

The sequence depicted in Figure 7.2 consists of the chords d° G c A♭ F D♭ b♭ E♭ A♭, containing a modulation from C minor to A♭ major, a modulation to what is considered a relatively close key. Both listeners and model yielded an extremely weak activation pattern for the first two chords, d° and G, although the focus for listeners after the second chord was weakly near C minor. The third chord, c, clarified this focus near C minor for both listeners and model, where it remained for the fourth and fifth chords, A♭; and f. The sixth chord, E♭, which is the tonic triad in the relative major of C minor (E♭ major) produced a strong focus on E♭ major for listeners and a shift in that direction for the model. The seventh chord, B♭, diffused this focus for both listeners and model before the new key of A♭ major clarified with the E♭ and A♭ chords in the last two positions (which are V–I in the A♭ major key).

Conclusion

Experimental studies suggest that the sense of tonality undergoes dynamic and subtle changes when a listener hears music. The sense of key develops and strengthens as certain cues appear, then may weaken or shift to a new key as subsequent events are sounded. An important step in understanding this process is a suitable means of representing such changes. Towards this end, we have developed a spatial representation based on psychological data. The distributed map of the SOM provided a visually accessible representation of these subtle dynamic changes. The key-finding models described here suggested that listeners' sense of key can be modelled quite well using tone distributions and tone transitions. Two models were formulated to incorporate various psychological phenomena, including durational accent as a function of tone duration, the duration of sensory memory, temporal-order asymmetries, and pitch streaming as a function of the distances between tones in pitch and time. The models accounted well for the results of an experiment with relatively simple and short chord sequences. Further tests of such models with more complex, extended, and musically realistic materials may point to additional factors, such as rhythm, meter, phrasing, and form, that may also influence the sense of tonality.

References

1. **Krumhansl, C. L.** and **R. N. Shepard** (1979) Quantification of the hierarchy of tonal functions within a diatonic context. *J. Exp. Psychol. Hum. Percept. Perform.* 5, 579–94.
2. **Krumhansl, C. L.** and **E. J. Kessler** (1982) Tracing the dynamic changes in perceived tonal organization in a spatial representation of musical keys. *Psychol. Rev.* 89, 334–68.
3. **Krumhansl, C. L.** and **P. Toiviainen** (2000) Dynamics of tonality induction, a new method and a new model. In C. Woods, G. Luck, R. Brochard, F. Seddon, and J.A. Sloboda (eds) *Proceedings of the Sixth International Conference on Music Perception and Cognition.* Keele, UK: Keele University, pp. 1504–13.
4. **Krumhansl, C. L.** (1990) *Cognitive Foundations of Musical Pitch.* New York: Oxford University Press.
5. **Kohonen, T.** (1997) *Self-organizing Maps.* Berlin: Springer-Verlag.
6. **Vos, P. G.** and **E. W. Van Geenen** (1996) A parallel-processing key-finding model. *Music Percept.* 14, 185–223.
7. **Vos, P. G.** and **M. Leman** (Eds) (2000) Tonality induction. Special issue of *Music Percept.*
8. **Leman, M.** (1995) A model of retroactive tone-center perception. *Music Percept.* 12, 439–71.
9. **Bharucha, J. J.** (1999) Neural nets, temporal composites, and tonality. In D. Deutsch (ed.) *The Psychology of Music*, 2nd edn. San Diego, CA: Academic Press, pp. 413–40.
10. **Fucks, W.** (1962) Mathematical analysis of the formal structure of music. *I R E Trans. Information Theory* 8, 225–8.

11. **Youngblood, J. E.** (1958) Style as information. *J. Music Theory* 2, 24–5.

12. **Knopoff, L.** and **W. Hutchinson** (1978) An index of melodic activity. *Interface* 7, 205–29.

13. **Krumhansl, C. L.** (1979) The psychological representation of musical pitch in a tonal context. *Cognit. Psychol.* 11, 346–74.

14. **Bregman, A. S.** (1990) *Auditory Scene Analysis.* Cambridge, MA: M.I.T. Press.

15. **Gjerdingen, R. O.** (1994) Apparent motion in music? *Music Percept.* 11, 335–70.

16. **Parncutt, R.** (1994) A perceptual model of pulse salience and metrical accent in musical rhythms. *Music Percept.* 11, 409–64.

17. **Darwin, C. J., M. T. Turvey,** and **R. G. Crowder** (1972) An auditory analogue of the sperling partial report procedure, evidence for brief auditory storage. *Cognit. Psychol.* 3, 255–67.

18. **Fraisse, P.** (1982) Rhythm and tempo. In D. Deutsch (ed.) *The Psychology of Music,* 1st edn. San Diego, CA: Academic Press, pp. 149–80.

19. **Treisman, A. M.** (1964) Verbal cues, language, and meaning in selective attention. *Am. J. Psychol.* 77, 206–19.

CHAPTER 8

LEARNING AND PERCEIVING MUSICAL STRUCTURES: FURTHER INSIGHTS FROM ARTIFICIAL NEURAL NETWORKS

BARBARA TILLMANN, JAMSHED J. BHARUCHA, AND EMMANUEL BIGAND

Abstract

Artificial neural networks expand our understanding of the acquisition and representation of knowledge of our environment and the influence of this knowledge on perception. In the present chapter, we review applications of artificial neural networks to music cognition, notably to the learning and perceiving of musical structures. We present a hierarchical self-organizing model that learns basic regularities of the Western tonal system by mere exposure and simulates tonal acculturation. After learning, the model simulates a variety of experiments dealing with the processing of tone, chord, and key relationships. It provides a parsimonious account of these data sets by postulating activation as the unifying mechanism underlying various cognitive tasks. The modelling of music cognition presented in this chapter is restricted to behavioural data. Nevertheless, the computational processes are based on fundamental neural constraints. Future developments of artificial networks simulating neuropsychological cases and establishing direct links to neural correlates will contribute to enhance our understanding of mechanisms of music perception.

Keywords: Music cognition; Connectionist modeling; Self-organization; Tonal acculturation

Introduction

Artificial neural networks are rooted in the biological structure of the neural system: they consist of a set of artificial neurons (units) that are linked via synaptic connections of different strengths. A unit does not represent one neuron, but simulates a population of neurons. The goal of artificial networks is not to describe neural anatomy and physiology, but to be founded on neural principles in order to simulate different levels of perceptual and cognitive processing. Recent developments in artificial networks establish correspondences to neural mechanisms by relating components of a model to brain structures, creating artificial lesions or suggesting biologically plausible networks (i.e. neurobiological models with autonomous and adaptive behaviour).

The present chapter reviews some artificial neural networks that have been proposed in auditory and music perception. Neural nets are helpful in understanding how we learn musical patterns by mere exposure, how these patterns might be represented and how this knowledge arising from acculturation influences perception. To date, applications of networks for music cognition have been restricted to behavioural data. However, future developments in combination with neuropsychological cases and brain imaging methods should make it possible to establish links to brain structures and neural circuitry for the investigation of music perception. These developments are in progress in other domains (e.g. language perception, visual perception, memory). In these domains, artificial neural networks are used not only to simulate cognitive processes and behavioural data, but to postulate correspondences to cerebral structures, their interactions and the effects of brain damage. For behavioural data, a variety of networks have been proposed in connectionist psycholinguistics for language acquisition, sentence processing, reading, and production (cf. Ref. 1 for a recent review). Well-known networks developed by McClelland and colleagues on visual word and speech perception[2–5] simulate a variety of behavioural data and generate numerous hypotheses for further behavioural experiments. The creation of 'artificial lesions' in neural net models simulating behaviour of healthy participants have enabled the simulation of neuropsychological cases, and have provided further insights into the normal functioning of the brain, possible representations of knowledge and the modularity of subprocesses (see Ref. 6 for a review). Simulations in computational neuropsychology have been proposed by eliminating network units or by weakening connections in order to model clinical cases of aphasia,[7–9] dyslexia[10,11] or semantic impairments.[12,13] For example, comparing the behaviour of damaged connectionist models to double-dissociations observed in the behaviour of brain-injured patients suggests that behavioural deficits arise from impairments of two types of lexical information (semantic and phonological) and explains past tense formation of English verbs without rules or symbolic mechanisms.[14,15]

In what follows, we briefly review some basics of neural net modelling and summarize the regularities underlying Western tonal music. Next, we present our recent work with Self-Organizing Maps (SOMs) as an example of neural networks providing further insights to music cognition. We then suggest some possible, though still speculative, future directions in which neural nets can help us further to investigate the processing of music, notably by simulating neuropsychological cases and establishing links to neural structures and circuitry.

Some basics of artificial neural networks

A principal advantage of artificial neural networks is their capacity to adapt in such a way that representations, categorizations or associations between events can be learned. Connectionist models have the characteristic that rules governing the materials are not explicit, but emerge from the simultaneous satisfaction of multiple constraints represented by the connections; these constraints can be learned by repeated exposure. This learning process is either supervised by an external teaching exemplar or unsupervised via passive exposure. In the present review, we focus on unsupervised learning algorithms that extract statistical regularities and encode events that often occur together. The competitive learning algorithm[16] is an unsupervised learning algorithm that provides the basis for learning in self-organizing maps[17,18] and ART (adaptive resonance theory) networks.[19,20] Unsupervised learning algorithms seem to be well suited to model music cognition, as acculturation to musical structures presumably occurs without supervision in listeners.

In an artificial neural network, a set of units is linked via synaptic connections of different strengths. The units are generally arranged into layers, with an input layer coding the incoming information. When a stimulus is presented to the model, the input units are activated. This activation is sent via the connections to units in other layers, and the strength of the transmitted activation is controlled by the strengths of the connections (i.e. weights). In parallel with biological networks, the learning process is defined as a modification of the connection weights. For the learning process, a set of training stimuli is presented repeatedly to the network. The network adapts its connections in such a way that it becomes sensitive to the underlying correlational structure between events of the training set. Before learning starts, all connections are generally set to random values, a state that represents the 'ignorance' of the model. Over the course of learning, the neural net units gradually become sensitive to different input events or categories. With the competitive learning algorithm, the specialization takes place by competition among the units.[16] When an input is presented to the network, the unit that is best able to represent it wins the competition and is allowed to learn the representation of this input even better. The unit's response will be subsequently stronger for this same input pattern and weaker for others. In a similar way, other units learn to respond selectively to other input patterns. The competitive learning algorithm is generalized in SOMs that contain a spatial layout of the units. In SOMs, the winning unit and its neighbour units learn. This learning process leads to topographic mappings between input data and neural net units on the map: For two similar input patterns, map units that respond maximally are located near each other. This mirrors principles of cortical information processing, such as spatial ordering in sensory processing areas (i.e. somatosensory, vision, audition). In the primary visual cortex, the orientation of stimuli to which cells respond best changes in an orderly fashion with nearby cells responding best to similar orientations.[21] In the auditory system, tonotopic organization is found at almost all major stages of processing (i.e. inner ear, auditory nerve, cochlear nucleus, auditory cortex), and the auditory cortex displays a tonotopic organization in which nearby cells respond best to similar frequencies.[22–25]

According to Kohonen,[26] the SOM algorithm parallels the adaptive processes underlying plasticity in biological networks: the theoretical definition of neighbourhood results in learning that is similar in consequence to lateral connections modelled by chemical processes. The principles of self-organization are general across domains, but input representations are domain specific. The SOMs have been applied to a variety of domains, including visual perception,[27] semantic processing[28] or auditory perception.[29,30] Mercado et al.[30] used an SOM to simulate experience-dependent reorganization of representation maps in auditory cortex. The network architecture was constrained by properties observed in auditory cortex and which include the modulating influences of the basal forebrain. The simulations allowed the authors to formulate hypotheses on neuromodulatory effects in auditory cortical plasticity and to suggest future simulations including other neural regions (e.g. hippocampus) in order to model effects on learning and memory. Recently, we used the SOM algorithm to simulate an example of cognitive plasticity, notably the cognitive capacity to extract underlying regularities and to become sensitive to musical structures and regularities via implicit and unsupervised learning processes.[31]

An overview of regularities underlying Western tonal music

Western tonal music is an example of a highly structured system in our environment. It contains a set of regularities (i.e. regularities of cooccurrence, frequency of occurrence, and psychoacoustic regularities) based on a limited number of elements. The Western tonal system that contains a three-level organization is based on a set of 12 tones (C-C#-D-D#-E-F-F#-G-G#-A-A#-B). The 12 tones are combined into subsets of seven tones, the scales. For each tone of a scale, chords (e.g. major or minor) are constructed by adding two notes—creating a second order of musical units. The tones in a scale and their associated chords define a third level of organization in the tonal system: the keys. Keys sharing numerous tones and chords are harmonically related, and the strength of harmonic relationship depends on the number of shared events. The seven tones that belong to the underlying scale are in-key tones, the remaining five tones are out-of-key tones. Similarly for chords, in-key chords are differentiated from out-of-key chords. Hierarchies of functional importance exist among tones and chords belonging to a given key: For example, chords built on the first, fifth, and fourth scale degrees (referred to as tonic, dominant, and subdominant, respectively) have more important functions than chords built on other degrees. From a psychological point of view, the hierarchically important events of a key act as stable cognitive reference points[32] to which others are anchored.[33] As the tonal system is based on a restricted set of events, the same event can define an in-key or an out-of-key event or can take different levels of functional importance (i.e. tonal stability)—always depending on the established key.

The three levels of musical units occur with strong regularities of cooccurrence. Tones and chords belonging to the same key are more likely to cooccur in a musical piece than tones and chords belonging to different keys. Changes between keys are more likely to occur between closely related keys than between less related ones. Also within-key hierarchies are strongly correlated with the frequency of occurrence of tones and chords in Western musical pieces. Tones and chords that have more important music-theoretic functions in a given key are used with higher frequency (and longer duration).[34–36]

Despite the complexity of the system, Western tonal listeners become sensitive to the musical structures by mere exposure to musical pieces obeying this system of regularities.[35–37] As the number of opportunities to listen to musical pieces is so great in everyday life, this implicit knowledge is plausibly learned by the same implicit processes as those investigated in the laboratory.[38–41] Behavioural and neurophysiological research has provided evidence that even nonmusician listeners are sensitive to the context dependency of musical events. The implicit knowledge embodies the functions of tones and chords in a key,[35,42–44] the relations between different keys,[45–48] and the change in tonal functions depending on the context.[49–53] The influence of this internalized representation has been reported for musical memory,[54–57] musical expectancies,[52,58–61] and with electrophysiological and brain imaging methods.[62–69]

Learning musical structures

The Western tonal system embodies strong regularities to which listeners become sensitive via mere exposure to musical pieces.[35–37] We proposed to simulate implicit learning processes of tonal regularities with SOMs and used the trained network to simulate experimental data on music perception via activation spreading through the learned representation.[31]

In these simulations, a hierarchical network with two SOMs was defined (i.e. a multi-layer hierarchical self-organizing map HSOM[70]). The input layer consisted of 12 units coding the 12 pitch classes. Each unit of this layer was connected to a second layer (a self-organizing map) that in turn was connected to a third layer (a second self-organizing map). Before learning started, the units of two layers were fully interconnected with connection weights set to random values. Four learning simulations that differed in training material and richness of input coding were realized. The first SOM was trained with a set of chords presented separately. The second SOM was trained with either groups of chords that belonged to the same key or short chord sequences. The short chord sequences represented more realistic harmonic material since they respected chord transitions and frequencies of occurrence in Western tonal music. In addition, each chord was weighted according to recency in order to mimic memory decay in short-term memory. All training material was coded by either a sparse input pattern (i.e. a unit is activated (set to '1') when a note is present in the chord, and set to '0' otherwise) or a richer input pattern that coded a chord as the weighted sum of subharmonics of the present pitch classes (as proposed in Refs 71 and 72).

Independent of training material and input coding, the network became sensitive to regularities underlying the musical material (i.e. chords, chord sets, chord sequences). The units of the first SOM became specialized in the detection of chords and the units of the second SOM in the detection of keys. Both layers showed a topological organization of the specialized units. In the chord layer, units representing chords that share tones (or subharmonics) were located close to each other on the map, but chords not sharing tones were not represented by neighbouring units. In the key layer, the units specialized in the detection of keys were organized in a circle: keys sharing numerous chords and tones were represented close to each other on the map and the distance between keys increased with decreasing number of shared events. The organization of key units reflects the music theoretic organization of the cycle of fifths: the more the keys are harmonically related, the closer they are on the cycle (and on the network map). After training with the rich input coding, also the chord layer showed a more global organization reflecting harmonic relationships: chords from one side of the circle of fifths are represented on one half of the map, the other side of the circle on the other half of the map.

After learning, the connection weights were not at random values any longer, but reflected the regularities of cooccurrence. With the sparse input coding, a chord unit was linked to three tone units, tones that are components of this chord, and a key unit was linked to six chord units, chords that belong to the key. In addition, for the simulations using chord sequences, the strength of the connections reflected the frequency of occurrence of chords in the sequences, and the tonic chord in a given key had stronger links than the other chords. For the simulations with chord sets, all connections between chord and key units had the same strength. In sum, specialized representational units were formed for combinations of musical events (tones, chords) that occur with great regularity. The self-organization leads to a hierarchical encoding in which tones occurring together are represented by chord units, and similarly, chords occurring together are represented by key units. Interestingly, the learned connections mirrored the pattern of connections that had been hardwired in a previously proposed music perception network (MUSACT[73]).

The trained HSOM networks were used as feedforward and reverberation systems. In a feedforward system, activation consisted of bottom-up information only. Consequently, activation of chord units reflected the number of component tones shared with the input: the more tones are shared, the stronger the unit is activated. In a reverberation system, phasic activation spreads between the units of the three layers until an equilibrium is reached.[73] After reverberation, the activation pattern reflects top-down influences of learned, schematic structures, and respects tonal relations: the activation of major chord units, for example, decreased monotonically with increasing distance on the circle of fifths. After reverberation, top-down processes overwrote influences of coding richness and the imposed activation pattern was analogous for sparse and rich input coding. Finally, activation patterns after reverberation for the four trained HSOM networks showed strong correlations with activation patterns of MUSACT ($0.984 < r < 0.999$). This outcome suggests that MUSACT's hard-wired structure can emerge from self-organization.

The hierarchical self-organizing map thus manages to learn Western pitch regularities. The input layer of the network was based on pitch classes, the 12 tones of the chromatic scale. In Western tonal music, these pitch classes are repeated over octaves in different pitch heights. The phenomenon of octave equivalence (i.e. tones separated by an octave are perceived as similar in pitch) permits the presentation of the tonal system as based on 12 events. The abstract pitch-class coding in the network was based on previous simulations of octave category learning. An SOM learned octave-equivalent pitch classes via mere exposure to spectral representations of tones.[74] In addition, it has also been shown that neural nets are able to learn the extraction of pitch height from frequency,[75–77] and to transform a spectral representation of an acoustic source into a spatial distribution of pitch strengths.[75] These models represent the application of neural nets to the learning of low-level processes in auditory perception (pitch extraction, octave equivalence). The HSOM model with its three organizational layers of tones, chords, and keys can be conceived of as subsequent to these simulated phases of auditory preprocessing.

In the music perception domain, other neural net models have been proposed to simulate the learning of higher-level organizations. In contrast to the HSOM network presented above, these models focused on either one or two organizational layers in music perception, as for example, models of chord classification[78] or melodic sequence learning.[79–81] Griffith[82] and Leman[72,83] used SOMs to simulate the learning of key representations based on either melodies,[82] chords[72] or recordings of real musical pieces which are preprocessed by an auditory module.[83] After training, the specialized units of the SOMs showed a topological organization of the detected key centres that reflects the harmonic distances between keys (as on the cycle of fifths) with the distances on the map. Leman's work provided evidence that higher order units of Western music (i.e. tonal centres) can be learned via passive exposure to a rich acoustic input. These models focused on the learning of tonal centres, but did not account for relations between tones, chords, and keys. Gjerdingen[84] proposed to simulate a more complex aspect of musical learning: the perception of musical style. An ART network[19,20] was trained to categorize and memorize stylistic features of Mozart pieces and the learned feature patterns were compared to music theoretic concepts.

Perceiving musical structures

In order to be compelling, a cognitive model of Western music should not only simulate the internalization of Western pitch regularities via mere exposure, but should also simulate the behaviour of listeners after having adapted to Western tonal music. Numerous connectionist models in music have not been developed to reflect cognitive processes and their predictions are not directly tested with behavioural data observed with human listeners. In Leman's work,[72] for example, musical pieces were presented to the network and tonal centre activation was compared with music theory analyses. In Ref. 83, a context followed by a chord was presented to the network and changes in activation patterns were correlated with probe-chord judgements of human listeners.[36] The activation changes simulated indirectly the differences in subjective judgements, but the network was not able to generate predictions for the chords themselves. A different approach to compare performance of network and human listeners has been proposed by Stevens[85] and Stevens and Latimer.[86,87] A network was trained to distinguish musical excerpts (standard) from modified excerpts. Results of simulations were compared with performance of human listeners and the influence of musical expertise was modeled by length of training. However, the model was explicitly restricted to a recognition task without the goal to simulate other tasks or a more general representation of tonal knowledge. Krumhansl et al.[80] compared performance of human listeners and SOM networks for the specific case of melodic expectation in Finnish spiritual folk hymns. Expertise was simulated by contrasting two SOM networks trained with either hymns or different finish folk songs. Activation patterns of the hymn SOM correlated more strongly with melodic continuation judgements of human expert listeners and suggested that this SOM became sensitive to tone distributions and tone transitions underlying the Finnish hymns.

In Tillmann et al.,[31] the HSOM network was tested for its capacity to simulate a variety of empirical data about perceived relations between and among tones, chords, and keys in Western tonal music. Simulations were run with the experimental material used in the empirical studies. The underlying rationale of the simulations was to test activation (spreading through a representation of tonal knowledge) as a mechanism unifying a range of cognitive tasks. The experimental material was presented to the model and the activation levels of network units were interpreted as levels of tonal stability.[a] The more a unit (i.e. a chord

---

[a] For event sequences, activation due to each event is accumulated and weighted according to recency.[73] The total activation of a unit is thus the sum of the stimulus activation, the phasic activation accumulated during reverberation and the decayed activation due to previous events.

unit, a tone unit) is activated, the more stable the musical event is in the corresponding context. For the experimental tasks, it was hypothesized that the level of stability affects performance (e.g. a more strongly activated, stable event is more expected or judged to be more similar to a preceding event).

For perceived relations between chords, the model succeeded in simulating data obtained with similarity judgements,[49,53] recognition memory,[49] harmonic priming[52,59,88,89] and electrophysiological measures.[69] Harmonic priming and ERP data provided evidence for the development of harmonic expectations in a prime context that then influence the processing of a target chord: a target is processed more slowly and less accurately and evokes a larger late-positivity component LPC, when it is unrelated to the context than when it is related. When the experimental material is presented to the network, activation levels of chord units mirrored patterns of processing in the priming task (e.g. with higher activation for chord units representing facilitated targets), and activation changes in chord units after the target mirrored the amplitude of the LPC (e.g. with stronger activation changes for distant key targets). Both human listeners and network are sensitive to changes in chord stability caused by key contexts. Further behavioural experiments have shown that human listeners perceive keys underlying a given context, detect modulation (i.e. temporary changes in key) occurring in a musical excerpt and have implicit knowledge of distances between keys.[46,47,90] A further set of HSOM simulations showed that activation levels of key units and activation changes over time mirror listeners' behavioural data. For example, the changes of activation patterns in key units were more important when the excerpt modulated to distantly related keys.[46] As activation accumulates in the network over time, the model also tracks the key changes in a sequence and simulates a dynamic aspect of tonality sensation.

The HSOM network also simulated behavioural data on the perceived relations between tones, even if it was trained with chords only and not with melodies. Notably, the activation levels of tone units simulate the stability profiles obtained in probe-tone ratings,[90] the patterns of similarity ratings[32] and memory for melodies.[56] For example, when human listeners rate the similarity of a tone pair presented after a tonal context, the ratings reflect the differences in tonal functions and show a perceived asymmetry with higher similarity for a pair ending on a stable tone. The activation levels and activation changes of the tone units mirrored these data sets.

Overall, the simulations showed that activation in the trained self-organizing network mirrored data of human participants in tonal perception experiments. This outcome suggests that the level of activation in tone, chord, and key units is a single unifying concept for human performance in different tasks.

General discussion

The HSOM network was presented as an application of artificial neural networks to further our understanding of learning and perceiving music. Based on self-organization (i.e. a general unsupervised learning algorithm), the structure of the network adapted to tonal regularities through repeated exposure to musical material. The network combines three levels of music perception which can be placed on the top of networks simulating lower perceptual processing steps (pitch extraction, octave equivalence). After training, the network simulates a large set of experimental data on perceived relations between tones, chords, and keys. These simulations proposed activation as a unifying mechanism for different cognitive tasks. A context activates the network and the activation state then influences the perception (i.e. expectation, perceived similarity, memory). The HSOM network provided a model not only for the learning of implicit knowledge about the tonal system, but also for a low-dimensional and parsimonious representation of tonal knowledge. For example, the network proposes a parsimonious account of the contextual dependency of musical functions of an event and the changes associated with different keys. One single event has not multiple instances of representation, but its corresponding function in a given key emerges from activation spreading in the system. As a consequence, events representing prototypes and anchor points in a given key do not have to be stored separately, but emerge from the activation levels. A further emerging property of the network relates to the identification of a key; the underlying key does not need to be inferred employing separate processing steps, but emerges from the activation pattern in the key units.

The network also offers a framework for generating new predictions for further behavioural studies on music perception. These studies and associated simulations could investigate the perception of tones, chords, and keys. The experimental material will be presented to the network and on the basis of the activation levels precise hypothesis can be derived for the performance of human listeners. For example, the studies could be related to key identification (e.g. number of notes necessary to establish a key, disturbing effect of an unrelated event), to key modulation (e.g. how long the trace of a key remains) or to the eventual link between activation decay and musical short-term memory span.

In the following, we point out two limitations of the HSOM network and discuss future developments of the model. A first limitation is the restriction to pitch structures only, and the second one is that the network is more abstract than brain structures and neural circuitry.

The simulations have focused on how regularities of the pitch dimension may be internalized through passive learning processes. Although pitch is the most obvious form-bearing dimension of Western tonal music, temporal regularities also contribute to listeners' perceptual experience. Temporal regularities include the sensation of meter (sensation of a regular succession of strong and weak beats superimposed over an isochronous pulse) and patterns of intervals creating rhythms perceived against the metrical background. Two frameworks have been proposed to account for the respective contributions of regularities of pitch and time in the perception of musical events.[91] A single-component model[92] suggests that temporal and harmonic accents are not processed independently, but are integrated and together guide the attention of the listener during the unfolding musical piece.[51,54,93,94] Based on neuropsychological cases (with double-dissociations of amelodia without arhythmia and vice versa), and experimental data,[91,95–98] Peretz and Kolinsky[91] proposed a two-component model suggesting independence between temporal and nontemporal information processing which are integrated only at a later stage. Two types of neural net architectures can be used to mimic these two theoretical approaches and to account for learning and perception of regularities in pitch and time. A single-component neural net may learn the two regularities conjointly without a supplementary integrative step, by adapting input codings of metrical information as proposed by Berger and Gang[99,100] or by Stevens and Wiles.[101] A two-component network may learn separately regularities of pitch (as in the HSOM[31]) and time (as proposed in Ref. 102), followed by a later integration step in order to simulate the development of expectations. The network modelling shall allow further investigation of how pitch and time are combined—a question that arises for learning, perception, and memorization (cf. Ref. 103 for visual stimuli). In addition, networks integrating both pitch and time create the possibility to study neuropsychological cases. The goal would be to simulate neuropsychological cases with amelodia without arythmia (and vice versa) by creating artificial lesions to the networks of normal perception (see Ref. 6 for applications in other domains).

Even if the HSOM model is conceived on an abstract level and not in relation to brain structures or neural circuitry, it can be a source of inspiration to generate hypotheses about the neural circuitry underlying music perception. For example, the self-organizing algorithm conforms to principles of cortical information processing, such as spatial ordering in sensory cortex or tonotopic organization in auditory cortex. The outcome of the simulations, together with aspects of cortical organization, leads to the question whether there exist higher order maps such as a tonotopic organization of key centres.

In the domain of music perception, simulations are restricted to learning and perception in combination with behavioural data. Future developments of networks, however, should also have the goal of suggesting simulations that make the bridge to actual neural structures and circuitry in the brain. In other domains, connectionist models in computational neurosciences are created on the bases of existing knowledge about cerebral structures and neural circuitry.[104,105] In visual perception, Otto et al.[105] investigated invariant object recognition (same object despite changes in size or location). The creation of the network was based on a set of neurophysiological constraints known about the ventro-lateral and dorsal-parietal pathways associated with the processing of object identification ('what') and spatial localization ('where'). Based on the simulations' outcome, the authors derived new predictions about interactions between the neural pathways and motivated neurophysiological, biological and behavioural experiments. Recently, the hypothesis of two types of pathways ('what', 'where') has been proposed for auditory perception.[106,107] Once more details are known about their functioning, simulations following the line proposed by Otto et al.[105] will enhance the understanding of their interaction and stimulate further explorations.

References

1. Christiansen, M. H. and N. Chater (2001) *Connectionist Psycholinguistics.* Westoirt, CT: Ablex.

2. McClelland, J. L. and D. E. Rumelhart (1981) An interactive activation model of context effects in letter perception: part 1. An account of basic findings. *Psychol. Rev.* 86, 287–330.

3. Rumelhart, D. E. and J. L. McClelland (1982) An interactive activation model of context effects in letter perception. part 2. *Psychol. Rev.* 89, 60–94.

4. McClelland, J. L. and J. L. Elman (1986) The TRACE model of speech perception. *Cognit. Psychol.* 18, 1–86.

5. Seidenberg, M. S. and J. L. McClelland (1989) A distributed, developmental model of word recognition and naming. *Psychol. Rev.* 96, 523–68.

6. Cohen, G., R. A. Johnston, and K. Plunkett (2000) *Exploring Cognition: Damaged Brains and Neural Nets: Readings in Cognitive Neuropsychology and Connnectionist Modelling.* Hove, East Sussex, UK: Psychology Press.

7. Dell, G. S. (1986) A spreading-activation theory of retrieval in sentence production. *Psychol. Rev.* 93, 283–321.

8. Dell, G. S., M. F. Schwartz, N. Martin, E. M. Saffran, and D. A. Gagnon (1997) Lexical access in aphasic and nonaphasic speakers. *Psychol. Rev.* 104, 801–38.

9. French, R. M. (1997) Selective memory loss in aphasics: an insight from pseudo-recurrent connectionist networks. In J. Bullinaria *et al.* (eds) *Connectionist Representations.* London: Springer, pp. 183–95.

10. Shallice, T. and D. Plaut (1992) From connectionism to neuropsychological syndroms. In J. Alegria *et al.* (eds) *Analytic Approaches to Human Cognition.* Amsterdam: Elsevier Science, North Holland, pp. 239–58.

11. Harley, T. A. (1993) Connectionist approaches to language disorders. *Aphasiology* 7, 221–49.

12. Farah, M. J. and J. L. McClelland (1991) A computational model of semantic memory impairment: modality specificity and emergent category specificity. *J. Exp. Psychol. Gen.* 120, 339–57.

13. Devlin, J. T., L. M. Gonnerman, E. S. Andersen, and M. S. Seidenberg (1998) Category-specific semantic deficits in focal and widespread brain damage: a computational account. *J. Cognitive Neurosci.* 10, 77–94.

14. Joanisse, M. F. and M. S. Seidenberg (1999) Impairments in verb morphology after brain injury: a connectionist model. *Proc. Nat. Acad. Sci.* 96, 7592–7.

15. Lavric, A., D. Pizzagalli, S. Forstmeier, and G. Rippon (2001) Mapping dissociations in verb morphology. *Trends in Cognitive Sci.* 5, 301–8.

16. Rumelhart, D. E. and D. Zipser (1985) Feature discovery by competitive learning. *Cognitive Sci.* 9, 75–112.

17. von der Malsberg, C. (1973) Self-organizing of orientation sensitive cells in the striate cortex. *Kybernetic* 14, 85–100.

18. Kohonen, T. (1995) *Self-Organizing Maps.* Berlin: Springer.

19. Grossberg, S. (1970) Some networks that can learn, remember and reproduce any number of complicated space-time patterns. *Studies Appl. Math.* 49, 135–66.

20. Grossberg, S. (1976) Adaptive pattern classification and universal recoding: I. parallel development and coding of neural feature detectors. *Biological Cybernetics* 23, 121–34.

21. Hubel, D. H. and T. N. Wiesel (1962) Receptive fields, binocular interaction, and functional architecture in the cat's visual cortex. *J. Physiol.* 160, 106–56.

22. Brugge, J. F. and R. A. Reale (1985) Auditory cortex. In A. Peters and E. G Jones (eds) *Cerebral Cortex: Association and Auditory Cortices.* New York, NY: Plenum Press.

23. Wessinger, C. M., M. H. Buonocore, C. L. Kussmaul, and G. R. Mangun (1997) Tonotopy in human auditory cortex examined with functional magnetic resonance imaging. *Human Brain Map.* 5, 18–25.

24. Howard, M. A. I., I. O. Volkov, P. J Abbas, H. Damasio, M. C. Ollendieck, and M. A. Granner (1996) A chronic microelectrode investigation of the tonotopic organization of human auditory cortex. *Brain Res.* 724, 260–4.

25. Bilecen, D., K. Scheffler, N. Schmid, K. Tschopp, and J. Seelig, (1998) Tonotopic organization of the human auditory cortex as detected by BOLD-FMRI. *Hearing Res.* 126, 19–27.

26. **Kohonen, T.** (1993) Physiological interpretation of the self-organizing map algorithm. *Neural Net.* 6, 895–905.

27. **Schyns, P. G.** (1991) A modular neural network of concept acquisition. *Cognitive Sci.* 15, 461–508.

28. **Ritter, H.** and **T. Kohonen** (1989) Self-organizing semantic maps. *Biological Cybernetics* 61, 241–54.

29. **Kohonen, T.** (1988) The 'neural' phonetic typewriter. *Computer IEEE* 21, 11–22.

30. **Mercado, E. I., C. E. Myers,** and **M. A. Gluck** (2001) A computational model of mechanisms controlling experience-dependent reorganization of representational maps in auditory cortex. *Cognitive, Affective & Behavioral Neurosci.* 1, 37–55.

31. **Tillmann, B., J. J. Bharucha,** and **E. Bigand** (2000) Implicit learning of tonality: a self-organizing approach. *Psychol. Rev.* 107 (4), 885–913.

32. **Krumhansl, C. L.** (1979) The psychological representation of musical pitch in a tonal context. *Cognit. Psychol.* 11, 346–74.

33. **Bharucha, J. J.** (1984) Anchoring effects in music: the resolution of dissonance. *Cognit. Psychol.* 16, 485–518.

34. **Budge, H.** (1943) *A Study of Chord Frequencies. Teacher College.* New York: Columbia University.

35. **Francès, R.** (1958) *La perception de la musique.* Paris: Vrin.

36. **Krumhansl, C. L.** (1990) *Cognitive Foundations of Musical Pitch.* Oxford, England: Oxford University Press.

37. **Dowling, W. J.** and **D. L. Harwood** (1986) *Music Cognition.* Orlando, Florida: Academic Press.

38. **Altmann, G.T., Z. Dienes,** and **A. Goode** (1995) Modality independence of implicitly learned grammatical knowledge. *JEP-LMC* 21, 899–912.

39. **Dienes, Z., D. Broadbent,** and **D. C. Berry** (1991) Implicit and explicit knowledge bases in artificial grammar learning. *JEP-LMC* 17, 875–87.

40. **Reber, A. S.** (1967) Implicit learning of artificial grammars. *J. Verbal Learning and Verbal Behavior* 6, 855–63.

41. **Reber, A. S.** (1989) Implicit learning and tacit knowledge. *J. Exp. Psychol. Gen.* 118, 219–35.

42. **Cuddy, L. L.** and **B. Badertscher** (1987) Recovery of tonal hierarchy: some comparisons across age and levels of musical expertise. *P&P* 41, 609–20.

43. **Hébert, S., I. Peretz,** and **L. Gagnon** (1995) Perceiving the tonal ending of tune excerpts: the roles of pre-existing representation and musical expertise. *Can. J. Exp. Psychol.* 49, 193–209.

44. **Tillmann, B., E. Bigand,** and **F. Madurell** (1998) Influence of global and local structures on the solution of musical puzzles. *Psychol. Res.* 61, 157–74.

45. **Bartlett, J. C.** and **W. J. Dowling** (1980) The recognition of transposed melodies: a key-distance effect in developmental perspective. *J. Exp. Psychol. Hum. Percept. Perform.* 6, 501–15.

46. **Cuddy, L. L.** and **W. F. Thompson** (1992) Asymmetry of perceived key movement in chorale sequences: converging evidence from a probe-tone analysis. *Psychol. Res.* 54, 51–9.

47. **Cuddy, L. L.** and **W. F. Thompson** (1992) Perceived key movement in four-voice harmony and single voices. *MP* 9, 427–38.

48. **Thompson, W. F.** and **L. L. Cuddy** (1989) Sensitivity to key change in chorale sequences: a comparison of single voices and four-voice harmony. *MP* 7, 151–68.

49. **Bharucha, J. J.** and **C. L. Krumhansl** (1983) The representation of harmonic structure in music: hierarchies of stability as a function of context. *Cognit.* 13, 63–102.

50. **Bigand, E.** (1993) The influence of implicit harmony, rhythm and musical training on the abstraction of 'tension-relaxation schemes' in a tonal musical phrase. *Contemporary Music Rev.* 9, 128–39.

51. **Bigand, E.** (1997) Perceiving musical stability: the effect of tonal structure, rhythm and musical expertise. *J. Exp. Psychol. Hum. Percept. Perform.* 21, 808–22.

52. **Bigand, E.** and **M. Pineau** (1997) Global context effects on musical expectancy. *P&P* 59, 1098–107.

53. **Krumhansl, C. L., J. J. Bharucha,** and **M. Castellano** (1982) Key distance effects on perceived harmonic structure in music. *P&P* 32, 96–108.

54. **Bigand, E.** and **M. Pineau** (1996) Context effects on melody recognition: a dynamic interpretation. *Current Psychol. of Cognit.* 15, 121–34.

55. **Cuddy, L. L., A. J., Cohen,** and **D. J. Mewhort** (1981) Perception of structure in short melodic sequences. *J. Exp. Psychol. Hum. Percept. Perform.* 7, 869–83.

56. **Dowling, W. J.** (1978) Scale and contour: two components of a theory of memory for melodies. *Psychol. Rev.* 85, 341–54.

57. **Dowling, W. J.** (1991) Tonal strength and melody recognition after long and short delays. *P&P* 50, 305–13.

58. **Bharucha, J. J.** and **K. Stoeckig** (1986) Reaction time and musical expectancy: priming of chords. *J. Exp. Psychol. Hum. Percept. Perform.* 12, 403–10.

59. **Bharucha, J. J.** and **K. Stoeckig** (1987) Priming of chords: spreading activation or overlapping frequency spectra? *P&P* 41, 519–24.

60. **Bigand, E., F. Madurell, B. Tillmann,** and **M. Pineau** (1999) Effect of global structure and temporal organization on chord processing. *J. Exp. Psychol. Hum. Percept. Perform.* 25, 184–97.

61. **Cuddy, L. L.** and **C. A. Lunney** (1995) Expectancies generated by melodic intervals: perceptual judgements of melodic continuity. *P&P* 57, 451–62.

62. **Besson, M.** and **F. Faieta** (1995) An Event-Related Potential (ERP) study of musical expectancy: comparison of musicians and nonmusicians. *J. Exp. Psychol. Hum. Percept. Perform.* 21, 1278–96.

63. **Besson, M., F. Faita,** and **J. Requin** (1994) Brain waves associated with musical incongruities differ for musicians and nonmusicians. *Neurosci. Lett.* 168, 101–5.

64. **Besson, M.** and **F. Macar** (1987) An Event-Related Potential analysis of incongruity in music and other non-linguistic context. *Psychophysiology* 24 (1), 14–25.

65. **Koelsch, S., T. Gunter,** and **A. D. Friederici** (2000) Brain indices of music processing: 'nonmusicians' are musical. *J. Cogni. Neurosci.* 12 (3), 520–41.

66. **Maess, B., S. Koelsch, T. Gunter,** and **A. D. Friederici** (2001) 'Musical syntax' is processed in the Broca's area: an MEG-study. *Nature Neurosci.* 4, 540–5.

67. **Regnault, P., E. Bigand,** and **M. Besson** (2001) Event-related brain potentials show top-down and bottom-up modulations of musical expectations. *J. Cognit. Neurosci.* 13, 241–55.

68. **Tillmann, B., P. Janata,** and **J. J. Bharucha** (2003) Inferior frontal cortex activation in musical priming. *Cognit. Brain Res.* 16(2), 145–61.

69. **Patel, A. D., E. Gibson, J. Ratner, M. Besson,** and **P. J. Holcomb** (1998) Processing syntactic relations in language and music: an event-related potential study. *J. Cognit. Neurosci.* 10, 717–33.

70. **Lampinen, J.** and **E. Oja** (1992) Clustering properties of hierarchical self-organizing maps. *J. Mathematical Imaging and Vision* 2, 261–72.

71. **Parncutt, R.** (1988) Revision of Terhardt's psychoacoustical model of the roots of a musical chord. *MP* 6, 65–94.

72. **Leman, M.** (1995) *Music and Schema Theory.* Berlin: Springer.

73. **Bharucha, J. J.** (1987) Music cognition and perceptual facilitation: a connectionist framework. *MP* 5 (1), 1–30.

74. **Bharucha, J. J.** and **W. E. Mencl** (1996) Two Issues in auditory cognition: self-organization of octave categories and pitch-invariant pattern recognition. *Psychol. Sci.* 7, 142–9.

75. **Cohen, M. A., S. Grossberg,** and **L. L. Wyse** (1995) A spectral network model of pitch perception. *J. Acoust. Soc. of Am.* 98, 862–79.

76. **Sano, H.** and **B. K. Jenkins** (1991) A neural network model for pitch perception. In N. Todd and G. Loy (eds) *Music and Connectionism.* Cambridge, MA: MIT Press, pp. 42–9.

77. **Taylor, I.** and **M. Greenhough** (1994) Modelling pitch perception with adaptive resonance theory artificial neural networks. *Connection Sci.* 6, 135–54.

78. **Laden, B.** and **D.H. Keefe** (1991) The representation of pitch in a neural net model of chord classification. In (P. Todd and G. Loy (eds) *Music and Connectionism.* Cambridge, MA: MIT Press, pp. 64–83.

79. **Bharucha, J. J.** and **N. Todd** (1989) Modelling the perception of tonal structures with neural nets. *Computer Music J.* 13, 44–53.

80. **Krumhansl, C. L., J. Louhivuori, P. Toivianinen, T. Jarvinen,** and **T. Eerola** (1999) Melodic expectation in Finnish spiritual folk hymns: converging evidence of statistical, behavioral and computational analyses. *MP* 17, 151–95.

81. **Page, M. A.** (1994) Modelling the perception of musical sequences with self-organizing neural networks. *Connection Sci.* 6, 223–46.

82. **Griffith, N.** (1994) Development of tonal centres and abstract pitch as categorizations of pitch use. *Connection Sci.* 6, 155–75.

83. **Leman, M.** and **F. Carreras** (1998) Schema and Gestalt: testing the Hypothesis of Psychoneural Isomorphism by computer simulation. In M. Leman (ed.) *Music, Gestalt, Computing.* Berlin: Springer, pp. 144–68.

84. **Gjerdingen, R. O.** (1990) Categorization of musical patterns by self-organizing neuronlike networks. *MP* 8, 339–70.

85. **Stevens, C.** (1992) *Derivation and Investigation of Features Mediating Musical Pattern Recognition.* Sydney: University of Sydney.

86. **Stevens, C.** and **C. Latimer** (1992) A comparison of connectionist models of music recognition and human performance. *Minds and Machines* 2, 379–400.

87. **Stevens, C.** and **C. Latimer** (1997) Music Recognition: an illustrative application of a connectionist model. *Psychol. of Music* 25, 161–85.

88. **Tekman, H. G.** and **J. J. Bharucha** (1998) Implicit knowledge versus psychoacoustic similarity in priming of chords. *J. Exp. Psychol. Hum. Percept. Perform.* 24, 252–60.

89. **Tillmann, B., E. Bigand,** and **M. Pineau** (1998) Effects of global and local contexts on harmonic expectancy. *MP* 16 (1), 99–117.

90. **Krumhansl, C. L., J. J. Bharucha,** and **E. J. Kessler** (1982) Perceived harmonic structures of chords in three related keys. *J. Exp. Psychol. Hum. Percept. Perform.* 8, 24–36.

91. **Peretz, I.** and **R. Kolinsky** (1993) Boundaries of separability between melody and rhythm in music discrimination: a neuropsychological perspective. *Q. J. Exp. Psychol.* 46A, 301–27.

92. Jones, M. R. and M. Boltz (1989) Dynamic attending and responses to time. *Psychol. Rev.* 96, 459–91.

93. Boltz, M. (1991) Some structural determinants of melody recall. *Memory and Cognition* 19, 239–51.

94. Boltz, M. (1993) The generation of temporal and melodic expectancies during musical listening. *P&P* 53, 585–600.

95. Palmer, C. and C. L. Krumhansl (1987) Independent temporal and pitch structures in determination of musical phrases. *J. Exp. Psychol. Hum. Percept. Perform.* 13, 116–26.

96. Palmer, C. and C. L. Krumhansl (1987) Pitch and temporal contributions to musical phrase perception: effects of harmony, performance timing, and familiarity. *P&P* 41, 505–18.

97. Peretz, I. (1990) Processing of local and global musical information in unilateral brain-damaged patients. *Brain* 113, 1185–205.

98. Peretz, I. and J. Morais (1989) La musique et la modularité. In S. McAdams and I. Deliege (eds) *La musique et les sciences cognitives.* Bruxelles: P. Mardaga, pp. 393–414.

99. Berger, J. and D. Gang (1997) A neural network model of metric perception and cognition in the audition of functional tonal music. In *Int. Computer Music Conference.* 1997 September, Thessaloniki, Greece.

100. Berger, J. and D. Gang (1998) A computational model of meter cognition during the audition of functional tonal music. In *Int. Computer Music Conference.* 1998 October, Ann Arbor, Michigan.

101. Stevens, C. and J. Wiles (1994) Tonal Music as a componential code: learning temporal relationships between and within pitch and timing components. In J. D. Cowan *et al.* (eds) *Advances in Neural Information Processing Systems,* vol. 6. San Francisco, CA: Morgan Kaufmann, pp. 1085–92.

102. Large, E. W. and J. F. Kolen (1994) Resonance and the perception of musical meter. *Connection Sci.* 6, 177–208.

103. Mayr, U. (1996) Spatial attention and implicit sequence learning: evidence for independent learning of spatial and nonspatial sequences. *JEP-LMC* 22, 350–64.

104. McClelland, J. L., B. L. McNaughton, and R. C. O'Reilly (1995) Why there are complementary learning systems in the hippocampus and neocortex: insights from the successes and failures of connectionist models of learning and memory. *Psychol. Rev.* 102, 419–57.

105. Otto, I., P. Grandguillaume, L. Bouthkhil, Y. Burnod, and E. Guigon (1992) Direct and indirect cooperation between temporal and parietal networks for invariant visual recognition. *Cognit. Neurosci.* 4, 35–57.

106. Rauschecker, J. P. and B. Tian (2000) Mechanisms and streams for processing of 'what' and 'where' in auditory cortex. *Proc. Nat. Acad. Sci.* 24, 11800–6.

107. Belin, P. and R. J. Zatorre (2000) 'What', 'where' and 'how' in auditory cortex. *Nature Neurosci.* 3, 965–6.

PART III

THE NEURONS OF MUSIC

CHAPTER 9

NEUROBIOLOGY OF HARMONY PERCEPTION

MARK JUDE TRAMO, PETER A. CARIANI, BERTRUND DELGUTTE, AND LOUIS D. BRAIDA

Abstract

Basic principles of the theory of harmony reflect physiological and anatomical properties of the auditory nervous system and related cognitive systems. This hypothesis is motivated by observations from several different disciplines, including ethnomusicology, developmental psychology, and animal behaviour. Over the past several years, we and our colleagues have been investigating the vertical dimension of harmony from the perspective of neurobiology using physiological, psychoacoustic, and neurological methods. Properties of the auditory system that govern harmony perception include (1) the capacity of peripheral auditory neurons to encode temporal regularities in acoustic fine structure and (2) the differential tuning of many neurons throughout the auditory system to a narrow range of frequencies in the audible spectrum. Biologically determined limits on these properties constrain the range of notes used in music throughout the world and the way notes are combined to form intervals and chords in popular Western music. When a harmonic interval is played, neurons throughout the auditory system that are sensitive to one or more frequencies (partials) contained in the interval respond by firing action potentials. For consonant intervals, the fine timing of auditory nerve fibre responses contains strong representations of harmonically related pitches implied by the interval (e.g. Rameau's fundamental bass) in addition to the pitches of notes actually present in the interval. Moreover, all or most of the partials can be resolved by finely tuned neurons throughout the auditory system. By contrast, dissonant intervals evoke auditory nerve fibre activity that does not contain strong representations of constituent notes or related bass notes. Furthermore, many partials are too close together to be resolved. Consequently, they interfere with one another, cause coarse fluctuations in the firing of peripheral and central auditory neurons, and give rise to perception of roughness and dissonance. The effects of auditory cortex lesions on the perception of consonance, pitch, and roughness, combined with a critical reappraisal of published psychoacoustic data on the relationship between consonance and roughness, lead us to conclude that consonance is first and foremost a function of the pitch relationships among notes. Harmony in the vertical dimension is a positive phenomenon, not just a negative phenomenon that depends on the absence of roughness—a view currently held by many psychologists, musicologists, and physiologists.

Keywords: Consonance; Dissonance; Harmony, musical; Intervals, musical; Perception of harmony; Psychoacoustics of harmony

Introduction

Why do some combinations of simultaneous tones sound more harmonious than others? Pythagoras's curiosity about the nature of harmony inspired some of the earliest experiments relating mathematics and physics to perceptual phenomena.[1] Approaching the problem from the perspective of neurobiology, we ask: Are there physiological and anatomical properties of the auditory system and related cognitive systems that determine the degree to which simultaneous notes sound harmonious?

We restrict our consideration of harmony to basic tenets articulated by Piston,[2] among others. Harmony has a vertical dimension and a horizontal dimension. The vertical dimension encompasses the relationships among simultaneous notes. By convention, *note* refers to a pitch in the musical scale, and *harmonic interval* refers to two notes sounded simultaneously (Figure 9.1A–D). When a note is played on a musical instrument, its pitch corresponds to the fundamental frequency (F_0) of the complex tone generated by the instrument. Some synthesizers and other types of equipment are capable of generating pure tones, in which case the pitch of the note corresponds to the frequency of the pure tone. Harmonic intervals are a type of *dyad*. Three or more notes played simultaneously make up a *chord*. Chords with three notes are called *triads*. The time window over which acoustic information is integrated in the vertical dimension spans about a hundredth of a second to a few seconds (e.g. sixteenth notes to tied whole notes at a tempo of 120 beats per min). The horizontal dimension encompasses successive tones (melodic intervals and melodic progressions) and successive harmonic intervals and chords (harmonic progressions). Certain intervals and chords are treated as consonant (e.g. fifths, major triads) and others as dissonant (e.g. minor seconds, diminished triads). Acknowledging that different psychologists have attached different perceptual attributes and meanings to the terms *consonance* and *dissonance*, we nonetheless find considerable agreement among music texts and dictionaries that consonant means harmonious, agreeable, and stable, and that dissonant means disagreeable, unpleasant, and in need of resolution.[2–5] Psychoacoustic experiments bear out semantic overlap among the terms *consonant, pleasant, beautiful,* and *euphonious.*[6,7]

These basic concepts apply to a wide range of musical styles enjoyed by people throughout much of the industrialized world: contemporary pop and theater (including rock, rhythm and blues, country, and Latin-American), European music from the Baroque, Classical, and Romantic eras (1600–1900), children's songs, and many forms of ritualistic music (e.g. church songs, processionals, anthems, and holiday music). The overlap in their harmonic structure incorporates commonalities in musical phonology and syntax.[8] In our view, the widespread popularity of Western pop taps into (1) universal competence in auditory functions needed to extract the pitch of a note and to analyse the harmonic relationships among different pitches, and (2) universal competence in cognitive functions that parse acoustic information and associate perceptual attributes with emotion and meaning. Experimental results suggest that similar perceptual attributes can be associated with similar emotions and social contexts across different cultures.[9,10] Moreover, listeners from different cultures often use similar cognitive schemata to structure the processing of pitch-sequences.[11,12]

Much has been written in the psychology literature about the terms *harmony, consonance,* and *dissonance.* At present, many psychologists and musicologists subscribe to Terhardt's[13] two-component model of *musical consonance,* which subsumes all these terms. One component is *sensory consonance,* the absence of annoying features, such as roughness, in both musical and nonmusical sounds. The other component, *harmony,* is based on music-specific principles that govern pitch relationships in melodic and harmonic progressions. Terhardt

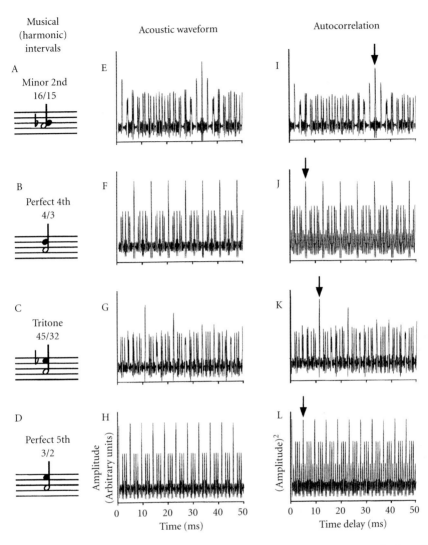

Figure 9.1 Acoustic representations of musical (harmonic) intervals in the time domain. *Left column* (A–D): Musical interval stimuli depicted in standard notation (G clef) below the name of each interval (e.g. minor second) and the F_0 ratio of its notes (16/15). *Middle column* (E–H): Acoustic waveforms of each interval. *Right column* (I–L): Autocorrelations of the acoustic waveforms. *Arrows* indicate the peaks corresponding to the period of each interval's 'missing' F_0.

asserts that 'sensory consonance...dominates the evaluation of single isolated chords...whereas harmony does not enter into the subject's response' (p. 282).[13]

With respect to terminology, we adhere in this discussion to the simple distinction between the vertical and horizontal dimensions of harmony. We restrict use of the terms *consonance* and *dissonance* to the vertical dimension and keep the term *harmony* supraordinate to them. We make no assumptions about the level of auditory processing (e.g. sensory, peripheral) where the perceptual attribute of consonance takes shape. We consider it likely that a listener's implicit (or explicit) knowledge about harmony in the horizontal dimension[14] bears on harmony perception in the vertical dimension.

In this paper, we present neurophysiological, neurological, and psychoacoustic evidence to support our contentions that (1) pitch relationships among tones in the vertical dimension influence consonance perception and (2) consonance cannot be explained solely by the absence of roughness. First, we review terminology and basic psychoacoustics pertinent to our subsequent discussion of experimental results. Second, we demonstrate that the harmonic relationships of tones in musical intervals are represented in the temporal discharge patterns of auditory nerve fibres. Third, we critically reevaluate the psychoacoustic literature concerning the consonance of isolated intervals and chords, paying particular attention to (1) the relationships among interval width, roughness detection thresholds, and consonance ratings; and (2) the predictions of roughness-based computational models about relative consonance as a function of spectral energy distribution. Finally, we discuss evidence that impairments in consonance perception following auditory cortex lesions are more likely to result from deficits in pitch perception than to deficits in roughness perception. This evidence highlights the dependence of so-called low-level perceptual processing on the integrity of the auditory cortex, the highest station in the auditory nervous system (Figure 9.2).

Psychoacoustics and neurophysiology of harmony

For authoritative reviews of the psychoacoustics of harmony, we refer the reader to Krumhansl,[14] Parncutt,[18] and Deutsch.[19] Here, only basic concepts and terminology pertinent to our subsequent discussion of psychoacoustic and neurophysiological experiments are covered.

Let us consider a modern restatement of Pythagoras's observation: The degree to which two simultaneous notes (a harmonic interval) sound consonant is determined by the simplicity of the ratio $x : y$, where x is the F_0 associated with one tone and y the F_0 of the other, lower tone. In musical terms, y is the root of the interval. x and y can take on any value between about 25 Hz and about 5 kHz. This upper limit coincides with (1) the upper F_0 of notes on a piccolo (~4500 Hz); (2) the upper F_0 for which octave similarity can be reliably judged;[20,21] and (3) the upper F_0 of strong phase locking by auditory nerve fibres—that is, the highest frequency at which neurons can fire in time with amplitude fluctuations in the acoustic waveform.[22,23] This convergence of facts from music, psychoacoustics, and physiology suggests that limitations in the phase-locking capacity of neurons in the auditory periphery constrain the range of note F_0s that are used in music and the way they are combined in the vertical dimension of harmony. Other authors have discussed the relationships among the temporal discharge patterns of auditory nerve fibres, fundamental pitch perception, octave equivalence, and the consonance of intervals formed by simple integer ratios.[24–29]

By convention, notes in popular Western music are tuned to the scale of equal temperament, which chunks the F_0 continuum into octaves (i.e. doublings of F_0) and each octave

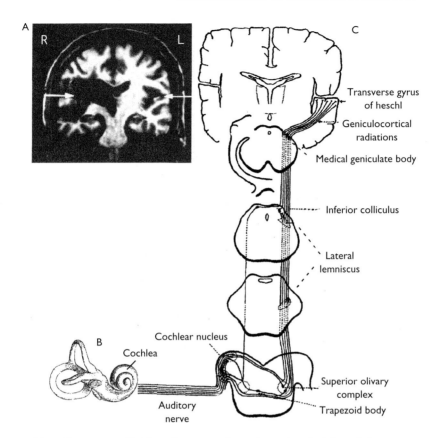

A
R   L

C

Transverse gyrus
of heschl

Geniculocortical
radiations

Medical geniculate body

Inferior colliculus

Lateral
lemniscus

Cochlear nucleus

B
Cochlea

Superior olivary
complex

Auditory
nerve

Trapezoid body

Figure 9.2 The auditory system. (A) Magnetic resonance image (coronal section) through the transverse gyri of Heschl and the superior temporal gyri of case MHS, who suffered bilateral infarction nine years earlier. *White arrows* point to the region of the transverse gyrus of Heschl in the right (R) and left hemispheres (L). The results of psychoacoustic experiments performed by MHS are shown in Figure 9.7. (B) The inner ear and the auditory nerve, the obligatory pathway from the cochlea to the cochlear nuclei in the lower brain stem. (C) Schematic of the central auditory pathway showing the main relay stations and projection patterns. Adapted from Tramo *et al.*[15] (A), Helmholtz[16] (B), and Davis[17] (C).

into 12 discrete, equal, logarithmic steps. Each step within the octave is called a semitone, and the F_0s of adjacent semitones differ by a factor of $2^{1/12}$, or about 6 per cent. The chromatic scale is made up of all 12 tones in the octave, whereas the major and minor (diatonic) scales are made up of partially overlapping sets of seven tones in the octave. Harmonic intervals and melodic intervals are named according to the scale relationship of the upper note to the lower note. Thus when the fifth note in the major or minor scale sits atop the first note on the scale, the interval is called a *fifth* (Figure 9.1D). The note named A_4 is assigned an F_0 value of 440 Hz. The letter name of each note corresponds to one of the 12 notes in the octave; the number of each note indicates the octave the note is in, with increments at each occurrence of C along the scale (e.g. ...A_4—$A\#_4$—B_4—C_5...). The frequency range over which pure tones are audible to humans extends from approximately E_0 (20.6 Hz) to E_{10} (21.1 kHz). For the purposes of this discussion, we will set y, the F_0 of the root of a harmonic interval, equal to 440 Hz (A_4).

In music theory, the interval formed by notes that are an octave apart (e.g. A_4 and A_5) is the most consonant interval, followed by the fifth (A_4 and E_5), fourth (A_4 and D_5), major third (A_4 and C#$_5$), and minor third (A_4 and C_5). In the scale of just intonation, these intervals correspond to $x:y$ ratios of 2:1, 3:2, 4:3, 5:4, and 6:5, respectively, consistent with Pythagoras's claim that the simplicity of the integer ratio correlates with perceived consonance. Combinations of some other notes on the scale between A_4 and A_5 have more complex $x:y$ ratios and sound dissonant. For example, the minor second and the tritone (also known as the augmented fourth, which, in equal-tempered tuning, is equivalent to the diminished fifth) have $x:y$ ratios of 16:15 and 45:32 (or approximately 7:5), respectively. The dependence of consonance on the simplicity of F_0 ratios tolerates small deviations from perfect integer relationships. For example, because the scale of equal temperament is based on equal logarithmic steps within each octave, a major third in this scale has a ratio of 5.04:4, not 5:4. This deviation amounts to 0.8 per cent. Even highly practised listeners participating in psychoacoustic experiments under ideal listening conditions cannot reliably detect a mistuned lower harmonic embedded within a harmonic complex tone if the deviation is less than 0.9 per cent (harmonics 1–12 at 60 dB SPL [sound pressure level] and isophase, $F_0 = 200$ Hz, duration ≤ 410 ms).[30] Moreover, conservatory students who excel at interval identification cannot reliably judge whether a mistuned major third composed of two harmonic complex tones has been stretched or compressed away from a perfect 5:4 ratio if the deviation is less than 1.2 per cent (each tone with harmonics 1–20 in isophase, first harmonic at 80 dB SPL, higher harmonics at a 6 dB decrease per octave, F_0 between 260 and 525 Hz, and duration = 1000 ms).[31]

All experimental studies that have used stimuli consisting of single, isolated, harmonic intervals formed by two complex tones (as would be the case if the intervals were sung or played on guitar or piano) show that listeners consistently perceive the fifth and fourth as more consonant than the minor second and tritone.[6,32–35] This convergence of results across study populations from different countries (United States, Germany, Japan), generations (1909–69), and musical backgrounds, combined with results obtained in infants from the United States[36] and European starlings,[37] motivates the hypothesis that common, basic auditory mechanisms underlie perceptual categorization of harmonic intervals as consonant or dissonant. However, there is disagreement about the nature of the underlying neural mechanisms, and few physiological experiments have systematically analysed responses to harmonic intervals at any level of the auditory nervous system.[25,27,38–41] Still, a large body of data is available on the responses of neurons to other types of complex tones in the auditory nerve,[42] cochlear nucleus,[43] inferior colliculus,[44,45] medial geniculate nucleus,[46] and auditory cortex[47–49] (Figure 9.2; only a few of the many available papers are cited here; for review see Ref. 50).

Neural coding of pitch relationships as a physiological basis of harmony

We synthesized simultaneous complex tones forming four musical intervals: the minor second (F_0 ratio = 16/15), perfect fourth (4:3), tritone (45:32), and perfect fifth (3:2,

Figure 9.1). Each of the two complex tones in the interval contained the first six harmonics with equal amplitude (60 dB SPL re: 20 μPa) and equal phase (cosine, Figure 9.3). Each interval had a duration of 200 ms (a bit shorter than an eighth note at a tempo of 120 beats per minute), including 5-ms rise and fall times. These stimuli are acoustically similar to the inputs into the computational models used by Plomp and Levelt,[51] Kameoka and Kuriyagawa,[35] and Hutchinson and Knopoff[52] to predict the consonance of complex-tone intervals on the basis of psychoacoustic data on puretone intervals.

Figure 9.1 illustrates two time-domain representations of our stimuli: the acoustic waveform, which plots sound pressure amplitude as a function of time (Figure 9.1E–H); and the autocorrelation of the waveform (Figure 9.1I–L). In the acoustic waveform of the

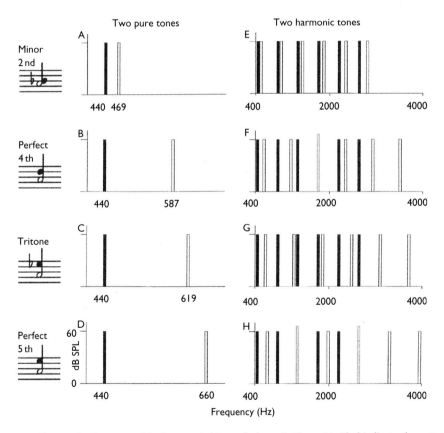

Figure 9.3 Line amplitude spectra of the four musical intervals shown in Figure 9.1. *Black* indicates the root and its harmonics, *white* the interval and its harmonics, and *gray* the frequencies at which harmonics of the root and interval overlap. (A–D) A minor second, perfect fourth, tritone, and perfect fifth composed of two pure tones. (E–H) The same intervals composed of two harmonic complex tones containing the first six harmonics at equal amplitude. These are the spectral domain representations corresponding to the time domain representations in Figure 9.1E–L.

most consonant interval, the perfect fifth, we see a regular pattern of major and minor peaks (Figure 9.1H). The pattern with one major peak and three minor peaks repeats every 4.55 ms ($1/x = 220$ Hz). This periodicity corresponds to the missing F_0 of a harmonic series containing energy at the second harmonic (440 Hz, A_4) and third harmonic (660 Hz, E_5), the F_0s of the notes actually present in the stimulus. Rameau's concept of the 'basse fondametale' (fundamental bass) in his *Treatise on Harmony*[53] is related to the missing F_0 of a harmonic interval.

Autocorrelation functions provide another representation of temporal regularities and irregularities embedded in acoustic waveforms (Figure 9.1I–L). Autocorrelation functions are computed by multiplying the waveform with a delayed copy of itself and integrating over time. A large value at a given delay indicates the presence of a dominant periodicity in the waveform whose period equals the delay. Like pitch percepts, but unlike acoustic waveforms, autocorrelation functions are stable despite changes in the relative phases of frequency components. In the autocorrelation functions plotted in Figure 9.1I–L, the periodicity at the upper limit of the x axis (50 ms) corresponds to 20 Hz, the lowest audible frequency.

In the autocorrelation function of the perfect fifth (Figure 9.1L), the first major peak again corresponds to the missing F_0, A_3 (220 Hz). The second major peak occurs at 9.09 ms, which corresponds to A_2 (110 Hz), the bass note an octave below. In fact, all the major peaks up to 50 ms correspond to the fundamental bass and its subharmonics (undertones) at A_2, D_2, A_1, and on down to A_0, the lowest note on the piano ($F_0 = 27.5$ Hz).

In between the major peaks is a set of three, evenly spaced, minor peaks. The first of these minor peaks occurs at 1.51 ms, which corresponds to E_5 (660 Hz), the upper note of the interval. The second minor peak occurs at 2.27 ms, which corresponds to A_4 (440 Hz), the root of the interval. The third minor peak occurs at 3.03 ms, which corresponds to E_4 (330 Hz), the octave below the fifth and the fifth above the fundamental bass at A_3.

Temporal regularities are also seen in the waveform and autocorrelation of the perfect fourth, the other consonant interval in our stimulus set (Figure 9.1F and J). Here the major peaks are at 6.82 ms (D_3, $F_0 = 146.7$ Hz) and 13.6 ms (D_2, $F_0 = 73.3$ Hz). Thus, in addition to a representation of the fourth, there is a representation of its inversion as a fifth with the implied root at D_3 and the fundamental bass at D_2. The autocorrelation function of the fourth is a bit more complicated than that of the fifth, as there are two more peaks between each pair of major peaks. In the first set of minor peaks, the following notes are represented: A_4 (the root), D_4 (the interval), A_3 (the octave below the root), and G_3 (the fifth below D_4, and the fourth of an interval rooted at D_3). Thus, we find representations of notes that function as fourths and fifths in the major and (all) minor scales of A and D.

In summary, the temporal fine structure of the perfect fifth and fourth contains representations of the two notes constituting the interval, plus harmonically related bass notes that are implied by the interval. In music, these bass notes support the deep structure of harmony. Parncutt[18] demonstrated experimentally that listeners associate major triads with pitches that are harmonically related to note F_0s, including the fundamental bass, plus the pitches of note F_0s actually in the stimulus. These pitches cannot be accounted for simply on the basis of combination tones (for review, see Ref. 54). Houtsma and Goldstein[55] showed that musicians can use missing F_0 pitches to identify melodic intervals (major and minor seconds and thirds), even when two upper harmonics are presented separately (dichotically) to each ear.

For the dissonant intervals in our stimulus set, the minor second and tritone, we find no such temporal regularity in the acoustic waveform and autocorrelation function. For the minor second (Figure 9.1I), the largest peak in the autocorrelation function occurs at 34.1 ms, which corresponds to a frequency of 29.3 Hz, and it decays rapidly into the background. This periodicity lies outside the range associated with strong periodicity pitch percepts (for review, see Ref. 56). In addition, we find multiple peaks between zero and the maximum peak. The largest of these is the first peak at 2.20 ms, which corresponds to mean of the note F_0s, 455 Hz. This pitch does not correspond to any of the notes in any scale that has A_4 in it. In short, there is no strong representation of any pitch below the note pitches in the interval, and the dominant pitch is off the scale. Both of these factors contribute to the dissonance of the minor second.

Likewise, the autocorrelation function of the tritone (Figure 9.1K) does not show a simple, regular pattern of peaks. The largest peak occurs at 11.4 ms, which corresponds to $F_0 = 88$ Hz, and it, too, decays into the background. This periodicity corresponds to a near coincidence between the fifth subharmonic of the root (440 Hz divided by 5) and the seventh subharmonic of the tritone (618.7 Hz divided by 7). It also lies close to F_2, which is related to the fundamental bass of an F dominant-seventh chord in its first inversion. Thus the autocorrelation function of the tritone implies a chord that is, in music theory, less consonant than the chords implied by the autocorrelation functions of the fifth and fourth.

To summarize, for the consonant intervals (the fifth and fourth), the pattern of major and minor peaks in the autocorrelation is perfectly periodic, with a period related to the fundamental bass. This pattern is obtained because these stimuli have a unique, clearly defined fundamental period. By contrast, for dissonant intervals (the minor second and tritone), no true periodicity is seen in the autocorrelation function. While some peaks occasionally stand out at specific delays, indicating a pseudoperiod, either there are no consistent peaks at multiples of this pseudoperiod, or the amplitudes of these peaks decay rapidly with increasing multiples of the pseudoperiod.

These observations suggest that the consonance of harmonic intervals reflects regularities in their temporal fine structure in the range of tenths to tens of milliseconds. Do neurons in the auditory system represent this information using a time code? Galileo,[57] who wrote about consonance while he was under house arrest for his work on the solar system, may have been the first to postulate that temporal coding in the auditory periphery was the physiological basis for consonance:

> Agreeable consonances are pairs of tones which strike the ear with a certain regularity; this regularity consists in the fact that the pulses delivered by the two tones, in the same interval of time, shall be commensurable in number, so as not to keep the ear drum in perpetual torment, bending in two different directions in order to yield to the ever-discordant impulses... The unpleasant sensation produced by [dissonances] arises, I think, from the discordant vibrations of two different tones which strike the ear out of time. Especially harsh is the dissonance between notes whose frequencies are incommensurable;...this yields a dissonance similar to the augmented fourth or diminished fifth [*tritono o semidiapente*]".
> (Ref. 57, 1638, pp. 103–4.)

To investigate the neural coding of consonance in the auditory periphery, we analysed the responses of over 100 cat auditory nerve fibres to the minor second, perfect fourth, tritone, and perfect fifth. Auditory nerve fibres are the central axons of spiral ganglion cells that synapse on cochlear nucleus neurons in the brain stem (Figure 9.2 for review, see Ref. 58). In humans, each auditory nerve contains about 30,000 auditory nerve fibres. Spiral ganglion cells also have peripheral axons that synapse on sensory receptors in the cochlea—the inner hair cells that ride atop the basilar membrane. Virtually all information about sound is transmitted from the ear to the brain via trains of action potentials fired by auditory nerve fibres.

When a minor second or some other interval is sounded, an auditory nerve fibre will increase the number of action potentials it fires only if it is sensitive to the frequencies present in the interval (Figure 9.4A). The time between consecutive action potentials in the train is called an *interspike interval* (ISI), and a plot of the number of times each ISI occurs in the spike train is called an *ISI histogram* (Figure 9.4B–E). We measured all the ISIs between all possible pairs of spikes (Figure 9.4A, ISI_1, ISI_2 ... ISI_N) with a precision of approximately one microsecond. The corresponding plot is called an *all-order ISI histogram*, which is equivalent to the autocorrelation of the spike train. The spike train of each fibre in the auditory nerve can be analysed in this way, and the resultant ISI histograms can be combined to show the ISI distribution in the entire population of auditory nerve fibres. Single-unit physiology experiments[59–61] and computational models[62] have shown that the first among the major peaks in the all-order ISI histogram computed from the entire auditory nerve fibre ensemble (the population ISI distribution) matches the fundamental period of complex tones and thus their periodicity pitch. This is essentially the time-domain equivalent of Terhardt's[63] spectrally based subharmonic sieve for virtual pitch extraction.

Figure 9.4B–E illustrates the population ISI distributions embedded in the spike trains fired by over 50 auditory nerve fibres in response to the minor second, fourth, tritone, and fifth. In the response to the fifth (Figure 9.3E), we see major peaks corresponding to the fundamental bass (A_3, 4.55 ms) and its subharmonics, just as we did in the acoustic waveform (Figure 9.1H) and the autocorrelation of the waveform (Figure 9.1L). Indeed, for all four intervals, the autocorrelation histograms of neural responses (Figure 9.4B–E) mirror the fine structure of acoustic information in the time domain (Figure 9.1).

Thus the peaks in the population ISI distribution evoked by consonant intervals reflect the pitches of each note, the fundamental bass, and other harmonically related pitches in the bass register. By contrast, the dissonant intervals (the minor second and tritone) are associated with population ISI distributions that are irregular. These contain little or no representation of pitches corresponding to notes in the interval, the fundamental bass, and related bass notes.

To obtain a physiological measure of the strength of the fundamental pitch of each interval relative to other pitches, we measured the number of intervals under the peak in the all-order ISI distribution corresponding to the missing F_0 (arrows in Figure 9.3B–E; bin width = 300 µs). We then divided that value by the value of y in each x bin from $x = 0–50$ ms. We found a high correlation ($r = 0.96$) between our physiological measure of fundamental pitch strength and previous psychoacoustic measures of the 'clearness' of musical intervals composed of two complex tones.[35]

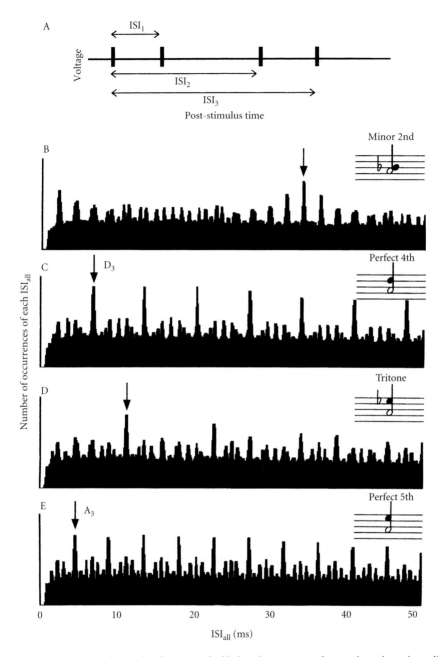

Figure 9.4 Interspike interval (ISI) distributions embedded in the responses of axons throughout the auditory nerve during stimulation with four musical intervals. (A) Schematic of a train of action potentials (or 'spikes', *vertical lines*) fired by an auditory nerve fibre when a musical interval is played. *Double arrows* demarcate some of the ISIs between pairs of spikes in the spike train. *ISI₁* refers to the first-order ISI, *ISI₂* and *ISI₃* to higher-order ISIs. All possible ISIs are in 'all-order' ISI histograms. (B–E) All-order ISI histograms showing ISIs embedded in the responses of 50 auditory nerve fibers to musical intervals composed of two complex tones (Figure 9.1E–H and Figure 9.3E–H). *Arrows* mark peaks in the ISI pattern that correspond to the missing F_0 of the interval. If the peak corresponds to a note on the scale, the name of the note is given.

In summary, the all-order ISI distribution embedded in auditory nerve fibre firing patterns contains representations of the pitch relationships among note F_0s that influence the perception of musical intervals as consonant or dissonant. The neural coding mechanisms that provide representations of these pitch relationships form part of the neurobiological foundation for the theory of harmony in its vertical dimension.

Neural coding of roughness as the physiological basis for harmony perception

Whereas pitch-based accounts treat consonance as a positive perceptual phenomenon associated with the presence of highly structured temporal information, roughness-based accounts treat consonance as a negative phenomenon associated with the absence of annoying perceptual attributes. Terhardt's notion that the consonance of isolated intervals and chords depends on the absence of roughness[13] echoes one of the main points in Helmholtz's[16,64] monumental work, *On the Sensations of Tone as a Physiological Basis for the Theory of Music*:

> As long as several simple tones of a sufficiently different pitch enter the ear together, the sensation due to each remains undisturbed in the ear, probably because entirely different bundles of [auditory] nerve fibers are affected. But tones of the same, or of nearly the same pitch, which therefore affect the same nerve fibers, do not produce a sensation which is the sum of the two they would have separately excited, but new and peculiar phenomena arise which we term interference...and beats[16] (p. 160)... Rapidly beating tones are jarring and rough...the sensible impression is also unpleasant[16] (p. 168). Consonance is a continuous, dissonance an intermittent tone sensation. The nature of dissonance is simply based on very fast beats. These are rough and annoying to the auditory nerve.[64] (Helmholtz 1863,[64] 1885.[16])

Because frequency selectivity throughout the auditory nervous system is finite, simultaneous pure tones that are separated by small frequency differences (ΔFs), such as a minor second (Figure 9.3A), cannot be separated or 'filtered out' from one another. Consequently, their waveforms are effectively summed, and the pitch of the tone combination matches their mean frequency.[65] The envelope of the summed waveform contains periodic amplitude fluctuations whose frequency equals ΔF (Figure 9.5, top). If these envelope fluctuations fall in the range of 20–200 Hz (the precise values depend on the frequencies of the two tones, Figure 9.6A), interruptions in continuous tone sensation are perceptible. These interruptions make the tone combination sound 'rough', analogous to the interruptions one feels on the fingertips when touching coarse sandpaper. At smaller frequency differences, and thus slower amplitude modulations, one perceives a single, continuous tone that is slowly fluctuating in loudness, or 'beating'. Auditory nerve fibres[38,39] (Figure 9.5, *bottom*), inferior colliculus neurons,[40,41] and populations of primary auditory cortex neurons[48] can fire in synchrony with amplitude fluctuations in the ΔF range associated with perception of roughness and beats.

The concept of *critical bandwidth* refers to the limits of ΔF over which frequency selectivity operates in the auditory system. Critical bandwidth has been estimated psychoacoustically in several ways that have yielded somewhat different results depending on the method (for reviews, see Refs 56 and 66). One estimate of critical bandwidth is based on the ΔF above which roughness disappears.

When musical intervals are composed of two complex tones (Figure 9.3E–H), the partials may interfere with one another and produce amplitude fluctuations at the corresponding ΔF. There is more interference between adjacent partials in the minor second and tritone (Figure 9.3E and G) than in the fourth and fifth (Figure 9.4F and H). Several computational models of consonance[16,35,51,52] assume that (1) the roughness generated by all the partials in the interval are added together (presumably by a central processor in the auditory brain stem or cortex), and (2) this total roughness determines the degree to which the interval is perceived as consonant.

Figure 9.6A shows Plomp and Steeneken's data on the relationships among the ΔF between two pure tones, the frequency of the lower tone (or root), and just-noticeable

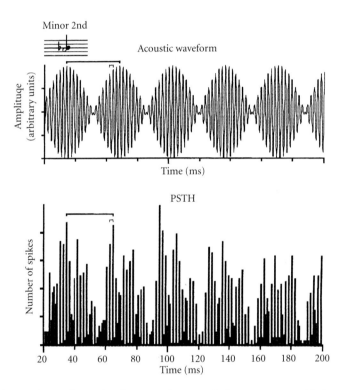

Figure 9.5 (*Top*) Acoustic waveform of a minor second composed of two pure tones with the root at A_4. *Thick bars* show the period of envelope fluctuations that render the minor second rough ($P = 1/\Delta F = 34.1$ ms). *Thin bars* show the period of fluctuations under the envelope that corresponds to the mean frequency of the tones and the pitch of the interval ($P = 2.20$ ms). (*Bottom*) Poststimulus time histogram (PSTH) showing the number of spikes fired by a single auditory nerve fibre during the steady state portion of its response to the minor second. Note that the global and local fluctuations in firing rate mirror those seen in the acoustic waveform of the minor second. This fibre was sensitive to frequencies at both the root and the interval at 60 dB SPL. Bin width = 1 ms. Number of stimulus repetitions = 100.

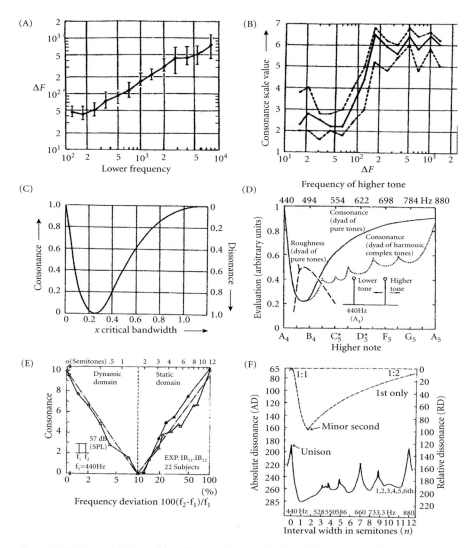

Figure 9.6 (A) Just-noticeable roughness (*line*) as a function of the frequency difference between two pure tones (ΔF) and the lower frequency of the tones. Tones were presented monaurally at 60 phons. The *bars* show the interquartile range of 20 subjects (musical background not given). (Adapted from Ref. 67 Figure 9.1, p. 883.) (B) Plomp and Levelt's data on consonance ratings as a function of ΔF for simultaneous pure tones with a mean frequency of 1000 Hz. Tones were presented in free field at 65 dB SPL. The *solid line* shows the mean consonance ratings of 10 subjects (musical background not given). *Dashed lines* show the interquartile range. (Adapted from Ref. 51 Figure 9.6, p. 554.) (C) Plomp and Levelt's idealized plot of the relationship between consonance and critical bandwidth. The *y* axis is in units of consonance (*left*) and dissonance (*right*). (From Plomp and Levelt[51] [Figure 9.10, p. 556]. Reproduced by permission.) (D) Terhardt's idealized plot showing the relationship of consonance and roughness to interval width (root at A_4, 440 Hz). The *solid line* shows consonance vs ΔF when the interval is composed of two pure tones. The *dotted line* shows consonance vs ΔF_0 when the interval is composed of two complex tones, each containing several lower harmonics. The *dashed line* shows the roughness of two pure tones as a function of ΔF. (From Terhardt[13] [Figure 9.1, p. 281]. Reproduced by permission.) (E) Kameoka and Kuriyagawa's data on consonance as a function of ΔF for simultaneous pure tones with the root at A_4 and intensities of 57 dB SPL. The *dashed line* is the mean performance of 22 audio engineers who performed the task twice (*solid lines* with *black* and *white triangles*). (From Kameoka and Kuriyagawa[72] [Figure 9.1, p. 1452]. Reproduced by permission.) (F) Kameoka and Kuriyzgawa's plot of dissonance as a function of interval width. The *dashed line* at the *top* shows the function when the interval is composed of two pure tones. The *solid line* at the *bottom* gives the calculated dissonance of an interval composed of two complex tones, each containing the first six harmonics at 57 dB SPL. (Adapted from Kameoka and Kuriyagawa,[35] Figure 9.8, p. 1465.)

roughness (line).[67] The data at $x = 500$ Hz would thus apply to the case of a harmonic interval composed of two pure tones with the root at B_4 ($x = 494$ Hz). The fifth of B_4, $F\sharp_5$, has a frequency of 741 Hz, so the ΔF between the root and the fifth is 247 Hz. According to Figure 9.6A, at $x = 500$ Hz, roughness disappears for ΔF values above 90–125 Hz. Therefore, the fifth should not be associated with roughness. Experimental studies agree that an isolated fifth composed of pure tones in this frequency register sounds 'consonant'[7,51] or 'pleasant'.[6,33] The pure-tone fifth is thus associated with the absence of roughness and with strong pitches associated with temporal regularities in its acoustic waveform and autocorrelation (similar to those described in the preceding section for a fifth composed of two harmonic complex tones; Figure 9.1H and L). The same set of observations applies to a perfect fourth composed of two pure tones.

Now consider the case of a minor second composed of two pure tones with the root at B_4 (494 Hz). Here, ΔF (between B_4 and C_5) is 33 Hz. This falls well within the range of noticeable roughness (Figure 9.6A). In fact, it lies near the ΔF associated with maximal roughness[67–69] (not shown). Experimental studies agree that a pure-tone minor second (and other tone combinations close to it) sounds 'dissonant'[7,51] or 'unpleasant'.[6,33]

The case of a tritone composed of two pure tones provides an interesting test of the roughness hypothesis. The ΔF between a tritone at F_5 and a root at B_4 is 201 Hz, well above the ΔF for just-noticeable roughness. Thus the fourth, tritone, and fifth are all above the roughness range. Does that mean they all have the same consonance?

Figure 9.6B shows Plomp and Levelt's data on consonance ratings as a function of ΔF for two pure tones whose mean frequency is 1000 Hz.[51] Because the y axis is an ordinal scale, not an interval or ratio scale, it is inappropriate to assume that equal distances reflect equal differences in consonance. It follows that $4 > y > 4$ is not to be taken as the categorical boundary for dissonance and consonance, respectively. In addition, because Plomp and Levelt intentionally avoided using standard intervals like the fourth and tritone (they were concerned that interval recognition would influence consonance ratings), it is difficult to estimate where on the curve these intervals would fall. These caveats aside, it is clear that all pure-tone combinations with ΔFs above approximately 150 Hz are consonant. This would apply to the fourth, tritone, and fifth with their roots in the vicinity of A_5. Tone combinations with $\Delta F_0 = 20$–80 Hz are dissonant; this would apply to a minor second with the root near A_5. Superficially, it would appear that we have a convergence between the disappearance of roughness at $\Delta F_0 = 150$–250 Hz (Figure 9.6A, interquartile range for a lower frequency of 1 kHz) and a steep increase in consonance ratings at $\Delta F_0 > 80$ Hz (at and above a minor third, Figure 9.6B). However, the ΔF associated with the highest mean consonance rating ($\Delta F \sim 180$ Hz) is within the range of noticeable roughness for many of Plomp and Steeneken's subjects.[67]

Beyond about $\Delta F = 180$ Hz, mean consonance ratings vary by only one rating point or less, but they are not perfectly flat (Figure 9.6B). One can discern alternating peaks and valleys out to about $\Delta F = 1200$ Hz. We estimated where the minor second, perfect fourth, tritone, and perfect fifth might fall on the interpolated lines drawn by Plomp and Levelt[51] (Figure 9.6B), and we estimated the frequency ratios and intervals that correspond to the peaks and valleys beyond $\Delta F = 1000$ Hz. The first peak is near 6:5, which would correspond to a minor third. The second peak falls close to 5:3, which would correspond to a major sixth (or inverted minor third). The ratio 5:3 could also be thought of as the fifth and third harmonics of a harmonic series corresponding to the third and first notes of a major triad in its second inversion. The third peak is at or close to a ratio of 3:1, which corresponds to the interval of a twelfth, that is, a root and a fifth in the octave above. High consonance ratings for the twelfth are also found in Plomp and Levelt's data for two pure tones with a mean frequency of 500 Hz[51] (not shown). The first valley between the first two peaks is near the tritone, and the second valley appears to be a mistuned octave, with a frequency ratio near 2.03:1.

Figure 9.6C shows Plomp and Levelt's idealized plot of the relationship between consonance and critical bandwidth[51] (the latter is defined here by loudness summation[70]). Note that the curve reaches an asymptote near the end of the *x* axis, at about one critical bandwidth. Thus a critical band account of consonance as the absence of roughness *cannot* apply to pure-tone intervals that are wider than a minor third or so.

Yet Terhardt's[13] idealized plot (Figure 9.6D) of the relationships among roughness, consonance, and pure-tone ΔF shows a monotonic increase in perceived consonance all the way out to the octave, well beyond the ΔF at which (1) roughness disappears (Figure 9.6A and D), (2) consonance ratings plateau (Figure 9.6B), and (3) loudness summation and masking effects are observed (Figure 9.6C; for review see Ref. 71). The representation of the psychoacoustic literature summarized in Figure 9.6D appears to draw upon Kameoka and Kuriyagawa's data showing increases in consonance well beyond the ΔF associated with disappearance of roughness[72] (Figure 9.6E). Although it is generally accepted that Kameoka and Kuriyagawa's work supports the idea that consonance is a function of roughness and critical bandwidth, comparisons of Figure 9.6A, C, and E reveal that their data actually argue against it, at least for musical interval widths greater than the ΔF for just-noticeable roughness.

The disagreement may arise from two sources. First, Kameoka and Kuriyagawa's Japanese audio engineers were instructed to judge tones for *sunda* (which they translate as 'clearness' in English) and *nigotta* ('turbidity').[72] Consequently, these listeners may have been rating different perceptual attributes than Plomp and Levelt's Dutch subjects, who were instructed to judge how 'consonant' [or *mooi* ('beautiful') or *welluidend* ('euphonious')] the intervals sounded.[51] Second, Kameoka and Kuriyagawa used an incomplete paired comparison paradigm—incomplete because only three or four adjacent intervals were paired for comparisons of relative consonance,[72] a much more restricted ΔF range than the one Plomp and colleagues used in their one-interval consonance rating paradigm.[7,51] When Kameoka and Kuriyagawa tried the method of magnitude estimation, presumably using all possible pairings, the task turned out to be 'rather difficult' for 'naive subjects'[72] (p. 1453), and they dropped it in favour of incomplete pairings. Comparing only adjacent intervals may have biased subjects to focus on differences they would not have otherwise attended to if all intervals had been paired with one another. The pattern of results suggests that pitch height, rather than absence of roughness, influenced consonance judgments beyond a minor third or so. Since the authors used these data to calculate the consonance of musical intervals formed by two complex tones (Figure 9.6F), they may have confounded roughness and pitch height in their predictions.

We reviewed previous studies that used isolated minor seconds, fourths, tritones, and fifths composed of two pure (or nearly pure) tones as experimental stimuli. Kaestner,[6] who used a *Stimmgabelklangen* to generate tones that were 'poor in over-tones', found that sub-jects judged the fourth to be slightly more 'pleasant' than the tritone. Malmberg,[32] who used tuning forks, found a more marked preference for the fourth over the tritone for judge-ments of 'blending', 'purity', and 'smoothness'. Pratt,[73] who used a Stern variator that may have produced weak overtones, found that the fourth was judged to be more 'pleasant', 'smoother', and more 'unitary' than the tritone. Brues,[74] using a Stern variator that pro-duced weak energy at the first overtone, found the fourth, tritone, and fifth were similar with respect to 'unitariness'. Guthrie and Morrill[75] used a Stern variator that produced 'very faint traces of the third partial' and reported that the fourth was judged to be more 'pleas-ant' than the tritone and of equal 'consonance'. Guernsey,[33] who used tuning forks, reported that nonmusicians, amateur musicians, and professional musicians found the fourth more 'pleasant' and 'smooth' than the tritone. Schellenberg and Trehub's recent experiments with nine-month-old babies are also relevant here.[76] When the upper pure tone of a repeating harmonic interval was flattened by one-fourth of a semitone, infants could detect the change if the interval was a fourth but not if it was a tritone. Their find-ings indicate that fourths provided a more stable background against which changes in tuning could be detected. All in all, these results indicate that the fourth, even when it is composed of two pure tones, is often perceived as more con-sonant than the tritone.

Another challenge for roughness-based accounts of consonance arises when we compare the consonance of pure-tone intervals and the consonance of complex-tone intervals. In Figure 9.6D, Terhardt[13] plots consonance ratings for pure-tone and complex-tone intervals on the same scale. In fact, Kameoka and Kuriyagawa's psychoacoustic data and calculations put them on different scales[35] (Figure 9.6F). Likewise, Plomp and Levelt use a dissonance scale from one to zero for their pure-tone data (Figure 9.6C) and a dissonance scale from six to zero for their complex-tone calculations (not shown).[51] Kameoka and Kuriyagawa's calculations predict that a minor second composed of two pure tones is more consonant than the unison of two complex tones with the first six harmonics at isoamplitude[35] (Figure 9.6F). Intuitively, this notion is untenable; however, direct comparisons between pure-tone intervals and complex-tone intervals have not been reported in the literature. We synthesized a pure-tone minor second and the unison of two complex tones (with the acoustic parameters specified by Kameoka and Kuriyagawa[35]) and asked several of our stu-dents to judge which of these two stimuli sounded more 'consonant'. These and Huron's (personal communication) informal observations raise the possibility that a combination of pitch height effects and loudness (shrillness), rather than or in addition to roughness, accounts for Kameoka and Kuriyagaw's predictions. For example, in the case of unison at A_4 (Figure 9.6F), spectral energy extends all the way up to 2200 Hz (fifth harmonic) and 2640 Hz (sixth harmonic), so there are high-frequency components that are greater in sen-sation level than the note F_0s. At the same time, ΔF (440 Hz) is higher than the highest ΔF associated with just-noticeable roughness when the root is at 2000 Hz (Figure 9.6A, interquartile range for $\Delta F \sim 250$–400 Hz^{67}).

In summary, the neural coding mechanisms that provide representations of roughness form part of the neurobiological foundation for the theory of harmony in its vertical dimension. However, our reappraisal of the psychoacoustic literature leads us to conclude that the dependence of consonance on the absence of roughness is overstated. We believe pitch relationships, as well as roughness, influence the perception of intervals and chords as consonant or dissonant in the vertical dimension.

Effects of auditory cortex lesions

Another approach to assessing the relative contributions of pitch and roughness to consonance perception might be to determine whether impairments in consonance perception caused by brain lesions are associated with deficits in one, the other, or both.

Consonance perception has been reported to be severely impaired following bilateral lesions of the auditory cortex.[15] In an experiment employing a one-interval, two-alternative, forced-choice paradigm, two types of stimuli were presented: a major triad, and a triad whose fifth was flattened by a fraction of a semitone. In each trial of the experiment, a young stroke patient, MHS, was asked if a single, isolated chord sounded 'in tune' or 'out of tune'. His response accuracy was 56 per cent, better than chance ($p < 0.05$), but more than two standard deviations below the mean of 13 normal controls (Figure 9.7A). Magnetic resonance imaging revealed that MHS's infarcts involved the primary auditory cortex in both hemispheres, all or almost all of the auditory association cortex in the right hemisphere, and about 20 per cent of the posterior auditory association cortex in the left hemisphere (Figure 9.2A). His pure-tone audiograms were within normal limits. Speech perception was impaired.

We subsequently compared MHS's performance on in-tune trials vs out-of-tune trials. If roughness perception were impaired, then MHS might make more errors in in-tune trials than out-of-tune trials. If frequency selectivity were coarsened and pitch perception impaired, then MHS might make more errors on in-tune trials. Consistent with the latter possibility, we found a marked response bias for out-of-tune judgments (Figure 9.7B). Two possible interpretations follow: (1) MHS was having difficulty extracting the pitches of chord frequency components and analysing their harmonic relationships; and/or (2) he heard more roughness in the chords than normals because his effective critical bandwidths were wider.

To assess whether MHS was having difficulty with frequency discrimination, we examined his performance on the Pitch Discrimination subtest of the Seashore Measures of Musical Talents.[77,78] This test uses the method of constant stimuli to measure one's ability to judge whether the second of two pure tones is higher or lower in pitch than the first tone. The ΔF between the tones gets smaller over successive blocks of trials. The tones were centred at 500 Hz, 600 ms in duration, and 600 ms apart, with an intensity of 35–40 dB above sensation level. Overall, MHS scored in the 15th percentile. His error pattern was again revealing. He performed poorly in the last third of the test, where the ΔFs between the tones were smallest. We subsequently measured pure-tone frequency difference thresholds for pitch discrimination using an adaptive procedure and a two-interval, two-alternative, forced-choice paradigm.[79] Whereas normal controls and patient controls had frequency difference thresholds corresponding to Weber fractions ΔF/mean frequency) of around 1 per cent, MHS's Weber fractions were over 10 per cent. In short, his ability to judge the direction of a pitch change was markedly impaired. A similar deficit has since been reported in patients with surgical lesions of the right primary auditory cortex and right anterior auditory association cortex.[80] We also found that perception of the missing F_0 of

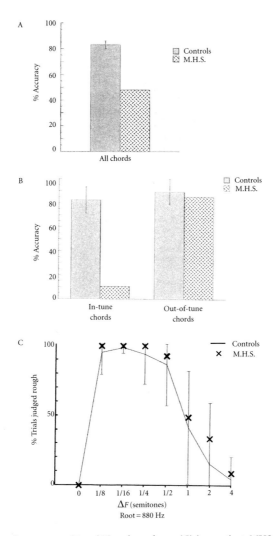

Figure 9.7   Perception of consonance (A and B) and roughness (C) in a patient, MHS, with bilateral lesions of auditory cortex (Figure 9.2A). (A) Data from Tramo et al.[15] showing response accuracy on a task that required MHS to determine whether a major triad was 'in tune' or 'out of tune'. (B) MHS's error rate as a function of stimulus condition. (C) Percentage of trials in which two simultaneous pure tones were judged to be fluctuating and rough (as opposed to steady and smooth) as a function of the $\Delta F\sharp$ between the tones. The mean (*line*) and standard deviation (*bars*) show the combined performance of 10 normal subjects and eight neurological patients who did not have bilateral lesions of auditory cortex. Three of the patients had chronic unilateral lesions of superior temporal cortex (left or right). and one had a lesion of the right inferior colliculus.

harmonic complex tones was impaired,[81] again consistent with observations in most right temporal lobectomy patients with partial or complete excisions involving the primary auditory cortex.[82] Taken together, these findings are consistent with the hypothesis that MHS's impaired consonance perception was related to deficits in pitch processing.

Was this increase in ΔF thresholds for pure-tone pitch discrimination associated with higher ΔF values for disappearance of roughness? We assessed MHS's ability to judge two simultaneous pure tones as 'steady and smooth' vs 'fluctuating and rough' using a one-interval, two-alternative, forced-choice paradigm and the method of constant stimuli. The lower tone was fixed at either 220 Hz (A_3) or 880 Hz (A_5), and the upper tone was above the root by a variable number of semitones: 0, 1/16, 1/8, 1/4, 1/2, 1 (a minor second), 2 (a major second), or 4 (a major third). Figure 9.7C shows the results when the root was at 880 Hz. When the tones were between 1/16 to 1/2 semitone apart, MHS, like controls, judged the combination as rough on > 80 per cent of trials. When the tones were zero, two, or four semitones apart, MHS and controls judged the combination to be rough on less than 20 per cent of trials. At one and two semitones apart, MHS's performance fell near the mean of controls, but there is too much variability in the normal data to meaningfully assess MHS's performance. Still, these observations mitigate the possibility that consonance perception was impaired because he heard more roughness in chords than normals.

In summary, MHS's bias to hear major triads as mistuned appears to be associated with impairments in pitch perception but not roughness perception. Consistent with our physiological data and review of the psychoacoustic literature, this pattern of lesion effects indicates that pitch relationships influence harmony perception in the vertical dimension.

Conclusions

Basic physiological and anatomical properties of auditory and cognitive systems determine why some combinations of simultaneous tones sound more harmonious than others. Distinctive acoustic features of consonant and dissonant intervals are translated into distinctive patterns of neural activity. A faithful representation of temporal regularities in the acoustic structure of consonant intervals exists in the population interspike interval (ISI) distribution of auditory nerve fibres. The most common ISIs in the distribution correspond not only to the pitches of note F_0s actually present in the consonant intervals, but also to the pitches of harmonically related notes in the bass register, such as the fundamental bass. By contrast, for dissonant intervals, the most common ISIs in the distribution do not correspond to one of the note F_0s, nor do they correspond to harmonically related notes. The relative strength of the missing F_0 in the population ISI distribution predicts the relative consonance of the minor second, perfect fourth, tritone, and fifth. Limits on the temporal precision and frequency selectivity of neurons throughout the auditory system constrain the range of note F_0s we can hear as strong pitches and how they are combined into intervals and chords. Implicit knowledge about the hierarchical relationships of pitches in a given tonal system is likely to exert cognitive influences on the degree to which intervals and chords sound consonant or dissonant, even when they are heard in isolation.

Representations of roughness exist in temporal patterns of neural activity at several levels of the auditory system. For the minor second, fourth, tritone, and fifth, the amount of 20- to 200-Hz temporal fluctuations in the firing patterns of auditory nerve fibres inversely correlates with perceived consonance. These representations of roughness are multiplexed with pitch representations in the spike trains of auditory nerve fibres. These two neural time codes operate over different time regimes. The fine timing of action potential firing with precision in the submillisecond range carries information about fundamental pitch. Periodic fluctuations in discharge rate with precision in the range of milliseconds to tens of milliseconds carry information about roughness.

Bilateral lesions of primary auditory cortex and auditory association cortex can lead to severe impairments in consonance perception, with a bias to judge well-tuned chords as out of tune. In our patient, MHS, impaired consonance perception was associated with severely impaired pitch perception, but roughness perception appeared to be normal or near normal.

We interpret our findings and the results of previous psychoacoustic experiments as evidence in favour of the hypothesis that harmony in the vertical dimension, like harmony in the horizontal dimension, is principally a function of the pitch relationships among tones, with roughness playing a secondary role. In light of these observations, and in view of the likelihood that cognitive representations of pitch hierarchies influence harmony perception in the vertical dimension, we urge that the terms *sensory consonance* and *sensory dissonance* be reconsidered.

Acknowledgements

This work was supported by NIH DC03382 (M.J. Tramo), DC03054 (P.A. Cariani), DC02258 (B. Delgutte), and DC00117 (L.D. Braida); and the McDonnell-Pew Program in Cognitive Neuroscience (M.J. Tramo). We gratefully acknowledge the instructive comments of David Cohen and Kay Shelemay of the Harvard Music Department; the technical support of Leslie Liberman of EPL, and David Lum, Andrew Grant, and Danielle Lemay of RLE; the graphics and manuscript assistance of Adda Kridler, Janelle Mallett, and Monique James; and, especially, our collaborators in the experimental studies cited here: Jamshed Bharucha, Martin McKinney, Michael Gazzaniga, Frank Musiek, Robert Zatorre, Carla Kovacs, Gaurav Shah, Eiling Yee. Special thanks go to Mark Smith and his family.

References

1. **Cohen, M. R.** and **I. E. Drabkin** (1948) *A Source Book in Greek Science.* New York: McGraw-Hill Book Company, Inc.

2. **Piston, W.** (1941/1987) *Harmony,* 5th edn. Revised and Expanded by Mark DeVoto. New York: W. W. Norton & Company, Inc.

3. **Apel, Willi,** (ed.) (1972) *Harvard Dictionary of Music,* 2nd edn. Cambridge, MA: Belknap Press of Harvard University Press.

4. **Randel, D. M.** (1986) *The New Harvard Dictionary of Music,* 3rd edn. Cambridge, MA: Belknap Press of Harvard University Press.

5. **Tyrrell, J.** and **S. Sadie** (eds) (2001) *The New Grove Dictionary of Music and Musicians,* 2nd edn. New York: Grove's Dictionaries, Inc.

6. **Kaestner, G.** (1909) Untersuchungen uber den Gefuhlseindruck unanalysieter Zweiklange. *Psychol. Studien.* 4, 473–504.

7. **Van de Geer, J. P., W. J. M. Levelt,** and **R. Plomp** (1962) The connotation of musical consonance. *Acta Psychologia* 20, 308–19.

8. **Bernstein, L.** (1976) *The Unanswered Question.* Cambridge, MA: Harvard University Press.

9. **Gundlach, R. H.** (1935) Factors determining the characterization of musical phrases. *Am. J. Psychol.* 47, 624–43.

10. **Balkwill, L.** and **W. F. Thompson** (1999) A cross-cultural investigation of the perception of emotion in music: psycho physical and cultural cues. *Music Percept.* 17, 43–64.

11. **Castellano, M. A., J. J. Bharucha,** and **C. L. Krumhansl** (1984) Tonal hierarchies in the music of north India. *J. Exp. Psychol. Gen.* 113, 394–412.

12. **Kessler, E. J., C. Hansen,** and **R. N. Shepard** (1984) Tonal schemata in the perception of music in Bali and in the west. *Music Percept.* 2, 131–65.

13. **Terhardt, E.** (1984) The concept of musical consonance: a link between music and psychoacoustics. *Music Percept.* 1, 276–95.

14. **Krumhansl, C. L.** (1990) *Cognitive Foundations of Musical Pitch.* New York: Oxford University Press.

15. **Tramo, M. J., J. J. Bharucha,** and **F. E. Musiek** (1990) Music perception and cognition following bilateral lesions of auditory cortex. *J. Cognit. Neurosci.* 2, 195–212.

16. **Helmholtz, H.** (1877/1954) *On the Sensations of Tone as a Physiological Basis for the Theory of Music.* Translated by A.J. Ellis, 1885. New York: Dover Publications, Inc.

17. **Stevens, S. S.** and **H. Davis** (1938/1983) *Hearing: Its Psychology and Physiology.* New York: American Institute of Physics, Inc.

18. **Parncutt, R.** (1989) *Harmony: A Psychoacoustical Approach.* Berlin: Springer-Verlag.

19. **Deutsch, D.** (ed.) (1999) *The Psychology of Music,* 2nd edn. San Diego, CA: Academic Press.

20. **Demany, L.** and **C. Semal** (1990) Harmonic and melodic octave templates. *J. Acoust. Soc. Am.* 88, 2126–35.

21. **Demany, L., C. Semal,** and **R. P. Carlyon** (1991) On the perceptual limits of octave harmony and their origin. *J. Acoust. Soc. Am.* 90, 3019–27.

22. **Kiang, N. Y. -S., T. Watanabe, E. C. Thomas,** and **L. F. Clark** (1965) *Discharge Patterns of Single Fibers in the Cat's Auditory Nerve.* Cambridge, MA: MIT Press.

23. **Rose, J. E., J. F. Brugge, D. J. Anderson,** and **J. E. Hind** (1967) Phase-locked response to low frequency tones in single auditory nerve fibers of the squirrel monkey. *J. Neuro-physiol.* 30, 769–93.

24. **Boomslitter, P.** and **W. Creel** (1961) The long pattern hypothesis in harmony and hearing. *J. Music Theory* 5, 2–31.

25. **Brugge J. F., D. J. Anderson, J. E. Hind,** and **J. E. Rose** (1969) Time structure of discharges in single auditory nerve fibers of the squirrel monkey in response to complex periodic sounds. *J. Neurophysiol.* 32, 386–401.

26. **Moore, B. C. J.** (1980) Neural interspike intervals and pitch. *Audiology* 19, 363–5.

27. **Rose, J. E.** (1980) Neural correlates of some psychoacoustic experiences. In D. McFadden (ed.) *Neural Mechanisms in Behavior.* New York: Springer-Verlag. pp. 1–37.

28. **Ohgushi, K.** (1983) The origin of tonality and a possible explanation of the octave enlargement phenomenon. *J. Acoust. Soc. Am.* 73, 1695–7.

29. **Patterson, R. D.** (1986) Spiral detection of periodicity and the spiral form of musical scales. *Psychol. Music* 14, 44–61.

30. **Moore, B. C. J., R. W. Peters,** and **B. R. Glasberg** (1985) Thresholds for the detection of inharmonicity in complex tones. *J. Acoust. Soc. Am.* 77, 1861–7.

31. **Vos, J.** (1982) The perception of pure and mistuned musical fifths and major thirds: thresholds for discrimination, beats, and identification. *Percept. and Psychophys.* 32, 297–313.

32. **Malmberg, C. F.** (1918) The perception of consonance and dissonance. *Psychol. Monogr.* 25, 93–133.

33. **Guernsey, M.** (1928) The role of consonance and dissonance in music. *Am. J. Psychol.* 40, 173–204.

34. **Butler, J. W.** and **P. G. Daston** (1968) Musical consonance as musical preference: a cross-cultural study. *J. Gen. Psychol.* 79, 129–42.

35. **Kameoka, A.** and **M. Kuriyagawa** (1969) Consonance theory part II: consonance of complex tones and its calculation method. *J. Acoust. Soc. Am.* 45, 1460–9.

36. **Zentner, M. R.** and **J. Kagan** (1998) Infants' perception of consonance and dissonance in music. *Infant Behav. and Dev.* 21, 483–92.

37. **Hulse, S., D. J. Bernard,** and **R. F. Braaten** (1995) Auditory discrimination of chord-based spectral structures by European starlings (Sturnus vulgaris). *J. Exp. Psychol. Gen.* 124, 409–23.

38. **Tramo, M. J., P. Cariani,** and **B. Delgutte** (1992) Representation of tonal consonance and dissonance in the temporal firing patterns of auditory nerve fibers. *Soc. Neurosci. Abstr.* 18, 382.

39. **Tramo, M. J., M. C. McKinney, P. A. Cariani,** and **B. Delgutte** (2000) Physiology of tonal consonance and dissonance. *Assoc. Res. Otolaryngol. Abstr.* 23, 275–6.

40. **McKinney, M. F., M. J. Tramo,** and **B. Delgutte** (2001) Neural correlates of musical dissonance in the inferior colliculus. In A. J. M. Houtsma *et al.* (eds) *Physiological and Psychophysical Bases of Auditory Function*. Maastricht, The Netherlands: Shaker Publishing, 71–7.

41. **McKinney, M. F., M. J. Tramo,** and **B. Delgutte** (2001) Neural correlates of the dissonance of musical intervals in the inferior colliculus. *Assoc. Res. Otolaryngol. Abstr.* 24, 54–55.

42. **Javel, E.** (1980) Coding of AM tones in the chinchilla auditory nerve: implications for the pitch of complex tones. *J. Acoust. Soc. Am.* 68, 133–146.

43. **Rhode, W. S.** (1995) Interspike intervals as a correlate of periodicity pitch in cat cochlear nucleus. *J. Acoust. Soc. Am.* 95, 2414–29.

44. **Schreiner, C. E.** and **G. Langner** (1988) Coding of temporal patterns in the central auditory nervous system. In *Auditory Function Neurobiological Bases of Hearing*. G. M. Edelman *et al.* (eds) New York: John Wiley & Sons pp. 337–61.

45. **Krishna, B. S.** and **M. N. Semple** (2000) Auditory temporal processing: responses to sinusoidally amplitude-modulated tones in the inferior colliculus. *J. Neurophysiol.* 84, 255–73.

46. **Preuss, A.** and **P. Muller-Preuss** (1990) Processing of amplitude modulated sounds in the medial geniculate body of squirrel monkeys. *Exp. Brain Res.* 79, 207–11.

47. **Bieser, A.** and **P. Muller-Preuss** (1996) Auditory responsive cortex in the squirrel monkey: neural responses to amplitude-modulated sounds. *Exp. Brain Res.* 108, 273–84.

48. **Fishman, Y. I., D. H. Reser, J. C. Arezzo,** and **M. Steinschneider** (2000) Complex tone processing in primary auditory cortex of the awake monkey. I. Neural ensemble correlates of roughness. *J. Acoust. Soc. Am.* 108, 235–46.

49. **Fishman, Y. I., D. H. Reser, J. C. Arezzo,** and **M. Steinschneider** (2000) Complex tone processing in primary auditory cortex of the awake monkey. II. Pitch versus critical band representation. *J. Acoust. Soc. Am.* 108, 247–62.

50. **Ehret, G.** and **R. Romand** (eds) (1997) *The Central Auditory System.* New York: Oxford University Press.

51. **Plomp, R.** and **W. J. M. Levelt** (1965) Tonal consonance and critical bandwidth. *J. Acoust. Soc. Am.* 38, 548–60.

52. Hutchinson, W. and L. Knopoff (1978) The acoustic component of Western consonance. *Interface* 7, 1–29.

53. Rameau, J.-P. (1722/1971) Treatise on Harmony. Translated by P. Gossett. New York: Dover Publications, Inc.

54. Wightman, F. L. and D. M. Green (1974) The perception of pitch. *Am. Sci.* 62, 208–15.

55. Houtsma, A. J. M. and J. L. Goldstein (1971) The central origin of the pitch of complex tones: evidence from musical interval recognition. *J. Acoust. Soc. Am.* 51, 520–9.

56. Moore, B. C. J. (1997) *An Introduction to the Psychology of Hearing.* San Diego, CA: Academic Press.

57. Galileo Galilei (1638/1954) *Dialogues Concerning Two New Sciences.* Translated by H. Crew and A. de Salvio, 1914. New York: Dover Publications.

58. Pickles, J. O. (1988) *An Introduction to the Physiology of Hearing.* London: Academic Press, Harcourt Brace Jovanovich, Publishers.

59. Cariani, P. A. and B. Delgutte (1996) Neural correlates of the pitch of complex tones. I. Pitch and pitch salience. *J. Neurophysiol.* 76, 1698–1716.

60. Cariani, P. A. and B. Delgutte (1996) Neural correlates of the pitch of complex tones. II. Pitch shift, pitch ambiguity, phase-invariance, pitch circularity, and the dominance region for pitch. *J. Neurophysiol.* 76, 1717–34.

61. Cariani, P. (1999) Temporal coding of periodicity pitch in the auditory system: an overview. *Neural Plast.* 6, 147–72.

62. Meddis, R. and M. J. Hewitt (1991) Virtual pitch and phase sensitivity of a computer model of the auditory periphery. II. Phase sensitivity. *J. Acoust. Soc. Am.* 89, 2883–94.

63. Terhardt, E. (1974) Pitch, consonance, and harmony. *J. Acoust. Soc. Am.* 55, 1061–9.

64. Helmholtz, H. L. F. (1863/1913) *Die Lehre von der Tonempfindungen als physiolo-gische Grundlage fur die Theorie der Musik,* 6th edn. Brauschweig: F. Vieweg, Quote translated by E. Terhardt,[13] pp. 283–4.

65. Dai, H. (1993) On the pitch of two-tone complexes. *J. Acoust. Soc. Am.* 94, 730–4.

66. Greenwood, D. D. (1991) Critical bandwidth and consonance in relation to cochlear frequency-position coordinates. *Hear. Res.* 54, 164–208.

67. Plomp, R. and H. J. M. Steeneken (1968) Interference between two simple tones. *J. Acoust. Soc. Am.* 43, 883–4.

68. Mayer, A. M. (1874) Researches in acoustics. *Am. J. Sci. Arts, 3rd Ser.* 8, 241–55.

69. Cross, C. R. and H. M. Goodwin (1891) Some considerations regarding Helmholtz's theory of consonance. *Am. J. Sci.* 58, 1–12.

70. Zwicker, E., G. Flottorp, and S. S. Stevens (1957) Critical band width in loudness summation. *J. Acoust. Soc. Am.* 29, 548–57.

71. Yost, W. A. (2000) Fundamentals of Hearing. San Diego, CA: Academic Press.

72. Kameoka, A. and M. Kuriyagawa (1969) Consonance theory part I: consonance of dyads. *J. Acoust. Soc. Am.* 45, 1451–9.

73. Pratt, C. C. (1921) Some qualitative aspects of bitonal complexes. *Am. J. Psychol.* 32, 490–515.

74. Brues, A. M. (1927) The fusion of non-musical intervals. *Am. J. Psychol.* 38, 624–38.

75. Guthrie, E. R. and H. Morrell (1928) The fusion of non-musical intervals. *Am. J. Psychol.* 40, 624–625.

76. Schellenberg, E. G. and S. E. Trehub (1996) Natural musical intervals: evidence from infant listeners. *Psychol. Sci.* 7, 272–7.

77. Tramo, M. J. (1990) Impaired perception of relative pure tone pitch following bilateral lesions of auditory cortex in man. *Soc. Neurosci. Abstr.* 16, 580.

78. Seashore, C. E., D. Lewis, and J. G. Saetveit (1960) *Seashore Measures of Musical Talents.* New York: The Psychological Corporation.

79. Tramo, M. J., A. Grant, and L. D. Braida (1994) Psychophysical measurements of frequency difference limens for relative pitch discrimination reveal a deficit following bilateral lesions of auditory cortex. *Soc. Neurosci. Abstr.* 20, 325.

80. Johnsrude, I. S., V. B. Penhune, and R. J. Zatorre (2000) Functional specificity in the right human auditory cortex for perceiving pitch direction. *Brain* 123, 155–63.

81. Bharucha, J. J., M. J. Tramo, and R. J. Zatorre (1993) Abstraction of the missing fundamental following bilateral lesions of auditory cortex. *Soc. Neurosci. Abstr.* 19, 1687.

82. Zatorre, R. J. (1988) Pitch perception of complex tones and human temporal-lobe function. *J. Acoust. Soc. Am.* 84, 566–72.

CHAPTER 10

INTRACEREBRAL EVOKED POTENTIALS IN PITCH PERCEPTION REVEAL A FUNCTIONAL ASYMMETRY OF HUMAN AUDITORY CORTEX

CATHERINE LIÉGEOIS-CHAUVEL, KIMBERLY GIRAUD, JEAN-MICHEL BADIER, PATRICK MARQUIS, AND PATRICK CHAUVEL

Abstract

One acoustic feature that plays an important role in pitch perception is frequency. Studies on the processing of frequency in the human and animal brain have shown that the auditory cortex is tonotopically organized: low frequencies are represented laterally whereas high frequencies are represented medially. To date, the study of the functional organization of the human auditory cortex in the processing of frequency has been limited to the use of either scalp-recorded auditory evoked potentials (AEPs), which have relatively poor spatial resolving power, or functional imagery techniques, which have poor temporal resolving power. The present study uses intracerebrally recorded AEPs to explore this topic in the primary and secondary auditory cortices of both hemispheres of the human brain. Recordings were carried out in 45 adult patients with drug-resistant partial seizures. In the right hemisphere, clear spectrally organized tonotopic maps were observed with distinct separations between different frequency-processing regions. AEPs for high frequencies were recorded medially, whereas AEPs for low frequencies were recorded laterally. In the left hemisphere, however, this tonotopic organization was less evident, with different regions involved in the processing of a range of frequencies. The hemisphere-related difference in the processing of tonal frequency is discussed in relation to pitch perception.

Keywords: Pitch perception; Auditory cortex; Neural processing

The ability to process pitch is of major importance to music and language perception. Although the acoustic cues necessary to the perception of pitch are mainly of a temporal nature, human subjects describe pitch as having a spatial dimension (i.e. musical scale). Traditionally, the literature on the processing of pitch in the human brain has been dominated by two main theories: one that postulates an exclusively tonotopic coding and another that is in favour of an exclusively 'temporal' coding.[1-3] Recently, however, Langner[4,5] has suggested that temporal information, coded at the subcortical level as spikes synchronized to the periodicity of the acoustic signal, is subsequently converted to spatial information coded in the form of tonotopic maps in the auditory cortex. This hypothesis is consistent with the finding that the temporal resolution of the auditory nerve[6] and inferior colliculus[7,8] may be higher than at the cortical level, where the temporal resolution of auditory information is possible only at frequencies below 100 Hz for the majority of neurons.[9,10] At the cortical level, pitch appears to be coded according to a frequency spectrum (i.e. tonotopically).

Experimental studies using single-unit recording techniques indicate that for most auditory neurons, a 'best frequency' (BF) can be determined at which a low-intensity auditory stimulus evokes the greatest electrophysiological response in a given region. The auditory cortex is said to be tonotopically organized because an ordered change in BFs occurs as one moves along the cortex. The auditory cortex is organized according to a frequency gradient, with low frequencies represented laterally and high frequencies represented medially.[11-18]

The tonotopic organization of the auditory cortex is best understood in nonhuman animals. The cytoarchitecture of the auditory cortex is not always uniform,[14] however, rendering the mapping of different tonotopic regions difficult. Merzenich and Brugge[12] have found that the auditory cortex in the superior temporal plane of the macaque can be subdivided into at least six distinct fields on the basis of cytoarchitectonic characteristics and BFs. Likewise, Reale and Imig[16] observed a tonotopic organization in six different auditory areas of the cat, and a similar tonotopic organization has been described in the albino rat.[18]

In humans, the use of noninvasive techniques such as magnetoencephalography (MEG) and positron emission tomography (PET) has shed some light on the functional organization of the auditory cortex with respect to frequency. In their PET study, Lauter et al.[19] observed that changes in regional cerebral blood flow induced by a high-frequency tone (4 kHz) were located deeper and more posteriorly in the temporal lobe than those induced by a low-frequency tone (500 Hz). In a similar vein, MEG studies on the tonotopic organization of N1 generators have shown that their estimated depth can vary as a function of frequency: higher frequencies involve more medial regions of the Heschl's gyrus (HGs), whereas lower frequencies involve more lateral areas.[20-24]

In a previous study,[25] using depth electrodes implanted in the HG of human subjects with medically intractable epilepsy, we identified four separable components of middle-latency auditory evoked potentials (MLAEPs), which peaked at approximately 30, 50, 60, and 80 ms. The sources of these components were definable, although some overlap was observed. In a recent MEG study, Pantev et al.[23] explored the sources of different middle-latency components as well as their distribution. In all subjects and for all the frequencies studied, only two components were consistently observed: the 30-ms 'Pam' component and the N1m. Also, a tonotopic organization was observed in the primary auditory cortex that mirrored that observed in the secondary cortex. The localization of Pam's source moved more superficially with higher frequencies, while the localization of the N1m's source moved progressively deeper with higher frequencies. The authors, however, did not consistently observe the

50-ms component, which is thought to be generated in the lateral part of the primary auditory cortex in close proximity to the neighboring secondary areas.

The present paper explores the tonotopic organization of the human auditory cortex using intracerebrally recorded evoked potentials studied as a function of anatomical recording site. The sensitivity of a neuronal population to a given frequency was determined from fluctuations in AEP amplitude between different recording sites in the primary auditory cortex and surrounding secondary areas like the planum temporale. Indeed, previous data suggest that the auditory cortex is tonotopically organized for frequency and that even several different tonotopic maps may be described for different cortical regions. But is this tonotopic organization the same in both left and right cerebral hemispheres? A substantial body of data suggests that the perception and processing of pitch is specific to a single hemisphere,[26] and hemisphere-related differences in the functional organization of the auditory areas underlying such processing are not inconceivable. The main objective of this study was to investigate the tonotopic organization of the human auditory cortex in both cerebral hemispheres.

Patients and methods

Intracerebral AEPs were recorded from 45 adult patients (aged 20–56 years) with medically intractable partial epileptic seizures of right and left temporal lobe origin (in 31 and 14 patients, respectively). These patients were undergoing stereo-electroencephalographic (SEEG) evaluation for the surgical relief of their seizures (for a description of this procedure, see Refs 27 and 28). Recordings were carried out in either the left or the right HG and right planum temporale, during which time subjects laid comfortably on a bed and remained vigilant and cooperative. All patients had previously given informed consent to participate in the study.

The anatomical localization of each implanted electrode was based on a stereotaxic procedure described elsewhere.[29–31] The three-dimensional coordinates of each electrode lead were defined and measured with respect to the temporal branch of the middle cerebral artery and allowed us to distinguish the primary from the secondary auditory areas in the different patients.[25,32]

The visualization of electrode tracks using stereotaxic MRI represents a means of confirming the anatomical localization of implanted sites and provides additional information on the anatomy of the HG in each subject (e.g. the presence of one or two gyri[33]). Such information can often be helpful in the interpretation of AEP data. MRI sections were cut along three spatial planes using bicommissural coordinates. Figure 10.1 shows the position of one electrode implanted orthogonally in the lateral part of the left HG.

Auditory stimulation

Auditory stimuli were tone bursts (with a 0.3-ms rise and decay time and a total duration of 30 ms) of different frequencies (ranging from 250 Hz to 4 kHz). These stimuli were generated using an SM 700 NICOLET auditory stimulator and presented at a rate of 0.7/s via TDH 39 earphones to the ear contralateral to the implanted site. Stimuli were presented in random order at an intensity of 70 dB SL (sensation level) for each subject.

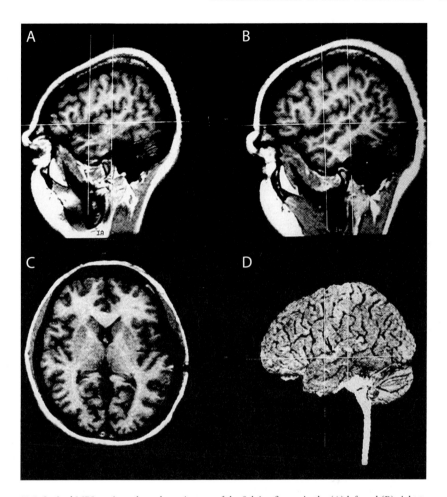

Figure 10.1 Sagittal MRI sections show the trajectory of the Sylvian fissure in the (A) left and (B) right temporal lobes. Note here the distinct shape of the end of the lateral sulcus (Sylvian fissure) on both sides (*white arrows*) and the longer length of the left planum temporale in this right-handed patient. The *three axes* of the bicommissural reference system (AC-PC, VAC, VPC) have been drawn. (C) The verticofrontal section shows the left Heschl's gyrus, and the *black arrow* indicates the trace of the electrode recorded from the auditory cortex. (D) On the surface view, the *arrow* shows the impact point of the same electrode.

Depth AEP recording and averaging

Intracerebral AEPs were recorded from all leads of an electrode (using an extra-cephalic reference looped around the neck) and were simultaneously amplified and bandpass filtered 1 Hz–1.5 kHz. Recording epochs lasted 350 ms with a prestimulus time of 35 ms, 10 per cent of the epoch. Two trials of 100 samples were administered to each subject. Variations (i.e. polarity inversions and/or changes in amplitude in AEPs) recorded from different leads were studied for each patient. Tonotopic maps were based on a comparison of the results obtained from patients with different anatomical recording sites.

The acquisition system was a Nicolet Pathfinder II with 16 acquisition channels and an 8-bit-resolution digital converter. Negative potentials were displayed as up and positive as down. Recordings of brainstem evoked potentials carried out before SEEG recordings confirmed that all the patients studied had normal afferent pathway conduction.

Temporospectral mapping

Data were stored on the hard drive of the computer and transferred via an asynchronous line to an IBM PC/AT. Off-line processing consisted of the construction of temporospectral maps, using a technique adapted from Rémond,[34] to depth recordings, particularly appropriate to the depth electrode geometry.[35,36]

Results

Primary and secondary areas were identified on the basis of component latency (for a description, see Ref. 25). The selectivity of an auditory area's response (and hence its BF was determined from frequency-related fluctuations in a component's amplitude and/or polarity inversions.

Recordings from the primary auditory cortex

Right hemisphere   Figure 10.2 shows AEPs recorded from 10 contiguous leads of an electrode implanted in the right auditory cortex of one patient. The first four leads recorded activity from the primary auditory cortex; the other six recorded activity from secondary areas. Tone bursts at different frequencies were presented to the patient's left ear. A triphasic N30/P50/N80 complex was recorded from the first four leads for which a polarity inversion was observed between leads 4 and 5, as well as a shift in latency between leads 6 and 10. AEPs recorded from lead 4 were highly sensitive to tonal frequency. For tones higher than 1 kHz, the amplitude of the 50- and 80-ms components progressively decreased until an isopotential response (note the polarity inversion between leads 3 and 5) was observed for tones at 4 kHz, suggesting that the cortical region at lead 4 has a high sensitivity for frequencies in the 4 kHz range. AEPs did not differ in terms of tonal frequency on any of the other leads.

It should be noted, of course, that the amplitude changes observed were never an all-or-none phenomenon, but were observed as increasing or decreasing from lead to lead in progressive steps. Also, unlike the 50- and 80-ms components, the amplitude of the 30-ms component did not appear to be frequency dependent.

Figure 10.3 is a temporospectral representation of AEPs recorded for different tonal frequencies from a second patient. In this figure, the amplitudes of the same three components (30, 50, and 80 ms) as for the first patient are shown for the three most responsive leads (2, 3, and 6 for different tonal frequencies). In each case, frequency is represented along the x-axis and latency along the y-axis. On lead 2, amplitude was maximal for tone bursts with the highest frequencies (3–4 kHz), although frequency-dependent fluctuations

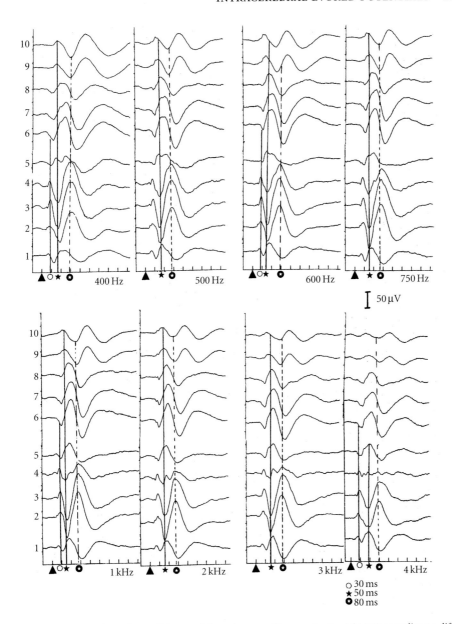

Figure 10.2 Recordings from the medial part of the primary auditory cortex in right HG according to different tonal frequencies. Each response corresponds to a monopolar recording of each lead of the electrode that is referenced to an extracephalic site. The leads are numbered from 1 to 10, from the medial to lateral part of the auditory cortex. Note the amplitude variations of the 50-ms component (indicated by the *star*) according to frequency (see comments in the text). The *arrow* indicates the onset of the stimulus. Recording time ends at 350 ms.

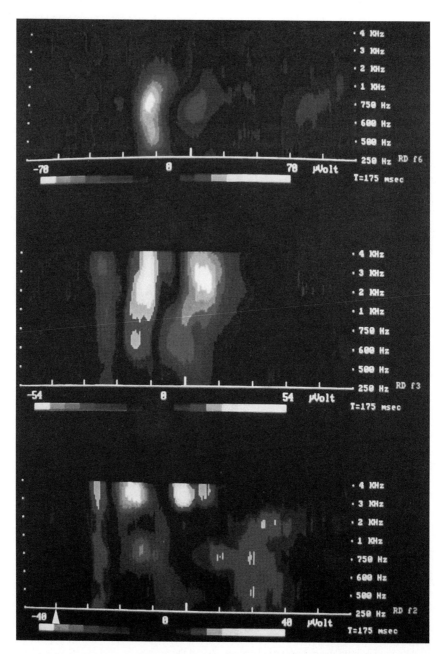

Figure 10.3 Temporospectral maps of amplitude variations of potentials recorded from the right primary auditory cortex (leads 2, 3, and 6). Time, related in abscissae, is reduced to 175 ms, full scale. On the ordinate axis, each *yellow dot* represents the frequency. Amplitude is represented by colour. A cubic spline interpolation is used in order to obtain a continuous potential line between the different frequencies. Each spatial /reconstruction gives a continuous map both in time and in frequency. *Dark colours* are values close to the neutral potential, and *bright colours* are used for the activity—*blue* represents negativity and *red* represents positivity. The *white arrow* indicates the beginning of the sound. (For comments see text.) (See Plate 1 in colour section.)

in amplitude were greater for the N50 and P80 components than for the N30. This was observed to an even greater extent on lead 3, where the amplitude of the N30 did not vary significantly according to tonal frequency, in spite of the highly significant fluctuations in P50 and N780 amplitude. On lead 3, the P50 and N80 were less sharply tuned and their amplitude was maximal at frequencies of 2–3 kHz. Lead 6 recorded neuronal activity in a region between the lateral part of the primary cortex and the medial part of the secondary cortex and yielded responses characterized, this time, by an almost complete absence of the 30-ms component. The N50 was the only component for which amplitude varied with tonal frequency. Its amplitude was maximal at 750 Hz.

Left hemisphere   The left-hand side of Figure 10.4 shows AEPs recorded from the left primary auditory cortex (leads 4 and 5) for different tonal frequencies. As was the case in the right primary cortex, a triphasic N30/P45/N100 complex was observed. P45 and N100 amplitude recorded from the left hemisphere, however, did not vary as a function of

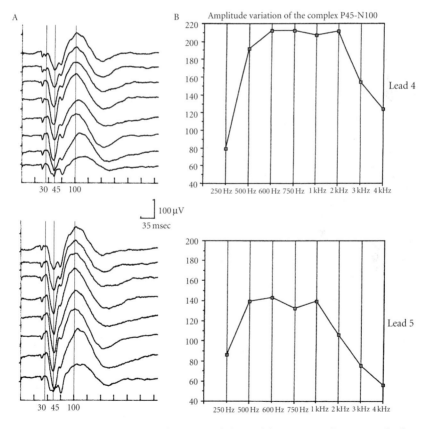

Figure 10.4   (A) Evoked responses recorded from the medial part of the primary auditory cortex (leads 4 and 5) in the left HG. (B) Graphs representing amplitude variations for the P45/N100 complex according to different tonal frequencies (ordinate axis: absolute amplitude expressed in μV; abscissa axis: tonal frequency). The frequencies vary from 250 Hz (*first line*) to 4 kHz (*last line*) (see comments in the text).

frequency, as shown on the right in the same figure. For these components, amplitude was maximal at a range of frequencies between 600 Hz and 2 kHz.

Recordings from the secondary auditory cortex in the left and right hemispheres

The secondary auditory areas studied were confined to an area anterior and lateral to the primary cortex, as previously identified in physiological[25,32] and morphological studies.[37,38] In this secondary area, frequency-dependent fluctuations in amplitude were observed for the 80-ms component. Figure 10.5 shows the localization of electrodes implanted in the right (left-hand side of figure) and left (right-hand side of figure) secondary auditory areas in 11 patients (six right; five left). The sagittal views (top) show the localization of each electrode, while the coronal views (below sagittal views) show the localization of those electrode leads yielding the greatest frequency-dependent fluctuations in amplitude. In the right hemisphere, a mediolateral as well as an anteroposterior distribution of BFs was observed for the 80-ms component. Neuronal populations sensitive to high frequencies (graphs A and E) 80-ms poststimulus onset were localized in the posterolateral part of right HG, while those sensitive to low frequencies (graph B) were localized in the anterolateral part of right HG. For the 80-ms component, high frequencies were also represented ventrally in an area adjacent to the lateral part of the primary cortex in the middle of right HG, overlapping the area in which low frequencies were represented for the 50-ms component.

The profile of amplitude curves for the right hemisphere was noticeably different from that for the left hemisphere. In the dorsolateral part of the left HG, the generators of the 80-ms component were most responsive over a range of high frequencies (1–4 kHz; graph B) or to two isolated sets of frequencies (500 Hz and 1–2 kHz; graph C); in the anterolateral part of left HG, this component was sensitive either to a range of low-to-medium frequencies (500 Hz–1 kHz) or to two isolated sets of frequencies (400 Hz and 1 kHz; graph D).

Figure 10.6 summarizes the main results. In the right primary cortex, the 30-ms component was not clearly tonotopic. A first tonotopic map is observed for the 50-ms component. A strict organization displaying high frequencies medially and low frequencies laterally is observed. A second map is observed for the 80- or 100-ms components generated in the secondary cortex. Neurons responsive to low frequencies were lateral to those responding to higher frequencies, but they were less finely tuned (broken line). Another map was observed for the 100-ms component generated in the planum temporale. High frequencies seemed to be more represented. On the left hemisphere, in the primary as well as in the secondary auditory cortex, the neurons were most sensitive to a range of frequencies (low or high). Nevertheless, the same tonotopic organization of the frequencies seems to be respected—high frequencies medially and low frequencies laterally represented.

Discussion

The present study suggests that the auditory cortex is composed of frequency-dependent tonotopic maps and that these maps are more complex than previously reported in surface EP studies.[20,21,23,39] Although the previously reported mediolateral tonotopic organization was also observed in this study, it was not robust for all AEP components recorded and was hemisphere specific.

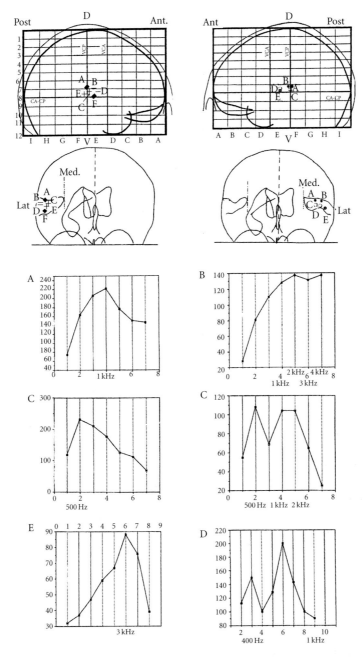

Figure 10.5 Mapping of amplitude variations for the 80-ms component (ordinate axis: absolute amplitude expressed in μV; abscissa axis: frequency) recorded from different loci of the lateral part of the right and left HG referenced to Talairach's proportional standard grid on the lateral view. On the frontal view, the depth of the most responsive lead of each patient is reported in the Heschl's gyrus. The frequencies vary from 250 Hz *(first line)* to 4 kHz *(last line)*. The *peak of the curve* corresponds to the CF (see comments in the text).

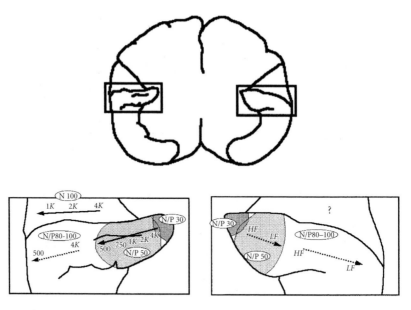

Figure 10.6 Schematic representation of the tonotopic maps recorded from the right and left auditory areas (see comments in the text).

In the primary auditory cortex, no frequency-dependent changes in amplitude or latency were observed for the earliest components (N13/P17) in either hemisphere. For the N30, only slight variations in amplitude were seen in response to tonal frequency, and most often its amplitude covaried with that of the 50-ms component. The amplitude of the 50-ms component was maximal for high frequencies (4 kHz) in medial regions of the primary cortex and for low frequencies (400–500 Hz) in lateral regions. Both mediolateral and anteroposterior organizations observed were marked by a progressive decrease in BFs toward the boundaries of the primary cortex.

The present data suggest the existence of an orderly, tonotopic representation of frequencies in the human primary auditory cortex, similar to that described in nonhuman animals.[13,40] In humans, BFs vary from 4 kHz medially to 400 Hz laterally for the 50-ms component. This range roughly corresponds to the frequency range useful for speech (this latter range actually begins near 250 Hz—a frequency at which a clear evoked response was difficult to obtain in this study). Studies exploring the auditory cortex of nonhuman primates have shed a great deal of light on the functional organization of the human auditory cortex, because its organization in primates appears to be similar to that in humans. In primates, BFs are represented in an orderly pattern in the primary auditory cortex and range from below 100 Hz to about 32 kHz, nearly the full frequency hearing range for primates. The lowest BFs are represented rostrally and laterally, whereas the highest BFs are found caudally and medially. Such an organization is thought to cover almost the entire auditory cortex, with all frequencies (except those at the extreme ends of the frequency hearing range) being represented.[2,16,41,42] The BFs observed in the present study were highly stable from patient to patient, in spite of the intersubject variability in localization and orientation of the primary auditory cortex.

In a recent study, Pantev et al.[23] observed a tonotopic organization of the human auditory cortex for the Pam component (corresponding to the 30-ms intracerebral AEP component); unlike the results of the present study, however, higher frequencies were represented more laterally than were lower frequencies. This discrepancy may be explained by the fact that, in the present study, only slight frequency-dependent fluctuations in amplitude were observed for the 30-ms component, compared to those observed for the P/N 50. Furthermore, the P1m (corresponding to the P/N 50 in this study), generated in the primary auditory cortex, was not systematically discernible in Pantev et al.'s study and has been shown in several MEG[44–46] and EEG studies to have highly variable scalp topography. With intracerebrally recorded AEPs, on the other hand, the P/N 50 is robust and can reach amplitudes of up to 150 μV.[25] It is also probable that two different overlapping tonotopic maps exist, each corresponding to either the 30- or the 50-ms component, and that different investigation techniques have differential capacities to explore these maps.

Frequency-dependent fluctuations in amplitude were also observed for the 80-ms component, which is generated in secondary auditory areas anterior and lateral to the primary cortex.[25] In the right hemisphere, a mediolateral as well as an anteroposterior tonotopic organization was seen, with high frequencies represented posteromedially and low frequencies represented anterolaterally. High frequencies were also represented ventrally in an area adjacent to the lateral part of the primary cortex, which was also the area in which low frequencies were represented for the 50-ms component. While the distribution of BFs was roughly similar for the 80-ms component in both hemispheres, this distribution was not as well defined in the left hemisphere, where neuronal populations were often found to respond to more than one frequency or over a broad range of frequencies. Neither Merzenich et al.[13] nor Reale and Imig,[16] however, found a clear tonotopic organization of the secondary cortex (AII) in their studies with nonhuman animals: several groups of neurons had multiple BFs or responded over a broad range of frequencies. Evoked responses from this area had longer latencies and were less well tuned than those from the primary cortex. [16,47] In their study, Merzenich et al.[14] reported that neurons in these secondary areas often responded over a broad range of frequencies and that the assignment of BFs was difficult, with two maxima often being observed. It is possible that a second harmonic distortion produced this 'double range' because the pairs of maxima in this study were often harmonically related.[48]

With respect to area 22, in the present study no tonotopic organization was observed in either hemisphere. This finding is consistent with data from animal studies using single-unit recordings[49] showing that neurons in nonprimary auditory areas in the macaque are not selectively responsive to pure tones, but respond only to frequency-centred sound bursts containing many frequencies.

One of the most significant findings in this study is the difference in the response selectivity of neurons in the right and left cerebral hemispheres. Neurons in the right auditory cortex were more sharply tuned to frequency than neurons in the homologous region of the left hemisphere. In a previous study, we showed that left auditory neurons were specifically sensitive to the temporal features of auditory information.[50]

As discussed earlier in this paper, the perceptual identity of a sound depends on both a sound's temporal structure as well as its spectral content. For example, periodic modulations of a sound's amplitude evoke a pitch percept. Taken together, the results from the numerous studies on the functional organization of the human auditory cortex suggest a different functional hemispheric asymmetry in the processing of spectral and temporal information. Frequency (i.e. spectral information) may be processed in HG of the right hemisphere, while temporal information may be processed in the left hemisphere. Not all data, however, is consistent with this idea. Using MEG, Langner et al.[51] found that periodicity pitch and frequency are arranged orthogonally in the human auditory cortex, with no differences observed according to hemisphere.

The asymmetry observed in the tonotopic organization of the right and left auditory cortices could underlie hemispheric specialization and could account for a fair amount of behavioural data obtained in studies on human auditory function. Robin et al.[52] found that left temporoparietal lesions impair the perception of temporal but not spectral auditory information; lesions in homologous regions of the right hemisphere were found to have the opposite effect. The lesions referred to in their study affected only the associative auditory areas, but such lesions could also disconnect the primary cortex from the rest of the brain.[53,54] Taken together with these findings, the present study's results suggest that the frequency analysis of sounds corresponds to the neural sharpening for neurons tuned to frequency. This mechanism could be conferred on the right auditory cortex, which plays an important role in the processing of pitch.[26,55] Auditory neurons in the left hemisphere, on the other hand, have been shown to be more selective for temporal pattern[50] than for spectral pattern. Such data are consistent with the results from studies with language-disordered subjects who have left-hemispheric lesions, suggesting that many of these patients are also impaired in auditory temporal perception.[56]

In conclusion, these results suggest that the processing of spectral information is carried out primarily in the right hemisphere, and the processing of the temporal aspects of auditory stimuli in the left auditory cortex.[50] Future research in this direction could not only provide insight into the cortical processes underlying speech and music perception, but may also help us better understand the psychoacoustic sequelae of cortical lesions.

Acknowledgements

The authors are grateful to Drs B. Devaux (Ste. Anne Hospital, Paris), A. Musolino (Clinica Neurochirurgica, Messina, Italy), and J.M. Scarabin (Pontchaillou Hospital, Rennes) for their collaboration.

References

1. **Whitfield, I. C.** (1970) Central nervous processing in relation to spatio-temporal discrimination of auditory patterns. In R. Plomp and Smoorenburg (eds) *Frequency Analysis and Periodicity Detection in Hearing.* Leiden: Sijthoff, pp. 136–52.

2. **Shamma, S. A.** (1985) Speech processing in the auditory system II: lateral inhibition and the processing of speech evoked activity in the auditory nerve. *J. Acoust. Soc. Am.* 78, 1622–32.

3. **Shamma, S. A.** (1986) Encoding the acoustic spectrum in the spatio-temporal responses of the auditory nerve. In B. C. J. Moore and R. D. Patterson (eds) *Auditory Frequency Selectivity.* New York: Plenum, pp. 289–96.

4. **Langner, G.** (1997) Neural processing and representation of periodicity pitch. *Acta Otolaryngol.* (Stockh.) 532, 68–76.

5. **Langner, G.** (1998) Neuronal periodicity coding and pitch effects. In P. W. Poon and J. F. Brugge (eds) *Central Auditory Processing and Neural Modeling.* New York: Plenum, pp. 31–41.

6. **Palmer, A. R.** (1982) Encoding of rapid amplitude fluctuations by cochlear nerve fibers in the guinea pig. *Acta Otolaryngol.* (Stockh.) 236, 197–202.

7. **Schreiner, C. E. and G. Langner** (1984) Representation of periodicity information in the inferior colliculus of the cat. *Abstr. Soc. Neurosci.* 10, 395.

8. **Langner, G. and C. E. Schreiner** (1988) Periodicity coding in the inferior colliculus in the cat. I: neuronal mechanisms. *J. Neurophysiol.* 60, 1799–822.

9. **Goldstein, M. H., F. De Ribaupierre, and G. H. Yeni-Komoshian** (1971) Cortical coding of periodicity pitch. In M. B. Sach (ed.) *Physiology of the Auditory System.* Baltimore, MD: National Education Consultants, pp. 299–306.

10. **Ribaupierre, F. De, M. H. Goldstein, and G. H. Yeni-Komoshian** (1972) Cortical coding of repetitive acoustic pulses. *Brain Res.* 48, 205–25.

11. **Goldstein, M. H., M. Abeles, M. R. Daly, and J. McIntosh** (1970) Functional architecture in cat primary auditory cortex: tonotopic organization. *J. Neurophysiol.* 33, 188–97.

12. **Merzenich, M. M. and J. F. Brugge** (1973) Representation of the cochlear partition on the superior temporal plane of the macaque monkey. *Brain Res.* 50, 275–96.

13. **Merzenich, M. M., P. L. Knight, and G. L. Roth** (1975) Representation of cochlea within primary auditory cortex in the cat. *J. Neurophysiol.* 38, 231–49.

14. **Merzenich, M. M., J. H. Kaas, and G. L. Roth** (1976) Auditory cortex in the grey squirrel: tonotopic organization and architectonic fields. *J. Comp. Neurol.* 166, 387–402.

15. **Phillips, D. P. and D. R. F. Irvin** (1981) Responses of single neurons in physiologically defined primary auditory cortex (A1) of the cat: frequency tuning and responses to intensity. *J. Neurophysiol.* 45, 16–34.

16. **Reale, R. A. and T. J. Imig** (1980) Tonotopic organization in auditory cortex of the cat. *J. Comp. Neurol.* 291, 192–265.

17. **Phillips, D. P. and S. S. Orman** (1984) Responses of single neurons in posterior field of cat auditory cortex to tonal stimulation. *J. Neurophysiol.* 51, 147–63.

18. **Sally, S. L. and J. K. Kelly** (1988) Organization of auditory cortex in the albino rat: sound frequency. *J. Neurophysiol.* 59, 1627–38.

19. **Lauter, J. L., P. Herscovitch, *et al.*** (1975) Tonotopic organization in human auditory cortex revealed by positron emission tomography. *Hear. Res.* 20, 199–205.

20. **Romani, G. L., S. J. Williamson, and L. Kaufman** (1982) Tonotopic organization of the human auditory cortex. *Science* 216, 1339–40.

21. **Pantev, C., M. Hoke, K. Lehnertz, *et al.*** (1988) Tonotopic organization of the human auditory cortex revealed by transient auditory evoked magnetic fields. *EEG Clin. Neurophysiol.* 69 160–70.

22. **Pantev, C., M. Hoke, K. Lehnertz, *et al.*** (1990) Identification of sources of brain neuronal activity with high spatiotemporal resolution through combination of neuromagnetic source localization (NMSL) and magnetic resonance imaging (MRI). *EEG Clin. Neurophysiol.* 75, 173–84.

23. Pantev, C., O. Bertrand, C. Eulitz, *et al.* (1995) Specific tonotopic organizations of different areas of the human auditory cortex revealed by simultaneous magnetic and electric recordings. *EEG Clin. Neurophysiol.* 94, 26–41.

24. Cansino, S., S. J. Williamson, and D. Karron (1994) Tonotopic organization of human auditory association cortex. *Brain Res.* 663, 38–50.

25. Liegeois-Chauvel, C., A. Musolino, J. M. Badier, P. Marquis, and P. Chauvel (1994) Evoked potentials recorded from the auditory cortex in human: evaluation and topography of the middle latency components. *EEG Clin. Neurophysiol.* 92, 204–14.

26. Zatorre, R. J., A. C. Evans, *et al.* (1992) Lateralization of phonetic and pitch discrimination in speech processing. *Science* 256, 846–9.

27. Bancaud, J., J. Talairach, *et al.* (1965) *La stéréoélectroencephalographie dans l'epilepsie: informations neurophysiopathologiques apportées par l'investigation fonctionnelle stéréotaxique.* Paris: Masson.

28. Bancaud, J., F. Brunet-Bourgin, P. Chauvel, *et al.* (1994) Anatomical origin of *déjà vu* and vivid 'memories' in human temporal lobe epilepsy. *Brain* 117, 71–90.

29. Szikla, G., G. Bouvier, T. Hori, and V. Petrov (1977) Angiography of the human brain cortex. In *Atlas of Vascular Patterns and Stereotactic Cortical Localization.* Berlin: Springer Verlag.

30. Musolino, A., J. Talairach, P. Tournoux, and O. Missir (1988) Comparative study between stereotactic angiography and magnetic resonance imaging (MRI) data on spatial organization of sulci and convolutions in man. Boll. *Lega Italiana contro Epilessia* 62/63, 51–6.

31. Musolino, A., P. Tournoux, O. Missir, and J. Talairach (1990) Methodology of *in vivo* anatomical study and stereo-electroencephalographic exploration in brain surgery for epilepsy. *J. Neuroradiol.* 17, 67–102.

32. Liegeois-Chauvel, C., A. Musolino, and P. Chauvel (1991) Localization of primary auditory area in man. *Brain* 114, 139–53.

33. Steinmetz, H., J. Rademacher, *et al.* (1989) Cerebral asymmetry: Mr planimetry of the human planum temporale. *J. Comput. Assist. Tomogr.* 13, 996–1005.

34. Remond, A. (1961) Integrated and topological analysis of the EEG *Clin. Neurophysiol.* 20 (Suppl.), 64–7.

35. Chauvel, P., P. Buser, J. M. Badier, *et al.* (1987) La 'zone épileptogène' chez l'homme: représentation des évènements intercritiques par cartes spatio-temporelles. *Rev. Neurol.* (Paris) 143(5), 443–50.

36. Badier, J. M. (1991) Etude de la localisation des sources cérébrales d'activité paroxystique par cartographie. Thèse de Doctorat. Université de technologie de Compiègne. Bertrand *et al.*

37. Braak, H. (1978) *Architectonics of the Human Telencephalic Cortex.* Berlin: Springer Verlag.

38. Galaburda, A. M. and F. Sanides (1980) Cytoarchitectonic organization of the human auditory cortex. *J. Comp. Neurol.* 190, 597–610.

39. Bertrand, O., F. Perrin, and J. Pernier (1971) Evidence for a tonotopic organization of the auditory cortex observed with auditory evoked potentials. *Acta Otolaryngol.* (Stockh.) 491 (Suppl.), 116–23.

40. Schreiner, C. E. and J. R. Mendelson (1990) Functional topography of cat primary auditory cortex: distribution of integrated excitation. *J. Neurophysiol.* 64, 1442–59.

41. Imig, T. J., M. A. Ruggero, L. M. Kitzes *et al.* (1977) Organization of auditory cortex in the owl monkey. *J. Comp. Neurol.* 171, 111–28.

42. Aitkin, L. M., M. M. Merzenich, D. R. F. Irvine, *et al.* (1986) Frequency representation in auditory cortex of the common marmoset. *J. Comp. Neurol.* 252, 175–85.

43. Imig, T. J. and R. A. Reale (1980) Patterns of cortico-cortical connections related to tonotopic maps in cat auditory cortex. *J. Comp. Neurol.* 192, 293–332.

44. Luethke, L. E., L. A. Krubitzer and J. H. Kaas (1988) Cortical connections of electro-physiologically and architectonically defined subdivisions of auditory cortex in squirrels. *J. Comp. Neurol.* 268, 181–203.

45. Reite, M., P. Teale, J. Zimmerman, *et al.* (1988) Source location of a 50 Msec latency auditory evoked field component. *EEG Clin. Neurophysiol.* 70, 490–98.

46. Makela, J. P., M. Hamalainen, R. Hari, and L. McEvoy (1994) Whole-head mapping of middle-latency auditory evoked magnetic field. *EEG Clin. Neurophysiol.* 92, 414–22.

47. Schreiner, C. E. and M. S. Cynader (1984) Basic functional organization of second auditory cortical field (AII) of the cat. *J. Neurophysiol.* 51, 1284–305.

48. Goldstein, M. H., J. L. Hall, and B. O. Butterfield (1968) Single unit activity in the primary auditory cortex of unanesthetized cats. *J. Acoust. Soc. Am.* 43, 444–55.

49. Rauschecker, J. P., B. Tian, *et al.* (1997) Serial and parallel processing in rhesus monkey auditory cortex. *Science* 268, 111–14.

50. Liegeois-Chauvel, C., J. De Graaf, V. Laguitton, *et al.* (1999) Specialization of left auditory cortex for speech perception in man depends on temporal coding. *Cereb. Cortex* 9, 484–96.

51. Langner, G., M. Sams, *et al.* (1997) Frequency and periodicity are represented in orthogonal maps in the human auditory cortex evidence from magnetoencephalography. *J. Comp. Physiol.* 181 (6), 665–76.

52. Robin, D. A., D. Tranel, and H. Damasio (1990) Auditory perception of temporal and spectral events in patients with focal left and right cerebral lesions. *Brain Lang.* 39, 539–55.

53. Pandya, D. N. and H. G. J. M. Kuypers (1969) Cortico-cortical connections in the rhesus monkey. *Brain Res.* 13, 13–36.

54. Pandya, D. N. and B. Seltzer (1982) Association areas of the cerebral cortex. *Trends Neurosci.* 5, 386–90.

55. Zatorre, R. J. (1988) Pitch perception of complex tones and human temporal-lobe function. *J. Acoust. Soc. Am.* 84, 566–72.

56. Tallal, P. and P. Newcombe (1978) Impairment of auditory perception and language comprehension in dysphasia. *Brain Lang.* 5, 137–52.

CHAPTER 11

THE NEURAL PROCESSING OF COMPLEX SOUNDS

TIMOTHY D. GRIFFITHS

Abstract

This chapter considers the temporal processing of complex sounds relevant to musical analysis. Functional imaging studies, using positron emission tomography (PET), functional magnetic resonance imaging (fMRI), and magnetoencephalography (MEG), and the psychophysical assessment of patients with lesions allow two different approaches to this. Functional imaging allows the determination of structures *normally involved* in temporal analysis, while patient studies allow inference about the *necessary* structures for temporal analysis. Both approaches suggest a hierarchal organization in the brain corresponding to the processing of music. The features of individual notes are analyzed in the pathway up to and including the auditory cortices, while higher-order patterns formed by those features are analyzed by distributed networks in the temporal lobe and frontal lobes distinct from the auditory cortices.

Keywords: Neural processing; Complex sounds; Musical analysis; Functional imaging

Introduction

This chapter might have been called 'The Neural Processing of Complex Sound *Features*'. *All* sound is processed by mechanisms for the analysis of simple acoustic features (intensity, frequency, onset), complex acoustic features (such as patterns of these simple features as a function of time), and semantic features (learned association of sound patterns and meanings). Here, I concentrate on the analysis of complex features likely to be important in musical analysis, below the level of semantic and affective processing. Such analysis is represented in the middle box in Figure 11.1.

For the analysis of music, analysis of temporal features is likely to be particularly important, although I would certainly not dismiss the role of spectral or spatial analysis. Temporal analysis can be considered at different levels that I will call fine temporal structure and higher-order temporal structure. Such a categorical distinction works well for music as a sound with a highly segmented structure. Fine temporal structure corresponds to temporal structure at the level of milliseconds or tens of milliseconds; this is a 'window' for the processing of the temporal regularity within individual notes that is relevant to complex pitch perception (see Refs 1 and 2 for discussion of mechanisms of pitch perception). Higher-order temporal structure corresponds to temporal structure at the level of patterns of the pitch, onset time, or duration of notes. This corresponds to a 'window' at

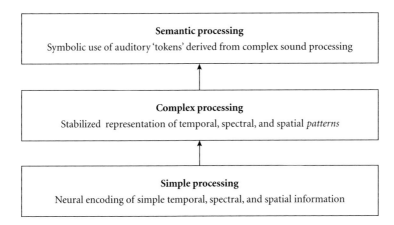

Figure 11.1 Modular representation of complex sound perception relevant to music.

the level of hundreds of milliseconds or seconds. Higher-order structure might itself be subdivided into 'local patterns' (e.g. single intervals) and 'global patterns' (e.g. contour) as used by Peretz and others.[3,4] For present purposes, higher-order structure simply means any structure formed by patterns of the features in individual notes. This categorical distinction of temporal structure is convenient when considering processing relevant to music. This is not the only way of considering the temporal processing of sound. In particular, I would point out approaches based on the modulation transfer function. Here, responses to modulation of the sound amplitude or frequency are considered as *continuous* functions of modulation rate. This approach has been used in human psychophysical work,[5–8] evoked-potential work,[9,10] and functional imaging work.[11,12]

In the human auditory system much work on mechanisms of temporal processing, particularly in the case of music, has focused on the auditory cortex and cortical networks involving the auditory cortices. However, the ascending auditory pathway (Figure 11.2) affords an extensive mechanism for the processing of complex signals before the cortex is reached. Subcortical mechanisms for the processing of temporally complex sound in the form of continuous modulation have been investigated in animals[13–15] and in man.[11] Little work has been carried out on the processing of segmented sound closer to music in the ascending pathway, especially in man. Because of the extensive cross-connections in the auditory pathway, bilateral lesions of the ascending pathway are needed to produce temporal deficits. Such lesions are rarely compatible with life, but do occur, for example, in multiple sclerosis.[16] Imaging of human auditory brain stem processing is technically limited in functional imaging techniques, including PET, fMRI, and MEG. I point this out primarily to declare an open mind about the existence of ascending processing systems for sound sequences such as music. The concentration in this chapter on cortical mechanisms simply reflects a lack of data, rather than any a priori limitation on such processing in the ascending pathway. Another area of future interest is cortical 'molding' of auditory processing in the ascending pathway that has been demonstrated in other species such as the bat.[17]

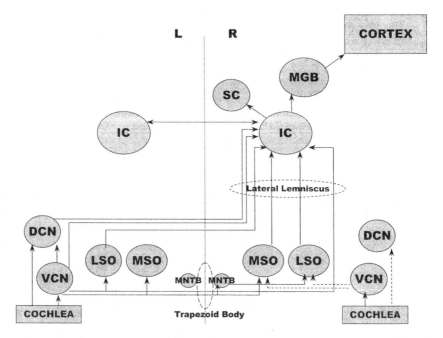

Figure 11.2 Simplified representation of ascending auditory pathway to the auditory cortex. This is based on animal and human studies (e.g. Refs 18 and 34) and demonstrates extensive processing of auditory information before the cortex is reached. For clarity, only the convergence of the input from both ears at the right-sided brain stem auditory nucleii is shown. A dorsal pathway, via the dorsal cochlear nucleus (DCN) and inferior colliculus (IC) is shown, which is involved in animals in the analysis of spectrally complex waveforms. The diagram also shows a ventral pathway, via the ventral cochlear nucleus (VCN), trapezoid body, and medial superior olive (MSO), thought to be important in animals for the analysis of spatial information. LSO = lateral superior olive, MNTB = medial nucleus of the trapezoid body, MGB = medial geniculate body, SC = superior colliculus.

The human auditory system[18] also contains a rich descending system that could mold behaviourally significant sounds such as music.

This chapter considers temporal processing in humans relevant to musical processing. I will consider functional imaging (using PET, fMRI, and MEG) and the psychophysical assessment of patients with lesions. Functional imaging allows the determination of structures *normally involved* in temporal analysis, and patient studies allow inference about the *necessary* structures for temporal analysis. For discussion of the extension of this approach above the level of acoustic pattern analysis, I refer the reader to Chapter 16 by Zatorre in this volume.

Lesion studies

Fine temporal structure

There have been a number of studies suggesting that the detection of sounds of different frequencies (as measured in the routine pure tone audiogram) depends on an intact ascending auditory pathway to at least one of the auditory cortices. The rare condition of cortical deafness occurs following lesions to both superior temporal lobes (see Ref. 19 for review). The perception of pitch, as opposed to the detection of a pure tone at a given frequency, has been investigated using complex stimuli where the pitch is not immediately determined by the spectral characteristics of the sound. Zatorre[20] used a stimulus where the pitch is determined by the 'missing fundamental' of the spectral representation. The stimulus in this experiment, considered in the frequency domain, is a harmonic series where the lower harmonics including the fundamental stimulus are removed. The pitch of this stimulus is determined by the missing fundamental, against the idea that for a pitch to be heard there needs to be a representation of that pitch in the stimulus spectrum. The determination of pitch by any frequency domain model requires a form of template fitting;[21] the spectrum still contains harmonics that are *spaced* by an amount equal to the fundamental frequency. Alternatively, the pitch of this stimulus might be explained by temporal domain models; the waveform of this stimulus has a periodicity equal to the reciprocal of the fundamental, both before and after removal of the lower harmonics. Using the missing fundamental stimulus Zatorre investigated the perception of this complex pitch in subjects with well-characterized lesions affecting the superior temporal lobes. Subjects with right lesions involving the primary auditory cortex had deficits in perception of this pitch, but not subjects with right superior temporal lobe lesions sparing the primary auditory cortex, or subjects with lesions of the left primary auditory cortex. This suggests a particular involvement of the right primary auditory cortex in complex pitch perception.

Patterson, Yost, and others have developed stimuli containing regular intervals where the pitch properties are most parsimoniously explained by the fine temporal rather than the spectral characteristics of the sound.[22,23] Of course, both characteristics are interchangeable at the stimulus level, but these stimuli are manipulated in such a way that spectral template models are difficult to apply because of the filtering properties of the auditory system. Iterated rippled noise (IRN) is one such type of regular interval sound produced by taking bandpass noise and adding it to itself in a delay-and-add cycle. With increasing delay-and-add cycles (or gain in each cycle) the stimulus becomes more regular, as shown by the increasing first peak in the autocorrelation spectrum. In parallel with this temporal change, a pitch emerges from the noise with a signal-to-noise ratio that parallels the degree of temporal regularity of the auditory signal. In contrast, the spectrum of the auditory signal retains its bandpass properties. It is therefore easier to infer in the case of this signal (than for the missing fundamental) that changes in perceived properties are due to the fine temporal structure rather than the spectral structure in the auditory signal (see Ref. 2 for more detailed discussion). Using this stimulus I investigated one of Peretz's patients, I.R., with apperceptive amusia following bilateral temporal lobe lesions[24] (see Chapter 13 by Peretz, this volume, for further discussion of amusia). This patient has normal appreciation of pitch but is unable to perceive musical sequences. She has an intact pathway up to and including the right primary auditory cortex, but effective 'isolation' of that cortex from other areas of cortex that are lesioned. Testing this patient with IRN showed that she had a normal threshold for the detection of this stimulus presented to both ears. Testing each ear separately with contralateral masking noise showed that her normal performance was entirely accounted for by the performance at the left ear, the predominant input to the intact right auditory cortex.

Taken together these two studies are consistent with the pathway up to and including the primary auditory cortex being a necessary and sufficient substrate for the perception of complex pitch. I have discussed these studies under the heading fine temporal structure; both studies can be interpreted in terms of a need for primary cortex (particularly on the right) to perceive fine temporal structure, but the missing fundamental work is equally consistent with a spectral template model. These data would be consistent with activity of the human primary cortex being a neural correlate of the conscious perception of complex pitch.[25] Such processing is important for the perception of the pitch of the individual notes produced by most musical instruments.

Higher-order temporal structure

Lesion studies can also allow inference about the detection of higher-order temporal patterns of segmented sounds, including music. A number of studies have looked at very simple tests of segmented sound processing in patients with auditory agnosias including amusia (see Ref. 19 for review). The tests used include gap detection and click-fusion threshold. Many studies have shown deficits, and been interpreted in terms of a temporal processing deficit, but conventional gap detection paradigms are confounded by the presence of spectral artifact in the stimulus (this is overcome in more refined paradigms such as those developed by Phillips[26]). Many of the patients in these studies had large bilateral lesions involving the superior temporal cortices, consistent with a role for the secondary and association areas of auditory cortex in this region being needed for the perception of this type of temporal pattern.

A deficiency in the evaluation of patients with auditory agnosia is the lack of a systematic battery of tests of sound sequence processing above the level of gap detection but below the level of actual musical sequences. Such a battery would have the potential to demonstrate 'generic' sound sequence mechanisms that might be relevant to a number of different sound processing disorders without higher-level confounds. A crude test of sequence discrimination in a patient, H.V., with amusia[27] suggested a loss of the perception of *rapid* but not slow sequences. This paralleled the phenomenology in a patient who had lost the ability to recognize and enjoy music with a high tempo. That patient had a unilateral lesion affecting the posterior superior temporal lobe and inferior parietal lobe, and the deficit in his case was less profound than in other cases reported following bilateral lesions.

Auditory agnosia can also be studied by a parallel approach based on the modulation transfer function as discussed earlier. In terms of the temporal 'window', the level of higher-order structure for patterns of notes (hundreds of milliseconds or seconds) parallels the level of low modulation rates (of tens of Hz or less). The patient with mild amusia discussed above (H.V.[27]) had a mild deficit in the detection of sinusoidal frequency modulation (FM) and amplitude modulation (AM) at a rate of 2 Hz. The dissociation between this and his profound deficit in the discrimination of rapid sequences of segmented sound was striking, and cautions against any universal approach in these patients based on modulation characterization. In contrast, the patient I.R., with a more marked amusia due to bilateral lesions, had a striking deficit in the detection of both AM and FM, particularly at low modulation rates (her threshold for 2-Hz sinusoidal AM was 11 times normal). Apart from demonstrating auditory deficits linked to the phenomenology, her case allows the inference that a single intact pathway to the right auditory cortex is not a sufficient substrate for the normal perception of modulation. The presence of normal processing of IRN by I.R. provides an important control to allow the exclusion of other possible causes of the deficit. The IRN task demanded similar attention and working memory for simple acoustic features using a similar two-alternative forced-choice paradigm. The presence of such dissociated deficits is critical to these studies,[28] and studies showing a general deficit in performance in a range of tasks do not allow such interpretation in terms of distinct perceptual processes.

In terms of the psychophysical examination of higher-order temporal processing in subjects with lesions, these studies suggest that the deficits are produced by temporal lobe lesions that involve superior temporal lobe areas beyond the primary auditory cortex. Additionally, subject I.R. has a large right frontal lesion implicating this area in the perception of sound sequences and low-rate modulation. More studies of such patients using detailed modern structural imaging and systematic psychoacoustic testing will characterize the necessary structures for higher-order temporal processing. Such studies will never be supplanted by functional imaging, from which *sufficient* processing mechanisms cannot be immediately inferred.

Functional imaging

Fine temporal structure

The missing fundamental stimulus has been used in MEG experiments[29,30] where a mapping of perceived pitch has been demonstrated. For reasons discussed above, this map cannot be interpreted unambiguously in terms of the temporal structure of the stimulus, as template models could also explain the perceived pitch. But the mapping of perceived complex pitch to auditory cortex, derived by whatever means, is convergent with the lesion data discussed above. In the study of Langner, distinct representations of the frequency and temporal domains were suggested, with different orientations in the superior temporal planum. This would allow extensive processing in auditory cortex of spectrotemporal properties such as pitch as well as spectral (timbre) and temporal (attack) instrument characteristics. These are all features of individual notes.

IRN has also been used in functional imaging experiments, with the aim of identifying brain areas where the brain activity varies as a function of the fine temporal regularity of the stimulus.[2] In an initial study with PET in collaboration with Patterson, such a relationship was demonstrated in both auditory cortices. On the right, a region of activation was demonstrated in the medial part of Heschl's gyrus, containing the primary auditory cortex. On the left, the activation was situated more laterally and may correspond to secondary auditory cortex; these asymmetries are of interest in view of the lesion data suggesting a particular involvement of the right primary auditory cortex in the processing of temporal regularity. The activity shown in the PET study was argued to correspond to neural activity occurring after temporal regularity is converted into a more stable code in the ascending pathway, a process called temporal integration. The study is critically dependent on this assumption, but not on the exact mechanism by which such temporal regularity is stabilized, the simplest possibility being based on autocorrelation as mentioned above.

Models for this temporal integration mechanism[31] allow it to occur at an early stage in the auditory pathway, perhaps as early as the cochlear nucleus, and ongoing work is being carried out with fMRI to further delimit it to brain stem structures.

The work using IRN therefore also supports the existence of a representation of temporal regularity in the auditory cortex, with closer control of the auditory spectrum than in the case of the missing fundamental.

Higher-order temporal structure

In the IRN experiment,[2] higher-order structure was also investigated. The individual notes with pitches determined by temporal regularity were presented as two pitch patterns: as a regular pitch 'staircase' and as novel diatonic melodies. We hypothesized that areas involved in the analysis of sound sequences would show greater activation as a function of the pitch strength of the individual notes for the melody condition than for the staircase condition. Sound sequence analysis represents an emergent property of the detection of the pitch of individual sounds, and areas involved in sequence analysis will show a more marked dependence on pitch strength for more complex pitch sequences like the melody condition. This was demonstrated in four areas, distinct from the primary auditory cortex, in both anterior temporal lobes near the poles and in the posterior superior temporal lobes. These areas are shown in Figure 11.3. A scheme is hypothesized, consistent with the data, where the temporal properties of the individual notes are extracted in the region of the primary auditory cortex before higher-order temporal properties of the stimulus sequence are analysed in the distinct network shown in Figure 11.3.

A subsequent study used PET to demonstrate areas involved in the processing of simple sequences that are not musical.[32] Here, simple six-element atonal sequences were presented to nonmusical subjects in order to demonstrate areas involved in the analysis of both pitch sequences and sequences of notes of different duration. Pairs of sequences were presented to subjects where either the pitch sequence, the duration sequence, neither, or both were varied between the two. During any scan, subjects were required to detect either changes in pitch sequence or duration sequence. The results showed, again, a network of activation distinct from the primary auditory cortex (in addition to activation in the primary auditory cortex in the principal comparison between the sound conditions and rest). Bilateral activation was demonstrated in the posterior superior temporal planum in the region of the planum temporale, and in both frontal opercula, with greater spatial extent of the clusters of activity demonstrated on the right. Highly significant activation was also demonstrated in both lobes of the cerebellum. The activation during the pitch sequence and duration sequence tasks was strikingly similar, and direct comparison of the two conditions showed no significant differences in activation. This would be consistent with a common mechanism for the two tasks at some level, consistent with some work in the musical domain.

These studies using 'submusical' stimuli, therefore, suggest the existence of networks for processing of higher-order structure in both temporal lobes that are distinct from the primary auditory cortices. The planum temporale is consistently activated in a number of studies, with less consistency in activation anterior to the primary auditory cortex. Activation anterior to the auditory cortex occurs in the anterior temporal lobe in the IRN

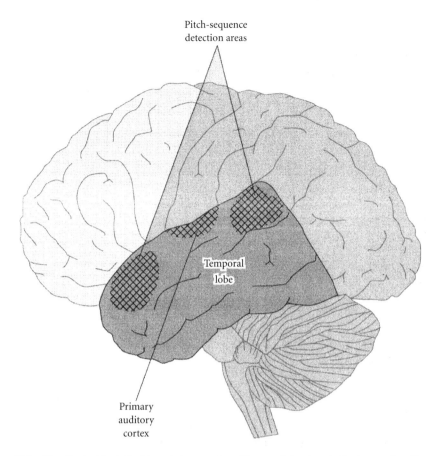

Pitch-sequence
detection areas

Temporal
lobe

Primary
auditory
cortex

Figure 11.3 Hypothesized basis for hierarchal processing of temporal structure in the temporal cortices suggested by the experiment using iterated rippled noise. The temporal structure within individual notes is processed in the pathway up to and including the primary auditory cortex, while pitch sequences are processed in the distinct areas shown. (Artist: © 1998, Bob Crimi. Reprinted with permission.)

study and frontal opercula in a number of other studies. The patterns of activation shown are similar to those demonstrated by studies using actual musical stimuli[33] (see also Chapter 16 by Zatorre, this volume), but show less striking lateralization. This suggests the possibility that the imposition of higher levels of cognitive processing in more musical studies contributes to the lateralization during musical processing.

Conclusion

Both studies of humans with brain lesions and functional imaging provide convergent evidence for the existence of a neural substrate for the processing of sound sequences that is hierarchal in organization. The pathway up to and including the primary auditory cortices may provide a sufficient mechanism for the processing of spectrotemporal features of individual sounds. Subsequent processing of higher-order temporal patterns formed by those individual sounds depends on processing in bilateral temperofrontal networks. These networks provide a first stage in the neural processing of music. Outstanding issues relate to the relationship between the elements of these networks and the perceptual attributes of the stimulus, the type of subject, and the type of task, to name but three.

References

1. Hartmann, W. M. (1997) *Signals, Sound, and Sensation*. New York: American Institute of Physics Press.
2. Griffiths, T. D., C. Buechel, R. S. J. Frackowiak, *et al.* (1998) Analysis of temporal structure in sound by the human brain. *Nat. Neurosci.* 1, 421–7.
3. Peretz, I. (1990) Processing of local and global musical information by unilateral brain-damaged patients. *Brain* 113, 1185–205.
4. Liegeois-Chauvel, C., I. Peretz, M. Babai, *et al.* (1998) Contribution of different cortical areas in the temporal lobes to music processing. *Brain* 121, 1853–67.
5. Zwicker, E. (1952) Die Grenzen der Horbarkeit der Ampiltudenmodulation und der Frequenzmodulation eines Tones. *Acustica Akust. Beih.* 3, 125–33.
6. Kay, R. (1982) Hearing of modulation in sounds. *Physiol. Rev.* 62, 894–975.
7. Moore, B. C. J. and A. Sek (1995) Effects of carrier frequency, modulation rate, and modulation waveform on the detection of modulation and the discrimination of modulation type (amplitude modulation versus frequency modulation). *J. Acoust. Soc. Am.* 97, 2468–78.
8. Wojczak, M. and N. F. Viemeister (1999) *Adaptation Produced by Amplitude Modulation. Abstr. 59.* St. Petersburg, FL: Association for Research in Otolaryngology.
9. Rees, A., G. G. R. Green, and R. H. Kay (1986) Steady-state evoked responses to sinusoidally amplitude-modulated sounds recorded in man. *Hear. Res.* 23, 123–33.
10. Stefanatos, G. A., G. G. R. Green, and G. G. Ratcliff (1989) Neurophysiological evidence of auditory channel anomalies in developmental dysphasia. *Arch. Neurol.* 46, 871–5.
11. Harms, M. P., J. R. Melcher, and R. Weisskoff (1998) Time courses of fMRI signals in the inferior colliculus, medial geniculate body, and auditory cortex show different dependencies on noise burst rate [abstract]. *Neuroimage* 7, S365.
12. Giraud, A. L., C. Lorenzi, J. Wable, *et al.* (1999) Temporal envelope representation in the human auditory cortex [abstract]. *Neuroimage* 9, S787.
13. Moller, A. R. (1974) Response of units in the cochlear nucleus to sinusoidally amplitude modulated tones. *Exp. Neurol.* 45, 104–17.
14. Rees, A. and A. R. Moller (1983) Responses of neurons in the inferior colliculus of the rat to AM and FM tones. *Hear. Res.* 10, 301–30.
15. Langner, G. and C. E. Schreiner (1988) Periodicity coding in the inferior colliculus of the cat. I. Neuronal mechanisms. *J. Neurophysiol.* 60, 1799–822.
16. Quine, D. B., D. Regan, K. I. Beverly, *et al.* (1984) Patients with multiple sclerosis experience hearing loss for shifts of tone frequency. *Arch. Neurol.* 41, 506–7.
17. Yan, W. and N. Suga (1998) Corticofugal modulation of the midbrain frequency map in the bat auditory system. *Nat. Neurosci.* 1, 54–85.

18. **Moore, J. K.** (1994) The human brainstem auditory pathway. In R. K. Jackier and D. E. Brackmann (eds) *Neurotology*. St. Louis, MO: Mosby, pp. 1–17.

19. **Griffiths, T. D., A. Rees,** and **G. G. R. Green** (1999) Disorders of human complex sound processing. *Neurocase* 5, 365–78.

20. **Zatorre, R.** (1988) Pitch perception of complex tones and human cerebral lobe function. *J. Acoust. Soc. Am.* 84, 566–72.

21. **Cohen, M. A., S. Grossberg,** and **L. Wyse** (1995) A spectral network model of pitch perception. *J. Acoust. Soc. Am.* 98, 862–79.

22. **Patterson, R. D., S. Handel, W. A. Yost,** *et al.* (1996) The relative strength of the tone and the noise components in iterated rippled noise. *J. Acoust. Soc. Am.* 100, 3286–94.

23. **Yost, W. A., R. Patterson,** and **S. Sheft** (1996) A time domain description for the pitch strength of iterated rippled noise. *J. Acoust. Soc. Am.* 99, 1066–78.

24. **Griffiths, T. D., V. Penhune, I. Peretz,** *et al.* (2000) Frontal processing and auditory perception. *NeuroReport* 11, 919–22.

25. **Frith, C., R. Perry,** and **E. Lumer** (1999) The neural correlates of conscious experience: an experimental framework. *Trends Cognit. Sci.* 3, 105–14.

26. **Phillips, D. P., T. L. Taylor, S. E. Hall,** *et al.* (1997) Detection of silent intervals between noises activating different perceptual channels: some properties of 'central' auditory gap detection. *J. Acoust. Soc. Am.* 101, 3694–705.

27. **Griffiths, T. D., A. Rees, C. Witton,** *et al.* (1997) Spatial and temporal auditory processing deficits following right hemisphere infarction: a psychophysical study. *Brain* 120, 785–94.

28. **Ellis, A.** and **A. W. Young** (1998) *Human Cognitive Neuropsychology*. Hove, Sussex, UK: Lawrence Erlbaum Associates.

29. **Pantev, C., M. Hoke, B. Lutkenhoner,** *et al.* (1989) Tonotopic organisation of the auditory cortex: pitch versus frequency representation. *Science* 242, 486–8.

30. **Langner, G., M. Sams, P. Heil,** *et al.* (1997) Frequency and periodicity are represented in orthogonal maps in the human auditory cortex: evidence from magnetoencephalography. *J. Comp. Physiol.* 181, 665–76.

31. **Patterson, R. D., M. H. Allerhand,** and **C. Giguerre** (1995) Time-domain modeling of peripheral auditory processing: a modular architecture and a software platform. *J. Acoust. Soc. Am.* 98, 1890–4.

32. **Griffiths, T. D., I. Johnsrude, J. L. Dean,** *et al.* (1999) A common neural substrate for the analysis of pitch and duration pattern in segmented sound? *Neuroreport* 18, 3825–30.

33. **Zatorre, R. J., A. C. Evans,** and **E. Meyer** (1994) Neural mechanisms underlying melodic perception and memory for pitch. *J. Neurosci.* 14, 1908–19.

34. **Irvine, D. R. F.** (1986) *The Auditory Brainstem. A Review of the Structure and Function of the Auditory Brainstem Processing Mechanisms.* Berlin: Springer-Verlag.

PART IV

MUSICAL BRAIN SUBSTRATES

CHAPTER 12

MUSIC AND THE NEUROLOGIST: A HISTORICAL PERSPECTIVE

JOHN C. M. BRUST

Abstract

Neurological disorders affecting musical function can produce either positive or negative symptoms. Positive phenomena include musicogenic epilepsy (seizures triggered by music), musical partial seizures (hallucinated music as the expression of the seizure), musical release hallucinations (nonepileptic musical hallucinations, usually associated with impaired hearing), and synesthesia (hallucinated colors triggered by musical tones). Negative phenomena comprise the amusias, which can be receptive, expressive, or both, and can selectively involve particular components of musical processing, including pitch, interval, contour, rhythm, meter, timbre, and emotional response. Amusia is often accompanied by aphasia, but each can occur in the absence of the other. Neurological disorders provide evidence that musical processing is multimodal and widely distributed in both cerebral hemispheres.

Keywords: Musicogenic seizures; Musical partial seizures; Release hallucinations; Amusia; Aphasia

Introduction

In nearly all right-handed people the left cerebral hemisphere is 'dominant' for propositional or analytic processing (exemplified by language), whereas the right hemisphere is more responsible for appositional or gestalt processing (exemplified by spatial manipulation and aspects of emotional expression or response). How the brain processes music has intrigued neurologists and psychologists for over a century. A straightforward answer would not be expected, for the components of music—for example, pitch, timbre, duration, loudness, and rhythm—are likely processed through separate circuits. Music can be both linear (e.g. melody) and nonlinear (e.g. chords), and different kinds of music make different intellectual and emotional demands on different kinds of listeners or performers.

The biological survival value of music remains an enigma. Darwin believed that musical 'calling systems' evolved into speech,[1] whereas Herbert Spencer believed that music evolved as a stylized form of speech.[2] Steven Pinker notes, 'Of [all] mental faculties . . . music . . . shows the clearest signs of not being [adaptive]',[3] yet in all cultures most people enjoy music. On the other hand, it takes severe mental retardation to prevent language acquisition, whereas musical aptitude ranges from tone deafness to Mozartian genius independently of other measures of intelligence.[4] Estimates of absolute pitch in the general population range from 1 in 1500 to 1 in 10,000.[5]

Clues as to how the brain processes music come from clinical case reports of patients with deranged musical function, from psychological testing of either normal or brain-damaged subjects, and, more recently, from studies using functional imaging (positron emission tomography [PET] and functional magnetic resonance imaging [fMRI]). Neurological symptoms can be positive or negative. Positive phenomena include musicogenic epilepsy, musical partial seizures, musical release hallucinations, and synesthesia. Negative phenomena include the amusias.

Positive phenomena

Musicogenic seizures are triggered by hearing music. Attacks typically begin with subjective distress, agitation, tachycardia, and tachypnea and may or may not generalize to grand mal. Victims are often musically talented but do not have to be. The stimulus can be quite specific—for example, classical vs popular music, or a particular piece. Reported triggers include the second movement of Beethoven's Symphony No. 5 and a sequence of church bells with a frequency range of less than one octave.[6,7] In one case seizures occurred only if the patient actively listened to the music. In another, seizures could be precipitated by background music of which the patient was barely aware. Seizures have been triggered by the voices of particular singers.[8] A two-year-old boy's seizures were precipitated by his own singing.[9] In another case seizures were triggered by playing 'Now Thank We All Our God' on the organ but not by hearing it, singing it, silently reading it, or silently playing the notes on the keyboard.[10] Lesions causing musicogenic epilepsy are usually in the temporal lobe, right more often than left.[11]

Musical partial seizures consist of hallucinated music, which can be of any type but tends to be stereotypic for a particular epileptic subject. Such patients are less likely than those with musicogenic epilepsy to be musically talented. In a reported series of 666 temporal lobe epileptics, 16 per cent had auditory hallucinations, the great majority of which were unformed (e.g. banging, ticking).[12] Formed hallucinations could be verbal, musical, or both. In a more detailed description of hallucinatory seizures precipitated by cortical electrical stimulation, subjective phenomena included a male chorus and orchestra singing 'White Christmas', a radio jingle, organ music, and an orchestra playing in a music hall, which was simultaneously visually hallucinated.[13] Seizures most predictably followed stimulation of the superior temporal gyrus, right more often than left. Interestingly, spoken words also followed either left or right hemispheric stimulation, and there was no topographical separation between areas precipitating voices and those precipitating music.

Visual or auditory hallucinations associated with impaired vision or deafness ('Charles Bonnet syndrome', release hallucinations) can consist of music; they most often affect elderly people with presbycusis. Neither dementia nor psychiatric disease need be present, and the hallucinations are often pleasurable rather than frightening or threatening. Some subjects sing along with the music, and some report that they can switch to another tune by consciously thinking about it. In some cases the pleasurable aspects of the music deteriorate over time, becoming distorted or too loud, or degenerating into tinnitus.[14,15] The pathophysiological basis of such hallucinations is uncertain; plausibly, reduced sensory input results in disinhibition of perception-bearing circuits, and perceptual traces are 'released'.

Synesthesia is an involuntary perception produced by stimulation of another sense. Thus, sounds produce the perception of colors. Geometric patters can occur, but more elaborate formed hallucinations do not. In some cases particular pitches produce the same colour; for example, C produced red, D green, and E blue in a boy with poor vision and musical talent (but not absolute pitch).[16] In addition to deafferentation, synesthesia is associated with hallucinogenic drug use (e.g. LSD) and, in one case, with a brain stem neoplasm. Many cases are idiopathic and noted in early childhood; some are familial. Women and left-handers are overrepresented, as are people who have difficulties with spatial relations.[17] Alexander Scriabin and Nicholai Rimsky-Korsakoff are believed to have had coloured-hearing synesthesia. The disorder, if it can be called that, is an example of unusually strong cross-modal association, but the physiological basis is otherwise unclear.

Negative phenomena: amusia and aphasia

Amusia is an acquired impairment of musical processing. As with aphasia—a comparable impairment of language—the problem can be expressive, receptive, or both, and the disorder cannot be explained by damage either to the articulatory apparatus or to primary receptor mechanisms. In other words, tongue paralysis is not expressive amusia, and deafness is not receptive amusia. Amusia and aphasia can occur together or each can occur in the absence of the other.

Since the nineteenth century, clinicians investigating the amusias have tended to adopt either a localizationist/anatomical or a holistic/psychological approach. Among the localizers, Henschen classified amusia as either motor or sensory and then identified 'centres' in the left cerebral hemisphere: singing resided in the pars triangularis of the third frontal convolution, musical reception in the temporal pole, note reading near the angular gyrus, and instrument playing at the foot of the second frontal convolution (with a separate centre for violinists).[18,19] Similarly, Kleist described motor and sensory amusia, each affecting either tone or melody. His anatomical localization included separate centers for singing and for whistling.[20]

Opposed to such rigid diagramming was Feuchtwanger, who considered music too complex to localize or even to restrict to one cerebral hemisphere.[21] Ustvedt noted the heterogeneity of amusic patients and the lack, in most reports, of premorbid baseline information or of standardized tests.[22] A review of such reports reveals that heterogeneity is indeed the rule and that the presence or absence of aphasia does not predict the type of amusia.

The first report of aphasia and relatively preserved musical ability was in 1745; the patient, who had right hemiparesis and speech limited to the word 'yes', could sing hymns if someone else sang along.[23] Similar cases include two children with nonfluent aphasia, one of whom could sing with words and the other without words;[24] a right-handed man with largely expressive aphasia following left hemispherectomy who could sing familiar songs with some errors in articulation but with little hesitation;[25] and a woman with transcortical aphasia (her verbal expression was limited to a few recurrent phrases, such as 'Hi, Daddy', but she had compulsively preserved speech repetition with echolalia) who could sing both old and newly taught songs.[26] Of 24 patients with Broca's aphasia and severely restricted speech output, 21 could sing (6 excellently), some sang only without words, some sang with paraphasic errors, and some needed help to get started.[27] A musically naïve patient with transcortical aphasia had hyperprosodic speech, whistled much of the time (including responses to questions), and listened to music much more often than before his illness.[28]

A professional pianist with Wernicke's aphasia, including alexia and agraphia for language, continued to play publicly; he could play unfamiliar melodies sung to him; reproduce heard chords; recognize dynamics, instruments, and intentional errors; and read a score nearly correctly.[29] A music professor with aphasia that included impaired speech comprehension and severe agraphia continued to write music.[30] The composer Shebalin developed Wernicke's aphasia with alexia and agraphia yet continued composing pieces 'which other musicians considered to be up to standard', including songs, quartets, choruses, and a symphony.[31] A conductor with global aphasia and ideomotor apraxia continued to conduct his orchestra.[32] A blind organist and composer who had written and read music in Braille developed Wernicke's aphasia and could no longer read or write language in Braille; yet he continued to read and write music in Braille.[33]

Cases of amusia plus aphasia are similarly diverse. A patient with anomia heard music as dissonant and voices, including his own, as too high pitched; he could neither sing nor reproduce rhythmic patterns.[34] Following surgery for a right frontal glioma, an accordionist had left hemiparesis and mild aphasia. Thereafter he sang 'wrong' and could no longer play his instrument (although he held it properly); he could correctly sing notes sung to him, but hearing them played on his accordion, he sang them a fourth too high or too low, and he could not imitate rhythm unless it was bound to a melody.[35] A violinist with absolute pitch had a stroke with right hemiparesis and Wernicke's aphasia, after which he had difficulty recognizing intervals, pitches, and rhythmic patterns; imitating heard rhythm; singing a melody previously unknown to him; and writing music spontaneously or to dictation.[36]

A man with probable Broca's aphasia was unable to identify popular songs or to sing melodies, but he could sing single tones and sequences without rhythm; rhythm recognition and production were completely lost whether presented visually, aurally, or tactilely.[37] A musician with primary progressive aphasia, unable any longer to read music, could improvise but did so repetitively and without completion; he could not write or copy music or reproduce rhythm, but he could reproduce fragments of melodies with a sense of meter.[38] A woman with computerized tomographic evidence of right perisylvian atrophy developed aprosodic speech and could not recognize the prosody (e.g. sad, glad, mad) of others; she could no longer sing even single notes or identify melodies, although she could tell which of two notes was higher, and she could read and write music.[39]

Maurice Ravel had progressive aphasia with alexia, agraphia, and ideomotor apraxia; 'musical thinking' was said to be intact—he recognized melodies and errors of rhythm and pitch and continued to listen to music critically—but he could no longer write or dictate music and thus could not compose the pieces he heard 'in his head'.[40,41] Following excision of a meningioma beneath the left temporal lobe, a young voice student had transcortical aphasia, alexia, and agraphia; she also had musical alexia and agraphia, yet she could still identify pitch, interval, melody, harmony, timbre, rhythm, and meter, and in a singing recital that included works in five languages, there were no apparent musical errors (although there may have been occasional paraphasic errors in the foreign languages).[42]

Cases of amusia without language disturbance are also heterogeneous; not surprisingly, in right-handers the lesions most often involve the right cerebral hemisphere. Reported symptoms include difficulty recognizing sounds as musical,[43] loss of a sense of rhythm,[44] hearing musical sounds 'out of tune',[45] and hearing both voices and music as monotonal.[46] Following a right temporoparietal infarct a man could no longer play the organ, yet other musical capabilities such as singing and imitating rhythm were intact ('expressive instrumental amusia').[47] Following a right temporal lobe infarct a man lost appreciation of timbre, including nonmusical sounds and people's voices; music sounded 'low and dull' with a kind of echo overlapping the sounds, and although he could recognize a guitar, a trumpet, or a drum, he could not recognize a violin, a piano, or an organ.[48]

A composer with right frontoparietotemporal infarction lost his emotional response to music and could no longer compose meaningfully; he could still compose serial music, '... but I have never been awed by the musical content of this style of composition'.[49] A man with a right temporoparietal vascular malformation had 'difficulty understanding the nuances of words and the inflections of sentences' and in understanding music; the relationship between a soloist and an accompanist became blurred, and there was a loss of aesthetic pleasure, yet there was no auditory agnosia, and he correctly recognized pitch, melody, timbre, harmony, and rhythm.[50]

A piano teacher with bilateral posterior cerebral atrophy of uncertain cause developed object-use apraxia and could no longer write or play the piano with two hands; her playing and singing were melodically disorganized and discontinuous, with poor rhythm and meter, and she read music note for note, with loss of 'global processing of pitch sequences'.[38] Following surgical clipping of bilateral middle cerebral artery aneurysms, a woman could no longer recognize or hum well-known tunes, and although she could tell if piano tones were the same or different, she could not tell if melodies were the same or different, whether melodic contour was preserved or violated, or whether a melody ended on the tonic or a nontonic; rhythm recognition and production were intact, however.[51]

Studies of brain-damaged populations

Studies involving groups of patients with either left or right cerebral hemispheric disruption have also been inconsistent. Subjects receiving right carotid artery amobarbital injection could not sing properly, with pitch more distorted than rhythm, but they recognized their errors and identified songs sung to them.[52] Patients who had undergone either left or right temporal lobectomy were studied using the Seashore Test of Musical Abilities, which measures discrimination of pitch, loudness, rhythm, duration, timbre, and tonal memory; right but not left lobectomy resulted in impaired recognition of timbre and tonal memory and a lesser degree of impairment involving pitch and rhythm.[53] A different testing instrument, the Musical Aptitude Profile, which involves tonal imagery (melody and harmony), rhythm (tempo and meter), and 'musical sensitivity' (phrasing, balance, and style) was used to study subjects with no musical training who had undergone either left or right temporal lobectomy; right-sided but not left-sided surgery resulted in impairment involving rhythm and sensitivity, not tonal imagery.[54]

Patients with either left or right temporal lobectomy were presented with spoken words, tunes without words, and words and tunes combined as an unfamiliar song. Left lobectomy resulted in impaired recognition of words alone, and right lobectomy resulted in impaired recognition of tunes alone, but either left or right lobectomy resulted in impaired recognition of melody combined with words.[55]

Several studies have compared local and global aspects of musical information processing in brain-damaged subjects. (For melody, pitch intervals are local, whereas melodic contour is global; for temporal patterns, rhythm is local, whereas meter is global.) In one study of patients with either right or left cerebral stroke, right hemispheric damage produced difficulty recognizing changes in either interval or contour, whereas left hemispheric damage produced difficulty only with intervals; either right or left hemispheric damage produced difficulty with rhythm but not with meter.[56] By contrast, although a similar study of patients following right or left cerebral corticectomy found comparable abnormalities involving interval and contour, either right or left hemispheric damage produced difficulty with meter, not rhythm.[57] In another study of patients with cerebral strokes, of eight patients with right-sided damage, five had impaired musical processing; of 12 patients with left-sided damage, nine had impaired musical processing. Right hemispheric damage caused abnormal processing of both contour and interval and of both meter and rhythm, whereas left hemispheric damage caused much more variable abnormalities: contour and interval could be affected alone or in combination, and meter and rhythm could be affected alone or in combination.[58]

Normal subjects recognize pitch even when the fundamental is missing if overtones are retained. This ability is lost following right temporal lobe damage that includes Heschl's gyrus.[59] Another study assessed the ability to recognize timbre derived either from spectral envelopes or from onset-offset times, and it was found that right temporal lobectomy produced greater impairment in either ability than did left temporal lobectomy.[60]

Following right but not left temporal lobectomy, patients had difficulty reproducing auditory but not visual rhythm; lesions producing such impairment encroached on the primary auditory cortex.[61]

In normal subjects the harmonic context established by a prime chord influences judgments of target chord intonation; in patients who had undergone corpus callostomy, this normal interaction was preserved in the right cerebral hemisphere but not the left.[62]

Studies of normal subjects

Paralleling clinical case reports and studies of brain-damaged subjects have been studies of musical processing in normal people. Space does not allow a detailed review of such investigations, the findings of which have often been as inconsistent as those of clinical reports. Early studies used the technique of dichotic listening, in which the two ears simultaneously receive different auditory information. In one such investigation musically naïve subjects appeared to have left ear advantage—that is, right cerebral hemispheric dominance—listening to melodies, whereas musically sophisticated subjects had right ear advantage; the findings were considered to reflect right hemispheric gestalt and emotional processing on the part of naïve listeners, in contrast to left hemispheric detailed analysis on the part of the musicians.[63] Other investigators, however, found no differences between musically sophisticated and musically naïve subjects,[64,65] and in some reports differences were found that seemed to depend on inherent musical aptitude,[66] age,[67] sex,[68] or right-ear advantage for higher pitch.[69,70] In one study the right hemisphere was used more for melody recognition when the tones had a complex timbre with rich overtones, again perhaps reflecting a right hemispheric advantage in dealing with simultaneous or gestalt, rather than linear or analytic, information.[71] It should be noted, however, that many investigators consider dichotic listening a highly unreliable technique for defining hemispheric functional 'dominance'.[72]

In normal subjects, functional imaging—positron emission tomography (PET) and functional magnetic resonance imaging (fMRI)—allows different components of musical processing to be assessed in real time. Such studies demonstrated that pitch recognition selectively activates the right prefrontal cortex, whereas active retention of pitch requires interaction of right frontal and right temporal cortices.[73,74] In another study, musical sight-reading, unlike reading words, activated the left occipitoparietal cortex, perhaps reflecting the dependence of musical reading on spatial location, in contrast to the dependence of word reading on feature detection.[75] In another study subjects listened to the same piece but were instructed to attend to different aspects of the music—for example, melody recognition, pitch, rhythm, or how many instruments were playing; even though the auditory information did not change with repeated trials, brain activation patterns were sharply altered by such changes in selective attention.[76]

As with brain-damaged patients, studies of normal subjects involve particular aspects of musical experience—auditory (pitch, harmony, timbre, interval, contour), visual (notational score, which includes real words; notes designated by letter but represented spatially, with duration indicated by appearance; purely musical symbols, such as rests, fermata, clef, crescendo, staccato, and repeat; and display of both simultaneous and sequential sounds), motor (performance, dance); memory; and emotion. Musical experience, however, is more than the sum of these parts. The multimodal components of musical processing cannot be sharply localized to one part of the brain or even to one cerebral hemisphere. The psychological whole that emerges from their interaction is even more widely distributed.

References

1. **Darwin, C.** (1871) *The Descent of Man, and Selection in Relation to Sex.* New York: Appleton.

2. **Spencer, H.** (1857/1951) The origin and function of music. In *Literary Style and Music.* New York: Philosophical Library.

3. **Pinker, S.** (1997) *How the Mind Works.* New York: W. W. Norton & Co.

4. **Gardner, H.** (1983) Musical Intelligence. In *Frames of Mind. The Theory of Multiple Intelligences*: New York: Basic Books, Inc. pp. 99–127.

5. **Profita, J.** and **T. G. Bidder** (1988) Perfect pitch. *Am. J. Med. Genet.* 29, 763–71.

6. **Critchley, M.** (1937) Musicogenic epilepsy. *Brain*, 60, 13–27.

7. **Poskanzer, C., E. Brawn,** and **H. Miller** (1962) Musicogenic epilepsy caused by only a discrete frequency band of church bells. *Brain* 85, 77–92.

8. **Brien, S. E.** and **T. J. Murray** (1984) Musicogenic epilepsy. *Can. Med. Assoc. J.* 131, 1255–8.

9. **Herskowitz, J., N. P. Rosman,** and **N. Geschwind** (1984) Seizures induced by singing and recitation. A unique form of reflex epilepsy in childhood. *Arch. Neurol.* 41, 1102–3.

10. **Wieser, H. G., H. Hungerbühler, A. M. Siegel,** and **A. Buck** (1997) Musicogenic epilepsy: review of the literature and case report with ictal single photon emission computed tomography. *Epilepsia* 38, 200–7.

11. **Sutherling, W. W., L. M. Hershman, J. Q. Miller,** *et al.* (1980) Seizures induced by playing music. *Neurol.* 30, 1001–4.

12. **Currie, S., K. W. G. Heathfield, R. A. Henson,** and **D. F. Scott** (1971) Clinical course and prognosis of temporal lobe epilepsy. A survey of 666 patients. *Brain* 94, 173–90.

13. **Penfield, W.** and **P. Perot** (1963) The brain's record of auditory and visual experience. *Brain* 86, 595–696.

14. **Ross, E. D., P. B. Jossman, B. Bell,** *et al.* (1975) Musical hallucinations in deafness. *J. Am. Med. Assoc.* 231, 620–1.

15. **Hammeke, T. A., M. P. McQuillen,** and **B. A. Cohen** (1983) Musical hallucinations associated with acquired deafness. *J. Neurol. Neurosurg. Psychiatry* 46, 570–2.

16. **Rizzo, M.** and **P. J. Eslinger** (1989) Colored hearing synesthesia: an investigation of neural factors. *Neurol.* 39, 781–4.

17. **Cytowic, R. E.** (1989) Synesthesia and mapping of subjective sensory dimensions. *Neurol.* 39, 849–50.

18. **Henschen, S. E.** (1925) Clinical and anatomical contributions on brain pathology. *Arch. Neurol. Psychiatry* 13, 226–49.

19. **Henschen, S. E.** (1926) On the function of the right hemisphere of the brain in relation to the left in speech, music, and calculation. *Brain* 49, 110–23.

20. **Kleist, K.** (1928). Gehirnpathologie und localisatorische Ergebnisse über Horstorungen, Gerauschtaubheiten und Amusien. *Monatsschr. Psychiatr. Neurol.* 68, 853–60.

21. **Feuchtwanger, E.** (1930) Amusie. Studien zur pathologischen Psychologie der akustischen Wahrnehmung und Vorstellung undihrer Strukturgebiete, besonders in Musik und Sprache. Berlin: Julius Springer.

22. **Ustvedt, H. J.** (1937) Ueber die unersuchung der musikalischen funktionen bei patienten mit gehirnleiden, besonders bei patienten mit aphasie. *Acta Med. Scand.* 86 (Suppl.), 1–737.

23. **Dalin, O.** (1745) Berättelse om en dumbe, som kan siumga. *Kung Sven Vetensk Acad Handlinger* 6, 114–15. Cited in Benton, A. K. and R. J. Joynt. (1960) Early descriptions of aphasia. *Arch. Neurol.* 3, 205–22.

24. **Jackson, J. H.** (1871) Singing by speechless (aphasic) children. *Lancet* 2, 430–1.

25. **Smith, A.** (1966) Speech and other functions after left (dominant) hemispherectomy. *J. Neurol. Neurosurg. Psychiatry* 29, 467–71.

26. Geschwind, N., F. A. Quadfasel, and J. M. Segarra (1968) Isolation of the speech area. *Neuropsychologia* 6, 327–40.

27. Yamadori, A., Y. Osumi, S. Masuhara, and M. Okubo (1977) Preservation of singing in Broca's aphasia. *J. Neurol. Neurosurg. Psychiatry* 40, 221–4.

28. Jacome, D. E. (1984) Aphasia with elation, hypermusia, musicophilia, and compulsive whistling. *J. Neurol. Neurosurg. Psychiatry* 47, 308–10.

29. Assal, G. (1973) Aphasie de Wernicke sans amusie chez un pianiste. *Rev. Neurol.* 129, 251–5.

30. Assal, G. and J. Buffet (1983) Agraphie et conservation de l'écriture musicale chez un professeur de piano bilingue. *Rev. Neurol.* 139, 569–74.

31. Luria, A. R., L. S. Tsvetkova, and D. S. Futer (1965) Aphasia in a composer. *J. Neurol. Sci.* 2, 288–92.

32. Basso, A. and E. Capitani (1985) Spared musical abilities in a conductor with global aphasia and ideomotor apraxia. *J. Neurol. Neurosurg. Psychiatry* 48, 407–12.

33. Signoret, J. L., P. Van Eeckhout, M. Poncet, *et al.* (1987) Aphasie sans amusie chez un organiste aveugle. *Rev. Neurol.* 143, 172–81.

34. Pötzl, O. and H. Uiberall (1937) Zur Patholgie der Amusie. *Wien Klin. Wochenschr.* 50, 770–5.

35. Botez, M. and N. Wertheim (1959) Expressive aphasia and amusia following right frontal lesion in a right-handed man. *Brain* 82, 186–202.

36. Wertheim, N. and M. Botez (1961) Receptive amusia: a clinical analysis. *Brain* 84, 19–30.

37. Mavlov, L. (1980) Amusia due to rhythm agnosia in a musician with left hemispheric damage: a non-auditory supramodal defect. *Cortex* 16, 331–8.

38. Polk, M. and A. Kertesz (1993) Music and language in degenerative disease of the brain. *Brain Cogn.* 22, 98–117.

39. Confavreux, C., B. Croisile, P. Garassus, *et al.* (1992) Progressive amusia and aprosody. *Arch. Neurol.* 49, 971–6.

40. Alajouanine, T. (1948) Aphasia and artistic realization. *Brain* 71, 229–41.

41. Henson, R. A. (1988) Maurice Ravel's illness: a tragedy of lost creativity. *Br. Med. J.* 296, 1585–8.

42. Brust, J. C. M. (1980) Music and language. Musical alexia and agraphia. *Brain* 103, 367–92.

43. Pittrich, H. (1956) Sensorische Amusie mit Paramusie nach rechtsseitger Temporalverletzung. Cited by Spreen, O., A. L. Benton and R. W. Fincham (1965) Auditory agnosia without aphasia. *Arch. Neurol.* 13, 84–92.

44. Pötzl, O. (1939) Zur Pathologie der Amusie. *Z. Neurol. Psychiatr.* 165, 187–95.

45. Jellineck, A. (1956) Amusia. On the phenomenology and investigation of central disorders of the musical functions. *Folia Phoniatr.* 8, 124–49.

46. Sidtis, J. J. and B. T. Volpe (1988) Selective loss of complex-pitch or speech discrimination after unilateral lesion. *Brain Lang.* 34, 235–45.

47. McFarland, H. R. and D. Fortin (1982) Amusia due to right temporoparietal infarct. *Arch. Neurol.* 39, 725–7.

48. Mazzucchi, A., C. Marchini, R. Budai, *et al.* (1982) A case of receptive amusia with prominent timbre perception defect. *J. Neurol. Neurosurg. Psychiatry* 45, 644–7.

49. Judd, T. L., A. Arslanian, L. Davidson, *et al.* (1979) A right hemisphere stroke in a composer. *Presented at International Neuropsychological Society.* February 2. New York.

50. Mazzoni, M., P. Moretti, L. Pardossi, *et al.* (1993) A case of musical imperception. *J. Neurol. Neurosurg. Psychiatry* 56, 322.

51. Peretz, I. and R. Kolinsky (1993) Boundaries of separability between melody and rhythm in music discrimination: a neuropsychological perspective. *Q. J. Exp. Psychol.* 46A, 301–25.

52. Gordon, H. W. and J. E. Bogen (1970) Hemispheric lateralization of singing after intracarotid sodium amylobarbitone. *J. Neurol. Neurosurg. Psychiatry* 37, 737–8.

53. Milner, B. (1962) Laterality effects in audition. In V. B. Mountcastle (ed.) *Interhemispheric Relations and Cerebral Dominance.* Baltimore: John Hopkins University Press. pp. 177–95.

54. Kester, D. B., A. J. Saykin, M. R. Sperling, *et al.* (1991) Acute effect of anterior temporal lobectomy on musical processing. *Neuropsychologia* 29, 703–8.

55. Samson, S. and R. J. Zatorre (1991) Recognition memory for text and melody of songs after unilateral temporal lobe lesions: evidence for dual encoding. *Q. J. Exp. Psychol: Learn Mem. Cogn.* 17, 793–804.

56. Peretz, I. (1990) Processing of local and global musical information by unilateral brain-damaged patients. *Brain* 113, 1185–205.

57. Liégois-Chauvel, C., I. Peretz, M. Babai, *et al.* (1998) Contribution of different cortical areas in the temporal lobes to music processing. *Brain* 121, 1853–67.

58. Schuppert, M., T. F. Münte, B. M. Wieringa, *et al.* (2000) Receptive amusia: evidence for cross-hemispheric neural networks underlying music processing strategies. *Brain* 123, 546–59.

59. Zatorre, R. J. (1988) Pitch perception of complex tones and human temporal lobe function. *J. Acoust. Soc. Am.* 84, 566–72.

60. Samson, S. and R. J. Zatorre (1994) Contribution of the right temporal lobe to musical timbre discrimination. *Neuropsychologia* 32, 231–40.

61. Penhune, V. B., R. J. Zatorre, and W. H. Feindel (1999) The role of auditory cortex in retention of rhythmic patterns as studied in patients with temporal lobe removals including Heschl's gyrus. *Neuropsychologia* 37, 315–31.

62. Tramo, M. J. and J. J. Bharucha (1991) Musical priming by the right hemisphere post-callosectomy. *Neuropsychologia* 29, 313–25.

63. Bever, T. G. and R. J. Chiarello (1974) Cerebral dominance in musicians and non-musicians. *Science* 185, 537–9.

64. Peretz, I. and J. Morais (1980) Modes of processing melodies and ear asymmetry in non-musicians. *Neuropsychologia* 18, 477–89.

65. Zatorre, R. J. (1979) Recognition of dichotic melodies by musicians and non-musicians. *Neuropsychologia* 17, 607–17.

66. Gaede, S. E., O. A. Parsons, and J. H. Bertera (1978) Hemispheric differences in music perception: aptitude vs. experience. *Neuropsychologia* 16, 369–73.

67. Wagner, M. T. and R. Hannon (1981) Hemispheric asymmetries in faculty and student musicians and non-musicians during melody recognition tasks. *Brain Lang.* 13, 379–88.

68. Shannon, B. (1984) Asymmetries in musical aesthetic judgements. *Cortex* 20, 567–73.

69. Deutsch, D. (1974) An auditory illusion. *Nature* 251, 307–9.

70. Deutsch, D. (1992) Paradoxes of musical pitch. *Sci. Am.* 267, 88–95.

71. Sidtis, J. J. (1980) On the nature of cortical function underlying right hemisphere auditory perception. *Neuropsychologia* 18, 321–30.

72. Sergent, J. (1993) Mapping the musician brain. *Hum. Brain Map.* 1, 20–38.

73. Zatorre, R. J., A. C. Evans, E. Meyer, *et al.* (1992) Lateralization of phonetic and speech discrimination in speech processing. *Science* 256, 846–9.

74. **Zatorre, R. J., A. C. Evans,** and **E. Meyer** (1994) Neural mechanisms underlying melodic perception and memory for pitch. *J. Neurosci.* 14, 1908–19.

75. **Sergent, J., E. Zuck, S. Terriah,** *et al.* (1992) Distributed neural network underlying musical sight-reading and keyboard performance. *Science* 257, 106–9.

76. **Platel, H., C. Price, J.-C. Baron,** *et al.* (1997) The structural components of music perception. A functional anatomic study. *Brain* 120, 229–43.

CHAPTER 13

BRAIN SPECIALIZATION FOR MUSIC: NEW EVIDENCE FROM CONGENITAL AMUSIA

ISABELLE PERETZ

Abstract

Brain specialization for music refers to the possibility that the human brain is equipped with neural networks that are dedicated to the processing of music. Finding support for the existence of such music-specific networks suggests that music may have biological roots. Conversely, the discovery that music may have systematic associations with other cognitive domains or variable brain organization across individuals would support the view that music is a cultural product. Currently, the evidence favours the biological perspective. There are numerous behavioural indications that music-specific networks are isolable in the brain. These neuropsychological observations are briefly reviewed here with special emphasis on a new condition, that of congenital amusia (also commonly referred to as tone-deafness).

The notion that music might have biological foundations has only recently gained legitimacy. Over the past 30 years, music has mostly been studied as a cultural product. Musicologists were analysing each musical system in the context of its specific culture. Neuroscientists and psychologists were viewing music as a convenient window to the general functioning of the human brain. However, neuropsychological observations have consistently and recurrently suggested that music might well be distinct from other cognitive functions, in being subserved by specialized neural networks. As such, music might be viewed as pertaining more to biology than to culture. The goal of the present paper is to review the neuropsychological evidence that supports the biological perspective.

Specialized neural networks for music processing

If music is biologically determined, then music is expected to have functional and neuro-anatomical specialization. That is, music is expected to be subserved by neural networks that are dedicated to its processing, in being unresponsive or inadequate for dealing with nonmusical input. Presently, support for the existence of such specialized neural networks is compelling. Most evidence in this regard derives from the functional examination of individuals whose brain condition is disturbed in highly selective aspects. The brain anomaly may either impair or spare musical abilities exclusively. It can be revealed in three types of conditions: (1) Acquired disorders; (2) Congenital disorders; and (3) Brain stimulation.

Acquired disorders

Acquired disorders refer to sequelae of a brain accident. Such injuries most frequently are subsequent to a cerebro-vascular accident at the adult age. In such cases, disorders are expected to reveal normal brain organization due to the fact that the disorders are constrained by the organization of the undamaged system, which was fully stabilized prior to the accident. Thus, the study of brain-damaged adults provides a unique opportunity to uncover the functional organization of the normal brain by a procedure akin to reverse engineering.

This research strategy is facilitated by the recurrent observation that brain damage does not affect cognition in its entirety, but rather, in particular aspects. Cognitive disorders can be highly selective. The selectivity of the disorder can take spectacular forms such as in brain-damaged composers who may lose their language and yet remain able to maintain their musical activities in their prior professional level.

> The most famous case is probably that of Shebalin, the Russian composer who, following successive vascular accidents occurring in his left hemisphere, suffered from severe disturbances of his language abilities. He remained aphasic for the rest of his life; he could neither understand nor speak intelligibly. Nevertheless, he continued to compose, notably completing his Fifth symphony, which Shostakovitch considered to be one of his most brilliant and innovative works.[1] Therefore, Shebalin displayed severe language deficits yet retained his musical skills to a remarkable degree.

This dissociation between language and music cannot simply be explained by the fact that these professional musicians were 'abnormally musical' from the start. Indeed, the reverse dissociation can also be observed, even in ordinary listeners. That is, persons devoid of any special talent, linguistic or musical, can experience spectacular losses of musical abilities, like losing the ability to recognize one's national anthem, without accompanying language difficulties.

> I have been fortunate to study in detail three such cases.[2,3] One of them, I.R., was a restaurant manager when she sustained bilateral brain damage as a consequence of successive surgeries in both sides of the brain for the clipping of ruptured aneurysms. Ten years post-onset, I.R. still suffers from severe and irreversible deficits in music perception and memory as a consequence of her brain damage.[3] Prior to her brain surgeries, music had great value to I.R. She was raised in a musically-inclined family since her only brother is a professional musician. Fortunately, I.R. did not lose her language skills. She understands speech perfectly and remains verbally fluent, being able to express herself quite effectively (see her poem recently published in French[3]).

Such musical disorders—called amusia in neurological terms—are not rare and are dissociable from disorders of language—that is, aphasia, as reviewed by Brust (Chapter 12, this volume). This recurrent finding suggests that most processing components that underlie language and music are not shared and are neuroanatomically separable.

Although dissociation between music and language has been reported in various spheres of activities, it remains that the two domains are rarely compared in analogous contexts. Hence, significant association between language and music might have escaped attention. It is important to examine music and language in similar tasks. One such simple task that the auditory system performs constantly and without effort, in both music and language domains, is sound pattern recognition. Hence, recognition of tunes and lyrics provide a sound basis for cross-domain comparisons.

In comparing recognition of spoken lyrics to the recognition of instrumental tunes, it has been possible to show that these auditory functions are not performed by a single auditory system but by separate ones, each being specialized for its particular domain.[4,5] For instance, auditory recognition of music appears to recruit mechanisms that are not implicated in speech recognition or in environmental sound recognition. Indeed, one can find brain-damaged cases whose unique symptom is the loss of the ability to recognize and memorize music. The patients retain the ability to recognize and understand speech as well as to identify common environmental sounds normally.[2,3,6-8] The deficit can be remarkably selective. For example, C.N. was unable to recognize hummed melodies coming from familiar songs above chance. Yet, she could perfectly recognize the lyrics accompanying the melodies that she failed to recognize.[7] Moreover, C.N. was able to recognize the voice of speakers[2] and the intonation of speech.[9] The existence of such a specific problem with music alongside normal functioning of other kinds of auditory abilities, including speech comprehension, suggests damage to processing components that are not only specific to the musical domain but also essential to the normal process of music recognition. We refer to this condition, which is a particular form of amusia, as *music agnosia*.[7]

The reverse condition, that corresponds to a selective sparing of music recognition, has been reported (see Table 13.1) but not yet well documented. Nevertheless, in the available cases,[10-12] the lesion spared music processing relative to both speech comprehension and environmental sound recognition that were both severely disturbed. Such cases suggest isolated sparing of music recognition abilities, hence complementing the music-specific deficits described above. Thus, the current evidence, summarized in Table 13.1, is indicative of the

Table 13.1 Case reports of selective impairment and of sparing in the recognition of music

Reports	Domain				Lesions
	Music	Speech (not prosody)	Environmental sounds	Voices	
Peretz et al.,[2] C.N. and G.L.	−	+	+	+	Bilateral temporal lobes
	−	+*	+	+	Bilateral temporal lobes
Peretz et al.,[3] I.R.	−	+	+	+	Bilateral temporal lobes and right frontal lobe
Griffith et al.[6]	−	+	+		Posterior right temporal lobe
Piccirili et al.[8]	−	+	+	+	Left superior temporal gyrus#
Laignel-Lavastine et al.[10]	+	−	−		Right temporal lobe
Godefroy et al.[11]*	+	−	−		Right posterior hemisphere
Mendez[12]	+	−	−		Right temporal lobe#

+ = normal recognition; − = impaired recognition.
* after or during recovery; # left-handed.

presence of specialized brain circuits for music recognition. These circuits are damaged in the cases of music agnosia and spared in the few cases who suffer from verbal agnosia coupled with agnosia for environmental sounds.

Congenital disorders

Further neuropsychological evidence that is indicative of brain specialization for music comes from congenital disorders. These disorders refer to unexpected failures or achievements in musical abilities in comparison to the general level of intellectual and socio-emotional functioning. These deficiencies are termed congenital since their presence can be detected very early in development. One such well-known condition corresponds to the 'music-savant syndrome' that can often be observed in autistic individuals. The etiology of autism is not yet known; however, its incidence is relatively high, with one to two cases out of every 1000 births (about the same rate as the Down syndrome). Autism is currently viewed as deriving from some brain anomaly because of its frequent association with other brain defect (e.g. epilepsy), its genetic transmission and its atypical cerebral functioning as measured by brain imaging studies.[13] More interestingly from our perspective, 1–10 per cent of autistic individuals might be qualified as musicians.[14] In effect, autistic subjects are generally more apt in the area of music than in other domains, such as language.[15] Several even become *musical savants*, a term which refers to the observation of high achievements in musical activities in individuals who are otherwise socially and mentally handicapped.

> A well-known case (described in more details by L. Miller[14]) is that of "Blind Tom". Blind Tom was a young blind slave who gave piano concerts at the White House and all around the world. While his language repertoire consisted of less than 100 words, his musical repertoire contained more than 5000 musical pieces. This "music-savant" was sold in 1850 during a slavery sale in Georgia. Blind Tom was sold along with his mother to Colonel Bethune. Until age 5, he did not say a word and manifested no other sign of intelligence than his remarkable interest for the musical performance given by the colonel's daughters. At age 4, he was playing Mozart sonatas, which he had heard. At age 6, he was able to improvise, and at age 7, he gave his first recital. In 1862, despite the fact that he did not know how to read music, he was able to play without errors 14 pages of an original composition that he had heard just once. Blind Tom gave recitals until age 53 when following the colonel's death, he had to end his career.

The mirror image of this condition corresponds to individuals who are musically inept, despite normal exposure to music, normal intelligence, and social adaptation. Such individuals are sometimes called *tone-deaf* (see Ref. 16 for the first report).

> Che Guevara was known to be "tune-deaf".[17] He was well aware of his handicap as the following anecdote illustrates. At a party, by prior arrangement, Alberto, his best friend, was required to give a poke to the Che every time a tango was played. At some point during the party, the orchestra played an agitated Brazilian shora that had been Alberto's favorite. Alberto wished to share his enthusiasm with the Che. But the Che, with his eyes on a woman across the room, believed Alberto's nudge to be a tango signal and took to the floor, dancing a slow and passionate tango with everyone else jiggling to the shora. Realizing something was wrong, Che Guevara came over to ask Alberto for advice, who was too convulsed with laughter to be able to explain.

We refer to these rare individuals as *congenital amusics*. The term reflects better the likelihood that there are multiple forms of music developmental disorders, as there are various patterns of acquired amusia resulting from brain accident (see Chapter 12, this volume, for an illustration of the heterogeneity of acquired amusias).

Unlike other developmental disorders such as *dysphasia* and *dyslexia, congenital amusia* has not received much scientific attention. One obvious reason for this neglect is that attention is generally directed at learning disabilities that affect language because of their wide educational implications. Moreover, music educators are reluctant to suspect the presence of congenital disorders because such a diagnosis may mean discontinuation of musical studies.[18] The other reasons are less pragmatic. As mentioned at the outset, many scientists conceive music as the product of a general-purpose brain organization. In that context, amusia is not a developmental disorder that is expected to occur in isolation. Rather, amusia is expected to result from intellectual and/or socioemotional dysfunctioning. However, as *Music-savants* suggest, music proficiency does not seem to depend on the normal development of the cognitive and affective system. Musical proficiency can be achieved while sociocognitive functioning is globally deficient. Therefore, one can expect to observe the reverse condition. That is, we should be able to find congenital amusics in whom musical competence does not match the level of achievement reached in sociocognitive spheres.

We actively searched for such amusic cases by means of various advertisements over the last five years. The early discovery of a textbook case (called Monica, reported in Ref. 19, and represented in Figure 13.1) who closely matched the two case descriptions available in the literature (i.e. Grant-Allen's case[16] and Geshwind's case[20]) has greatly contributed to the advancement of the study. Since then, the presence of *amusia* has been confirmed in 21 adults and studied in detail in 11 of them.[21] All are self-declared 'musically impaired'. However, self-declaration does not suffice. Nonmusicians are prone to complain about their musical deficiencies, in general. Therefore, we selected only subjects who exhibited clear-cut performance deficits on our screening musical battery.[22–24] Furthermore, in order to exclude extraneous causalities, we carefully selected participants who had no psychiatry or neurological history and who possessed a solid level of education. To ensure adequate stimulation and to exclude lack of interest or of motivation, only volunteers who had experienced unsuccessful attempts at learning music during childhood were considered.

Up to now, we have found 21 individuals who exhibited a pattern of performance that unambiguously indicated the presence of a receptive musical disorder. Their results are represented in Figure 13.1 with two tests that allow comparisons of results on the melodic and temporal dimension because the tests are very close in structure. One test serves to evaluate the use of melodic cues (one altered note that modifies either pitch directions, key or pitch intervals) and the other to assess the use of rhythmic cues (one altered note that modifies rhythmic grouping by a change in duration values) in the discrimination of two successive short musical sequences as 'same or different'. The same set of novel but conventional musical phrases served in both types of tests.

Examination of the data in Figure 13.1 is informative in several aspects. First, most controls are confined to the right top quarter and do no overlap with amusics' performance. This confirms the usefulness of our screening battery to detect the presence of a music receptive disorder. Second, and more importantly, all amusic participants score below the normal range in the discrimination of musical stimuli that differ on the melodic dimension

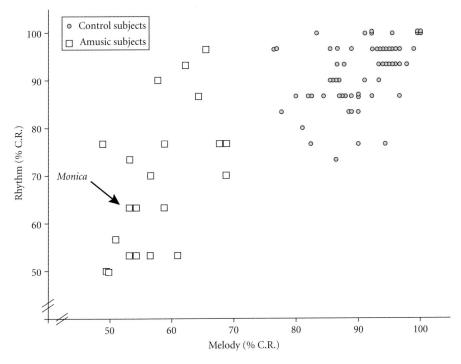

Figure 13.1   Percentage of correct responses obtained by 21 congenital amusics relative to the normal distribution (constituted by 60 nonmusicians, age range: 14–74 years; education range: 7–20 years) in two series of tests of the montreal battery of evaluation of amusia[17–19] assessing melodic change discrimination (abscissa) and rhythmic change discrimination (ordinate axis). Chance level is at 50 per cent of correct responses.

while a majority of them succeed to discriminate the same stimuli when these differ in temporal structure. None of the amusic subjects is experiencing an isolated deficit on the rhythmic dimension. This difficulty in detecting pitch-related changes extends to dissonance for which amusics show little sensitivity.[21] The defect also extends to the detection of an anomalous pitch inserted in an otherwise conventional melody.[21] We propose that one likely origin for congenital amusia is related to a deficiency in musical pitch recognition.[19,21]

The deficit seems limited to music. Amusic subjects retain the ability to process non-musical material as well as their matched controls. In one set of tests originally designed for music agnosic patients,[7] amusic participants, and their matched controls are presented with standard memory recognition tasks that only differ by the domain from which the test items are taken. In the music memory test, subjects are presented with 20 instrumental tunes (taken from familiar songs) to memorize. The melodies are then represented among 20 unstudied (but equally familiar) melodies that are randomly mixed. The subject is requested to indicate which melodies were heard in the study phase. For comparison purposes, in the lyrics and the environmental sound tests, subjects are given similar opportunities to learn and recognize 20 spoken lyrics (taken from the same familiar songs) and 20 environmental sounds (e.g. a barking dog), respectively. The three tests are performed in different sessions.

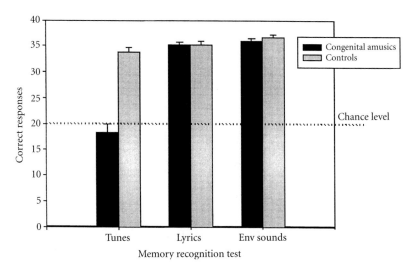

Figure 13.2   Number of correct responses obtained by 12 amusics and 20 matched controls in the memory recognition of studied melodies, lyrics, and environmental sounds. Error bars represent standard error from the mean. Chance level is at 20 correct responses.

As can be seen in Figure 13.2, amusics' performance is at chance in the music test whereas their scores are fairly high and lie within normal limits for nonmusical material, be they song lyrics or environmental sounds. The results clearly show the music specificity of the disorder.

   In conclusion, congenital amusia appears as a new class of learning disabilities that are domain specific. Affected individuals appear to be born without the essential wiring elements for developing a normally functioning system for music, while achieving a high degree of proficiency in their professional and social life. This impairment seems to result, at least in some cases, from a more elemental problem that makes the individual unable to hear the pitch-relevant variations in music. Although it seems unlikely that a single defective mechanism, such as a pitch defect, is responsible for the proper operation of all processing components that subserve musical functions, it may be the case that a single essential defective component brings the development of the musical system to a halt. In this perspective, fine-grained pitch perception might be an essential component around which the musical system develops in a normal brain.[19]

   The existence of congenital amusia coupled with the music-savant syndrome strongly suggests the presence of early pressures for the normal development of neural networks that are dedicated to music. Identification of these neural bases as well as of their associated heritability should provide crucial elements in the debate surrounding the existence of biological foundations for musicality.

Brain stimulation

Investigations with epileptic patients provides the third source of evidence that speaks for the existence of neural networks that are dedicated to music. Indeed, in a few individuals, music will be the exclusive trigger of the pathological firing of neurons conductive to the epileptic crisis. This form of epilepsy is called *musicogenic epilepsy*[25] (see also Brust, Chapter 12, this volume) and suggests that the epileptogenic tissue lies in a neural region that is tied to music processing.

> The British neurologist Macdonald Critchley[26] describes one regular visit of an epileptic patient who reports that hearing music exclusively provoked her attacks. The patient specified that music of the "popular" type had not effect, only "classical" music did, while confessing she had no particular preference for this kind of music. She was subsequently admitted to the hospital and, despite her discomfort, was presented with various kinds of music. The only record of classical music possessed by the experimenters, which contained "la valse des fleurs" de Tchaikovsy, immediately provoked a seizure with generalized convulsive movements, frothing of the lips and cyanosis. (Ref. 26, pp. 344–5).

During musicogenic epileptic seizures, abnormalities in electrical activity (recorded from the scalp) are generally observed at the temporal lobes, with a slight bias towards the right one (see Ref. 25 for a recent review). Thus, some processing component that is exclusively related to music must be located in those regions.

The direct application of electric stimulation to the brain of epileptic patients yields to a similar conclusion. *In vivo* electric stimulation of particular areas of the auditory associative cortex of awake patients may produce highly vivid *musical hallucinations.*[27] These provoked hallucinations suggest that the stimulation be applied to circuits that contain memories of musical experiences.

> Penfield & Perot report stimulating a particular region of the first right temporal circumvolution. The patient then says: "I hear music". The experimenters then repeat the stimulation, without telling the patient, who immediately says, "I hear the music again. It is like the radio". When asked what tune she was hearing, she said she did not know but it was familiar. The stimulation is again repeated and the patient shouts: "I hear it". The electrode was kept in place and the patient is asked to describe what she hears. The patient hummed the tune quite distinctly. The song comes out so clearly that one of the nurses recognizes "Rolling along together". The patient agreed that this sounded like the words in the song. (Ref. 27, case #5, p. 620)

The left, and slightly more often, right temporal regions are prone to evoke such musical experiences. The fact that musical memories can be exclusively elicited in individuals with no musical training underscores once again brain specialization for music.

In summary, the patient-based approach converges on one precise point: neuronal networks that are situated in or close to the superior temporal gyrus participate in music perception and memory in a decisive and exclusive manner. Presently, there is little evidence for music specificity coming from the study of normal brains (but see Chapters 15 and 18, this volume, for recent data).

Localization of the music-specific networks

Precise localization of the music-specific networks is essential when biological determinism is at issue. Finding brain specialization for music is not sufficient. Brain specialization for music may just result from the recruitment of a free neural space in the infant's brain. Music could modify that space to adjust it to its processing needs and hence be associated to neural specialization. This type of specialization does not require prewiring. It may occur as a response to early cultural pressures. In that case, a variable localization and distribution of the musical networks can be expected across individuals. Depending on the moment, quality, and quantity of exposure, various brain spaces might be mobilized. Thus, if music is a brain 'squatter', localization should vary capriciously across members of the same culture.

In contrast, biological functions are expected to be prewired. A prewired organization is expected to exhibit consistency in localization. For example, the primary auditory areas (located in the Heschl's gyri) are systematically buried in the sylvian fissure; this holds for all humans. Similarly, if brain specialization for music is pre-wired, then the music-specific networks are expected to have a relatively *fixed* arrangement. That is, brain implementation of music networks should be similar in the vast majority of humans, nonmusicians, and musicians alike. Moreover, this organization is not expected to vary as a function of the musical culture considered. Musical functions are expected to be similarly implemented in the brain of an isolated Pacific Islander, a Chinese opera singer, and a Western fan of rap music. This brain localization hypothesis can be easily tested with the new brain imagery techniques.

However, the demonstration of a similar brain organization for music in all humans remains elusive. Localization of the brain substrates underlying music has been an enduring problem for more than a century. In my view, the only consensus that has been reached today about the cerebral organization underlying music concerns pitch contour processing. The vast majority of studies point to the superior temporal gyrus and frontal regions on the right side of the brain as the responsible areas for processing pitch contour information.[28] However, it remains to be determined if this mechanism is music specific, since the intonation patterns of speech seem to recruit similarly located, if not identical, brain circuitries.[9,29]

Similarly, assuming comparable brain organization in musicians and nonmusicians may sound controversial, since there is strong evidence that musical training has a sizable effect on cortical morphology (see Chapter 24, this volume) and activity (see Chapters 25 and 26, this volume). It remains to determine to what extent these changes due to musical training are merely quantitative or rather represent qualitative modifications. In other words, it will be important to qualify the effect of training on brain organization. Presently, music training does not seem to distribute musical modules differently in the neural space of the expert compared to the ordinary listener, as a specialization by default would predict. Yet, the relevant evidence is still scarce.

Clearly, what is needed at the present stage is a grid that allows specification of the processing mechanisms that are essential for music appreciation. Once these essential ingredients have been identified, their respective localization may be tracked down in the brain of musicians and nonmusicians of different musical cultures. The research agenda involved is dense and will only be briefly sketched in section 'What is the content of the music-specific neural networks?'.

What is the content of the music-specific neural networks?

The music-specific neural networks should correspond to a common core of musical abilities that is acquired by all normally developing individuals of the same culture. This common core should also be universal, in forming the essence of the musical competence acquired by members of all cultures. This universal competence can hopefully be reduced to a few essential processing components that represent the germ of brain specialization for music. In this perspective, there is no need for all musical abilities to have initial specialization. Brain specialization for a few mechanisms that are essential to the normal development of musical skills should suffice.

I am proposing that the two anchorage points of brain specialization for music are the encoding of pitch along musical scales and the ascribing of a regular beat to incoming events. The notion that a special device exists for tonal encoding of pitch has been developed in previous papers[30] and will thus not be elaborated further. Similarly, the notion that regularity might be fundamental to music appreciation is slowly emerging[31] (e.g. Chapter 2, this volume), although its specificity to music is rarely addressed.

Universality of musical scales and of pulse regularity is another issue that has received very little attention from ethnomusicologists. As mentioned earlier, ethnomusicologists cautiously avoid generalization across musical cultures. Yet, the plausibility of considering pitch scales and regularity as music universals has increased in recent years.[32]

In contrast, developmental psychologists have made significant progress in identifying plausible musical universals. Infants' studies have largely confirmed the presence of precocious sensitivity to musical scales and to temporal synchronicity in auditory processing. For example, 6- to 9-month-old infants exhibit enhanced discrimination in a consonant interval context compared to a dissonant one;[33] they also exhibit learning preferences for musical scales.[34] In most musical cultures, musical scales make use of unequal pitch steps. Infants already show a sensitivity bias towards musical scales, since they have been shown to be better at detecting a small pitch change in an unequal-step scale than in an equal-step scale (see Chapter 1, this volume). On the time dimension, infants prefer music that is subject to an isochronous temporal pulse. For instance, like adults, 4-month-old infants are biased towards perceiving regularity; they exhibit sensitivity to slight disruptions of temporal isochrony[31] (Chapter 2, this volume). All of these aspects of auditory pattern processing suggest the presence of innate learning preferences.

In conclusion, appreciation of music fits well with the product of a specialized cortical arrangement that is present and functional early in human development. Hence, music does not seem to be a game for the mind, for the neurons or for the senses. Music seems to serve needs that are so important to humans that their brain has dedicated some neural space to its processing. It remains to demonstrate that these music-specific networks are fulfilling needs that are not optional but have adaptive value.

Acknowledgements

This chapter is based on studies supported by grants from the Canadian Institute of Health Research and the Canadian Natural Science and Engineering Research Council.

References

1. Luria, A., L. Tsvetkova, and J. Futer (1965) Aphasia in a composer. *J. Neurolog. Sci.* 2, 288–92.

2. Peretz, I., R. Kolinsky, M. Tramo, L. Labrecque, C. Hublet, and G. Demeurisse (1994) Functional dissociations following bilateral lesions of auditory cortex. *Brain* 117, 1283–301.

3. Peretz, I., S. Belleville, and S. Fontaine (1997) Dissociations entre musique et langage après atteinte cérébrale: un nouveau cas d'amusie sans aphasie. *Revue Canadienne de Psychologie Expérimentale* 51, 354–67.

4. Peretz, I. (1993) Auditory agnosia: a functional analysis. In S. McAdams and E. Bigand (eds) *Thinking in Sound. The Cognitive Psychology of Human Audition*. New York, NY: Oxford University Press, pp. 199–230.

5. Polster, M. and S. Rose (1998) Disorders of auditory processing: evidence for modularity in audition. *Cortex* 34, 47–65.

6. Griffiths, T., A. Rees, C. Witton, P. Cross, R. Shakir, and G. Green (1997) Spatial and temporal auditory processing deficits following right hemisphere infarction: a psychophysical study. *Brain* 120, 785–94.

7. Peretz, I. (1996) Can we lose memories for music? The case of music agnosia in a non-musician. *J. Cognitive Neurosci.* 8, 481–96.

8. Piccirilli, M., T. Sciarma, and S. Luzzi (2000) Modularity of music: evidence from a case of pure amusia. *J. Neurol. Neurosurgery Psychiatry* 69, 541–5.

9. Patel, A. D., I. Peretz, M. Tramo, and R. Labrecque (1998) Processing prosodic and musical patterns: a neuropsychological investigation. *Brain Lang.* 61, 123–44.

10. Godefroy, O., D. Leys, A. Furby, J. De Reuck, C. Daems, P. Rondepierre, B. Dabachy, J.-F. Deleume, and A. Desaulty (1995) Psychoacoustical deficits related to bilateral subcortical hemorrhages: a case with apperceptive auditory agnosia. *Cortex* 31, 149–59.

11. Laignel-Lavastine, M. and T. Alajouanine (1921) Un cas d'agnosie auditive. *Revue Neurologique* 37, 194–8.

12. Mendez, M. (2001) Generalized auditory agnosia with spared music recognition in a left-hander. Analysis of a case with a right temporal stroke. *Cortex* 37, 139–50.

13. Bailey, A., W. Phillips, and M. Rutter (1996) Autism: towards an integration of clinical, genetic, neuropsychological, and neurobiological perspectives. *J. Child Psychol. Psychiatry* 37, 89–126.

14. Miller, L. (1989) *Musical Savants. Exceptional Skill in the Mentally Retarded*. Hillsdale, NJ: Erlbaum.

15. Heaton, P., B. Hermelin, and L. Pring (1998) Autism and pitch processing: a precursor for savant musical ability? *Music Percept.* 15, 291–305.

16. Grant-Allen (1878) Note-deafness. *Mind* 10, 157–67.

17. Taibo II, P. I. (1996) *Ernesto Guevara, también conocido como el Che*. Buenos Aires: Planeta.

18. Kazez, D. (1985) The myth of tone deafness. *Music Educators J.* 71, 46–7.

19. Peretz, I., J. Ayotte, R. Zatorre, J. Mehler, P. Ahad, V. Penhune, and B. Jutras (2002) Congenital amusia: a disorder of fine-grained pitch discrimination. *Neuron* 33 (13), 185–91.

20. Geschwind, N. (1984) The brain of a learning-disabled individual. *Annals of Dyslexia* 34, 319–27.

21. Ayotte, I., I. Peretz, and K. Hyde (2002) Congenital amusia: a group study of adults afflicted with a music-specific disorder. *Brain* 125, 1–14.

22. **Peretz, I.** (1990) Processing of local and global musical information by unilateral brain-damaged patients. *Brain* 11, 1185–205.

23. **Liégeois-Chauvel, C., I. Peretz, M. Babaï, V. Laguitton,** and **P. Chauvel** (1998) Contribution of different cortical areas in the temporal lobes to music processing. *Brain* 121, 1853–67.

24. **Ayotte, J., I. Peretz, I. Rousseau, C. Bard,** and **M. Bojanowski** (2000) Patterns of music agnosia associated with middle cerebral artery infarcts. *Brain* 123, 1926–38.

25. **Wieser, H. G., H. Hungerbühler, A. Siegel,** and **A. Buck** (1997) Musicogenic epilepsy: review of the literature and case report with ictal single photon emission computed tomography. *Epilepsia* 38, 200–7.

26. **Critchley, M.** (1977) Musicogenic epilepsy. In M. Critchley and M. Henson (eds) *Music and the Brain.* London: W. Heinemann, pp. 344–53.

27. **Penfield, W.** and **P. Perot** (1963) The brain's record of auditory and visual experience. *Brain* 86, 595–696.

28. **Peretz, I.** (2000) Music perception and recognition. In B. Rapp (ed.) *The Handbook of Cognitive Neuropsychology.* Hove: Psychology Press, pp.519–40.

29. **Zatorre, R. J., A. C. Evans, E. Meyer,** and **A. Gjedde** (1992) Lateralization of phonetic and pitch processing in speech perception. *Sci.* 256, 846–9.

30. **Peretz, I.** and **J. Morais** (1989) Music and modularity. *Contemporary Music Rev.,* 4, 277–91.

31. **Drake, C.** (1998) Psychological processes involved in the temporal organization of complex auditory sequences: universal and acquired processes. *Music Percept.* 16, 11–26.

32. **Arom, S.** (2000) Prolegomena to a biomusicology. In N. Wallin, B. Merker, and S. Brown (eds) *The Origins of Music.* Cambridge: MIT press, pp. 27–9.

33. **Schellenberg, E. G.** and **S. Trehub** (1996) Natural musical intervals: evidence from infants listeners. *Psycholog. Sci.* 7, 272–7.

34. **Trehub, S., G. Schellenberg,** and **S. Kamenetsky** (1999) Infants' and adults' perception of scale structure. *J. Exp. Psychol.: Hum. Percept. Perform.* 25, 965–75.

CHAPTER 14

CEREBRAL SUBSTRATES FOR MUSICAL TEMPORAL PROCESSES

SÉVERINE SAMSON AND NATHALIE EHRLÉ

Abstract

Music as well as language consists of a succession of auditory events in time, which require elaborate temporal processing. Although several lines of evidence suggest that the left dominant hemisphere is predominantly involved in the processing of rapid temporal changes of speech, very little is known about the cerebral substrates underlying such auditory temporal processes in music. To investigate this issue, we examined epileptic patients with either left (LTL) or right (RTL) temporal-lobe lesions as well as normal control subjects (NC) in two different tasks involving the processing of time-related (temporal) information. By manipulating inter-onset interval (IOI) in a psychophysical task, as well as in a task of detection of rhythmic changes in real tunes, we studied the processing of temporal microvariations in music. The first task assessed anisochrony (or irregularity) discrimination of sequential information according to different presentation rates (between 80 and 1000 ms IOI). For all subjects, an effect of tempo was obtained, thresholds were lower for the 80 ms IOI than for longer IOIs. Furthermore, there was a specific impairment of rapid anisochrony discrimination (80 ms IOI) for LTL patients as compared to RTL and NC subjects, but no deficit was observed for longer IOI. These findings suggest the specialization of LTL structures in processing rapid sequential auditory information. The second task involved the detection of inter-onset interval increments in familiar monodic tunes. Performance was measured for two increments (easy vs difficult to detect according to cognitive expectation) to assess the effect of cognitive expectation using a forced-choice paradigm (changed vs unchanged melody). The results showed that LTL patients but not RTL were impaired as compared to NC subjects in the increment detection. However, all groups showed differences between the two levels of difficulty, suggesting that top-down processing remains functional. These findings suggest that LTL structures are predominantly involved in perceiving time-related perturbations in familiar tunes as well as in isochronous sequences, extending to the musical domain findings previously reported in speech.

Introduction

Music as well as language consists of a succession of auditory events in time, which require elaborate temporal processing. In the present study, we will consider the temporal coding of musical information which plays an important role in performing and perceiving rhythm. This time-related processing concerns a large range of time frames that may implicate different forms of information processing. In the neuropsychological domain, simple auditory sequences and musical patterns have been used to investigate the cerebral structures underlying musical temporal processes. Studies reported in the literature will be reviewed first. Then, experimental findings that we obtained in two different studies will be reported to clarify the role of the left (LTL) as opposed to the right temporal lobe (RTL) structures in processing subtle temporal variations within a range of 10–100 ms.

Temporal processing in simple auditory sequences

Several studies have explored time-related processing by using simple auditory sequences. In this domain, several paradigms classically used in experimental psychology have been adapted to neuropsychology. In a seminal paper, Efron[1] investigated the ability of brain-damaged patients to judge the temporal order of two-tones of different frequencies separated by a silent interval. The results showed that aphasic patients with left-hemisphere lesions required longer intervals (between 140 and 400 ms) to discriminate temporal order than nonaphasic patients with right-hemisphere lesion or normal subjects (75 ms interval). It was therefore suggested that the left hemisphere structures generally thought to be involved in language processing may also contribute to the temporal analysis of fast auditory sequential information. Subsequently, Tallal and Newcombe[2] provided convergent evidence by demonstrating that selective damage to the left but not to the right hemisphere disrupted the ability to process two-tones separated by a short interval (300 ms or less between the tones). Importantly, neither left- nor right-hemisphere damaged subjects were affected when longer intervals were used. This finding has been reproduced with similar paradigms and generalized to other tasks involving gap detection or perception of simulaneity and succession.[3–7] One case report of an amusic patient (HV) seems to contradict previous results since a deficit in temporal order processing of rapid patterns was observed in presence of a right-hemisphere lesion.[8] However, the authors noted that the cortical lesion of this patient was associated with an underlying bilateral white matter lesion which may have caused bilateral cortical deafferentation. Such a cerebral dysfunction, that presumably involved the left hemisphere, might have been responsible for the disruption of rapid temporal processing explaining therefore the apparent contradiction between the results.

However, inconsistent results were reported in studies investigating the perception of duration. Indeed, results of different studies have shown that impairments in this perceptual ability have been observed in patients with unilateral lesions implicating the right or the left hemisphere,[9] in a case of auditory agnosia following a bilateral cerebral dysfunction[10] as well as in patients with RTL lesions.[11] These findings suggest that the perception of continuous signals, as opposed to discrete events, depends on different processing involving distinct neural substrate.

Except for the perception of duration, the results previously reviewed suggest that left-hemisphere structures are predominantly involved in the processing of rapid sequential information. Recent electrophysiological results indicate that this function can be linked to auditory cortices of the LTL. By recording intracerebral evoked potentials to syllables in the right and the left human auditory cortices, Liégeois-Chauvel and her collaborators[12] demonstrated a specialization of the left auditory cortex for speech perception that depends on rapid temporal coding (within a few tens of milliseconds). If the left temporal cortex is dominant for fine grained time-related processing of language, it seems plausible to hypothesize that it would also be important for such temporal processing in music.

Temporal processing in musical sequences

Parallel to the previously reported studies using simple auditory sequences, several studies investigated temporal processes in musical sequences. It has been suggested that temporal processing, of which musical rhythm would be an example, is best performed by the functions of the dominant left hemisphere. However, the evidence reported in the literature provide little support for this hypothesis. Few studies investigating the perception of dichotically presented stimuli in normal listeners usually report a right ear advantage which is supposed to reflect left-hemisphere predominance for the perception of temporally complex nonspeech stimuli,[13–16] but this perceptual asymmetry has not always been obtained.[17] Similarly, studies carried out in brain damaged subjects have not systematically documented a deficit in rhythmic tasks in the presence of a left-hemisphere lesion. Although evidence supporting left-hemisphere involvement in rhythm have been reported in a few studies carried out in unilateral brain damaged subjects,[18,19] other studies have demonstrated the contribution of right-hemisphere structures and/or a bilateral cerebral involvement in rhythm discrimination.[20–25] Two studies have even failed to report deficits in rhythm discrimination after unilateral temporal lobe resection.[11,26] However, the use of musical stimuli for which familiarity and rhythmical complexity are extremely variable make the comparison between studies difficult. Based on these seemingly contradictory results obtained in lesion studies, it seems impossible to conclude that left-hemisphere structures are predominantly involved in musical rhythm.

One functional neuroimaging study investigated the temporal processing of musical patterns[27] but interpretation of the results in this study is made difficult because of methodological factors. Using Positron Emission Tomography in normal subjects, an increase of cerebral blood flow was obtained in left inferior Broca's area and in left insula when rhythmic and pitch judgement conditions were compared. Although this finding was interpreted by the authors as evidence supporting left-hemisphere superiority for temporal processing, it seems impossible to attribute these foci of activation to a purely temporal processing. Indeed, many other nontemporal aspects related to the task demands and to the stimuli, that differ between the two compared conditions, might have contributed to these metabolic changes.

In cognitive psychology, it has been proposed that the perception of rhythmic grouping, consisting of a sequential organization of relative durations of tones and silent intervals, should be differentiated from the perception of metre, referring to the underlying perceived beat marking off equal duration units.[28–31] Neuropsychological studies have demonstrated a dissociation between these two components involved in subjective organization of temporal patterns,[23,26,32] but this dissociation has not been systematically observed.[20] Moreover, no indication in favour of a lateralized deficit in metrical processing has been reported.

Based on this review, we can assume that the left-dominant hemisphere and more specifically the temporal lobe plays an important role in the processing of simple auditory sequences requiring rapid timing variations ranging from 10 to 100 ms. However, this left-hemisphere superiority has not been consistently demonstrated in studies using musical sequences. Although precise timing information is not usually reported in such studies, the description of the stimuli indicates that the manipulated temporal information refers to slower changes resulting, for example, from the permutation of two notes. As previously emphasized, left-hemisphere damage affected the processing of fast but not slow temporal information explaining therefore why left cerebral lesions do not systematically interfere with time-related judgement involved in musical sequences (which usually concerned longer temporal information superior to 200 ms[33]).

To try to clarify the role of the LTL in fast temporal coding in music, we examined the consequences of unilateral temporal lobe dysfunction in processing rapid sequential information. In this chapter, we present evidence supporting the hypothesis that LTL structures are predominantly involved in auditory temporal processes within the 10–100 ms time frame. For this purpose, inter-onset interval (IOI) was manipulated in a psychophysical task of anisochrony discrimination by using simple auditory sequences, as well as in a detection task involving rhythmic changes in real tunes.

Perception of inter-onset increment in simple auditory sequences: anisochrony discrimination

As frequently suggested, an important component of the rhythmic subjective structure is its underlying isochrony (i.e. a regular beat), which corresponds to musical metre (or tempo). In its simplest form, the metre can be expressed as a series of regular sounds. In the present study, we designed an experiment based on anisochrony perception which refers to the ability to differentiate a regular from an irregular sequence of sounds. The goal of this experiment was to test the effect of tempo on anisochrony (or irregularity) discrimination in patients with unilateral temporal lobe dysfunction, using an adaptive procedure. The rate of presentation or tempo (defined by the IOI separating the sounds in the sequence) was systematically manipulated to compare anisochrony discrimination using different tempos.

The anisochrony paradigm is very adequate for looking at temporal processing. As indicated by the results of experiments carried out in normal subjects,[34] anisochrony discrimination remains unaffected by duration or number of tones but it is influenced by tempo or presentation rate. By using sequences presented at various tempos ranging from 80 ms (fast) to 1000 ms (slow) IOI, it allows to compare perception of fast to slow sequential information without changing the task demands. Results obtained in normal listeners also showed that the discrimination thresholds for the anisochronous sequences were proportional to the size of the IOI for tempos between 300 and 1400 ms, whereas sensitivity deteriorated for IOIs of 80 ms as compared to slower tempos. This finding corroborates the assumption of different processes for temporal stimuli inferior or equal to 200–300 ms compared to longer ones.[35–37]

Furthermore, the paradigm that we designed uses an adaptive procedure which offers the opportunity to determine precise and fine individual thresholds which represent sensitive measures of perceptual abilities. In particular, the use of such a method in neuropsychology improves the chance of documenting subtle perceptual difficulties in brain-injured patients that could not be detected by classical paradigms involving fixed levels of stimulation common to all subjects.

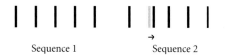

Sequence 1   Sequence 2

Figure 14.1 Example of the two sequences presented at one trial in the anisochrony discrimination task.

Two successive sequences of five tones with the same frequency, intensity, duration and attack, and decay time were presented on each trial (one regular and one irregular). The subject had to decide if the irregular sequence was in the first or second position (see Figure 14.1). Five conditions with an IOI of 80, 300, 500, 800, or 1000 ms were prepared in order to test the effect of tempo on anisochrony discrimination. The anisochrony was introduced by delaying either the second or the fourth sound of the isochronous sequence. To obtain reliable measures of anisochrony discrimination, a psychophysical procedure developed by Levitt[38] was used to determine the minimum temporal shift necessary for each individual to discriminate the regular from the irregular sequence. The size of the first shift corresponded to 10 per cent of the base interval (i.e. 50 ms for an IOI of 500 ms). The threshold of the shift detection was determined by an adaptive procedure in which the subject's response on one trial determined the size of the shift on the next trial. The perceptual threshold was then expressed as a percentage of the base IOI to allow comparison with other differential thresholds reported in the literature. Further details about the methods are provided in another paper.[39]

Eighteen patients with medically intractable epilepsy, candidates for surgical treatment at La Salpêtrière hospital (Paris) as well as a group of normal control subjects ($n = 6$), participated in this study. They all presented medial temporal lobe epilepsy associated with lateralized hippocampal sclerosis as identified by magnetic resonance imaging (MRI). None of them suffered from language disturbances and language function was lateralized in the left-hemisphere for all subjects. These patients were divided into two groups: those with right hippocampal atrophy ($n = 8$) and those with left hippocampal atrophy ($n = 10$).

According to the literature, we hypothesized that the thresholds of patients with LTL lesions would be significantly higher than the thresholds of patients with RTL lesions or normal control subjects for tempos with IOIs at or below 300 ms. In contrast, no specific deficit was predicted for slower tempos with IOIs greater than 300 ms. Finally, we predicted that for all subjects the thresholds obtained for the fastest tempo (80 ms) would be higher than those obtained for slower tempos (≥300 ms) as indicated by previous results in normal listeners.

In keeping with our predictions, the results displayed in Figure 14.2 clearly showed that anisochrony discrimination thresholds for the rapid tempo (80 ms IOI) were significantly higher for the patients with LTL dysfunction (mean threshold: 27.5 per cent) than for the patients with RTL dysfunction (17.7 per cent) and for the normal control subjects (16.4 per cent). However, there were no differences between the groups for the slower tempos (from 300 to 1000 ms IOI). This finding is compatible with results of aphasic patients with left-hemisphere lesion[1,2,4] and provides strong evidence suggesting that fast auditory sequential information processing depends specifically on the integrity of LTL structures.

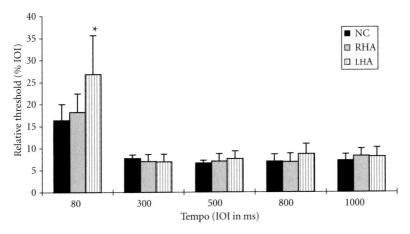

Figure 14.2   Relative thresholds of the three groups of subjects (LHA = left hippocampal atrophy, RHA = right hippocampal atrophy and NC = Normal controls) for Inter Onset Intervals (IOI) of 80, 300, 500, 800, and 1000 msec. The bars represent the standard error of the mean.

In addition, an effect of tempo was systematically obtained for all the subjects. The thresholds for very rapid sequences (80 ms IOI = 21.43 per cent) were always higher than the thresholds obtained with slower tempos ranging from 300 to 1000 ms IOI (7.6 per cent on average), for which the different thresholds remained proportional to IOI. This finding confirmed results of a previous study carried out in healthy subjects[34] and is in agreement with the assumption that brief auditory information is processed differently from longer information.[35–37]

In a previous paper,[39] we proposed that the decreased sensitivity observed for the fastest tempo could be related to an auditory memory saturation. According to echoic memory studies (Ref. 40; see Ref. 41 for a review), acoustic properties of sounds necessitate a 200–300 ms delay following the presentation of a tone to be adequately retained. This time delay was obviously shorter for the fastest tempo (80 ms IOI). Indeed, the interval between the two sequences to be discriminated was twice the base interval, in order to maintain isochrony across the trial. Thus, the inter-sequence interval for the fastest tempo (80 ms IOI) was 160 ms whereas a minimum of 600 ms separated the sequences for the other tempos. Therefore, a saturation of echoic memory could have been responsible for the observed difference between the thresholds of the fasted tempo and the slower tempos, because the inter-sequence interval would be too short to allow consolidation of the first sequence. If such an explanation is validated in the future, the deficit documented in patients with LTL dysfunction in fast sequential auditory perception could be interpreted as an echoic memory dysfunction. Although an eventual relation between a temporal processing dysfunction and an auditory memory deficit in dysphasic children has already been suggested by Tallal and collaborators,[42] the possible link between an echoic memory dysfunction and an anisochrony discrimination deficit of fast auditory information in patients with LTL lesion remains to be clarified.

It is also possible that the decreased temporal sensitivity for the rapid tempo is related to a difficulty to determine if the irregular sequence was the first or the second one suggesting deficit in the temporal order processing. Although this judgement was not affected when slower tempos were presented, it becomes more difficult to make such a judgement in rapid sequences (subjects sometimes having trouble to separate the sequences *per se*). This additional constraint might have penalized more strongly patients with LTL dysfunction than the other subjects.

In previous studies, rapid temporal processing deficits were usually reported in language-impaired subjects (Ref. 43 for review). Results of the present investigation extend this finding to patients presenting a limited LTL lesion without associated massive language disorders, indicating that time-related disturbances are not necessarily associated with language disturbances. However, the present results differ from the data obtained in language-impaired subjects since in this latter case, subjects presented a deficit with a slower tempo (300 ms IOI) while the subjects with LTL dysfunction did not present any difficulties in this condition. It seems that the severity of the sequential auditory deficit observed in patients with or without verbal deficit varies. Although these divergent results could be explained by methodological differences between the studies, it is also possible that the severity of the temporal deficits could be correlated to the severity of verbal deficits. The patients tested in the present study might be situated at one end of the continuum, showing limited temporal processing deficits and relatively preserved verbal abilities, while dysphasic or dyslexic subjects could be located at the other end, with more severe temporal deficits and more severe language deficits. Conversely, it is also possible that rapid sequential temporal processing can be disturbed without affecting language functions, which would suggest that they depend on distinct neural substrates. Future research will be necessary to determine whether the same underlying mechanism is responsible for the deficit observed in epileptic and dysphasic patients.

Perception of inter-onset increment in musical sequences: temporal microstructure of familiar tunes

The goal of this study was to extend to the musical domain the role of the LTL in processing small timing variations. As emphasized in the introduction, it seems that the perception of small timing differences within a musical sequence has not been investigated in neuropsychology. To explore this issue, we designed a task involving the detection of inter-onset interval increments in familiar monodic tunes improving therefore the ecological validity of the task.

Several descriptive studies showed that performers considerably modify the temporal structure as noted in the score when interpreting a piece of music (for review, see Ref. 44), a piece being never played exactly as it is written in the score. However, music played in this way seems perfect to the listeners, suggesting that we are expecting these temporal changes. Such temporal microvariations occur at specific locations and are supposed to reflect the subjective temporal structure of music. It has been demonstrated that consequently, a listener is expecting these musical microvariations in perceiving musical excerpts.[45] In an experimental study using classical pieces of music (microstructural expectations), Repp

showed that increment detection accuracy was correlated with the temporal microstructure profiles of expert performances suggesting that temporal increments of an interval
which is usually lengthened are more difficult to detect than temporal increments of intervals for which no microvariations were introduced. In the cognitive literature, two hypothesis, which are not mutually exclusive, have been proposed to explain variations in the
accuracy detection. A top-down hypothesis suggests that listeners' expectations reflect
expressive performance of temporal microvariations[45] whereas a bottom-up hypothesis
indicates that some expectations may be due to psychoacoustical characteristics of the
stimulus.[44]

Based on these observations, we designed an experiment involving the detection of
inter-onset interval increments introduced in musical sequences to test perception of these
temporal microvariations in patients with unilateral temporal lobe lesions. The musical
excerpts used were very familiar in order to generate high expectations and to prevent bias
due to each listeners' musical background.

In the experimental task, half of the trials consisted of the presentation of a score (played
exactly as it is written in the score) version of a familiar tune whereas the other half consisted of a modified version of the tune in which one inter-onset interval was increased by
25 per cent, producing an increment of 10–140 ms (mean = 85 ms; standard deviation = 62 ms) depending on the size (or duration) of the modified interval within the tune.
The subject's task was to decide whether the presented trial corresponded to the mechanical or to the modified version of the excerpt using a two-alternative forced choice paradigm. Two types of inter-onset interval were introduced. One type corresponds to expected
increments and the other one corresponds to unexpected increments. The level of expectation was determined by results of previous studies detailed elsewhere.[46] Basically, the
recording of pianists' performances were compared to a score (or computerized) version of
each selected tune to allow the analysis of temporal microstructure. The results of this
experiment allowed the identification of one interval that was systematically lengthened in
pianists' recordings as compared to metrical version, and another interval that was systematically preserved. Inter-onset interval increments were thus introduced at these specific locations and it was hypothesized that temporal increments located at 'lengthened intervals'
would be more difficult to detect than temporal increments located at 'preserved intervals'
since listeners would be expecting temporal increments in the first but not in the second
condition. The ability to distinguish these two types of inter-onset increments was subsequently tested in a perceptual task confirming therefore the relevance of this temporal
manipulation in normal nonmusician listeners. Based on these results, we designed an
experimental task to evaluate the ability to detect subtle temporal changes by taking into
account implicit knowledge of the rhythmical structure underlying musical listening. By
manipulating temporal increments and cognitive expectations, especially in regard to the
temporal (or rhythmic) dimension, it was possible to assess bottom-up as well as top-down
processing involved in musical rhythm perception.

Twenty-two patients who had undergone a right ($n = 11$) or a left ($n = 11$) temporal
lobe resection for the relief of medically intractable epilepsy as well as 14 normal control
subjects were tested in this experiment. None of the patients presented language disorders
or suffered from extra temporal lesions. Language was lateralized on the left side in all

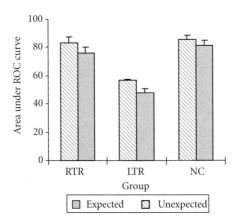

Figure 14.3 Detection accuracy derived from the area under the receiver operating curve (ROC) of the three groups of subjects (LTR = left temporal resection, RTR = right temporal resection and NC = Normal controls) for expected and unexpected inter onset increments. The bars represent the standard error of the mean.

subjects. As opposed to the previous study, the patients were tested post-operatively. The temporal resection includes the medial temporal lobe structures (hippocampal and surrounding cortex) and in some patients, the excision involves the temporal pole as well.

Considering the predominant contribution of LTL structures in processing rapid sequential information, we expected a deficit in detecting microtemporal variations in familiar tunes in patients with LTL lesion. In this study, the task of detection of temporal increments required no tonal judgment, for which the RTL is usually needed.[47–50] We therefore postulated adequate performance for patients with RTL lesion. Moreover, an effect of level of expectation of inter-onset interval was predicted for normal subjects and for patients with RTL lesion. If this effect reflects a perceptually driven processing, it should disappear in patients with LTL lesion, otherwise it might be also present in this patient group.

The results of this study are displayed in Figure 14.3 which represents detection accuracy of the three groups of subjects for expected and unexpected inter-onset increments. An area under the receiver operating curve (ROC) derived from the number of hits and false alarms was computed for each subject. As predicted, a significant deficit in detecting inter-onset increments was obtained in patients with LTL lesion as compared to subjects with RTL lesion and normal subjects, these two latter groups being not different. This deficit characterizing patients with LTL lesion cannot be attributed to difficulty in identifying the tunes since all the subjects were able to adequately recognize the melodies. The results of this study suggest that the ability to detect an inter-onset increment introduced in very well known tunes depends on the integrity of LTL structures, extending to the musical domain the previously reported role of the LTL in rapid sequential processing.

Moreover, the results showed that it is more difficult to detect expected than unexpected temporal increments for all the subjects indicating therefore that top-down processing remains functional for the three groups of subjects. Moreover, it means that expectations of nonmusician listeners were identical to those of pianists, extending to the simple monodic familiar tunes findings reported with polyphonic classical stock pieces.[45]

Although patients with LTL lesion presented a clear deficit in perceiving temporal microvariations, they seem to be able to generate temporal expectations to the same extent as healthy subjects.

To summarize, the results of this study illustrate a dissociation between a selective deficit in fine grained temporal sensitivity whereas temporal expectations seem to be relatively spared in the presence of LTL lesions, suggesting that top-down (or descending) processing may function independently from bottom-up (or ascending) processing. In addition, these data indicate that top-down processing involved in the temporal perception of musical information can still be preserved despite disrupted bottom-up processing.

Conclusion

The experiments reported in this paper were designed to test the hypothesized role of LTL structures to musical temporal processing. We focused our interest on the perception of brief sequential information ranging from few tens to hundreds of milliseconds by comparing results obtained with very simple auditory sequences and real musical excerpts. In keeping with our predictions, the data reported in this paper suggest that LTL structures are predominantly involved in perceiving inter-onset interval increments in familiar tunes as well as in isochronous sequences, extending to the musical domain findings previously reported in speech.[12,43]

The patients included in both studies had lesions located within the medial temporal lobe structures and more specifically in the hippocampus. It remains difficult to know if the deficit could be attributed to the hippocampal lesion or to a more global dysfunction of the temporal neocortical structures. Evidence from a functional cerebral imaging study (Positron Emission Tomography with 18 Fluorodeoxyglucose, FDG-PET) carried out in a similar population of epileptic subjects indicates that the temporal lobe dysfunction associated with unilateral hippocampal sclerosis is not restricted to the hippocampus but extends to include the anterior part of the temporal neocortex corresponding to the temporal pole.[51] Although the structural lesion is apparently limited to the hippocampal formation, it does not mean that the connections between the medial temporal lobe structures and the neocortex or the surrounding and external temporal cortex *per se* remain functional. The present data does not allow to differentiate the role of the hippocampus from the contribution of the adjacent cortical areas in auditory sequential information processing. However, it seems relevant to suggest that abnormal metabolism reported in these surrounding cortical structures reflects a temporal lobe dysfunction or an interruption of the hippocampo-neocortical loop that may be responsible for the deficits obtained in our patients with LTL dysfunction.

In the present studies, the time-related deficit following LTL lesion was reproduced in two different tasks involving purely temporal stimuli as well as multidimensional musical sequences in the context of an adaptive or a fixed level paradigm, respectively. Despite numerous methodological differences, the results of these two studies provide strong support for the selective sensitivity of LTL structures in processing rapid time-related events. Indeed, the two methodologies require the detection of subtle temporal variations which was made possible by the use of regular sequences or very familiar tunes producing strong temporal expectations. It is therefore tempting to consider that a single mechanism, depending on the processing of very brief sequential events, is responsible for impairments obtained in both tasks.

However, it is too early to assume that such impairments can be explained by a unique deficit. We already suggested that deficit in anisochrony discrimination of rapid sequences can also result from the saturation of sensory memory or from an inability to judge the temporal order. Such a hypothesis should be tested in the future to elucidate the nature of the deficit characterizing subjects with LTL dysfunction.

Acknowledgements

We are also indebted to Xavier Gangand for programming the experiments. This research was supported by a grant from Contrat d'objectif Région Nord—Pas de Calais: 'Motricité et Cognition' (France) and by GIS 'Dysfonctionnement de la Cognition'.

References

1. **Efron, R.** (1963) Temporal perception, aphasia and déjà vu. *Brain*, 86, 403–24.

2. **Tallal, P.** and **F. Newcombe** (1978) Impairment of auditory perception and language comprehension in dysphasia. *Brain and Language* 5, 13–24.

3. **Lackner, J. R.** and **H. L. Teuber** (1973) Alterations in auditory fusion thresholds after cerebral injury in man. *Neuropsychologia* 11, 409–15.

4. **Mills, L.** and **G. B. Rollman** (1980) Hemispheric asymmetry for auditory perception of temporal order. *Neuropsychologia* 18, 41–7.

5. **Robin, D. A., D. Tranel,** and **H. Damasio** (1990) Auditory perception of temporal and spectral events in patients with focal left and right cerebral lesions. *Brain and Language*, 39, 539–55.

6. **Sherwin, L.** and **R. Efron** (1980) Temporal ordering deficits following anterior temporal lobectomy. *Brain and Language* 11, 195–203.

7. **Swisher, L.** and **I. J. Hirsh** (1972) Brain damage and the ordering of two temporally successive stimuli. *Neuropsychologia* 10, 137–52.

8. **Griffiths, T. D., et al.** (1997) Spatial and temporal auditory processing deficits following right-hemisphere infarction. *Brain*, 120, 785–94.

9. **Musiek, F. E., J. A. Baran,** and **M. L. Pinheiro** (1990) Duration pattern recognition in normal subjects and patients with cerebral and cochlear lesions. *Audiol.* 29, 304–13.

10. **Albert, M. L., et al.** (1972) A case study of auditory agnosia: linguistic and non-linguistic processing. *Cortex* 8, 427–43.

11. **Milner, B.** (1962) Laterality effects in audition. In V. Mountcastle (ed.) *Interhemispheric Relations and Cerebral Dominance*, Baltimore: John Hopkins University Press, pp. 173–201.

12. **Liégeois-Chauvel, C., et al.** (1999) Specialization of left auditory cortex for speech perception in man depends on temporal coding. *Cereb Cortex* 9, 484–96.

13. **Gordon, H.** (1978) Left-hemisphere dominance for rhythmic elements in dichotically-presented melodies. *Cortex*, 14, 58–70.

14. **Halperin, Y., I. Nachshon,** and **A. Carmon** (1973) Shift of ear superiority in dichotic listening to temporally patterned nonverbal stimuli. *J. Acousti. Soc. Am.* 53, 46–50.

15. **Papçun, G., et al.** (1974) Is the left-hemisphere specialized for speech, language and/or something else? *J. Acoust. Soc. Am.* 55, 319–27.

16. **Robinson, G. M. and D. J. Solomon** (1974) Rhythm is processed by the speech hemisphere. *J. Exp. Psychol.* 102, 508–11.

17. **Peretz, I. and J. Morais** (1980) Modes of processing melodies and ear asymmetry in non-musicians. *Neuropsychologia* 18, 447–89.

18. **Mavlov, L.** (1980) Amusia due to rhythm agnosia in a musician with left-hemisphere damage: a non-auditory supramodal defect. *Cortex* 16, 331–8.

19. **Prior, D. A., G. Kinsella, and J. Giese** (1990) Assessment of musical processing in brain-damaged patients: implications for laterality of music. *J. Clinical Exp. Neuropsychol.* 12, 301–12.

20. **Kester, D., et al.** (1991) Acute effect of anterior temporal lobectomy on musical processing. *Neuropsychologia* 29, 703–8.

21. **Michel, F., F. Peronnet, and B. Schott** (1980) A case of cortical deafness: clinical and electro-physiological data. *Brain and Language* 10, 367–77.

22. **Penhune, V. B., R. J. Zatorre, and W. H. Feindel** (1999) The role of auditory cortex in the retention of rhythmic patterns as studied in patients with temporal lobe removals including Heschl's gyrus. *Neuropsychologia* 37, 315–31.

23. **Peretz, I.** (1990) Processing of local and global musical information by unilateral brain-damaged patients. *Brain* 113, 1185–205.

24. **Reitan, R. M. and D. Wolfson** (1989) The Seashore rhythm test and brain functions. *The Clinical Neuropsychologist* 3, 70–8.

25. **Shapiro, B. E., M. Grossman, and H. Gardner** (1981) Selective musical processing deficits in brain damaged populations. *Neuropsychologia* 19, 161–9.

26. **Liégeois-Chauvel, C., et al.** (1998) Contribution of different cortical areas in the temporal lobes to music processing. *Brain* 121, 1853–67.

27. **Platel, H., et al.** (1997) The structural components of music perception. A functional anatomical study. *Brain* 120, 229–43.

28. **Dowling, W. J. and D. Harwood** (1986) *Music Cognition.* New York, NY: Academic Press.

29. **Povel, D. J.** (1981) Internal representation of simple temporal patterns. *J. Exp. Psychol: Hum. Percept. and Perform.* 7, 3–18.

30. **Povel, D. J. and P. Essens** (1985) Perception of temporal patterns. *Music percept.*, 2, 411–40.

31. **Repp, B. H.** (1995) Detectability of duration and intensity increments in melody tones: partial connection between music perception and performance. *Percept. Psychophy.* 57, 1217–32.

32. **Polk, M. and A. Kertesz** (1993) Music and language in degenerative disease of the brain. *Brain and Cognit.* 22, 98–117.

33. **Fraisse, P.** (1982) Rhythm and tempo. In D. Deutsch (ed.) *The Psychology of Music.* New York: Academic Press, pp. 149–78.

34. **Ehrlé, N. and S. Samson** (1996) Détection de l'irrégularité temporelle: influence de la durée et du tempo. In F. Anceaux and J. M. Coquery (eds) *Sciences Cognitives, Individus et Société. Actes du 6ème Colloque de l'Association pour la Recherche Cognitive.* Villeneuve d'Ascq, pp. 209–14.

35. **Michon, J. A.** (1964) Studies on subjective duration: I. Differential sensitivity in the perception of repeated temporal intervals. *Acta Psychol.* 22, 441–50.

36. **Nakajima, Y., G. ten Hoopen, and R. Van der Wilk** (1991) A new illusion of time perception. *Music Percept.* 8, 431–48.

37. ten Hoopen, G., *et al.* (1995) Auditory isochrony: time shrinking and temporal patterns. *Percept.* 24, 577–93.

38. Levitt, H. (1971) Transformed up-down methods in psychoacoustics. *J. Acoust. Soc. Am.* 49, 467–77.

39. Ehrlé, N., S. Samson, and M. Baulac (2001) Processing of rapid auditory information in epileptic patients with left temporal lobe damage without dysphasia. *Neuropsychologia* 39, 525–31.

40. Massaro, D. W. (1972) Preperceptual images, processing time and perceptual units in auditory perception. *Psycholog. Rev.* 79, 124–45.

41. Cowan, N. (1984) On short and long auditory stores. *Psycholog. Bull.* 96, 341–70.

42. Tallal, P., R. L. Sainburg, and T. Jernigan (1991) The neuropathology of developmental dysphasia: behavioral, morphological, and physiological evidence for a pervasive temporal processing disorder. *Reading and Writing: an Interdisciplinary Journal* 3, 363–77.

43. Tallal, P., S. Miller, and R. H. Fitch (1993) Neurobiological basis of speech: a case for the preeminence of temporal processing. *Annals of the New York Academy of Sciences* 682, 27–47.

44. Penel, A. and C. Drake (1998) Sources of timing variations in music performance: a psychological segmentation model. *Psycholog. Res.* 61, 12–32.

45. Repp, B. H. (1992) Probing the cognitive representation of musical time: structural constraints on the perception of timing perturbations. *Cognit.* 44, 241–81.

46. Ehrlé, N. (1998) Traitement temporel de l'information auditive et lobe temporal. Ph.D. Thesis. France: University of Reims.

47. Samson, S. and R. J. Zatorre (1988) Melodic and harmonic discrimination following unilateral cerebral excision. *Brain and Cognit.* 7, 348–60.

48. Johnsrude, I., B. B. Penhune, and R. J. Zatorre (2000) Functional specificity in the right human auditory cortex for perceiving pitch direction. *Brain* 123, 155–63.

49. Zatorre, R. J. (1988) Pitch perception of complex tones and human temporal-lobe function. *J. Acoust. Soc. Am.* 84, 566–72.

50. Zatorre, R. J. and S. Samson (1991) Role of the right temporal neocortex in retention of pitch in auditory short-term memory. *Brain* 114, 2403–17.

51. Semah, F. *et al.* (1995) Is interictal temporal hypometabolism related to mesial temporal sclerosis? A positron emission tomography/magnetic resonance imaging confrontation. *Epilepsia* 36, 447–56.

CHAPTER 15

CEREBRAL SUBSTRATES OF MUSICAL IMAGERY

ANDREA R. HALPERN

Abstract

Musical imagery refers to the experience of 'replaying' music by imagining it inside the head. Whereas visual imagery has been extensively studied, few people have investigated imagery in the auditory domain. This chapter reviews a program of research that has tried to characterize auditory imagery for music using both behavioural and cognitive neuroscientific tools. I begin by describing some of my behavioural studies of the mental analogues of musical tempo, pitch, and temporal extent. I then describe four studies using three techniques that examine the correspondence of brain involvement in actually perceiving vs imagining familiar music. These involve one lesion study with epilepsy surgery patients, two positron emission tomography (PET) studies, and one study using transcranial magnetic stimulation (TMS). The studies converge on the importance of the right temporal neocortex and other right-hemisphere structures in the processing of both perceived and imagined nonverbal music. Perceiving and imagining songs that have words also involve structures in the left hemisphere. The supplementary motor area (SMA) is activated during musical imagery; it may mediate rehearsal that involves motor programs, such as imagined humming. Future studies are suggested that would involve imagery of sounds that cannot be produced by the vocal tract to clarify the role of the SMA in auditory imagery.

Keywords: Musical imagery; Behavioural studies; Cognitive neuroscience

Introduction

Many people experience the sounds of music in two distinct but related manners. Listening to live or recorded music is, of course, the way we commonly think of enjoying music. However, many people also report that they can reexperience music by imagining it in their heads. This can be pleasurable or not, depending on the circumstances, but in either case, the experience appears to be a vivid one, even among people untrained in music. In fact, I am often asked how to 'stop' a tune from obsessively intruding into everyday thoughts. Highly trained musicians report that they can use auditory imagery to help them in their everyday tasks, such as 'hearing' music as they read musical notation.

In recent years, I have studied the characteristics of this auditory imagery experience, initially from a behavioural perspective and more recently from a cognitive neuroscientific perspective. I have been most interested in the auditory imagery experiences of untrained or moderately trained musicians, although many interesting questions derive from considering experts as well. My paradigms and experimental logic have been derived partly from the more extensive literature in visual imagery; other approaches have been created anew as the need arose. In studying any mental imagery, the challenge is to externalize what is essentially an internal experience to examine what it means to have, in the case of musical imagery, a 'tune inside the head'.

Behavioural approach

In the 1980s, I carried out an extensive series of experiments with young adult college students to explore how auditory imagery of music may be characterized. I explored the mental representation of *tempo*[1,2] and *pitch*[3] in familiar songs. To study representation of tempo, I asked participants to set their preferred tempo for a familiar tune being played on a computer. The program allowed continuous adjustments of tempo until the tune sounded right to the listeners. I then asked them to imagine the same tunes and set a metronome to the imagined tempo. Tempo settings were highly correlated in the perception and imagination tasks. I also showed that people can manipulate the tempo of an imagined song, within limits, to make it 'sound' very fast or very slow. Finally, I showed that musicians showed impressive consistency when asked to tap out the tempo of an imagined song on one day and again two to five days later (average standard deviation = 1.4 metronome settings over four attempts), although nonmusicians were somewhat less consistent.

In the domain of pitch, I asked people to imagine familiar songs and hum the starting note corresponding to their auditory image of the song. In a second task, I asked people to think of the starting note of a familiar song and select that note from a piano keyboard (all the tunes were popular folk or children's songs, unlikely to have been heard with any particular starting note in the past). Once again, consistency of pitch production or selection was impressive for musically unselected participants, even over a delay of several days (average standard deviation = 1.25 semitones for production, two semitones for selection over four attempts). Finally, I asked people to rate how similar a played note was to the opening note of a tune they had imagined and produced a few days earlier. The person's own preferred note was rated quite highly, as were starting notes a major third lower, minor third higher, and a perfect fifth higher than the preferred notes (these are all musically coherent intervals). However, subjects rated notes only one semitone higher or lower than their preferred note as dissimilar to their imagined pitch, showing a fairly acute sense of pitch representation.

These behavioural tasks seem to show a veridical representation of characteristics particular to music. However, I also explored the *extension in time* that is characteristic of almost all auditory stimuli and thus ought to be captured in auditory imagery. I explored this temporal aspect in the subsequent cognitive neuroscientific studies of auditory imagery for music.

To begin, I modified a paradigm introduced in visual imagery by Kosslyn *et al.*[4] In that study, they asked people to learn a map of an imaginary island. Pairs of features on the island were presented, and subjects had to 'mentally scan' between them. Latencies to do so were highly correlated with actual distance between the features on the map, suggesting that the mental representation was preserving an analogue of space.

To extend this paradigm to musical imagery,[5] I selected a number of familiar songs where unique lyrics fell on specified beats of the tune. For instance, the first line of the American national anthem, 'The Star Spangled Banner,' is 'Oh, say can you see by the dawn's early light?' In the most relevant study in that series, I presented the title of the song, followed by one lyric from the first line of the song, followed by the second lyric. The task was mental pitch comparison: Was lyric 2 higher or lower in pitch than lyric 1? No singing or humming was allowed. The lyrics were either close together ('Oh' and 'can') or far apart in the actual tune ('Oh' and 'dawn's'). I found that this was a difficult task for my musically unselected subjects; nevertheless, reaction times increased nearly linearly as the separation in beats between the two lyrics increased. Subjects reported using auditory imagery to accomplish the task, even though they were not instructed to do so. The consistency of reaction time data with this report strongly suggested to me that this task had captured the extension in time of auditory imagery for music.

Cognitive neuroscientific approach

The behavioural studies cited above have in common the logic that if responding to an imagined stimulus resembles responding to a perceived stimulus, we may conclude that imagery is a particularly vivid and veridical form of mental representation. However, this comparison between imagery and perception may be strengthened by examining the similarities in neural underpinnings of the two processes. This approach is complementary to the behavioural approach in that at least to some extent behavioural responses might be influenced by external influences such as demand characteristics or experimenter expectancies.[6] However, it is unlikely that people can influence their own brain structures or activities. We may thus look to similarities in the brain loci involved in auditory imagery and perception to gain a better perspective on the processing of similarities and differences in the two types of tasks. An argument for this approach is well articulated by Farah[7] for the visual domain.

The strongest hypothesis is of course that the brain areas would be identical in auditory imagery and perception. This may serve as a guiding null hypothesis, but we would not in reality expect this amount of overlap; people other than those hallucinating can tell the difference between imagining and hearing a song. However, the extent of overlap may tell us how similarly the brain processes hearing and imagining hearing. Brain areas uniquely active in imaging tasks can by extension inform us as to the additional or alternative processing demands imposed in imagery by having to, in effect, create as well as perceive the stimulus.

As noted above, the approach has been reasonably successful in the visual domain. For instance, Kosslyn et al.[8] used positron emission tomography (PET) to measure brain activity during parallel perceptual and imagined visual tasks. They found quite a few areas activated in common, even to the extent that varying the size of the presented object and varying the size of an imagined object activated similar brain areas in similar ways. Few people have looked at auditory imagery using parallel perceptual and imagery tasks. However, the neural structures responsible for some aspects of musical perception are well defined. My partner for most of the studies described in the following sections has been

Robert Zatorre. When we began our first study, he and Samson, among others, had already established that a number of musical tasks are impaired after lesions in the right temporal neocortex.[9-12] Thus our initial hypothesis was that the same region would be involved in musical imagery tasks that resembled musical perceptual tasks.

What follows are brief descriptions of a series of studies using three different cognitive neuroscience techniques to investigate the cerebral substrates of musical imagery. The first is a lesion study, which can give information about the necessary involvement of some brain areas in an activity. The next two studies use PET paradigms to investigate brain areas that are active in auditory imagery for verbal and nonverbal songs, respectively. Finally, I describe a study using transcranial magnetic stimulation (TMS) that returns to the logic of the lesion studies, in that a brain area in normal people is disrupted for a brief time and the ensuing decrements in performance are measured.

Lesion study

My first study with Zatorre[13] examined the effect of right temporal lobectomy on performance of a mental pitch comparison task that I described earlier.[5] Participants were patients having undergone surgical excision of the anterior portion of the right or left temporal lobe (excluding the primary auditory cortex) for relief of intractable epilepsy. We tested the patients either two weeks after surgery (approximately two-thirds of the patients), or at follow-up medical appointments a year or more after surgery. A control group consisted of age- and education-matched neurologically normal individuals. Preoperative testing insured that the patients had typical language representation. All participants were familiar with the songs we used, and they all passed a brief test of pitch discrimination ability.

The imagery task was essentially the one described earlier. Participants saw a title of a song, for instance, 'Jingle Bells', followed by the first line of the song, with two words in capital letters, such as 'Dashing through the SNOW, in a one-horse open SLEIGH'. They decided if SLEIGH was higher or lower in pitch than SNOW, and pressed a button to answer. The parallel perception task, which was always presented first, was the same except that the song, sung with lyrics, was actually presented to participants from a digitized sound file while they made their judgement. Accuracy and reaction times were recorded. The reaction time pattern replicated the pattern I had shown earlier[5] of increasing latency with increasing distance in beats between the lyrics, although accuracy turned out to be the measure of interest here.

Accuracy results are shown in Figure 15.1. It is clear that the imagery task was more difficult than the perception task, as expected. It is also clear that the right temporal lobectomy group was impaired relative to controls on both the imagery and perception tasks, to an equal extent, whereas the left temporal lobectomy group was impaired on neither.

This pattern was consistent with our hypothesis that the right temporal lobe is an important mediator of musical imagery, as it has been shown to be for musical perception. We considered which particular aspect of the task was most likely to have been subserved by the right temporal lobe. All participants passed a simple tone discrimination task, so a

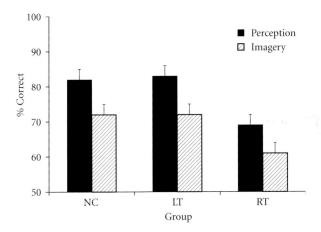

Figure 15.1 Mean per cent correct, plus standard error, for normal control subjects (NC), patients with left temporal lobe excision (LT), and patients with right temporal lobe excision (RT) in perception and imagery tasks in the lesion study.

deficit in pitch comparison itself was unlikely to be the cause of the group's impairment. Furthermore, this group was impaired in the perception task, when the tune did not need to be generated from memory, making memory retrieval unlikely to be the right temporal lobe's crucial contribution. Thus we concluded that the right temporal deficit is likely to be primarily due to a difficulty in remembering the (imagined) pitches to be compared.

PET studies

Lesion studies allow one to draw conclusions about the areas *crucial* to perform certain tasks. They do not, however, allow any conclusions about what brain areas are *active* in the tasks, whether or not they are crucial. Lesion studies also are confined to the particular excisions made available by accidents of nature or deliberate surgery. If we want to study the somewhat broader question of what areas throughout the brain are active during imagery and perception tasks, then functional brain imaging technology is a useful addition to our investigations. Another advantage of brain imaging techniques is that neurologically normal participants can be studied, in contrast to the neurologically abnormal people studied, by definition, in lesion work. In our next study, Zatorre and I[14] used PET to observe the changes in cerebral blood flow (CBF) as participants performed musical imagery tasks similar to the ones already described.

In this approach, tasks are set up in a series so that more complex tasks include elements of the simpler tasks presented to subjects. Subtracting the activation observed in the simpler task from that observed in the more complex task allows one to isolate activation unique to the critical components of the more complex task. For instance, in almost any cognitive task, the brain activation due to the simple registration of auditory or visual stimuli, and the motor activation involved in pressing buttons, are not of major interest. Therefore, control tasks are often presented that involve simply seeing or hearing a stimulus and pressing a button in response. Subtracting activation due to these lower-level components gives a better indication of the mental work involved in the tasks of more interest.

In our study, we presented the imagery and perception tasks that we used previously,[14] except we presented single words instead of complete first lines from the songs. A third task was meant to control for such simpler tasks as visual perception and button pressing. This visual baseline presented pairs of words used in the imagery and perception task, but each pair member came from a different song. For each pair presented on the screen, participants had to judge which one was longer in length and press a button for their choice. Because the pairs were scrambled, we assumed listeners would not be reminded of songs; thus auditory imagery should not be activated. But over the course of the baseline condition, all words used in the main task would be seen. All songs were very familiar to the subjects, who were 12 healthy right-handed young adults. Most had some musical training but none were serious musicians.

All participants underwent a magnetic resonance imaging (MRI) scan in order to allow us to later localize CBF activity to the appropriate anatomy for each person. For the test session, the three tasks were explained and there was a short practice session. After being placed in the scanner, the subjects received an injection of radioactively labelled water ($H_2^{15}O$) required to index the CBF activity, and performed the visual baseline task. This was then repeated for the perception task and then the imagery task, in that order.

As expected, people were more accurate on the perception task than the imagery task, and once again reaction times in both imagery and perception increased as a function of distance between the lyrics in the real tunes. The analysis then proceeded by subtracting the activation shown in the baseline task from the perception task and also the baseline task from the imagery task. A graphic representation of the results is shown in panel I of Figure 15.2. Here we see in the upper part of panel I that the primary auditory area (located in superior temporal gyrus, or STG) is quite active when listening to sounds, as one would expect. More interesting is the fact that several areas of the STG adjacent to the primary auditory cortex (secondary auditory cortex) are also active when people were just imagining the sounds (lower part of panel I). Panel II shows several other areas of correspondence between the imagery and perception tasks: several areas in the frontal lobe were active in both tasks, as was one area in the parietal lobe. Panel III shows activity in the supplementary motor area (SMA, involved in motor planning) in both tasks, stronger in imagery than perception. When we subtracted the activity in the perception task from that in the imagery task, only four brain areas were unique to imagery, two of which are pictured in panel IV. These two areas, the thalamus and inferior frontopolar areas, are known to be involved in memory functions, and may be associated with the extensive memory demands attached to the imagery task.

The results of this study supported several of our earlier ideas but also raised new questions. Consistent with our lesion study,[13] several areas of the temporal lobe classified as secondary auditory cortex were activated when people were carrying out mental pitch comparisons, in the absence of any overt auditory stimulation. Thus we concluded that the right STG is both *active* during such tasks (shown by the PET study), as well as *necessary*

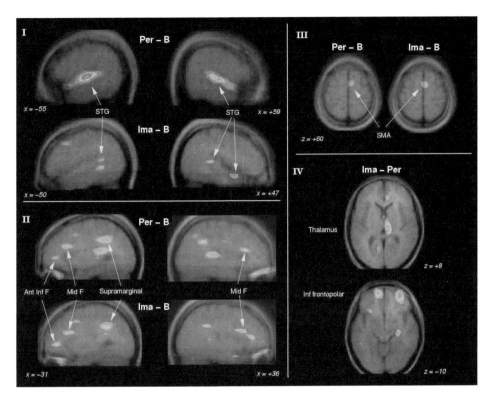

Figure 15.2 Brain areas showing activation in the perception minus baseline, imagery minus baseline, and imagery minus perception conditions of the verbal tune PET study. (See Plate 2 in colour section.)

for carrying out the task successfully (shown by the lesion study). We were also not surprised by the areas of activation in the frontal lobes. Activation in frontal areas similar to the ones seen here was found by Zatorre et al.[15] in a PET study in which participants had to judge relative pitches of notes in novel (perceived) tunes, and in a study where the pitches of spoken syllables were compared.[16]

Two results were more unexpected. First, contrary to the literature cited earlier that consistently showed right-sided asymmetries in brain activation during music processing,[15] and deleterious consequences of right-sided lesions for music processing,[9–13] here almost all the activated areas were bilateral, except for right-sided activation in the thalamus. A second unexpected finding was the strong activation of the SMA during imagery even though subjects were not actually producing any motor movements. Both these findings might be related to the fact that the stimulus songs all had words, which participants had to access during the tasks. The left frontal regions have been implicated in various overt verbal tasks,[17,18] so that the bilateral activation seen here might be reflecting the dual nature of the stimulus to be processed (words plus music). Activation of the SMA has been observed when subjects are asked to generate internal speech[19] and to overtly vocalize music.[20] Thus the SMA activation observed here in our imagery task may reflect a subvocal rehearsal process of either words or music to support performance on an otherwise difficult task.

In light of these issues, our next PET study[21] used only nonverbal tunes. We were interested to see whether removing words from our task would lead to more right-sided activation than we saw earlier, consistent with various findings in the music perception literature. We also wanted to see if SMA would be active even when potential rehearsal devices would not involve words. Finally, we wanted to try a different type of imagery task to see if our results would generalize over paradigms.

To this end, we developed a stimulus pool of tunes that were familiar but did not have lyrics. These included movie and television themes, classical excerpts, and miscellaneous tunes such as the Westminster (Big Ben) chimes. In our main task (cue/imagery) we played the first few notes of a theme as a cue, and asked participants to imagine the theme to the end of its first phrase (this task and the materials had been presented to people in advance of scanning to familiarize them with task parameters). To have a behavioural index of auditory imagery, the played excerpts differed in length. If subjects were carrying out instructions as we intended, latency to press the button should increase from our shortest (2.2 s on average) to longest excerpts (6.2 s on average).

We also had some control tasks. For these, we took the first few notes of each real tune, and scrambled the note order so that the cue did not elicit a memory of any real tune. In the control task for simple listening and button pressing we presented these 'fake' cues and simply had people press a button after each one (control). A second control task involved imagery but no retrieval from long-term memory. In this task, we presented the fake cue and asked for people to simply reimagine it immediately after presentation (control/imagery). The subtraction of interest for current purposes is the cue/imagery minus the control task.

As previously, PET scanning was undertaken in conjunction with an MRI to provide anatomical localization of CBF activation for each person. Eight healthy, right-handed young adults participated, who had from 3 to 16 years of musical training. The conditions were presented in order of control, cue/imagery, and control/imagery.

As predicted, the average time to press a button indicating imaging of the tune was complete in the cue/imagery condition varied proportionally to the length of the tune. Thus we are confident that subjects were following our imagery instructions. The results of the cue/imagery minus control subtraction are shown in Figure 15.3. As in our previous study,[14] we found activation in the secondary auditory cortex (marked STG), although this time the activation was in the right but not left temporal lobe. We also found activation in several regions of the frontal lobe (inf F), most of which were more prominent on the right than the left side. Finally we once again found strong activation in the SMA.

We thus confirmed several findings from our study with verbal tunes:[14] areas normally concerned with processing of auditory information are recruited even when the auditory information is internally generated. This occurred even with a different behavioural task and different songs than had been used earlier. We also confirmed the activity of the SMA in our task. The fact that this area was active even though no verbal rehearsal could logically have been taking place suggests that the SMA is involved with some kind of subvocal

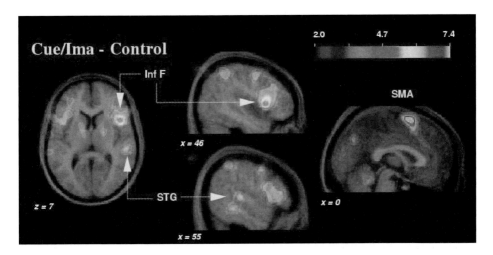

Figure 15.3 Brain areas showing activation in the cue/imagery minus control subtraction in the nonverbal tune PET study. (See Plate 3 in colour section.)

humming strategy during the imagery generation. The frontal areas activated here are also approximately the same as some of the frontal areas seen in our previous task. Because the current task did not require extensive involvement of working memory (mental pitch comparison was not required, merely internal scanning of the tune), it is likely that the areas in common in our two studies reflect retrieval from musical semantic memory rather than working memory.

The major new contribution here was that once words were removed from the stimulus and the task, we found prominent right-sided asymmetry in the areas active in the imagery task. The temporal lobe activation is consistent with our lesion study[13] that showed similar decrements from right-sided temporal lobectomy in both imagery and perception tasks. Thus we conclude that this area is both active in and necessary to the support of musical imagery tasks. The second right-sided asymmetry involved a region in the frontal lobes. This area, on the left, has been implicated in retrieval from verbal semantic memory,[22] suggesting that retrieval from semantic memory may be lateralized depending on the type of material. Another right-sided asymmetry was found in activation of the thalamus, a subcortical area involved in memory among other functions. In our earlier PET study,[14] that activation was above our statistical threshold; here it was just below the threshold and thus was not pictured with our main results. However, we can take this as at least suggestive evidence that a circuit involving temporal, frontal, and subcortical areas on the right are important in imagined music processing.

Transcranial magnetic stimulation

The final study in the series I am reviewing is currently unpublished, and was conducted in partnership with Alvaro Pascual-Leone, Fumiko Maeda, and Gottfried Schlaug. TMS is a noninvasive method of affecting underlying brain tissue by application of a magnetic pulse to the outside of the skull. The pulse is discharged via a coil that can be placed on the skull overlying the brain area of interest, using external anatomical landmarks, or in our case an MRI of each subject, to locate the areas of interest. A high-frequency series of pulses (10–20 Hz) has been shown to excite the underlying brain tissue, and low-frequency (1-Hz) sequences have been shown to inhibit the underlying tissue.[23] The inhibition is temporary, and the technique is safe for most people, although some discomfort may be experienced by the tapping sound the coil makes. Precautions are taken to exclude people with a history of seizure, as well as people who would be excluded from any study involving MRI, such as anyone with metal implants in the skull. The excitatory aspect of TMS is of interest to clinicians and researchers in the treatment of mental illness such as depression.[24] The inhibitory function of low-frequency TMS is of interest to researchers in that a temporary 'lesion' can be created in otherwise normal people, and subsequent effects on behaviour can be studied.

TMS has already been used to investigate visual imagery. Kosslyn, Pascual-Leone, and colleagues[25] showed that an application of 10 min of 1-Hz TMS to the visual cortex impaired later performance of both a visual perception and equivalent visual imagery task. They took this as evidence, in accord with lesion logic, that the primary visual cortex is necessary for performance of the visual imagery task, strengthening the argument that visual perception and imagery are mediated by common structures.

In our TMS study, we selected three brain areas that had been shown to be active during auditory imagery in my previous work, plus one control area. We also wanted to look at auditory imagery for both verbal and nonverbal tunes, as some different brain areas were shown to be active for these two types of tasks. To this end, we needed an auditory imagery task that would be suitable for both types of tunes. We modified a task used by Smith,[26] in which participants are given the title of a familiar tune and then asked about a pitch relationship between two notes indexed by ordinal position. In our case, we asked participants to judge whether the second note of a given tune was higher or lower than its first note. Verbal and nonverbal tunes could both be tested, and we intermixed the two types in the test.

The general outline of a session was to administer the auditory imagery task as a pretest. We then determined each person's motor threshold, or the lowest amount of energy that, when applied to the skull overlying the hand area of the motor cortex, just made the person's finger twitch. Each person received TMS at 90 per cent of that value. Administration of 10 min of 1-Hz TMS to a designated brain area ensued, followed immediately by another auditory imagery task as a posttest (using different tunes for pretest and posttest). When more than one brain area was investigated in a single session, 30 min of rest intervened between testing different brain areas, to allow the effects of the TMS to dissipate entirely.

Participants were nine right-handed adults with average age of 34, all of whom had some musical background (four were active musicians). Each person underwent an MRI scan before the TMS session. This allowed us to locate, using anatomical measurements, the areas of interest to us. The control area we selected was primary visual cortex (coil placed at the back of the skull), which had not been implicated in auditory imagery tasks before. The three experimental areas were the SMA (top of the skull a little more than midway towards the back), and the left and the right auditory cortex (above and slightly behind the top of the ear in most people). Because of the anatomy of the auditory cortex, we could not localize our coil placement exactly on secondary auditory cortex. We located the coil instead as near as possible on the primary auditory cortex, with the assumption that the TMS activation would also likely affect the secondary cortex that is immediately adjacent to that area. Our prediction was that after 10 min of low-frequency stimulation, performance overall (in accuracy and/or time) would decrease for the experimental but not for the control areas. We made a further prediction that both left and right auditory cortex stimulation would impair processing of verbal tunes, but that the right auditory cortex stimulation would only impair nonverbal tunes.

Brain areas were tested in different orders for each person. However, as early results seemed to indicate that stimulation to the SMA was showing no effect, three volunteers did not receive SMA stimulation, in an effort to reduce subject time and discomfort. Thus all results except those for SMA were based on nine subjects; those for SMA were based on six subjects.

Accuracy was quite high in the task, so results concentrated on reaction times. Figure 15.4 shows the results for each brain area for the verbal and the nonverbal tasks, both before and after TMS stimulation. The nonverbal tunes are a little less familiar to people, and thus they were responded to on average more slowly than the verbal tunes. Inspection of the four panels shows that in accord with the prediction, the TMS made no difference when applied to the visual cortex. But, surprisingly, TMS made no significant difference when applied to SMA and left auditory cortex. The lower right panel does show a predicted effect: TMS applied to right auditory cortex slowed down responses to the imagery task, but only for the nonverbal tunes.

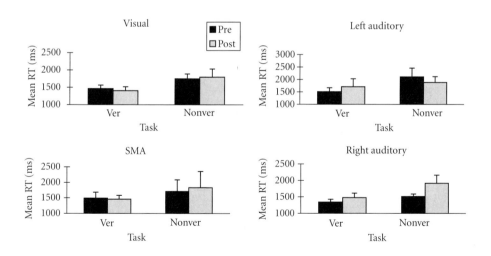

Figure 15.4 Mean reaction time before and after TMS for the verbal (Ver) and nonverbal (Nonver) imagery tasks, after application to the visual cortex, supplementary motor area (SMA), left auditory cortex, and right auditory cortex.

Stimulation to the two auditory areas were the most comparable in terms of subjective experience: the coil clicks were rather loud in the ear, and some jaw muscles were activated by the stimulation. Thus we compared those two areas statistically in an analysis of variance, using the three factors of tune (verbal, nonverbal), area (left, right auditory) and test (pre-, post-); all factors were within subjects. The main effect of tune was significant, $F(1, 8) = 6.24$, $p < 0.05$, but the crucial three-way interaction of tune, area, and test just failed to reach significance, $F(1, 8) = 3.26$, $p = 0.10$. Because of the strong prediction about these areas, we made a specific comparison of the pre- and posttests after right auditory stimulation. The comparison was not significant for verbal tunes, but was for nonverbal tunes, Newman–Keul's $t = 4.173$, $p = 0.05$.

As far as I know, this study was the first use of TMS to investigate auditory areas. As mentioned above, the coil had to be localized over primary auditory cortex, which in my previous studies was not activated in auditory imagery tasks. Thus we were relying on the somewhat weaker collateral activation to the secondary auditory cortex to show inhibition in the areas of more interest to us. Therefore, although the results were not as statistically strong as we would like, the increase in latency to nonverbal tunes after nonverbal tunes only is consistent with the pattern of data shown in our PET study with nonverbal tunes.[21] The isolation of this effect to non-verbal tunes is particularly notable, because the verbal tunes were tested in the same session with the same subjects, and did not elicit the inhibition.

The lack of effect after SMA stimulation, after strong activation of this area shown in two PET studies, is more puzzling. Null effects are always hard to interpret, but two possibilities suggest themselves. One is methodological: the neural fibres subserving SMA bend as they move ventrally from the skull surface, and it may be that our particular configuration of coil type and its placement simply did not activate the area sufficiently. On the other hand, it is possible that although SMA provides useful rehearsal mechanisms during auditory imagery tasks, it may not be an area that *must* be involved in such tasks. The task used here required retrieval of the tune once a title was given, but only the first two notes had to be retrieved. Perhaps SMA is more useful when auditory imagery tasks that extend more in time are required, such as 'scanning' between two notes several beats apart[14] or 'playing' several seconds of a familiar tune inside one's head.[21] Pilot versions of the TMS task, in fact, asked subjects to compare the first and third notes, which might involve SMA to a greater extent; this could be tried in the future (although accuracy rates would be lower, making interpretation of reaction times more problematic).

Conclusions and directions

The studies just reviewed seem to converge on the general idea that parts of the cortex specialized for processing actual sound are also recruited to process imagined sound. Furthermore, the particular structures processing imagined music bear some similarity to those processing heard music. Specifically, the right temporal lobe has been shown to be active in, and necessary for, adequate performance on both perceived and imagined pitch comparison tasks derived from previously known music. This structure may be especially important for processing music that does not have words, when the left temporal structures cannot be recruited for verbal processing.

The role of the SMA remains unclear, in several respects. Because of our failure to disrupt imagery processing with TMS inhibition, we are not sure if a fully functioning SMA is necessary for good performance on musical imagery tasks. The strong activation of SMA shown by PET in both verbal and nonverbal auditory imagery tasks suggests that 'internal humming' may at least be helpful to maintain an auditory image over time.

This latter point can be subjected to test by devising auditory imagery tasks in which internal humming would not be helpful or even possible to support the task. One domain to investigate would be imagery for environmental sounds. Intons-Peterson[27] has shown that people can generate images of everything from volcanoes erupting to wind chimes tinkling, and make mental comparisons on subjective loudness of these sounds. As people cannot possibly produce most of these sounds, it would be useful to find a task that shows activation in secondary auditory areas (which we can, by now, use as a tentative correlate of the subjective state of auditory imagery) and see if SMA is also activated.

An alternative domain to explore might be that of timbre. Crowder[28] demonstrated in several behavioural paradigms that people asked to imagine timbres of different instruments can do so. He gave people a sine wave of a particular pitch and asked them to imagine it in an instrument timbre. A second tone was then presented in an actual timbre at the same or a different pitch and subjects had to say if the pitch was the same or different as the first note. People were slower to confirm that two pitches were the same if the imagined and perceived timbres did not match. As people cannot produce the sounds of guitars and clarinets, SMA support should not be necessary if it is providing a motor rehearsal program. Timbre imagery tasks would also have the advantage of providing us a lateralization hypothesis, as Samson and Zatorre[11] showed the importance of the right temporal lobe in timbre tasks. Thus brain imaging studies using either PET or functional magnetic resonance imaging in these domains should help us clarify the role of the SMA in auditory imagery tasks.

Acknowledgements

I thank the National Science Foundation and the McDonnell-Pew Program in Cognitive Neuroscience for support of this research.

References

1. **Halpern, A. R.** (1988) Perceived and imagined tempos of familiar songs. *Music Percept.* 6, 193–202.

2. **Halpern, A. R.** (1992) Musical aspects of auditory imagery. In D. Reisberg (ed.) *Auditory Imagery.* Hillsdale, NJ: Lawrence Erlbaum, pp. 1–27.

3. **Halpern, A. R.** (1989) Memory for the absolute pitch of familiar songs. *Mem. Cognit.* 17, 572–81.

4. **Kosslyn, S. M., T. M. Ball,** and **B. J. Reiser** (1978) Visual images preserve metric spatial information: evidence from studies of image scanning. *J. Exp. Psychol. Hum. Percept. Perform.* 4, 47–60.

5. **Halpern, A. R.** (1988) Mental scanning in auditory imagery for tunes. *J. Exp. Psychol. Learn. Mem. Cognit.* 14, 434–43.

6. **Intons-Peterson, M. J.** (1983) Imagery paradigms: how vulnerable are they to experimenters' expectations? *J. Exp. Psychol. Learn. Mem. Cognit.* 10, 699–715.

7. **Farah, M. J.** (1988) Is visual imagery really visual? Overlooked evidence from neuropsychology. *Psychol. Rev.* 95, 307–17.

8. **Kosslyn, S. M., N. M. Alpert, W. L. Thompson** *et al.* (1993) Visual mental imagery activates topographically organized visual cortex: PET investigations. *J. Cognit. Neurosci.* 5, 263–87.

9. **Zatorre, R. J.** (1985) Discrimination and recognition of tonal melodies after unilateral cerebral excisions. *Neuropsychologia* 23, 31–41.

10. **Zatorre, R. J.** (1988) Pitch perception of complex tones and human temporal-lobe function. *J. Acoust. Soc. Am.* 84, 566–72.

11. **Samson, S.** and **R. J. Zatorre.** (1994) Contribution of the right temporal lobe to musical timbre discrimination. *Neuropsychologia* 32, 231–40.

12. **Zatorre, R. J.** and **S. Samson.** (1991) Role of the right temporal neocortex in retention of pitch in auditory short-term memory. *Brain* 114, 2403–17.

13. **Zatorre, R. J.** and **A. R. Halpern.** (1993) Effect of unilateral temporal-lobe excision on perception and imagery of songs. *Neuropsychologia* 31, 221–32.

14. **Zatorre, R. J., A. R. Halpern, D. W. Perry** *et al.* (1996) Hearing in the mind's ear: a PET investigation of musical imagery and perception. *J. Cognit. Neurosci.* 8, 29–46.

15. **Zatorre, R. J., A. C. Evans,** and **E. Meyer** (1994) Neural mechanisms underlying melodic perception and memory for pitch. *J. Neurosci.* 14, 1908–19.

16. **Zatorre, R. J., A. C. Evans, E. Meyer,** and **A. Gjedde** (1992) Lateralization of phonetic and pitch processing in speech perception. *Science* 256, 846–9.

17. **Smith, E. E., J. Jonides,** and **R. A. Koeppe** (1996) Dissociating verbal and spatial working memory using PET. *Cereb. Cortex* 6, 11–20.

18. **Gabrieli, J. D. E., J. E. Desmond, J. B. Demb** *et al.* (1996) Functional magnetic resonance imaging of semantic memory processes in the frontal lobes. *Psychol. Sci.* 7, 278–83.

19. **Paulesu, E., C. D. Frith,** and **R. S. J. Frackowiak** (1993) The neural correlates of the verbal component of short-term memory. *Nature* 362, 342–5.

20. **Perry, D., M. Petrides, B. Alivasatos** *et al.* (1993) Functional activation of human frontal cortex during tonal working memory tasks. *Soc. Neurosci. Abst.* 19, 843.

21. **Halpern, A. R.** and **R. J. Zatorre** (1999) When that tune runs through your head: a PET investigation of auditory imagery for familiar melodies. *Cereb. Cortex* 9, 697–704.

22. **Nyberg, L., R. Cabeza,** and **E. Tulving** (1996) PET studies of encoding and retrieval. *Psychol. Bull. Rev.* 3, 135–48.

23. **Walsh, V.** and **M. Rushworth** (1999) A primer of magnetic stimulation as a tool for neuropsychology. *Neuropsychologia* 37, 125–35.

24. **Pridmore, S.** and **R. Belmaker** (1999) Transcranial magnetic stimulation in the treatment of psychiatric disorders. *Psychiatry Clin. Neurosci.* 53, 541–8.

25. **Kosslyn, S. M., A. Pascual-Leone, O. Felician** *et al.* (1999) The role of area 17 in visual imagery: convergent evidence from PET and rTMS. *Science* 284, 167–9.

26. **Smith, J. D., M. Wilson,** and **D. Reisberg** (1995) The role of subvocalization in auditory imagery. *Neuropsychologia* 33, 1433–54.

27. **Intons-Peterson, M. J.** (1980) The role of loudness in auditory imagery. *Mem. Cognit.* 8, 385–93.

28. **Crowder, R. G.** (1989) Imagery for musical timbre. *J. Exp. Psychol. Hum. Percept. Perform.* 15, 472–8.

CHAPTER 16

NEURAL SPECIALIZATIONS FOR TONAL PROCESSING

ROBERT J. ZATORRE

Abstract

The processing of pitch, a central aspect of music perception, is neurally dissociable from other perceptual functions. Studies using behavioural-lesion techniques as well as brain imaging methods demonstrate that tonal processing recruits mechanisms in areas of the right auditory cortex. Specifically, the right primary auditory area appears to be crucial for fine-grained representation of pitch information. Processing of pitch patterns, such as occurs in melodies, requires higher-order cortical areas, and interactions with the frontal cortex. The latter are likely related to tonal working memory functions that are necessary for the on-line maintenance and encoding of tonal patterns. One hypothesis that may explain why right-hemisphere auditory cortices seem to be so important to tonal processing is that left auditory regions are better suited for rapidly changing broad-band stimuli, such as speech, whereas the right auditory cortex may be specialized for slower narrow-band stimuli, such as tonal patterns. Evidence favouring this hypothesis was obtained in a functional imaging study in which spectral and temporal parameters were varied independently. The hypothesis also receives support from structural studies of the auditory cortex, which indicate that spectral and temporal processing may depend on interhemispheric differences in grey/white matter distribution and other anatomical features.

Keywords: Hemispheric functional specialization; Pitch processing; Pitch patterns

How does the nervous system analyze and make sense of information coming from the environment? This central question in contemporary neuroscience has been addressed from many perspectives in the last two decades. In the auditory domain, a great deal of effort has gone into understanding the way in which the human brain processes speech sounds. Given the importance of speech and spoken language to human communication and behaviour, this is not surprising. It is interesting, however, to consider other aspects of auditory information processing that may help to round out the picture. Increasingly, music is being recognized as an important component of human activity that may help us to gain insight into the functional organization of the human brain. It may be argued that the perception, encoding, and reproduction of musical sounds requires neural mechanisms that are at least as complex as those for speech; indeed, it seems likely that speech and music must engage the most cognitively demanding aspects of auditory processing. It may further be argued that these two classes of stimuli are uniquely human, making it particularly relevant to study them in the context of understanding those aspects of brain organization that are most relevant to human cognition and behaviour. Finally, an overarching theme of chapters presented in this volume is that music can and should be viewed as a biological phenomenon, not merely a cultural artifact; from this perspective, therefore, it is not only meaningful but even imperative to seek out the neural processes that may allow human beings to engage in the diverse array of behaviours we term music.

All of these considerations set the stage for the studies from my laboratory and from others that will be described in this chapter. The recent development of brain imaging techniques, coupled with more traditional behavioural approaches, has allowed for rapid developments in the field. A great deal of closely related information on music and brain function is presented in many of the other chapters in this volume, particularly in those by Besson, Griffiths, Halpern, Pantev, Parsons, Peretz, Samson, Schlaug, and Tervaniemi. The studies to be discussed in the present chapter focus specifically on aspects of tonal processing and their neural substrates. The underlying theme of the research approach is that by studying these processes we will achieve a more complete understanding not only of the auditory nervous system, but of the human brain in general. The idea that neural systems may display functional specializations is generally well accepted in cognitive neuroscience. The work described in this chapter therefore also has a goal of identifying these specializations in order to determine the extent to which musical processes depend on dedicated neural circuitry or may form part of shared neural architecture. In this context, another important feature of brain organization, hemispheric functional specialization, is also crucial, and will be important in understanding the pattern that emerges.

In order to make sense of a complex phenomenon such as music, it is necessary, at least as a starting point, to focus on a specific aspect; in the present set of studies, I have chosen to explore the processing of pitch, which is to say pitch information as used for musically relevant processes. This choice is motivated by the fact that pitch appears to be a central aspect of all music. Although other aspects of music, such as temporal organization for rhythm, for example, may play an equally important role, it is difficult to conceive of a musical system of any type that does not involve the patterning of pitches. Moreover, pitch processing is amenable to study not only because the physical parameters of sounds associated with pitch are relatively well understood and easily manipulated, but also because it affords us the opportunity to analyse different levels of processing. Thus, in what follows I will consider first of all studies examining relatively low-level aspects of pitch processing, such as pitch discrimination; second I will discuss higher-order aspects, including pitch patterns. Finally, I will present some anatomical findings that may be relevant to understanding the nature of the functional specializations that the other studies have uncovered.

Basic aspects of pitch processing

To begin, let us consider a relatively simple aspect of a musically relevant function: the ability to distinguish sounds on the basis of their pitch. The neural basis for the encoding of pitch has been studied for some time. Indeed, much neurophysiological work both in the periphery and in the central nervous system has examined the processing of frequency information (see Chapter 9, this volume). One of the salient features of the auditory nervous system, in fact, is that a tonotopic organization exists from the earliest level of the periphery, at the basilar membrane, to many fields within the auditory cortex. This topographic organization along the frequency axis points to the importance of pitch information in auditory processing generally. However, does the cortex carry out some essential function in the representation of pitch information? Several classic studies in experimental animals with bilateral destruction of auditory cortical areas have suggested that simple pitch discrimination remains unaffected, indicating that earlier levels of processing, in the midbrain or thalamus, for example, may be sufficient.[1–3] However, the nature of the pitch processing task appears to be critical in answering this question.

In a recent study from my lab, Johnsrude *et al.*[4] explored the specificity of pitch discrimination using a behavioural-lesion technique. We tested patients who had undergone surgical excision in the auditory cortex in the right or left temporal lobe; the patients' lesions were classified according to magnetic resonance imaging (MRI) as extending or not into Heschl's gyrus (HG), which contains the primary auditory cortex (see Ref. 5 for description of a lesion quantification procedure, and Figures 16.1 and 16.2). A simple psychophysical 'staircase' discrimination task was used, with pairs of pure tones to determine the threshold or minimal frequency separation needed to achieve a certain level of performance. Two separate tasks were administered. In the first, the two tones were either identical or different in pitch, and the subject answered accordingly. In the second task, the

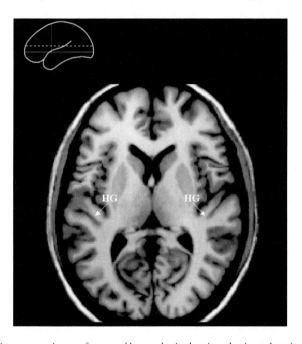

Figure 16.1 Magnetic resonance image of a normal human brain showing a horizontal section through the region of Heschl's gyrus, marked HG. The orientation and level of the horizontal section is indicated by the *dashed line* in the *inset*.

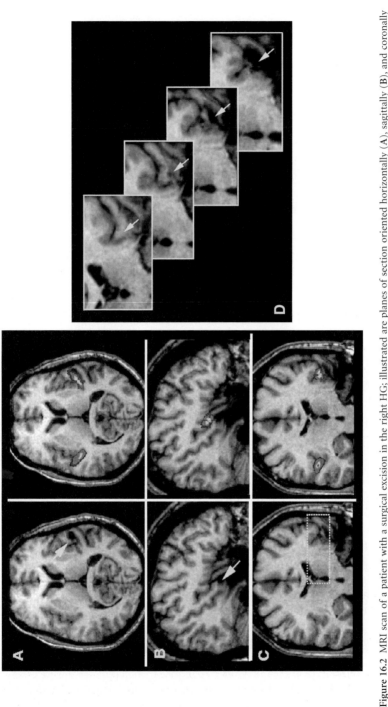

Figure 16.2 MRI scan of a patient with a surgical excision in the right HG; illustrated are planes of section oriented horizontally (A), sagittally (B), and coronally (C). The left side of panels A, B, and C show the patient's scan alone, with an *arrow* indicating the region of excision/undercutting. The images on the *right side of* panels A, B, and C show the patient's scan coregistered with an anatomical probabilistic map of HG derived from normal individuals (Ref. 44). The *crosshairs* indicate the same position in the standardized space as the *arrow*. Note the correspondence between the position of HG as determined from the map and the patient's partially excised HG region. The *yellow box* in panel C indicates the region of the removal pictured in close-up in panel D, which illustrates the transition from intact, to undercut, to fully excised tissue (coronal sections taken at 3-mm intervals, posterior to anterior). *Arrows* again correspond to the *crosshairs* in the other panels and indicate the location of the HG region. (See Plate 4A–D in colour section.)

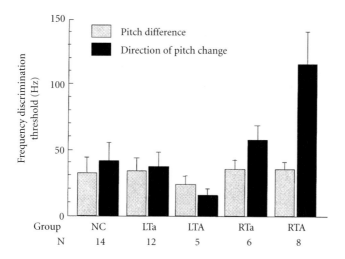

Figure 16.3 Mean frequency difference discrimination thresholds observed in two pitch discrimination tasks in patients with right or left (RT or LT) temporal-lobe excision, extending into the region of HG (A) or sparing this area (a). The simple discrimination thresholds were not different across the groups. Thresholds in the direction-of-pitch-change task were significantly higher in the RTA group than in any of the other groups. (Reproduced with permission from Ref. 4).

two tones always differed, and the subject's task was to indicate if the second tone was higher or lower than the first. The tones themselves were identical across the two tasks. The idea here is that whereas the simple pitch discrimination task merely requires that a difference be noted, the second, pitch-direction task requires that the tones be discriminated and ordered along some underlying pitch scale.

The findings (Figure 16.3) indicated several interesting dissociations. First, the patients with lesions within the left temporal lobe were quite unimpaired as compared to control participants on either task, regardless of the extent of excision with HG. Second, the patients with damage to the right temporal lobe but excluding HG also had normal thresholds. The group of subjects with right HG damage, however, showed a fourfold increase in their pitch thresholds, but only for the pitch-direction task; they were normal on the simple pitch discrimination task. The findings are thus quite specific in indicating that only a certain restricted lesion in the right temporal lobe has an effect, and then only on a particular task. Thus, one may conclude that the right primary auditory area plays a special role not simply in discriminating one pitch from another, but in some aspect of organizing the sounds according to their pitch. This aspect of pitch organization, it is argued, is essential for any musical use of pitch information. Interestingly, all but one of the patients in question were able to perform the task itself; it was only the threshold that was abnormally high. This aspect of the result suggests that a much coarser level of pitch organization still exists in these patients, which may be mediated by left auditory cortex, a point to which we shall return below.

These results are consistent with those of a much earlier study[6] in which patients with right temporal lobe excisions with encroachment onto Heschl's gyri had significant difficulties with a missing-fundamental pitch discrimination task but not with the identical task when the fundamental frequency was present. Patients with more anterior right temporal lobe damage, or those with similar damage on the left were unimpaired. Both studies thus point to a specificity for basic aspects of pitch processing, indicating a special role for areas in or adjacent to the right primary auditory cortex in these functions. Several other studies have added weight to this idea, although the degree of anatomical specificity has not always been possible; nonetheless, many authors have observed that the right temporal cortex plays a particularly important role for processing of pitch and of spectral pattern information.[7–11]

More recently, functional imaging studies have begun to add important new evidence to our emerging view of the functional organization of the human brain. Among the many advantages of techniques, such as positron emission tomography (PET) and functional magnetic resonance imaging (fMRI), is that they provide a noninvasive means of obtaining anatomically accurate information about the cerebral areas that change their neural activity as a function of stimulus or task parameters. Thus, these techniques provide critical complementary evidence to the data derived from more traditional behavioural studies. However, whereas activation studies can identify the sites of neural activity associated with a particular function, they cannot determine the degree to which necessary computations are carried out. Conversely, only lesion techniques or stimulation techniques (such as transcranial magnetic stimulation, see, Chapter 26, this volume) can provide information about essential areas, but they are constrained by various other limitations. Clearly, whenever converging evidence can be obtained from a variety of methods, the conclusions that can be drawn will be correspondingly stronger.

Several recent studies have examined pitch processing using functional imaging techniques. One relevant piece of evidence in favour of a special role for the right auditory cortex in pitch processing comes from PET studies of pitch production. Perry et al.[12] compared a condition in which subjects repeatedly produced a single vocal tone of constant pitch to a control in which they heard synthetic tones at the same rate. Increased cerebral blood flow (CBF) was noted in several motor areas, but within the superior temporal gyrus (STG), only right-sided activations were noted in both primary and secondary auditory cortices. The authors interpret this finding as a reflection of the specialization of the right auditory cortex for pitch perception. They argue that accurate perception of the pitch of one's own voice is required during singing in order to use feedback to maintain the desired pitch. Additional findings in favour of this conclusion come from regression analyses performed on these data, in which the accuracy of the subjects' singing was measured, and the degree of pitch excursion was covaried against CBF in the whole brain volume.[13] Strikingly, a region of covariation was identified in the right HG, such that increased CBF was observed with increasing pitch deviation. This result confirms the special role played by this region in pitch processing and suggests that a feedback mechanism may indeed be operative to maintain consistency of vocalized pitch.

Processing of pitch patterns

The initial phase of pitch analysis set the stage for processing of pitch patterns. The relationships between individual tones form the basis for the most fundamental aspect of musical processing: the encoding and recognition of melodies. Melodic patterns, in turn, may be investigated at many different levels of analysis, from the basic interval relationships between tones to the semantic networks that are important for long-term representations of familiar tunes, and the output mechanisms necessary for singing or playing them. Here, we shall concentrate on the way in which auditory cortical systems are engaged in perception of melodies. One critical consideration in this respect is that all melodic perception (indeed, all auditory perception) involves working memory mechanisms. Since sounds unfold over time, in order to compute the relationships between successive events, an on-line retention system is evidently necessary. In the case of even a brief melody, this would mean that relationships between tones have to be computed and maintained over periods ranging from seconds to minutes in order to achieve a relatively stable and coherent internal representation.

Many studies of melodic perception with brain-lesioned individuals have demonstrated that damage to the right STG often leads to behavioural deficits in discrimination tasks,[7,14–16] although most of these studies have also noted that damage to the equivalent structures on the left may also lead to some degree of impairment. Indeed, Peretz *et al.*[17] (see also Chapter 13, this volume) have noted that patients with bilateral lesions that involve portions of the STG and frontal cortical structures demonstrate much more severe disturbances in melodic tasks than most patients with unilateral damage. In fact, in each of the cases that Peretz and her colleagues have studied, the patients did not appear to show the specific musical deficit until after a second lesion had occurred, implying that unilateral damage had had at most only a mild effect not noted by the patients or their families. This point is important in that it suggests that the putative hemispheric specializations that are one theme of this chapter are likely to be relative rather than absolute.

The relative importance of right-hemisphere STG mechanisms has been demonstrated specifically for tonal working memory in two studies from our laboratory. In one,[18] we adapted a paradigm first developed by Deutsch[19] in which a target and a comparison tone are to be compared for pitch; the tones are either separated by a brief silent interval or by a series of interfering random tones. Deutsch had shown that memory for tones was relatively specific because it was not disrupted by other sounds, but only by other tones (see also Ref. 20). When this tonal working-memory task was administered to temporal-lobectomy patients, performance was significantly worse following damage to the right than to the left temporal cortex for the interference task. On the other hand, unlike the studies of basic pitch processing discussed above, there was no difference in degree of behavioural deficit as a function of encroachment onto HG. Thus, areas of auditory cortex outside of the primary zone are most likely to be involved in this function. Finally, it was also noted that right frontal cortical excisions produced an impairment similar to that seen in the right temporal patients, a point that is taken up below.

To follow up on the question of tonal working memory function, Zatorre *et al.*[21] used PET to test 12 volunteer nonmusicians with unfamiliar melodies and noise bursts that had been constructed so as to approximate the acoustic characteristics of the melodies. Four conditions were run; subjects were asked to (1) listen to the noise bursts; (2) listen to the melodies without explicit instruction; (3) listen to the same melodies and compare the pitch of the first and second notes (two-note condition); and (4) listen to the melodies and compare the pitch of the first and last notes (first/last condition).

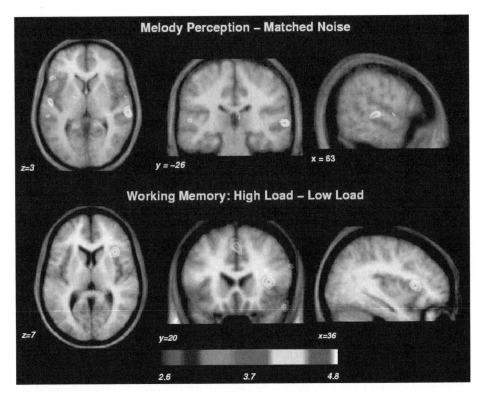

Figure 16.4 Selected PET CBF activation sites associated with processing of tonal melodies. The figures show averaged PET subtraction images superimposed on a corresponding section of an average anatomical MRI. (*Top*) Horizontal, coronal, and sagittal views through a focus located in the right superior temporal gyrus representing a significant blood flow increase while subjects listened to a series of short, unfamiliar tonal melodies, as compared with a baseline condition in which they listened to noise bursts that were acoustically equated to the melodies. Also visible in the horizontal section is a region of significant activity in the left temporal cortex. (*Bottom*) Horizontal, coronal, and sagittal views through a focus in the right frontal/opercular region showing activity associated with making judgements about the pitch of the first and last notes of the tonal sequences as compared to making judgements about the first two notes. Data reanalysed from Zatorre *et al.*[21] (See Plate 5 in colour section.)

The comparison of listening to melodies minus noise permits examination of the cerebral regions specifically active during processing of novel melodies. The principal result indicated a significant CBF increase in the right superior temporal gyrus, anterior to the primary auditory cortex; a weaker CBF increase was also observed in the left STG. A reanalysis of these data with a smaller reconstruction filter and improved image registration[22] indicates that the right STG activation is in the ventrolateral aspect of the gyrus (Figure 16.4). These findings point to differential activation of primary vs secondary auditory areas within the STG, depending on the stimulus features. Caution must still be exercised in interpreting the results, for the noise bursts clearly differ from the melodies on a number of dimensions (e.g. periodicity, frequency modulation, and spectral composition). It remains to be established, therefore, which specific features of the melodies may lead to the observed pattern of

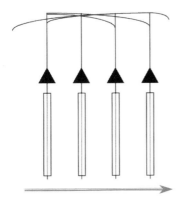 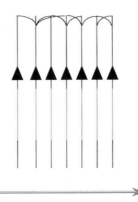

Figure 16.5 Cartoon depiction of putative differences in anatomical structure between left and right auditory cortical areas. *Triangles* and *lines* represent individual neurons with differing degrees of myelination (thicker on the left). Neurons on the left are larger than those on the right, have wider spacing across tonotopically organized cortex, and are more widely interconnected. These structural features would lead to relatively fast conduction but poor spectral resolution on the left, and to poorer temporal resolution but greater sensitivity to fine spectral differences on the right.

activation. The finding of an activation within the right STG while listening to melodies fits in well with the lesion data, however, and likely reflects the specialization of neuronal networks within the right secondary auditory cortices for perceptual analysis of tonal information.

Zatorre *et al.*[21] also examined working memory for pitch by subtracting the passive condition from the two-note condition, which resulted in significant activation within the right frontal lobe (both inferiorly and superiorly). The first/last minus passive melodies subtraction yielded a large number of cortical and subcortical activation sites in both hemispheres, including a focus in the right inferior frontal cortex identical to that observed in the two-note condition. A comparison not reported in the original study pits the first/last condition against the two-note condition. The advantage of this contrast is that both involve pitch comparisons, the main difference being the degree of working memory load. The interesting finding here (Figure 16.4) is once again an area of increased blood flow in the right inferior frontal region, though not in the same location as in the other subtractions. The pattern of results from these conditions therefore implicates frontal-lobe mechanisms in effecting pitch comparisons, with a particularly important contribution from right-frontal regions. It should be recalled, however, that in the first/last minus passive melody comparison, a large number of separate foci of CBF change were seen over a wide swath of cortical and subcortical territory; this finding perhaps reflects the complexity and increased cognitive demands of the task, which was also manifested in increased error rate and slower reaction times.

One may speculate that the numerous frontal lobe sites observed might be associated with successful performance of distinct aspects of the task. The findings of Perry *et al.*[23] are directly relevant to this issue; they observed CBF increases with a rightward asymmetry in dorsolateral frontal areas while subjects were engaged in an auditory tonal working memory task that required them to monitor a sequence of tones. This finding suggests a functional dissociation between the cognitive act of monitoring information as opposed to holding sensory information in working memory. Perry *et al.*[23] suggest a hierarchical view, compatible with other evidence,[24] such that right inferior lateral frontal areas are important for maintenance of tonal information, whereas dorsolateral frontal areas are required for higher-level functions such as monitoring the contents of working memory. This conclusion would be in accord with the lesion study described earlier,[18] as well as with PET studies[25] that also indicated increased activity in the right frontal cortex during pitch judgements on speech syllables.

Several other imaging studies over the past few years have supported the idea that the right secondary auditory cortex may be particularly important in processing tonal patterns (but see Chapter 10, this volume, for evidence that the story is more complicated).The results of Démonet *et al.*[26,27] are relevant, since tone judgement tasks were used, in which subjects were required to detect pitch changes of tones within a sequence, and the difference in activity pattern between the tonal task and a language task was examined. The findings were consistent with data presented above, implicating the right auditory cortical areas in tonal processes, since foci were observed in posterior right STG and middle temporal areas. More recently, Binder *et al.*[28] reported whole-brain fMRI data using an active tone judgement task. This task, which required subjects to discriminate two pitches during a series of tones (which ranged from 3 to 7 tones in length) and then to make a judgement pertaining to the entire series of tones, emphasized not only pitch perception but also maintenance of simple pitch information in working memory. When this task was compared to an active task involving semantic categorization of words, stronger activation associated with the tone task was observed in the posterior STG bilaterally, the supramarginal region bilaterally (but much more on the right), the right posterior middle temporal gyrus, premotor cortex bilaterally (also much more on the right), and right superior parietal cortex.[28] These right temporoparietal foci are in agreement with the right posterior STG, middle temporal, and inferior parietal foci reported by Démonet in their tone-speech comparisons.[26,27]

A further source of relevant evidence comes from studies of musical imagery (reviewed by Halpern, Chapter 15, this volume). Those studies, including both behavioural-lesion experiments and functional imaging,[29–31] have indicated that a greater role is played by secondary auditory cortical areas on the right than on the left not only in perceptual tasks involving judgements of real melodies, but also in imaginal tasks in which subjects are invited to imagine a well-known tune in 'the mind's ear'. These studies, together with additional recent neuroimaging findings pointing in the same general direction,[32–34] provide additional evidence for a special role of several right-hemispheric cortical regions in various aspects of tonal pattern processing.

Hemispheric differences in spectral processing

Much of the evidence presented above converges towards the conclusion that hemispheric specialization exists in the processing of pitch information, with right auditory cortical areas playing a more prominent role than left. Moving beyond the mere fact that differences do exist, it is critical to pose the question of why such lateralization might have evolved. One classic way of thinking about hemispheric differences, favoured, for example, by investigators such as Teuber or Sperry, is in terms of complementary functional specialization—that is, that hemispheric processing advantages emerge because they confer some advantage over shared processing, since each hemispheric system can specialize in one domain, thus leading to an overall enhancement for the organism as a whole.

If we think about the data presented earlier in this chapter within this context, it seems obvious that the two domains for which the auditory cortices in each hemisphere have become specialized are, roughly, speech and tonal patterns. A bit of additional reflection suggests a unifying hypothesis to explain these complementary functional specializations: speech and tonal stimuli differ in their acoustic structure, and hence in their processing requirements. Whereas the analysis of speech requires good temporal resolution to process rapidly changing energy peaks (formants) that are characteristic of many speech consonants (see, for example, the work of Tallal *et al.*[35]), it can be argued that tonal processes instead require good frequency resolution. In a truly linear system, temporal and spectral resolution are inversely related, so that improving temporal resolution can only come at the expense of degrading spectral resolution and vice versa. This tradeoff naturally arises from a fundamental physical constraint in acoustic processing: better resolution in the frequency domain can be obtained only at the expense of sampling within a longer time window, hence degrading temporal resolution; conversely, high resolution in the temporal domain entails a degraded spectral representation. The auditory nervous system is, of course, a highly nonlinear and distributed system; yet, it may also respect this fundamental computational constraint, such that in the left auditory cortex the high temporal resolution needed to process speech imposes an upper limit on the ability to resolve spectral information, and vice versa for the right auditory cortex. To put it more simply, the hypothesis is that there may be a tradeoff in processing in temporal and spectral domains, and that auditory cortical systems in the two hemispheres have evolved a complementary specialization, with the left having better temporal resolution, and the right better spectral resolution.

According to the foregoing idea, therefore, the hemispheric differences we see in the tonal perception literature reviewed above might reflect this more fundamental level of functional organization. If this hypothesis is correct, then we ought to be able to obtain evidence for differential response within left and right auditory cortices by manipulating temporal and spectral parameters of an auditory stimulus, even if it is not particularly perceived as speech or music. A recent functional imaging study from our lab[36] set out to do just that using a parametric approach. Rather than looking for differences in cerebral blood flow between a control and an activation condition, we examined the functional changes in the brain that correlated with a given input parameter. This approach can be particularly powerful since it helps to isolate brain activity that is specifically related to the parameter of interest. We first created nonverbal stimuli that varied independently and systematically along two dimensions, one temporal, the other spectral. The stimuli were merely a series of pure tones that varied in frequency and duration; in one set of conditions the frequency change was held constant and the temporal rate became faster across scans, while in the other set of conditions the rate was held constant and the frequency differences became finer across scans. We predicted that increasing the rate of temporal change would preferentially recruit left auditory cortical areas, while increasing the number of spectral elements would engage right auditory cortical regions.

The results of greatest relevance for the present discussion were that cerebral blood flow in a region of the left auditory cortex showed a greater response to increasing temporal than spectral variation, whereas a symmetrical area on the right showed the reverse pattern. A third area in the right superior temporal sulcus also showed a significant response to the spectral parameter but showed no change to the temporal parameter. Thus, the data supported the hypothesis that corresponding regions of the auditory cortex in the two hemispheres have different sensitivity to temporal and spectral information. Neurophysiological recordings in macaque monkeys have shown that auditory cortical neurons are highly sensitive to both spectral and temporal features of sounds simultaneously, and that they exhibit complex response functions.[37–39] It has also been shown that neurons in the belt region of the macaque auditory cortex are optimally responsive to stimuli of specific bandwidths, hence demonstrating sensitivity to a spectral parameter.[40] As well, Eggermont[41] noted that in two primary fields of the cat there was an inverse relation between bandwidth and temporal resolution, consistent with our proposal.

Additional evidence that left auditory cortical units have higher temporal resolution comes from recent depth-electrode recordings within Heschl's gyri[42] showing that the responses within the left auditory cortex encode the voice-onset time of a consonant, whereas the right auditory cortex did not show sensitivity to this temporal parameter. Even more striking consistency is offered by additional data from the same investigators (Chapter 10, this volume), who showed that intracortically recorded auditory evoked potentials were more sharply tuned to frequency in the right auditory cortex than in the left, as predicted by the hypothesis that resolution in the frequency and time domains are different in the two hemispheres.

This hypothesis has also received support from a PET study by Belin *et al.*,[43] in which the rate of formant transitions in a pseudospeech sound—not perceived as speech—was varied from 40 to 200 ms. CBF changes in the left auditory region were found for both types of stimuli, indicating a capacity for processing spectral change over a wide range of durations; by contrast, regions in the right auditory cortex responded only to the slower rates, and not to the faster rate. Thus, the right auditory cortex seems unable to respond to fast formant transitions, whereas the homologous area on the left is better able to track rapidly changing acoustic information that would be relevant for speech processing. Finally, it is also relevant to recall the findings of Robin *et al.*,[9] who studied auditory discrimination in brain-damaged patients. They too found that damage to association cortices in the right hemisphere resulted in spectral but not temporal processing deficits, while the converse was observed after left-hemispheric damage.

Anatomical considerations

One advantage of the hypothesis presented above is that it offers a unifying framework to understand some of the functional characteristics of the auditory nervous system that allow us to be able to process speech and tonal patterns. This model raises an important question, however: How are these functional differences instantiated in the brain? That is, can we find any evidence in the structure of the auditory cortex that would not only support the existence of processing differences but would also suggest how these differences are implemented?

Some answers to these questions are provided by recent anatomical data from our laboratory[44] and from other investigators. Unlike the functional techniques described above, the aim of this research was to characterize the structural features (shape, volume, and position) of the human primary auditory cortical region *in vivo*. The approach taken was to use MRI scans from groups of normal right-handed volunteer subjects and to label the region of HG

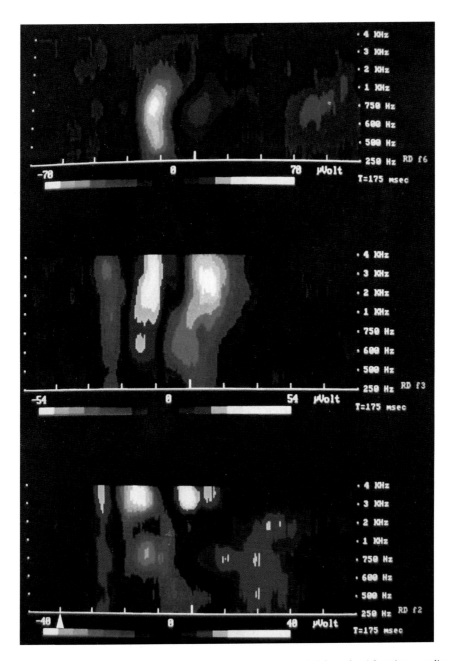

Plate 1 Temporospectral maps of amplitude variations of potentials recorded from the right primary auditory cortex (leads 2, 3, and 6). Time, related in abscissae, is reduced to 175 ms, full scale. On the ordinate axis, each yellow dot represents the frequency. Amplitude is represented by colour. A cubic spline interpolation is used in order to obtain a continuous potential line between the different frequencies. Each spatial /reconstruction gives a continuous map both in time and in frequency. Dark colors are values close to the neutral potential, and bright colors are used for the activity—blue represents negativity and red represents positivity. The white arrow indicates the beginning of the sound.

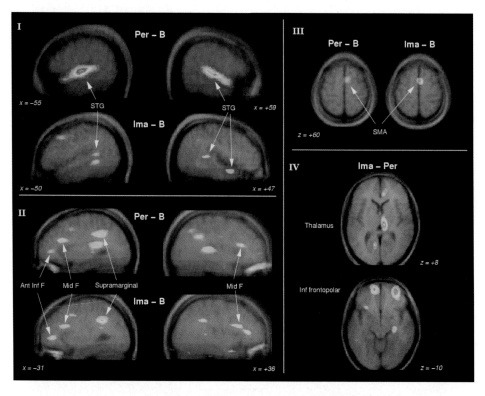

Plate 2 Brain areas showing activation in the perception minus baseline, imagery minus baseline, and imagery minus perception conditions of the verbal tune PET study.

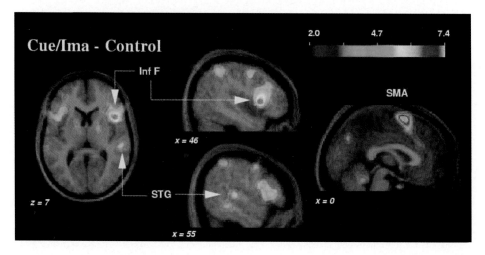

Plate 3 Brain areas showing activation in the cue/imagery minus control subtraction in the nonverbal tune PET study.

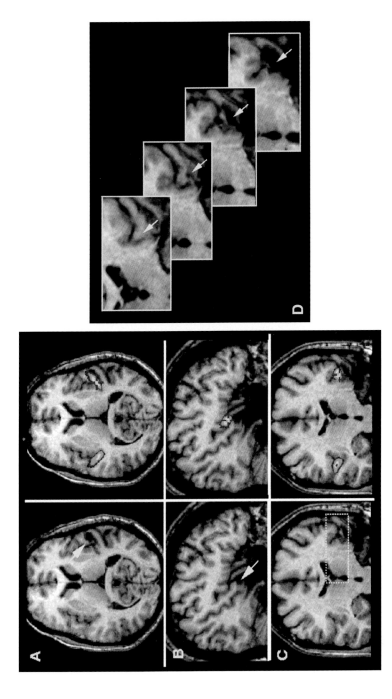

Plate 4 MRI scan of a patient with a surgical excision in the right HG; illustrated are planes of section oriented horizontally (A), sagittally (B), and coronally (C). The left side of panels A, B, and C show the patient's scan alone, with an *arrow* indicating the region of excision/undercutting. The images on the *right side* of panels A, B, and C show the patient's scan coregistered with an anatomical probabilistic map of HG derived from normal individuals (Ref. 44). The *crosshairs* indicate the same position in the standardized space as the *arrow*. Note the correspondence between the position of HG as determined from the map and the patient's partially excised HG region. The *yellow box* in panel C indicates the region of the removal pictured in close-up in panel D, which illustrates the transition from intact, to undercut, to fully excised tissue (coronal sections taken at 3-mm intervals, posterior to anterior). *Arrows* again correspond to the *crosshairs* in the other panels and indicate the location of the HG region.

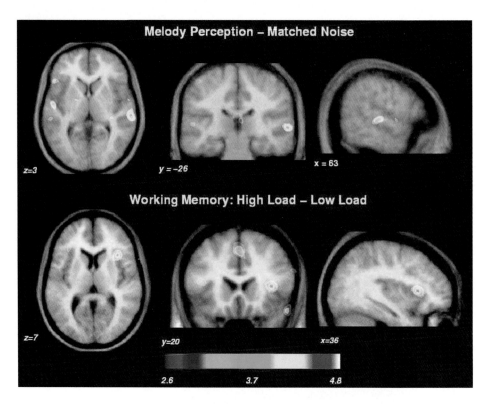

Plate 5 Selected PET CBF activation sites associated with processing of tonal melodies. The figures show averaged PET subtraction images superimposed on a corresponding section of an average anatomical MRI. (*Top*) Horizontal, coronal, and sagittal views through a focus located in the right superior temporal gyrus representing a significant blood flow increase while subjects listened to a series of short, unfamiliar tonal melodies, as compared with a baseline condition in which they listened to noise bursts that were acoustically equated to the melodies. Also visible in the horizontal section is a region of significant activity in the left temporal cortex. (*Bottom*) Horizontal, coronal, and sagittal views through a focus in the right frontal/opercular region showing activity associated with making judgements about the pitch of the first and last notes of the tonal sequences as compared to making judgements about the first two notes. Data reanalysed from Zatorre *et al*.

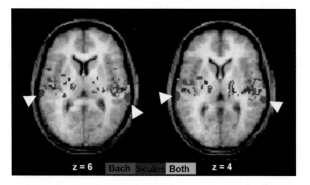

Plate 6 Significant blood flow activations in auditory (temporal) cortex specific to playing the Bach score (*red*), specific to playing scales (*blue*), and common to both performances (*cyan*). These are logical contrasts of Bach vs rest and scales vs rest shown in group-averaged PET images overlaid on anatomical magnetic resonance images (MRIs). The z-values indicate the axial height of the brain volume relative to the Talairach and Tournoux stereotactic atlas. Throughout, left side of brain images shows the left side of the brain, and vice versa.

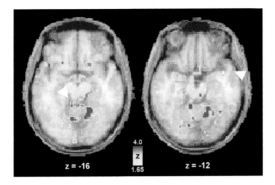

Plate 7 Correlated blood flow activations in right anterior auditory cortex and left cerebellum (see *arrows*) as subjects played the Bach score. These are group-averaged PET images for Bach (contrasted with rest) overlaid on anatomical MRIs. PET data are *z*-scores displayed on a colour scale ranging from 1.65 (*yellow*; $p < 0.1$) to 4.0 (*red*; $p < 0.0001$).

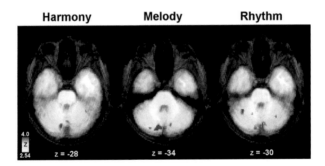

Plate 8 Significant blood flow activations in the cerebellum as musicians sight-read a J. S. Bach chorale score and listen for performance errors in harmony, melody, or rhythm. These are group-averaged PET images for each task (contrasted with passive listening control) overlaid on anatomical MRIs. PET data are *z*-scores displayed on a colour scale ranging from 1.96 (*yellow*; $p < 0.05$) to 4.0 (*red*; $p < 0.0001$).

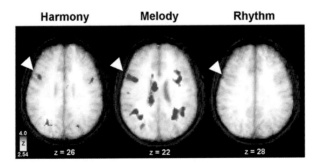

Plate 9 Activations in different subareas of a major cytoarchitectonic area of frontal cortex (BA 44) as musicians sight-read a J. S. Bach chorale score and listen for performance errors in harmony, melody, or rhythm. These are group mean PET images for each task (contrasted with passive listening control) overlaid on MRIs. PET data are *z*-scores displayed on a colour scale ranging from 2.54 (*yellow*; $p < 0.01$) to 4.0 (*red*; $p < 0.0001$).

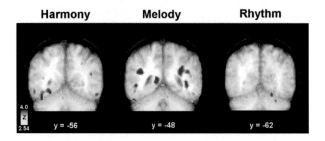

Plate 10 Activations in different subareas of auditory cortex as musicians sight-read a J. S. Bach chorale score and listen for performance errors in melody, harmony, or rhythm. These are group mean PET images for each task (contrasted with passive listening control) overlaid on MRIs. PET data are *z*-scores displayed on a colour scale ranging from 2.54 (*yellow; p* < 0.05) to 4.0 (*red; p* < 0.0001).

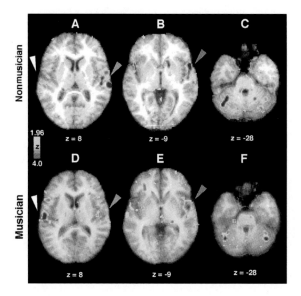

Plate 11 Activations in superior and middle temporal cortex (A, B, D, and E) and in cerebellum (C and F) as nonmusicians and musicians discriminate pitch sequences. These images show group mean PET data for each task (contrasted with rest) overlaid on MRIs. PET data are *z*-scores displayed on a colour scale ranging from 1.96 (*yellow; p* < 0.1) to 4.0 (*red; p* < 0.0001).

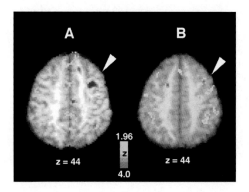

Plate 12 Activations in left medial frontal cortex (BA 9) for nonmusicians (A) as compared to musicians (B) during the discrimination of musical tempi. Shown are group mean PET images for each task (contrasted with rest) overlaid on MRIs.

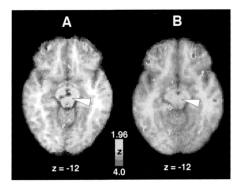

Plate 13 Activations in midbrain for nonmusicians (A) as compared to musicians (B) during the discrimination of musical pattern. These are group-averaged PET images for each task (contrasted with rest) overlaid on anatomical MRIs.

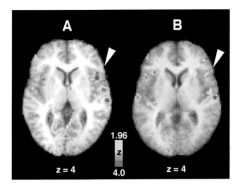

Plate 14 Activations in right inferior frontal cortex (BA 47) for nonmusicians (A) as compared to musicians (B) during discrimination of musical meter. Shown are group-averaged PET images for each task (contrasted with rest) over-laid on anatomical MRIs.

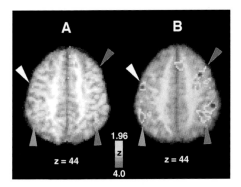

Plate 15 Activations in bilateral medial frontal cortex (BA 9) and bilateral inferior parietal cortex (BA 40) for musicians (B) as compared to nonmusicians (A) during the discrimination of sequence durations. Shown are group-averaged PET images for each task (contrasted with rest) overlaid on anatomical MRIs.

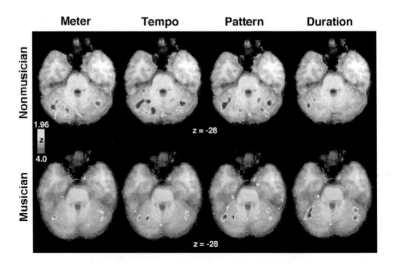

Plate 16 Activations in posterior cerebellum as nonmusicians and musicians discriminate meter, tempo, pattern, and duration. Shown are group-mean PET images for each task (contrasted with rest) overlaid on MRIs.

Plate 17 Anecdotal evidence reports superior musical abilities in blind individuals. *Left*: Stevie Wonder. From: *The Rolling Stone. Illustrated History of Rock and Roll*. A. DeCurtis, J. Henke, H. George-Warren (eds) New York: Random House, p. 294. *Right*: Wolfgang Amadeus Mozart, though not blind, possibly suffered from strabismic amblyopta, reducing vision in one or both eyes by an unknown amount. Portrait attributed to Kymli of Mannheim, Germany, 1783 (held in a private collection).

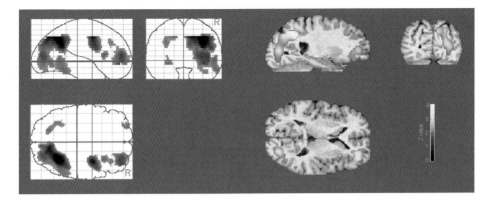

Plate 18 Results of PET scanning in congenitally blind subjects during localization of sounds presented via headphones in virtual auditory space (data from Ref. 19). Areas in the occipital cortex that are driven by visual stimuli in sighted individuals are now activated during sound localization. Note that the right hemisphere seems to profit more from the expansion of auditory into visual territory. The 'rewiring' seems to be mediated by the parietal cortex, consistent with studies on visually deprived animals.

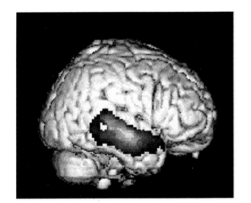 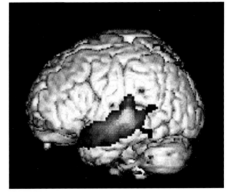

Plate 19 Auditory cortical activation while listening to music. Averaged group results of functional magnetic resonance imaging are shown. While the processing of music by the right cerebral hemisphere has often been emphasized (as opposed to language, which is thought to be processed primarily on the left), it is now generally accepted that different aspects of music are processed by *both* hemispheres.

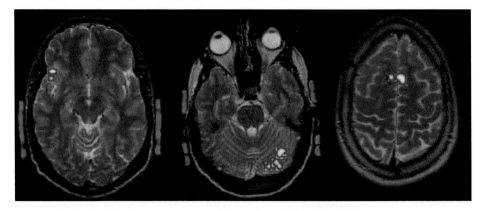

Plate 20 Results of functional magnetic resonance imaging during anticipatory imagery of music. The axial sections from individual subjects are displayed in radiological coordinates showing the left side of the brain on the right and vice versa. Imagery leads to activation of anterior regions of auditory cortex in the right hemisphere (in conjunction with right inferior frontal regions; panel on the left of the figure). This emphasizes the role of sensory cortices in mental imagery. However, brain regions outside auditory cortex, such as the cerebellum (left cerebellar hemisphere; middle panel) and the anterior cingulate bilaterally (right panel), are also activated, demonstrating their role in cognitive processing.

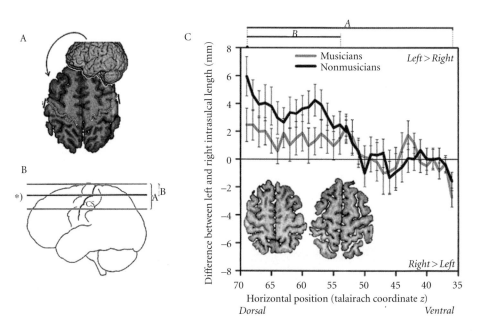

Plate 21 (A) The intrasulcal length of the posterior bank of the precentral gyrus (ILPG) was measured in horizontal slices (parallel to the AC–PC plane) from the deepest point of the central sulcus following the contour line of the precentral gyrus to a lateral surface tangent that connected the crests of the pre- and postcentral gyrus. (B and C) We differentiated a dorsal and a ventral subregion. The dorsal subregion roughly corresponds to the location of the functional hand motor area. We found prominent differences in the intrasulcal length of the precentral gyrus in the dorsal subregion between musicians and nonmusicians. Musicians had more symmetrical lengths which was due to a disproportional increase in length of the nondominant hemisphere.

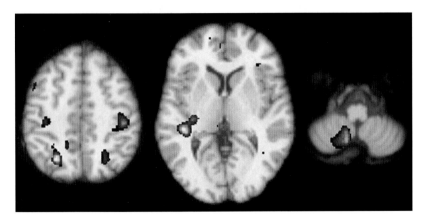

Plate 22 Preliminary findings of a voxel-by-voxel morphometric study comparing a group of 15 male musicians with 15 male nonmusicians. Three axial slices show significant differences ($p < 0.05$ corrected) between musicians and nonmusicians superimposed on corresponding T1-weighted structural images. Yellow and red voxels indicate more gray-matter concentration in the musicians, blue voxels indicate more gray matter concentration in the nonmusicians.

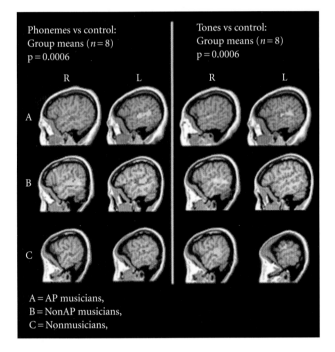

Plate 23 Results of a fMRI experiment aimed to investigate the functional significance of the increased leftsided anatomical PT asymmetry in AP musicians. Three groups of subjects were examined: AP musicians, nonAP musicians, and nonmusicians. A phoneme memory task and a tone memory task were contrasted with a rest condition. Suprathreshold voxels showing significant task related activity changes were superimposed on a representative sagittal anatomical image of right and left hemisphere. AP musicians showed prominent left superior temporal lobe activation during the tone memory task that was not seen in the other two groups. The cerebral activation pattern of the phoneme memory task was similar between the three groups.

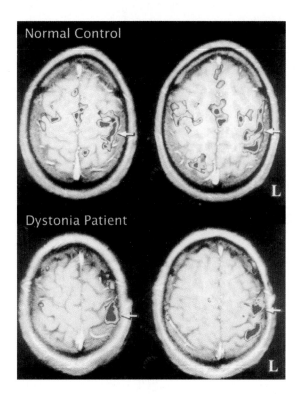

Plate 24 The bold fMRI images of a normal and dystonic guitar player executing right hand arpeggios in the scanner are displayed. Note the greater activation of the sensorimotor cortex (*arrows*) and the lack of activation of premotor and supplementary motor cortices in the dystonic patient. Modified from Ref. 40.

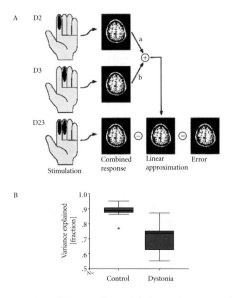

Plate 25 (A) Schematic representation of the experimental design and representative fMRI data in one subject. Sensory stimulation was applied to the index (D2) or middle (D3) finger alone or to both fingers at the same time (D23) while the fMRI bold signal was recorded. A linear approximation of the fMRI signal associated with combined stimulation of D2 and D3 was calculated and substracted from the measured signal, giving rise to the 'error' of 'variance'. (B) Variance results in graphic form for all control subjects and patients with dystonia. Modified from Refs 46 and 47.

(Figure 16.1) using interactive pixel-marking software that permits simultaneous viewing in all three planes of the section. The result of greatest relevance pertains to the estimates of the volume of HG, which was found to be significantly greater on the left than on the right in two independent samples of 20 subjects each.[44] Most interesting of all was that the differences in volume were found to be confined to the white matter underlying HG, and not to the volume of cortical tissue (grey matter) within the structure (this effect may be seen qualitatively in the MRI shown in Figure 16.1). This finding suggests an anatomical asymmetry that arises from a difference in the volume of fibres that carry information to and from the primary auditory cortex and surrounding regions.

Although an MRI cannot reveal details of the underlying neuronal organization, the greater degree of white matter on the left could be consistent with the notion of greater speed of processing on the left, if the white-matter volume measures are related to degree of myelination. That is, a greater degree of left-sided myelination could lead to faster transmission of acoustically relevant information, because it is well established in neurophysiology that more heavily myelinated fibres transmit neuronal impulses more quickly. Confirmation that the left auditory cortical regions are indeed more heavily myelinated comes from a recent postmortem electron microscopy study showing that the myelin sheath is thicker in the left than in the right posterior temporal cortex.[45] As well, Hutsler and Gazzaniga[46] reported larger left- than right-layer IV pyramidal cells in the human auditory cortex, which would also lead to faster time constants.

In addition to the idea that left auditory cortical fibres are more heavily myelinated, there is also evidence for other hemispheric differences in the structural organization of the auditory cortex that are broadly consistent with the hypothesis presented above. For example, Seldon[47] reported that cortical columns in the left auditory cortex were more widely spaced than those on the right. Galuske et al.[48] recently found that clusters of neurons were spaced more widely in the left posterior temporal cortex, with more long-range intrinsic connections between these clusters. These features could be compatible with a greater degree of integration across tonotopically organized cortical areas on the left than on the right, hence leading to a relative degradation of spectral resolution on the left. Conversely, neurons in the right auditory cortex would have structural features that would enhance spectral resolution (much as shown by Liégeois-Chauvel, Chapter 10, this volume) because they would be smaller, with fewer myelinated inputs, therefore perhaps more tightly packed together; and would integrate over narrower frequency regions. These characteristics would also result in poorer temporal resolution.

Concluding comments

We have seen how a variety of different methods and techniques point towards a general conclusion about the way in which the auditory nervous system processes information relevant for our ability to process speech and tonal sounds. These two domains of auditory processing are, of course, at the core of our uniquely human abilities to communicate. It is perhaps no coincidence that abilities to process both speech and music arise precociously in development and follow relatively fixed developmental sequences (see Chapter 1, this volume). It is perhaps also not irrelevant that both speech communication and tonal patterns appear to be ubiquitous across all human cultures (see Chapters 4 and 5, this volume).

The general approach we have defended, to view music within a biological framework, thus would seem to make sense of these disparate observations, if musical perceptual abilities—and by extension musical production abilities—are seen as emerging from functional and structural features of our nervous system. There is a final point that should perhaps be addressed, however, and this concerns the origins of music. Without entering into the controversies and speculations of this field of scholarship (see Chapter 5, this volume), perhaps it is sufficient to point out that the approach offered here would provide a relatively parsimonious account. In order to understand the emergence of music, it might be sufficient to assume only one set of evolutionary pressures: the need to communicate verbally. If the specialization of the left auditory cortex discussed above reflects the nervous system's adaptation to this selective pressure, then all we need to assume is that the complementary structural and functional changes of the two hemispheres arose as a consequence of this specialization (see also Ref. 49 for further discussion).

The ideas presented in this chapter, or indeed in this entire volume, will ultimately be shown to be correct, or at least partially so, or in error by the usual slow and meandering path of science. Regardless of the details, however, the hope is that by viewing music as a phenomenon worthy of scientific study, we will enhance both our understanding of music within our species, as well as the workings of our nervous system that make music possible.

Acknowledgements

I wish to thank all my colleagues and students who contributed to the research described in this chapter. Funding for the work has been provided by grants from the Canadian Institutes of Health Research, the McDonnell-Pew Cognitive Neuroscience Program, and the International Foundation for Music Research.

References

1. **Evarts, E. V.** (1952) Effect of auditory cortex ablation on frequency discrimination in monkey. *J. Neurophysiol.* 15, 443–8.

2. **Heffner, H. E.** and **B. Masterton** (1978) Contribution of auditory cortex to hearing in the monkey (*Macaca mulatta*). In D. J. Chivers and J. Herbert (eds) Recent Advances in Primatology, vol. 1, *Behaviour*. New York: Academic Press.

3. **Jerison, H. J.** and **W. D. Neff** (1953) Effect of cortical ablation in the monkey on discrimination of auditory patterns. *Fed. Proc.* 12, 237.

4. **Johnsrude, I. J., V. B. Penhune,** and **R. J. Zatorre** (2000) Functional specificity in right human auditory cortex for perceiving pitch direction. *Brain* 123, 155–63.

5. **Penhune, V., R. Zatorre,** and **W. Feindel** (1999) The role of auditory cortex in retention of rhythmic patterns in patients with temporal-lobe removals including Heschl's gyrus. *Neuropsychol.* 37, 315–31.

6. **Zatorre, R. J.** (1988) Pitch perception of complex tones and human temporal-lobe function. *J. Acoust. Soc. Am.* 84(2), 566–72.

7. **Milner, B. A.** (1962) Laterality effects in audition. In V. Mountcastle (ed.) Interhemispheric Relations and Cerebral Dominance. Baltimore, MD: Johns Hopkins Press, 177–95.

8. Divenyi, P. and A. Robinson (1989) Nonlinguistic auditory capabilities in aphasia. *Brain Lang.* 37, 290–326.

9. Robin, D. A., D. Tranel, and H. Damasio (1990) Auditory perception of temporal and spectral events in patients with focal left and right cerebral lesions. *Brain Lang.* 39, 539–55.

10. Samson, S. and R. J. Zatorre (1994) Contribution of the right temporal lobe to musical timbre discrimination. *Neuropsychol.* 32, 231–40.

11. Sidtis, J. J. and B. T. Volpe (1988) Selective loss of complex-pitch or speech discrimination after unilateral lesion. *Brain Lang.* 34, 235–45.

12. Perry, D. W., R. J. Zatorre, M. Petrides, *et al.* (1999) Localization of cerebral activity during simple singing. *NeuroReport* 10, 3979–84.

13. Perry, D., R. Zatorre, and A. Evans (1996) Co-variation of CBF during singing with vocal fundamental frequency. *NeuroImage* 3(3), S315.

14. Liégeois-Chauvel, C., I. Peretz, M. Babaï, *et al.* (1998) Contribution of different cortical areas in the temporal lobes to music processing. *Brain* 121, 1853–67.

15. Samson, S. and R. J. Zatorre (1988) Melodic and harmonic discrimination following unilateral cerebral excision. *Brain Cogn.* 7, 348–60.

16. Zatorre, R. J. (1985) Discrimination and recognition of tonal melodies after unilateral cerebral excisions. *Neuropsychol.* 23, 31–41.

17. Peretz, I., R. Kolinsky, M. Tramo, *et al.* (1994) Functional dissociations following bilateral lesions of auditory cortex. *Brain* 117, 1283–301.

18. Zatorre, R. J. and S. Samson (1991) Role of the right temporal neocortex in retention of pitch in auditory short-term memory. *Brain* 114, 2403–17.

19. Deutsch, D. (1970) Tones and numbers: specificity of interference in short-term memory. *Science* 168, 1604–5.

20. Semal, C., L. Demany, K. Ueda, *et al.* (1996) Speech versus nonspeech in pitch memory. *J. Acoust. Soc. Am.* 100, 1132–40.

21. Zatorre, R. J., A. C. Evans, and E. Meyer (1994) Neural mechanisms underlying melodic perception and memory for pitch. *J. Neurosci.* 14(4), 1908–19.

22. Zatorre, R. and J. Binder (2000) Functional and structural imaging of the human auditory system. In A. Toga and J. Mazziota (eds) *Brain Mapping: The Systems.* Los Angeles: Academic Press, 365–402.

23. Perry, D. W., M. Petrides, B. Alivisatos, *et al.* (1993) Functional activation of human frontal cortex during tonal working memory tasks. *Soc. Neurosci. Abstr.* 19, 843.

24. Petrides, M. (1995) Functional organization of the human frontal cortex for mnemonic processing: evidence from neuroimaging studies. *Ann. N.Y. Acad. Sci.* 769, 85–96.

25. Zatorre, R. J., A. C. Evans, E. Meyer, *et al.* (1992) Lateralization of phonetic and pitch processing in speech perception. *Science* 256, 846–9.

26. Démonet, J.-F., F. Chollet, S. Ramsay, *et al.* (1992) The anatomy of phonological and semantic processing in normal subjects. *Brain* 115, 1753–68.

27. Démonet, J.-F., C. Price, R. Wise, and R. S. J. Frackowiack (1994) A PET study of cognitive strategies in normal subjects during language tasks. *Brain* 117, 671–82.

28. Binder, J., J. Frost, T. Hammeke, *et al.* (1997) Human brain language areas identified by functional magnetic resonance imaging. *J. Neurosci.* 17, 353–62.

29. Zatorre, R. J. and A. R. Halpern (1993) Effect of unilateral temporal-lobe excision on perception and imagery of songs. *Neuropsychol.* 31(3), 221–32.

30. Zatorre, R. J., A. R. Halpern, D. W. Perry, *et al.* (1996) Hearing in the mind's ear: a PET investigation of musical imagery and perception. *J. Cognit. Neurosci.* 8(1), 29–46.

31. Halpern, A. R. and R. J. Zatorre (1999) When that tune runs through your head: a PET investigation of auditory imagery for familiar melodies. *Cereb. Cortex* 9, 697–704.

32. Griffiths, T. D., I. S. Johnsrude, J. L. Dean, *et al.* (1999) A common neural substrate for the analysis of pitch and duration pattern in segmented sound? *NeuroReport* 10, 3825–30.

33. Hugdahl, K., K. Bronnick, S. Kyllingsbaek *et al.* (1999) Brain activation during dichotic presentations of consonant-vowel and musical instrument stimuli: a 15O-PET study. *Neuropsychol.* 37, 431–40.

34. Tervaniemi, M., S. Medvedev, K. Alho, *et al.* (2000) Lateralized automatic auditory processing of phonetic versus musical information: a PET study. *Hum. Brain Map* 10, 74–9.

35. Tallal, P., S. Miller, and R. Fitch (1993) Neurobiological basis of speech: a case for the preeminence of temporal processing. *Ann. N.Y. Acad. Sci.* 682, 27–47.

36. Zatorre, R. and P. Belin (2001) Spectral and temporal processing in human auditory cortex. *Cereb. Cortex* 11, 946–53.

37. de Charms, R. C., D. T. Blake, and M. M. Merzenich (1998) Optimizing sound features for cortical neurons. *Science* 280, 1439–43.

38. Phillips, D. P. (1993) Representation of acoustic events in the primary auditory cortex. *J. Exp. Psychol.: Hum. Percept. Perform.* 19(1), 203–16.

39. Steinschneider, M., C. Schroeder, J. Arezzo, *et al.* (1995) Physiologic correlates of the voice onset time boundary in primary auditory cortex of the awake monkey: temporal response patterns. *Brain Lang.* 48, 326–40.

40. Rauschecker, J. P., B. Tian, and M. Hauser (1995) Processing of complex sounds in the *Macaque* nonprimary auditory cortex. *Science* 268, 111–4.

41. Eggermont, J. (1998) Representation of spectral and temporal sound features in three cortical fields of the cat. Similarities outweigh differences. *J. Neurophysiol.* 80, 2743–64.

42. Liégeois-Chauvel, C., J. de Graaf, V. Laguitton, *et al.* (1999) Specialization of left auditory cortex for speech perception in man depends on temporal coding. *Cereb. Cortex* 9, 484–96.

43. Belin, P., M. Zilbovicius, S. Crozier *et al.* (1998) Lateralization of speech and auditory temporal processing. *J. Cognit. Neurosci.* 10, 536–40.

44. Penhune, V. B., R. J. Zatorre, J. D. Macdonald, *et al.* (1996) Interhemispheric anatomical differences in human primary auditory cortex: probabilistic mapping and volume measurement from magnetic resonance scans. *Cereb. Cortex* 6, 661–72.

45. Anderson, B., B. D. Southern, and R. E. Powers (1999) Anatomic asymmetries of the posterior superior temporal lobes: a postmortem study. *Neuropsychiatry Neuropsychol. Behav. Neurol.* 12, 247–54.

46. Hutsler, J. and M. Gazzaniga (1996) Acetylcholinesterase staining in human auditory and language cortices—regional variation of structural features. *Cereb. Cortex* 6, 260–70.

47. Seldon, H. (1981) Structure of human auditory cortex. II: axon distributions and morphological correlates of speech perception. *Brain Res.* 229, 295–310.

48. Galuske, R., W. Schlote, H. Bratzke, *et al.* (2000) Interhemispheric asymmetries of the modular structure in human temporal cortex. *Science* 289, 1946–9.

49. Justus, T. and J. Bharucha (2002) Music perception and cognition. In H. Pashler and S. Yantis (eds) *Steven's Handbook of Experimental Psychology: Vol. 1. Sensation and Perception.* New York: John Wiley and Sons.

CHAPTER 17

EXPLORING THE FUNCTIONAL NEUROANATOMY OF MUSIC PERFORMANCE, PERCEPTION, AND COMPREHENSION

LAWRENCE M. PARSONS

Abstract

This chapter highlights findings by my colleagues and me in four neuroimaging and neurological studies of music performance, perception, and comprehension. These investigations elucidate the neural subsystems supporting musical pitch, melody, harmony, rhythm, tempo, meter, and duration. In a positron emission tomography (PET) study of pianists, a memorized performance of a musical piece was contrasted with that of scales to localize brain areas specifically supporting music. A second PET study assayed brain areas subserving selectively the comprehension of harmony, melody, and rhythm. Musicians sight-read a score while detecting specific melodic, harmonic, or rhythmic errors in its heard performance. In a third PET study, musicians and nonmusicians discriminated pairs of rhythms with respect to pattern, tempo, meter, or duration. Data in these studies implicated the cerebellum in nonmotor, nonsomatic, sensory, or cognitive processing. In a fourth study, neurological patients with degeneration of the cerebellum were found to be impaired in fine discrimination of pitch. Overall, these data suggest that the neural systems underlying music are distributed throughout the left and right cerebral and cerebellar hemispheres, with different aspects of music processed by distinct neural circuits. Also discussed are key issues for interpreting the role in music of brain areas implicated in neuroimaging studies.

Keywords: Cerebellum; Neuroimaging studies; Musical performance; Harmony; Melody; Rhythm

In the last decade researchers in the cognitive sciences, experimental psychology, behavioural neurology, ethology, and neuroimaging have significantly advanced the scientific understanding of music, after a long period of slower progress.[1–14] It is not possible to review these important and exciting advances here (see other chapters in this volume for a sampling of such work). This chapter complements these advances by reviewing findings by my colleagues and me in four recent neuroimaging and neurological studies of music performance, perception, and comprehension. These investigations were attempts to elucidate the neural subsystems supporting major components of music—specifically, pitch, melody, harmony, rhythm, tempo, meter, and duration.

Functional neuroanatomy of musical performance

Our first experiment focused on musical expression or performance. This experiment, conducted in collaboration with Peter Fox, Donald Hodges, and Justine Sergent, attempted to clarify and extend a pioneering functional neuroimaging study of right-handed piano performance of a sight-read musical score.[15] In this early study, positron emission tomography (PET) was used to measure regional cerebral blood flow, an index of neural activity, in performing pianists. Among the main findings of this study was the observation that cortical areas distinct from, but adjacent to, those underlying language operations were activated during sight-reading. The relationship between music and language has continued to be a target of fruitful investigations.[16–20]

In our study, which built upon the foregoing results, we used PET to study bimanual piano performance of memorized music.[21] By recording brain activity when both hands were equally and concurrently producing music, we examined neural systems in both cerebral hemispheres when the left and right sides were fully involved in performance. In the prior study, although the score was read with both eyes and piano output was heard with both ears, only the right hand performed the music. This feature of the study left unclear which particular right hemispheric areas may be involved in music performance.

In addition, by eliminating musical score reading from scanned task performance, we examined brain activation during a more purely musical performance. Sight-reading a score during performance adds an additional cognitive load not directly related to music *per se*. Indeed, there is a strong belief among musicians that a fully memorized piece, one performed without score reading, engenders a distinctly deeper understanding of the music and more satisfying realization of the piece in performance.

We furthermore contrasted brain activity during the piano performance of a musical piece by J. S. Bach with that during the two-handed performance of scales. Our intent was to reveal the outline of brain areas that are specifically involved in the cognitive, perceptual, and emotional representation and performance of effective, strongly engaging music *per se*. The Bach and scales performances here required movements of nearly comparable frequency and complexity from each hand. (However, the Bach required somewhat more complicated, finely controlled fingering than the scales, and we expected this to be reflected in different patterns of activity when Bach and scales brain states were directly contrasted.)

After giving informed consent, eight right-handed professional musicians participating in three PET conditions performed three times in pseudorandom order (Figure 17.1). In the Bach condition, the third movement of the Italian Concerto (BMV 971) was performed from memory. Scales were executed synchronously (from memory) with both hands at a pace approximating that of the Bach performance. Subjects performed on a full-sized Yamaha P-132 electronic piano and heard the sounds they produced. In all conditions, subjects' eyes were closed and covered.

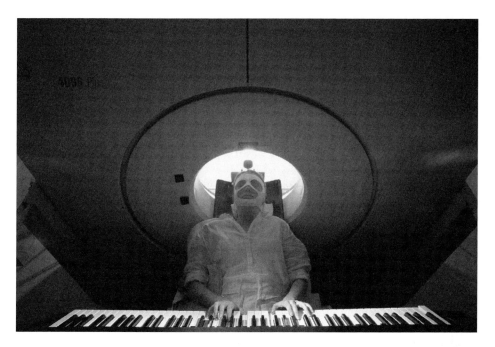

Figure 17.1 A pianist in a positron emission tomography (PET) scanning session[21] performing the third movement of the Italian Concerto by J. S. Bach. Photograph by Dr Stephan Elleringmann (Aurora/Bilderberg).

PET images, obtained by the ^{15}0-bolus method, were coregistered on each participant's MRI image and spatially normalized.[22–27] The grand-mean image for each task was compared to control, forming grand-mean images of the task-induced changes in brain activity ($p < 0.001$). Grand-mean images were converted to z-score images using the population variance.[28] Activation loci were identified by 3-D center-of-mass address, peak-voxel intensity, and z-value, cluster size, and statistical significance.[29] Response coordinates were interpreted[30] in accordance with the Talairach and Tournoux stereotaxic atlas[23] and confirmed with coregistered group-mean MRI.

Only a brief summary of some of the principal findings can be presented here. I will focus on the auditory cortex (the temporal lobe). This is where we detected the primary difference in neural activation for Bach and for scales, as indicated in the analysis of the direct contrast between activity in the two conditions. As illustrated in Figure 17.2, many of the activations were in the anterior secondary auditory association areas, in Brodmann's areas (BA) 22, 21, and 20. Overall, the performance of the Bach activated the temporal lobe more strongly than did the performance of scales. Scales performance activated middle temporal areas bilaterally, with more on the left than on the right (Figure 17.2). By contrast, the performance of the Bach activated superior, middle, and inferior temporal areas bilaterally, with more on the right than on the left.

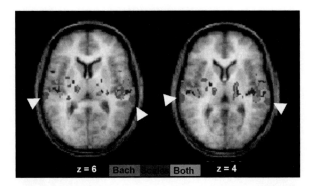

Figure 17.2   Significant blood flow activations[21] in auditory (temporal) cortex specific to playing the Bach score (*red*), specific to playing scales (*blue*), and common to both performances (*cyan*). These are logical contrasts of Bach vs rest and scales vs rest shown in group-averaged PET images overlaid on anatomical magnetic resonance images (MRIs). The z-values indicate the axial height of the brain volume relative to the Talairach and Tournoux stereotactic atlas.[23] Throughout, left side of brain images shows the left side of the brain, and vice versa. (See Plate 6 in colour section.)

The stronger activation in the right auditory cortex for the performance of the Bach is consistent with a variety of neuropsychological and neuroimaging results indicating that areas in right auditory association cortex are involved in the reception and expression of melody.[31–36] These findings suggest that some of the important areas specifically representing the higher-order representations of musical meaning, particular in performance, lie in these regions of temporal cortex.

Unexpectedly, there was also strongly correlated activation during the performance of the Bach (Figure 17.3) between right anterior temporal areas (BA 22, superior temporal gyrus) and left posterior lateral cerebellum ($r = + 0.77$, $p < 0.001$). Because left cerebellum has its primary connectivity with right cerebral cortex, we hypothesize that during the performance of the Bach, activation in right auditory cortex is related to that in left cerebellum. There was a corresponding, but less robust, correlation between left temporal areas and right posterior cerebellum. This contralateral coactivation of the auditory temporal cortex and lateral cerebellum suggests that they form a distributed circuit of processing. This cerebellar activity appears to be effectively dissociated from motor components and thus appears to contradict the traditional assumption that the cerebellum possesses only motor functions. It is unclear from the present data what function this temporal-cerebellar circuit performs for higher-order representations of music. Interestingly, there is a rapidly growing set of neuroimaging and neurological findings indicating that the cerebellum possesses functions other than those classically attributed to it. These new data suggest that the cerebellum is involved in some way in a variety of sensory and cognitive tasks.[37–45] The present findings, and others discussed below, appear to extend this new view of cerebellar function to the perceptual representation of music.

In summary, these data assist in outlining some of the neural systems that support musical performance and understanding. These findings appear to confirm or extend other neuroimaging and neurological observations and pave the way for new, more focused, research.

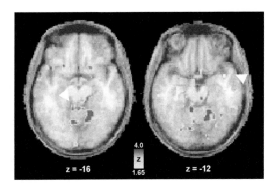

Figure 17.3 Correlated blood flow activations in right anterior auditory cortex and left cerebellum (see *arrows*) as subjects played the Bach score.[21] These are group-averaged PET images for Bach (contrasted with rest) overlaid on anatomical MRIs. PET data are *z*-scores displayed on a colour scale ranging from 1.65 (*yellow*; $p < 0.1$) to 4.0 (*red*; $p < 0.0001$). (See Plate 7 in colour section.)

Functional neuroanatomy of the comprehension of harmony, melody, and rhythm

We pursued these results in our second functional neuroimaging study, in which we attempted to map the brain basis of the comprehension of individual principal components of music *per se*.[46] Using the same PET methodology as in our first study, my colleagues and I imaged eight right-handed, male Ph.D. faculty musicians (none of whom participated in our first study). These subjects are experts at monitoring musical scores while listening for accurate performance. Each subject was competent on several instruments, with primary specializations in either winds, strings, voice, or keyboard.

During the experiment, these subjects detected errors in a computer-generated instrumental performance of unfamiliar Bach chorales as they read the corresponding score. The subjects made no overt response during a trial; rather they acknowledged covertly the location and presence of specific errors. The errors, which we implanted on each trial, were exclusively either rhythmic, harmonic, or melodic. The errors occurred unpredictably every two to three beats. On rhythm trials, errors occurred only in the performed rhythm of a note in one of the four voices but were otherwise correct. The rhythm errors changed either the duration or onset of a written note only (leaving unchanged the other aspects of rhythm such as meter and tempo). On melody trials, errors perturbed a written note in the highest voice by raising or lowering it a chromatic half step; otherwise they were accurate. On harmony trials, the errors could occur in any one of the four voices but were otherwise correct. The harmony errors perturbed the written note by raising or lowering it a chromatic half step. Pilot studies were used to develop stimuli that equated for difficulty across the three conditions. In prescan and postscan performance, subjects were accurately detecting approximately 80 per cent of the errors in each task.

After practicing the tasks, each subject was scanned performing each of the following five trials twice in pseudorandom order. On harmony, rhythm, and melody trials, subjects sight-read the score while listening to its errorful performance. On passive listening trials, subjects listened to a chorale performed without errors; they were not reading a score. On each scanned trial of the harmony, rhythm, melody, and passive listening tasks, subjects heard a different Bach chorale. On rest baseline control trials, subjects fixated on a fixation point (neither reading a score nor listening to music). The image data during the primary three tasks were contrasted with those from listening to the errorless performance of a Bach chorale without reading a score, as well as to the rest baseline control. Analyses were conducted as described earlier for our preceding PET study.

To highlight some of our principal findings, the melody, harmony, and rhythm conditions each showed a distinct pattern of distributed, statistically significant brain activity compared to passive listening control ($p < 0.001$). Often, each condition activated different subareas of a particular major brain area. In broad anatomical terms, score reading and comprehension of melodic, rhythmic, and harmonic features of a piece were supported by processes in both cerebral hemispheres. More specifically, melodic comprehension activated each hemisphere equally, whereas harmonic and rhythmic comprehension activated more of the left hemisphere than the right one. In addition, the rhythm condition activated comparatively few brain areas outside the cerebellum.

All three tasks strongly activated bilateral cerebellum, primarily the lateral hemispheres, with little overlap in activated area across the three tasks (Figure 17.4). Given the lack of explicit (and apparently implicit) movement, this cerebellar activity is likely related to sensory or cognitive processing, not to motoric processing (see below). Furthermore, activation of cerebellum in the rhythm condition was twice that in harmony and melody conditions. An involvement of the cerebellum in some way in processing rhythm is consistent with recent neurological and neuroimaging data.[42,47–49] Cerebellar activations during the processing of melody and harmony are relatively novel findings but are consistent with data above from our first study and with other recent studies showing lateral cerebellar activation for processing of tonal information (see later).

One area commonly activated by the harmony, melody, and rhythm tasks was in right fusiform gyrus. Because score reading was a central process common to all three conditions,

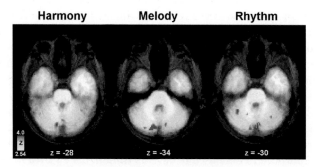

Figure 17.4   Significant blood flow activations in the cerebellum as musicians sight-read a J. S. Bach chorale score and listen for performance errors in harmony, melody, or rhythm.[46] These are group-averaged PET images for each task (contrasted with passive listening control) overlaid on anatomical MRIs. PET data are z-scores displayed on a colour scale ranging from 1.96 (*yellow*; $p < 0.05$) to 4.0 (*red*; $p < 0.0001$). (See Plate 8 in colour section.)

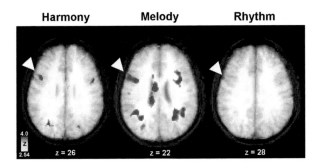

Figure 17.5 Activations in different subareas of a major cytoarchitectonic area of frontal cortex (BA 44) as musicians sight-read a J. S. Bach chorale score and listen for performance errors in harmony, melody, or rhythm.[46] These are group mean PET images for each task (contrasted with passive listening control) overlaid on MRIs. PET data are z-scores displayed on a colour scale ranging from 2.54 (*yellow*; $p < 0.01$) to 4.0 (*red*; $p < 0.0001$). (See Plate 9 in colour section.)

the observed right fusiform activation may implicate that area in the visual processing of musical notes. Such a function would be analogous to visual word processing by left fusiform.[50–53] These implied parallel locations for comparable reading functions in music and language are consistent with other functional and structural correspondences.[16–20]

Each of the three conditions activated different subareas of two major areas in frontal cortex, a lateral region, BA 6, and an inferior lateral region, BA 44/45 (Figure 17.5). These activations were bilateral, although stronger on the left side. In both of these major areas, the rhythm task activated superior subareas, the melody task activated inferior subareas, and the harmony task activated subareas between those two activations. These two major areas are currently associated with sequencing motor behaviour and with recognizing actions.[54–59] However, there was no activation detected in supplementary motor area (SMA) medial BA 6, as has been found in neuroimaging studies of song imagery.[7] In addition, there was no activation in primary motor areas. Therefore, the activation of these areas in the present conditions does not seem related to motor preparation as such, whether for subvocal singing or for imagined playing of an instrument. It is possible that these activations are involved in translating the notes to abstract motor-auditory codes. Such a translation process may be a natural component of expert score reading.

The melody, harmony, and rhythm tasks each also produced distinct patterns of activity in auditory cortex (Figure 17.6). During the melody condition, there were strong activations in secondary auditory association areas, specifically in bilateral superior (BA 22) and bilateral, strongly right, middle temporal (BA 21) cortex. The harmony task produced bilateral activation, more on the left side than the right, in middle (BA 21 and 20), posterior (BA 37), and superior (BA 22) temporal cortex. The rhythm condition produced only minor activation in left inferior (BA 20) and bilateral middle (BA 21) temporal cortex. Superior temporal activation for melodic and harmony tasks, but not rhythmic processing, is consistent with neuropsychological data showing that superior temporal lesions spare rhythmic processing but cause impaired melodic perception.[6,11,60] The activation of such secondary auditory regions bilaterally during these comprehension tasks is also in accord

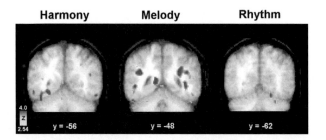

Figure 17.6   Activations in different subareas of auditory cortex as musicians sight-read a J. S. Bach chorale score and listen for performance errors in melody, harmony, or rhythm.[46] These are group mean PET images for each task (contrasted with passive listening control) overlaid on MRIs. PET data are z-scores displayed on a colour scale ranging from 2.54 (*yellow*; $p < 0.05$) to 4.0 (*red*; $p < 0.0001$). (See Plate 10 in colour section.)

with bilateral activation of those areas during the perception or performance of musical pieces and scales in our prior PET study.

The distributed pattern of activations observed in this investigation delineates some of the neural systems subserving musical comprehension. This study may provide an early glimpse of the functional neuroanatomy of expert musicians' comprehension of musical structure. These data confirm or extend prior understanding of the distributed system of brain areas supporting pitch and melody perception, auditory mental imagery, unimanual piano performance from a sight-read score, and bi-manual piano performance of a memorized score. These findings are also consistent with and complement those reported in a contemporaneous neuroimaging study by Platel, Price, Baron *et al.*[10] in which nonmusicians attended to either the timbre, melody, or rhythm properties of random-order, nonmusical tone sequences. Interestingly, the latter study reported that musical timbre, not studied here, was subserved by areas in right superior frontal, middle frontal, and precentral cortex.

The foregoing results suggest that music as a whole is represented in mechanisms widely distributed throughout the brain. However, different parts of the brain are activated when one pays close attention to different aspects of a piece of music. This observation is perhaps not surprising since music is a complex, multifaceted stimulus and activity. At the same time, the data illustrate the power of directed attention to change brain activity. The data also suggest that the specific subareas of major areas, such as cerebellum, and frontal and temporal cortex, perform different functions for particular subtasks of musical comprehension. More generally, the distributed neural system for musical comprehension revealed here can be compared in further studies to the better-known distributed neural systems for language tasks. Such studies can begin to identify independent and shared neural mechanisms for music and language and evaluate the scope of application for specific neural mechanisms.

Functional neuroanatomy of musical rhythm

The next study builds upon the findings of the preceding studies and aims to provide a more complete account of the functional neuroanatomy of the mental representation of musical rhythm. We examined the selective perception of individual principal components of musical rhythm—that is, pattern (phrasing), tempo, meter, and duration. In addition, in order to explore the effect of musical talent and training on the neural systems supporting musical rhythm perception, expert musicians were compared to nonmusicians.

Studies of brain-damaged patients have reported that the perception of rhythm can be impaired without affecting melodic processing, suggesting that there is a distinct neural system for the representation of rhythm.[61] Some studies have been in-conclusive as to whether rhythm was a left hemispheric or bilateral neural process.[62,63] Interestingly, recent fMRI data suggest that memory for familiar, regular rhythms (with whole-number interval ratios) is supported by left frontal (BA 6) and parietal cortex and right anterior cerebellum.[48] On the other hand, these data suggested that memory for more unfamiliar rhythms (with fractionated interval ratios) was supported by right prefrontal, frontal (BA 6), and parietal areas, along with bilateral posterior cerebellum.

The involvement of the cerebellum in the processing of musical rhythm is consistent with data from our second PET study (see earlier) and those of two other studies.[10,42] This implication is congruent with neurological findings that cerebellar patients are impaired at the fine perception of temporal features of auditory stimuli.[47]

Involvement of parietal and prefrontal cortex in rhythm processing[48] is also consistent with data from our second PET study. In addition, this activity is congruent with recent neurological data implicating an inferior parietal-prefrontal circuit that supports time-dependent attention and working memory functions necessary for perception of duration of auditory stimuli.[64] Of particular note in this context is a study of unilateral temporal corticectomy patients in which evidence was found for a dissociation between the areas processing meter as opposed to rhythm pattern, with anterior superior temporal areas implicated for meter.[11]

In the present study, Michael Thaut and I explored the principal components of rhythm: duration, pattern, tempo (dynamically increasing or decreasing rate), and meter (e.g. the differing periodicities of 3/4, 4/4, 5/4, 5/8, 7/8, and 9/8). Using the same PET methods as in our preceding studies, we imaged nonmusicians and musicians, making covert discriminations of pairs of rhythmic auditory patterns. Each scanned set of trials required the subject to focus on a single one of four principal components of rhythm. We also included a pitch discrimination control task in which subjects compared pairs of auditory sequences. In the pitch discrimination task it was possible for a single note to vary in pitch in one member of the stimulus pair. The pitch discrimination stimuli possessed a metronomic rhythm (i.e. all notes had the same duration). As a control task, the pitch stimuli required comparable auditory perception, working memory, and comparison and decision processes as the rhythm tasks, without requiring the processing of rhythmic features of duration, meter, tempo, or pattern.

Participating in the study were five musicians, with (at least) an undergraduate university degree in music, and five nonmusicians, with no music training or performance experience beyond childhood. All 10 subjects were right-handed adult males. The stimuli (apart from the pitch control) were always 440-Hz computer-generated piano timbre sounds of 231- or 462-ms duration. The interval between tones in a stimulus sequence was a multiple of 231 ms. The stimuli on the duration, pattern, and pitch control trials were modeled on the standardized Seashore Test.[65] The stimuli on the tempo and meter trials were modeled on the Gordon Musical Aptitude Profile.[66] These stimulus materials were adjusted (i.e. in tempo or accentuation) so that the stimuli on the tempo, phrasing, duration, meter, and pitch control trials were as similar as possible. Different conditions varied with respect to the exact nature of the task being performed, with stimuli being in almost all respects constant across conditions. Although tempo, pattern, and meter stimuli had more tones per sequence, between 9 and 12 events, approximately the same total number of tones per scanned interval were presented in the duration task as in the tempo, pattern, and meter tasks. A 'different' trial contained the same number of events (and accents) and was of the same total duration as the 'same' trials (by playing them at different tempi), except in the duration condition. In the pitch task, the tone alternated between 415, 440, and 466 Hz in sequences of 12 462-ms (quarter note) tones, without rests. Across all conditions, the intersequence interval was 1000 ms, and the intertrial interval was 1750 ms; the trial time was 14 s on average.

Stimuli were adjusted to produce comparable mean accuracy of musicians and of non-musicians on each task. Each subject subsequently performed 11 PET trials: two trials each of the pattern task, duration task, meter task, tempo task, and pitch control task, as well as one rest trial. The subject's eyes were closed on all trials. During each 60 s of task there were four covert discrimination judgments. For half of the trials, the pair of stimuli was identical. After the PET session, subjects replicated the trials from the PET session, overtly indicating their responses. Their average performance across the latter trials confirmed that task difficulty was equated across conditions and across groups.

To highlight some of our principal findings, for both nonmusicians and musicians, distinct patterns of brain activity were detected for the discrimination of pitch and each musical rhythm. There were also distinct differences between nonmusicians and musicians during each discrimination.

For pitch (contrasted with rest), superior temporal areas (BA 21/22) were activated on the right in nonmusicians and on the left in musicians (Figure 17.7A and D). However, middle and inferior temporal areas (BA 21/20) were activated on the right in both groups (Figure 17.7B and E). These temporal activations confirm prior neurological and neuro-imaging studies, including those for the comprehension of melody above.[6,7,11,34-36]

There were also strong cerebellar activations during pitch (Figure 17.7C and F), again confirming our earlier PET data. The cerebellar activations are not likely related to motor activity since no overt motor activity occurred and there was little or no activity detected in neocortical motor areas. Instead, the cerebellar activity seems to support perceptual or cognitive processing of pitch (or melody). Interestingly, the nonmusicians showed strong predominantly left-sided activation in posterior lateral cerebellar hemispheres (Figure 17.7C). The left cerebellum projects to the right cerebral cortex, so the activation in left cerebellum is likely supporting the right temporal activation for pitch. However, musicians showed bilateral cerebellar activation (Figure 17.7F), apparently supporting bilateral temporal activation.

The key rhythm-specific activations were as follows. First, certain activations were generally present for each rhythm task and for both nonmusicians and musicians, such as basal ganglia and cingulate cortex. The cingulate activations are likely involved in attention functions required in the task.[67-70]

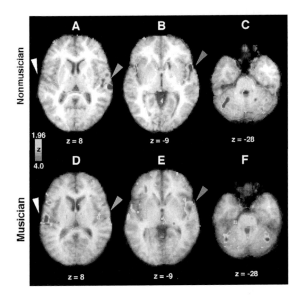

Figure 17.7   Activations in superior and middle temporal cortex (A, B, D, and E) and in cerebellum (C and F) as nonmusicians and musicians discriminate pitch sequences.[49] These images show group mean PET data for each task (contrasted with rest) overlaid on MRIs. PET data are z-scores displayed on a colour scale ranging from 1.96 (*yellow*; $p < 0.1$) to 4.0 (*red*; $p < 0.0001$). (See Plate 11 in colour section.)

For the tempo, pattern, and meter discriminations, there was a tendency for activation to be detected in nonmusicians that was not present for musicians. For tempo discrimination, nonmusicians showed activation in right medial frontal cortex (BA 9) and bilateral posterior lateral cerebellum, but this activation was very much weaker or absent in musicians (Figures 17.8 and 17.12). For pattern discrimination, nonmusicians showed activation in midbrain and bilateral posterior lateral cerebellum; however, this activation was absent and weaker in musicians (Figures 17.9 and 17.12). For meter discrimination, nonmusicians showed activation in right inferior frontal cortex (BA 47) and bilateral posterior lateral cerebellum (Figure 17.10 and 17.12), with little or no such activation in these areas for musicians. By contrast, during duration discrimination musicians showed bilateral medial frontal cortex (BA 9), bilateral inferior parietal cortex (BA 40), and strong activation in bilateral posterior lateral cerebellum (Figures 17.11 and 17.12). These activations were absent or very much weaker in nonmusicians.

As with pitch discrimination, the strong cerebellar activations during rhythm discriminations are not likely due to motoric processing *per se* but to a role in supporting non-motor sensory or cognitive processing.[38–45] In addition, in the meter, tempo, and pattern discriminations, cerebellar activity is much stronger for nonmusicians than for musicians, but the reverse is true for the duration discrimination. Interestingly, musicians found discriminating the duration of rhythmic sequences more novel than discriminating meter, tempo, and pattern. By contrast, the nonmusicians found discriminating the overall duration of rhythmic sequences less novel than discriminating other rhythm features. Thus, the

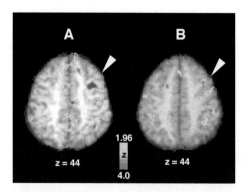

Figure 17.8 Activations in left medial frontal cortex (BA 9) for nonmusicians (A) as compared to musicians (B) during the discrimination of musical tempi.[49] Shown are group mean PET images for each task (contrasted with rest) overlaid on MRIs. (See Plate 12 in colour section.)

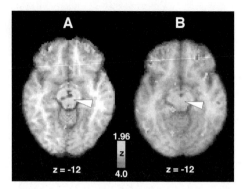

Figure 17.9 Activations in midbrain for nonmusicians (A) as compared to musicians (B) during the discrimination of musical pattern.[49] These are group-averaged PET images for each task (contrasted with rest) overlaid on anatomical MRIs. (See Plate 13 in colour section.)

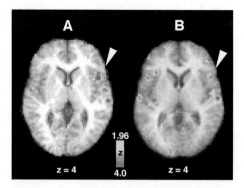

Figure 17.10 Activations in right inferior frontal cortex (BA 47) for nonmusicians (A) as compared to musicians (B) during discrimination of musical meter.[49] Shown are group-averaged PET images for each task (contrasted with rest) over-laid on anatomical MRIs. (See Plate 14 in colour section.)

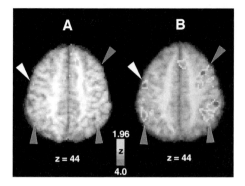

Figure 17.11   Activations in bilateral medial frontal cortex (BA 9) and bilateral inferior parietal cortex (BA 40) for musicians (B) as compared to nonmusicians (A) during the discrimination of sequence durations.[49] Shown are group-averaged PET images for each task (contrasted with rest) overlaid on anatomical MRIs. (See Plate 15 in colour section.)

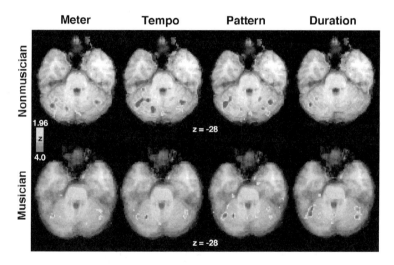

Figure 17.12   Activations in posterior cerebellum as nonmusicians and musicians discriminate meter, tempo, pattern, and duration.[49] Shown are group-mean PET images for each task (contrasted with rest) overlaid on MRIs. (See Plate 16 in colour section.)

increase in cerebellar activation appears to be associated with greater novelty of rhythm discrimination, consistent with other neuroimaging findings[71] and new hypotheses of cerebellar function.[37]

The activations in prefrontal cortical areas BAs 9, 10, and 47 are likely supporting working memory processes.[48] The activation in prefrontal and inferior parietal areas follows similar indications in the recent neurological study of tone duration discrimination.[64] We speculate that activations in temporal, frontal, and midbrain may be involved in processing the temporal grouping structure of rhythms.

These findings suggest some key brain areas in the distributed neural circuits underlying the perceptual/cognitive representation of central aspects of musical rhythm. These data suggest that distinct brain areas subserve musical meter, tempo, pattern, and duration. In addition, the results confirm that the neural subsystems underlying pitch discrimination are distinct from those subserving the elements of rhythm discrimination. The differences in activated brain areas for nonmusicians and musicians likely reflect differences in strategy, perceptual skill, and cognitive representation of the components of musical rhythm and pitch.

Neurology of pitch discrimination

In the foregoing review of neuroimaging and neurological studies of music, the cerebellum appears to be involved in some way in nonmotor, nonsomatic sensory or cognitive processing. This kind of conclusion is supported by many other recent neuroimaging and neurological findings.[37–45,73] Such findings challenge classical motor theories of cerebellar function and have created an environment in which researchers are increasingly questioning the extent to which the cerebellum is involved in motor control. Although in most cases, new alternative proposals are described as an extension of the role of the cerebellum in motor coordination itself, others, who have been driven primarily by new neuroimaging results, are proposing radically different functions for this structure.

James Bower and I, and our colleagues, have been using neuroimaging of tactile and cutaneous sensory and motor tasks to test the hypothesis that the cerebellum is involved in monitoring and optimizing the acquisition of information in various sensory modalities.[72–74] A direct prediction of this hypothesis is that damage to the cerebellum will impair performance on sensory tasks, especially those in which successful performance depends on sensory information processing at a very fine time scale. We evaluated this prediction for auditory perception by examining for the first time the effect of global cerebellar degeneration on auditory pitch discrimination in (nonmusician) patients.[75] This strictly auditory task does not depend on overt motor behaviour, as do other sensory tasks.

Fifteen patients and 15 healthy control subjects (matched in age and education) performed a pitch discrimination task measuring difference thresholds. The patients suffer from pancerebellar degeneration caused by hereditary, idiopathic, paraneoplastic, or postinfectious pancerebellitis. The degree of cerebellar degeneration in these patients, as confirmed by examinations of pancerebellar ataxia and anatomical imaging, ranged from minimal to severe, and included mild- and moderate-grade cases of ataxia. Patients and controls mostly had normal loudness thresholds; some had mild hearing loss in the 4000–8000 Hz range.

On each pitch discrimination trial, subjects decided whether a comparison tone was higher or lower than a preceding 500 Hz standard. All tones had suprathreshold loudness (80 dB) and 400 ms duration; the standard was followed 400 ms later by the comparison pitch. The tones were composed of the fundamental, three times the fundamental frequency at a 50 per cent amplitude, and five times the fundamental at a 25 per cent amplitude. The difference threshold estimation procedure used was PEST.[76,77] Subjects performed 60 trials, with threshold trials from above and below the standard pitch, mixed

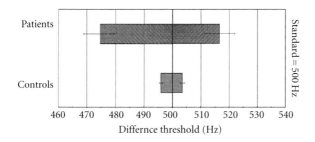

Figure 17.13   Average lower and upper difference discrimination thresholds for auditory pitch in pancerebellar degeneration patients and healthy controls.[75]

together in pseudorandom order. Each subject also performed two control tasks, the WAIS-III Digit Memory Span task, assessing auditory working memory capacity, and a simple auditory detection reaction time task, assessing simple motor reaction time for detecting audible sounds.

As shown in Figure 17.13, patients' pitch discrimination thresholds were on average 5.5 times that for controls ($p < 0.0001$). The degree of impairment was correlated ($r = +0.70$, $p < 0.003$) with the severity of patients' pancerebellar ataxia. Furthermore, the sizes of patients' pitch discrimination thresholds were uncorrelated with their loudness thresholds for the standard tone ($r = +0.02$, $p < 0.79$) and for the wider range from 125 to 8000 Hz ($r = +0.06$, $p < 0.22$). Patient and control groups did not differ on digit span memory or auditory detection reaction time.

As a group, then, patients with pancerebellar degeneration, but no other neurological conditions, show strongly impaired pitch discrimination. However, the degree of impairment for individuals is proportional to the severity of their pancerebellar ataxia. The severity of the pancerebellar ataxia (e.g. with symptoms in gait, speech, limb, and eye behaviour) is assumed to be indicative of the degree of pancerebellar atrophy. Although these data do not indicate the location of auditory processing regions in the cerebellum, it is assumed that atrophy in auditory regions of the cerebellum is proportional to the pancerebellar ataxia. Such atrophied auditory regions are assumed to be responsible for the pitch discrimination impairment. These cerebellar patients' auditory abilities are intact in a fundamental way, as indicated by reasonably normal auditory loudness thresholds. This observation is consistent with the idea that primary sensory processing is subserved in appropriate regions of cerebral cortex, which are spared in these patients. However, patients' loudness thresholds (ranging from normal hearing to mild hearing loss) are uncorrelated with the degree of their pitch discrimination impairment. Central to the idea of cerebellar involvement in sensory data acquisition is the suggestion that cerebellar effects would be most clearly evident in tasks that require highly optimized sensory data. In the current case, it seems reasonable to assume that the simple detection of the presence of a tone is unlikely to require the same quality sensory data as the fine discrimination of pitch.

Thus, these results suggest that the cerebellum has a fundamental supporting role in the information processing necessary for fine auditory discrimination. This conclusion is consistent with cerebellar activations reported in recent neuroimaging studies involving pitch or melody processing.[46,49] The pattern of coupled pitch and ataxia measures, and decoupled pitch and loudness measures, suggests that the role of the cerebellum is to monitor and optimize the acquisition of information in sensory modalities (audition). Patients and controls did not differ in digit span memory. This indicates that the differences between patients and controls in pitch discrimination were very likely not due to any working memory deficits that may possibly be associated with cerebellar damage.

An important independent corroboration of the implications of these data is provided by a recent study examining cerebellar degeneration patients' performance on a variety of visual tasks.[43] The authors report that the patients were impaired selectively for the detection of visual motion, speed, and direction, as dissociated from eye movement control and from any other attentional, memory, or cognitive task components. It should be noted that there are also neurological studies suggesting that the cerebellum may be instrumental in other nonmotor behaviours. These behaviours include judging the timing of events, solving perceptual and spatial reasoning problems, and generating words according to a semantic rule.[47,78–83] In terms of the sensory acquisition hypothesis we are testing, however, impairments in these specific tasks may be more related to the dependence of these tasks on well-controlled information processing (e.g. sensory acquisition) than to different specific roles for the cerebellum in each of those behaviors.

General issues in interpreting brain activations

Given the rapid emergence of promising new neuroimaging methods for the study of music performance, perception, and cognition, it may be useful in the present volume to discuss current and general methodological issues for interpreting the role of activated brain areas in the processing of music. Mapping elementary operations onto particular brain areas and mapping those operations/areas onto system-level models of specific musical and other cognitive tasks requires a convergence across paradigms (behavioural tasks) and independent experiments. No single task or paradigm used in neuroimaging or neurological investigations can isolate an elementary operation. Likewise, no single group of subjects (i.e. one study's sample) can fully capture the location and distribution of a brain area in a population. Thus, mapping localized operations entails sifting through multiple studies.

In functional neuroimaging, for example, the analysis of multiple studies, or metanalysis, can be rigorously and quantitatively performed[84] because the data are customarily reported in stereotaxic coordinates.[23,30] A growing number of rigorous metanalyses with important implications for mapping operations and systems, as well as for psychological models, are being conducted. For example, such analyses have been performed in motor processes and supplementary motor areas,[85] in oculomotor control and frontal eye fields,[86] in speech motor-sensory processes and the mouth area of primary motor-sensory cortex,[87,88] in visual information processing,[89–91] in visual attention,[91] and in memory.[92] Improved methods for such meta-analyses are currently being developed and validated.[84,87,88,93] Using such quantitative stereotactic-based metanalyses will yield important insights into the relationship between neural mechanisms supporting music and those supporting other cognitive processes.

As an aside, it should be noted that mapping neural mechanisms and systems will be advanced more efficiently if, whenever possible, the coordinate-based analyses just described replace analyses based only on lower resolution measures such as hemisphere, lobe, sulcus, gyrus, and, eventually, Brodmann area. Interestingly, close analysis suggests that much of the seemingly large variability in structure-function correlations remarked upon by some researchers using surface-based anatomical landmarks may vanish when the frame of analysis shifts to stereotactic coordinate-based analysis.[88]

Be that as it may, hypothesizing an operation (or computation) for an area requires a principled analysis of cognitive and behavioural processes and tasks. In spite of efforts in the cognitive sciences, there is no formal language in which to capture component operations that fractionate a task, including musical ones. A useful first step in that development would be for circumscribed communities of researchers studying a particular operation, area, or paradigm(s) in music processing to settle on an effective common vocabulary, with an eye towards establishing a working standard vocabulary with researchers studying other specific operations, areas, or paradigms. At the present time, this is rarely done, and apparently never in a concerted fashion. Standardized component models will be of great benefit for the process of mapping operations down to brain areas and up to system-level tasks in order to compare music and other cognitive processes.

Another significant point with regard to these goals is that whenever possible the operation hypothesized for a brain area should be consistent with its underlying microcircuitry. This is also rarely done in cognitive neuroscience. Take, for example, the case of hypothesizing operations for the cerebellum. The cerebellum has a uniform microcircuitry throughout, so until proved otherwise, we should assume that it performs a uniform operation, even if that operation may be performed on different kinds of information (as consistent with connectivity). Of course, even the most widely accepted facts about microcircuitry in an area can change from time to time. In the case of the cerebellum, David Marr's model of cerebellar function[94] was shown to be inconsistent with the underlying microcircuitry some time after its publication (although it continued to be influential).

Finally, there is a misguided tendency when interpreting neuroimaging data to assume that every activated area is directly involved in the cognitive or behavioural task eliciting it. A parallel tendency leads to the assumption that every cognitive or behavioural process affected by damage to a particular brain area necessarily implicates direct involvement of that area in those processes. As our sophistication in the computational and neural sciences grows, we will likely recognize that there are a range of indirect roles a mechanism might assume.

Consider again the cerebellum. The cerebellum is thought by various researchers to be directly involved in a variety of cognitive and behavioural processes. However, the consequences of injury to, or absence of, the cerebellum are often not fully appreciated. Although 70–80 per cent of the neurons in the brain are packed tightly in the cerebellum, the symptoms are mild and transient in cases when nearly all of it is removed. Likewise, persons born without a cerebellum show few impairments. These observations imply that the function of the cerebellum is subtly supportive and not necessary. On the hypothesis of cerebellar function that my colleagues and I are testing,[37,73] a brain with a healthy cerebellum is assumed to be optimized for operations necessary for fine sensory acquisition.

Furthermore, a brain without a cerebellum is viewed as subtly suboptimal, whereas a brain with a damaged cerebellum can range from mildly to very suboptimal, depending on degree and location of damage. In the more debilitating cases, the assumption is that a damaged cerebellum is causing other brain areas to operate on the basis of corrupted, noisy, poorly acquired and controlled sensory information. More generally, there may be a number of brain areas (such as basal ganglia or cingulate) with comparably indirect supporting roles in other cognitive or behavioural processes. Clearly, careful neurological studies (and, in some cases, transcranial magnetic stimulation studies) can assist in dissociating shades of involvement of a brain area in a particular psychological process.

Conclusion

Musical experiences intricately and deeply engage the mind and the whole brain. Details of this process are being unveiled by new scientific advances well represented in this volume. Although many challenges lie ahead for fully understanding the biological foundations of music, the tools for meeting at least a fair share of those challenges appear to be in hand.

Acknowledgements

I am grateful to the following collaborators for their stimulating, intelligent assistance with the studies discussed in this chapter: Peter Fox, Donald Hodges, James Bower, Jeremy Schmahmann, Stephen Grill, Michael Thaut, Bruno Repp, Michael Martinez, and John Tennison. I also thank our subjects, musicians, and patients for their gracious participation in support of basic research. The work described in this article was supported by the EJLB Foundation, the National Association for Music Merchants (now the International Foundation for Music Research), the Texaco Foundation, a State of Colorado Center of Excellence Award, and NIH (NINDS) Grant NS3710901A1.

References

1. Lerdahl, F. and R. Jackendoff (1983) *A Generative Theory of Tonal Music*. Cambridge, MA: MIT Press.
2. Dowling, W. and D. Harwood (1986) *Music Cognition*. Orlando, FL: Academic Press.
3. Krumhansl, C. (1990) *Cognition Foundations of Musical Pitch*. Oxford: Oxford University Press.
4. Repp, B. H. (1992) Probing the cognitive representation of musical time: structural constraints on the perception of timing pertubations. *Cognition* 44, 241–81.
5. Sergent, J. (1993) Mapping the musician brain. *Hum. Brain Map.* 1, 20–38.
6. Peretz, I., R. Kolinsky, M. Tramo, *et al.* (1994) Functional dissociations following bilateral lesions of auditory cortex. *Brain* 117, 1283–301.
7. Zatorre R. J., A. R. Halpern, D. W. Perry, *et al.* (1996) Hearing in the mind's ear: a PET investigation of musical imagery and perception. *J. Cognit. Neurosci.* 8, 29–46.
8. Deliege, I. and J. Sloboda (1997) *Perception and Cognition of Music*. Wicyita, KS: Psychology Press.
9. Palmer, C. (1997) Music performance. *Annu. Rev. Psychol.* 48, 115–38.

10. Platel, H., C. Price, J. C. Baron, *et al.* (1997) The structural components of music perception. *Brain* 120, 299–43.

11. Liegeois-Chauvel, C., I. Peretz, M. Babai, *et al.* (1998) Contribution of different cortical areas in the temporal lobes to music processing. *Brain* 121, 1853–67.

12. Pantev, C., R. Oostenveld, A. Engelien, *et al.* (1998) Increased auditory cortical representation in musicians. *Nature* 392, 811–14.

13. Blood, A. J., R. J. Zatorre, P. Bermudes, *et al.* (1999) Emotional responses to pleasant and unpleasant music correlate with activity in paralimbic brain regions. *Nat. Neurosci.* 2, 382–7.

14. Wallin, N. L., B. Merker, and S. Brown (eds) (1999) *The Origins of Music.* Cambridge, MA: MIT Press.

15. Sergent, J., E. Zuck, S. Terriah, *et al.* (1992) Distributed neural network underlying musical sight-reading and keyboard performance. *Sci.* 257, 106–9.

16. Besson, M. and F. Faita (1995) An Event Related Potential (ERP) study of musical expectancy: comparison of musicians with non-musicians. *J. Exp. Psychol.: Human Percept. Perform.* 21, 1278–96.

17. Patel, A. D. and I. Peretz (1997) Is music autonomous from language? A neuropsychological appraisal. In I. Deliege and J. Sloboda (eds) *Perception and Cognition of Music.* Wichita, KS: Psychology Press.

18. Besson, M., F. Faita, I. Peretz, *et al.* (1998) Singing in the brain: independence of lyrics and tunes. *Psychol. Sci.* 9, 494–8.

19. Patel, A. D., E. Gibson, J. Ratner, *et al.* (1998) Processing syntactic relations in language and music: an event-related potential study. *J. Cognit. Neurosci.* 10, 717–33.

20. Patel, A. D., I. Peretz, M. Tramo, *et al.* (1998) Processing prosodic and musical patterns: a neuropsychological investigation. *Brain Lang.* 61, 123–44.

21. Parsons, L. M., P. T. Fox, J. S. Sergent, *et al.* Neural systems underlying musical piano performance from memory. Submitted.

22. Fox, P. T., M. A. Mintun, M. E. Raichle, *et al.* (1984) A noninvasive approach to quantitative functional brain mapping with $H_2{}^{15}O$ tissue activity. *J. Nucl. Med.* 30, 141–9.

23. Talairach, J. and P. Tournoux (1988) Co-planar Stereotaxic Atlas of the Human Brain. New York: Thieme Medical Publishers.

24. Fox, P. T., M. A. Mintun, E. M. Reiman, *et al.* (1988) Enhanced detection of focal brain responses using inter-subject averaging and change-distribution analysis of subtracted PET images. *J. Cereb. Blood Flow Metab.* 8, 642–53.

25. Woods, R. P., S. R. Cherry, and J. R. Mazziotta (1992) Rapid automatic algorithm for aligning and reslicing PET images. *J. Comp. Assist. Tomogr.* 17, 536–46.

26. Woods, R. P., J. C. Mazziotta, and S. R. Cherry. (1993) MRI-PET registration with automated algorithm. *J. Comput. Assisted Tomogr.* 17, 536–46.

27. Lancaster, J. L., T. G. Glass, B. R. Lankiplli, *et al.* (1995) A modality-independent approach to spatial normalization of tomographic images of the human brain. *Hum. Brain Map.* 3, 209–23.

28. Fox, P. T. and M. A. Mintun (1989) Noninvasive brain mapping by change-distribution analysis of averaged PET images of $H_2{}^{15}O$ tissue activity. *J. Nucl. Med.* 30, 141–9.

29. Xiong J., J. H. Gao, J. L. Lancaster, *et al.* (1996) Clustered pixels analysis for functional MRI activation studies of the human brain. *Hum. Brain Map.* 3, 287–301.

30. Lancaster, J. L., M. G. Woldorff, L. M. Parsons, *et al.* (2000) Automatic Talairach labels for functional brain mapping. *Hum. Brain Map.* 10, 120–31.

31. **Zatorre, R. J.** (1988) Pitch perception of complex tones and human temporal-lobe function. *J. Acoust. Soc. Am.* 84, 566–72.

32. **Zatorre, R. J. and S. Samson** (1991) Role of the right temporal neocortex in retention of pitch in auditory short-term memory. *Brain* 114, 2403–17.

33. **Zatorre, R. J., A. C. Evans, E. Meyer, et al.** (1992) Lateralization of phonetic and pitch discrimination in speech processing. *Sci.* 256, 846–9.

34. **Zatorre, R. J., A. C. Evans, and E. Meyer** (1994) Neural mechanisms underlying melodic perception and memory for pitch. *J. Neurosci.* 14, 1908–19.

35. **Griffiths, T. D., C. Buchel, R. S. J. Frackowiak, et al.** (1998) Analysis of temporal structure in sound by the human brain. *Nature Neurosci.* 1, 422–7.

36. **Perry, D. W., R. J. Zatorre, M. Petrides, et al.** (1999) Localization of cerebral activity during simple singing. *NeuroReport* 10, 3979–84.

37. **Bower, J. M.** (1997) Is the cerebellum sensory for motor's sake, or motor for sensory's sake: the view from the whiskers of a rat? In C. I. de Zeeuw, P. Strata, and J. Voogd (eds) *Progress in Brain Research.* New York: Elsevier, pp. 483–516.

38. **Jueptner, M., S. Ottinger, S. J. Fellows, et al.** (1997) The relevance of sensory input for the cerebellar control of movements. *Neuroimage* 5, 41–51.

39. **Parsons, L. M. and P. T. Fox.** (1997) Sensory and cognitive functions. In J. D. Schmahmann (ed.) *The Cerebellum and Cognition.* New York: Academic Press, pp. 255–72.

40. **Schmahmann, J. D.** (ed.) (1997) *The Cerebellum and Cognition.* New York: Academic Press.

41. **Desmond, J. and J. Fiez** (1998) Neuroimaging studies of the cerebellum: language, learning, and memory. *Trends Cognit. Sci.* 2, 355–62.

42. **Penhune, V. B., R. J. Zatorre, and A. C. Evans** (1998) Cerebellar contributions to motor timing: a PET study of auditory and visual rhythm reproduction. *J. Cognit. Neurosci.* 10, 752–65.

43. **Thier, P., T. Haarmeier, S. Treue et al.** (1999) Absence of a common functional denominator of visual disturbances in cerebellar disease. *Brain* 122, 2133–46.

44. **Parsons, L. M., D. Denton, R. Shade et al.** (2000) Neuroimaging evidence implicating cerebellum in support of sensory/cognitive processes associated with thirst. *Proc. Natl. Acad. Sci. USA* 97, 2332–6.

45. **Tesche, C. D. and J. Karhu** (2000) Anticipatory cerebellar responses during somatosensory omission in man. *Hum. Brain Map.* 9, 119–42.

46. **Parsons, L. M., D. A. Hodges, and P. T. Fox** The brain basis of the comprehension of musical harmony, rhythm, and melody. Submitted.

47. **Ivry, R. and S. Keele** (1989) Timing functions of the cerebellum. *J. Cognit. Neurosci.* 1, 136–52.

48. **Sakai, K., O. Hikosaka, S. Miyauchi et al.** (1999) Neural representation of a rhythm depends on its interval ratio. *J. Neurosci.* 19, 10074–81.

49. **Parsons, L. M. and M. Thaut** Functional neuroanatomy of musical rhythm, meter, tempo, and duration. Submitted.

50. **Petersen, S. E., P. T. Fox, M. I. Posner et al.** (1989) Positron tomographic studies of the processing of single words. *J. Cognit. Neurosci.* 1, 153–70.

51. **Mazoyer, B. M., N. Tzourio, and V. Frak et al.** (1993) The cortical representation of speech. *J. Cognit. Neurosci.* 5, 467–79.

52. **Stromswold, K., D. Caplan, N. Alpert et al.** (1996) Localization of syntactic comprehension by positron emission tomography. *Brain Lang.* 52, 452–73.

53. **Price, C.** (1998) The functional anatomy of word comprehension and production. *Trends Cognit. Sci.* 2, 281–8.

54. **Kurata, K.** (1993) Premotor cortex of monkeys—set-related and movement-related activity reflecting amplitude and direction of wrist movements. *J. Neurophysiol.* 73, 836–54.

55. **Passingham, R. E.** (1993) *The Frontal Lobes and Voluntary Action.* New York: Oxford University Press.

56. **Kurata, K.** (1994) Information processing for motor control in primate premotor cortex. *Behav. Brain Res.* 61, 135–42.

57. **Jackson, S. R.** and **M. Husain** (1996) Visuomotor functions of the lateral pre-motor cortex. *Curr. Opin. Neurobiol.* 6, 788–95.

58. **Rizzolatti, G., L. Fadiga, M. Matellii, et al.** (1996) Localization of grasp representations in human by PET: I. Observations versus execution. *Exp. Brain Res.* 111, 246–52.

59. **Carey, D. P., D. I. Perrett,** and **M. W. Oram** (1997) Recognizing, understanding, and reproducing action. In F. Boller and J. Grafman (eds.) *Handbook of Neuropsychology,* vol. 11. Amsterdam: Elsevier, pp. 111–29.

60. **Thompson, W. F.** (1994) Sensitivity to combinations of musical parameters: pitch with duration, and pitch pattern with durational pattern. *Percept. Psychophys.* 56, 363–74.

61. **Peretz, I.** and **R. Kolinsky** (1993) Boundaries of separability between melody and rhythm in music discrimination: a neuropsychological perspective. *Q. J. Exp. Psychol.* 46, 1283–301.

62. **Peretz, I.** (1990) Processing of local and global musical information by unilateral brain-damaged patients. *Brain* 113, 1185–205.

63. **Polk, M.** and **A. Kertesz** (1993) Music and language in degenerative disease of the brain. *Brain Cognit.* 22, 98–117.

64. **Harrington, D. L., K. Y. Haaland,** and **R. T. Knight** (1998) Cortical networks underlying mechanisms of time perception. *J. Neurosci.* 18, 1085–95.

65. **Seashore, C. E.** (1938) *The Psychology of Music.* New York: McGraw-Hill.

66. **Gordon, E. E.** (1965) *Musical Aptitude Profile.* Boston: Houghton-Mifflin.

67. **Corbetta, M., F. M. Miezin, S. Dobmeyer, et al.** (1991) Selective and divided attention during visual discriminations of shape, color, and speed: funtional anatomy by PET. *J. Neurosci.* 11, 2383–402.

68. **Grasby, P. M., C. D. Frith, K. J. Friston, et al.** (1993) Functional mapping of brain areas implicated in auditory/verbal memory function. *Brain* 116, 1–20.

69. **Shallice, T., P. Fletcher, C. D. Frith, et al.** (1994) Brain regions associated with acquisition and retrieval of verbal episodic memory. *Nature* 368, 633–5.

70. **Doyon, J.** (1997) Skill learning. In J. D. Schmahmann (ed.) *The Cerebellum and Cognition.* New York: Academic Press pp. 273–94.

71. **Corbetta, M., G. L. Shulman, F. M. Miezin, et al.** (1995) Superior parietal cortex activation during spatial attention shifts and visual feature conjunction. *Science* 270, 802.

72. **Liu, Y., Y. Pu, J. H. Gao, et al.** (2000) The human red nucleus and lateral cerebellum in cooperative roles supporting sensory discrimination. *Hum. Brain Map.* 10, 147–59.

73. **Parsons, L. M, J. M. Bower, J. H. Gao, et al.** (1997) Lateral cerebellar hemispheres actively support sensory acquisition and discrimination rather than motor control. *Learn. Mem.* 4, 49–62.

74. **Gao, J. H., L. M. Parsons, J. M. Bower, et al.** (1996) Cerebellum implicated in sensory acquisition and discrimination rather than motor control. *Science* 272, 545–7.

75. **Parsons, L. M., J. D. Schmahmann, S. Grill, et al.** Neurological evidence implicating the cerebellum in fine auditory discriminations. Submitted.

76. **Taylor, M. and C. Creelman.** (1967) PEST: efficient estimates of probability functions. *J. Acoust. Soc. Am.* 41, 782–7.

77. **Pentland, A.** (1980) Maximum likelihood estimation: the best PEST. *Percept. Psychophys.* 28, 377–9.

78. **Bracke-Tolkmitt, R., A. Linden, G. M. Canavan, et al.** (1989) The cerebellum contributes to mental skills. *Behav. Neurosci.* 103, 442–6.

79. **Fiez, J. A., S. E. Petersen, M. K. Cheney, et al.** (1992) Impaired nonmotor learning and error-detection associated with cerebellar damage—a single case study. *Brain* 115, 155–78.

80. **Grafman, J., I. Litvan, S. Massaquoi, et al.** (1992) Cognitive planning deficits in patients with cerebellar atrophy. *Neurology* 42, 1493–6.

81. **Courchesne, E., J. Townsend, N. A. Akshoomoff, et al.** (1994) Impairment in shifting attention in autistic and cerebellar patients. *Behav. Neurosci.* 108, 848–65.

82. **Horak, F. B. and H. C. Diener** (1994) Cerebellar control of postural scaling and central set in stance. *J. Neurophysiol.* 72, 479–93.

83. **Daum, I., S. Graber, and H. Ackermann** (1998) Cognitive Neuroscience Abstracts Annual Meeting Program: Supplement, *J. Cognit. Neurosci.* 113, 15.

84. **Fox, P. T., L. M. Parsons, and J. L. Lancaster** (1998) Beyond the single study: function/location metanalysis in cognitive neuroimaging. *Curr. Opin. Neurobiol.* 8, 178–87.

85. **Picard, N. and P. L. Strick** (1996) Motor areas of the medial wall: a review of their location and functional activation. *Cereb. Cortex* 6, 342–53.

86. **Paus, T.** (1996) Location and function of the human frontal eye-field: a selective review. *Neuropsychologia* 34, 475–83.

87. **Fox, P. T., J. L. Lancaster, A. Huang, et al.** (1999) Functional volume modeling: scaling for group size in averaged images. *Hum. Brain Map.* 8, 143–50.

88. **Fox, P. T., A. Huang, L. M. Parsons, et al.** (2000) Location-probability profiles for the human primary-motor mouth representation. *Neuroimage* 13, 196–201.

89. **Shulman, G. L., M. Corbetta, and R. L. Buckner, et al.** (1997) Top-down modulation of early sensory cortex. *Cereb. Cortex* 7, 193–206.

90. **Shulman, G. L., M. Corbetta, and R. L. Buckner, et al.** (1997) Common blood flow changes across visual tasks: I. Increases in subcortical structures and cerebellum but not in nonvisual cortex. *J. Cognit. Neurosci.* 9, 623–46.

91. **Shulman, G. L., J. L. Fiez, M. Corbetta, et al.** (1997) Common blood flow changes across visual tasks: II. Decreases in cerebral cortex. *J. Cognit. Neurosci.* 9, 647–62.

92. **Buckner, R. L. and S. E. Petersen** (1996) What does neuroimaging tell us about the role of prefrontal cortex in memory retrieval? *Semin. Neurosci.* 8, 47–55.

93. **Fox, P. T., J. L. Lancaster, L. M. Parsons, et al.** (1997) Functional volume modeling. *Hum. Brain Map.* 5, 306–11.

94. **Marr, D.** (1969) A theory of cerebellar cortex. *J. Physiol. (Lond.)* 202, 437–70.

CHAPTER 18

COMPARISON BETWEEN LANGUAGE AND MUSIC

MIREILLE BESSON AND DANIELE SCHÖN

Abstract

Similarities and differences between language and music processing are examined from an evolutionary and a cognitive perspective. Language and music cannot be considered single entities; they need to be decomposed into different component operations or levels of processing. The central question concerns one of the most important claims of the generative grammar theory, that is, the specificity of language processing: do the computations performed to process language rely on specific linguistic processes or do they rely on general cognitive principles? Evidence from brain imaging results is reviewed, noting that this field is currently in need of metanalysis of the available results to precisely evaluate this claim. A series of experiments, mainly using the event-related brain potentials method, were conducted to compare different levels of processing in language and music. Overall, results favour language specificity when certain aspects of semantic processing in language are compared with certain aspects of melodic and harmonic processing in music. By contrast, results support the view that general cognitive principles are involved when aspects of syntactic processing in language are compared with aspects of harmonic processing in music. Moreover, analysis of the temporal structure led to similar effects in language and music. These tentative conclusions must be supported by other brain imaging results to shed further light on the spatiotemporal dynamics of the brain structure–function relationship.

Keywords: Language and music; Music and language; Event-related brain potentials; Brain imaging

Introduction

Once, a long time ago [. . .] it so happened that people took to uncivilized ways, were ruled by lust and greed, behaved in angry and jealous ways with each other [. . .]. Seeing this plight, Indra and other gods approached god Brahma and requested him to give the people a toy, but one which could not only be seen, but heard, and this should turn out a diversion (so that people gave up their bad ways).

A. Rangacharya, *Introduction to Bharata's Natya-Sastra*[1]

One main function of language is communication. Linguistic communication encompasses widely diverse uses of language, from the running of everyday life and basic interactions between individuals (*'Give me the salt, please'.*) to the esthetics of words, their combination in poetry (*'Come what come may/Hours and time run/Through the roughest day'*, Shakespeare), and the telling of stories. Language is also necessary for expression of rational thought and organization of human societies. It may well have evolved from the need for social bonding between individuals belonging to the same group.[2] Language also permits projections into the past and into the future and is necessary for the transmission of knowledge.[3] While these characteristics, among others, make language specific to *Homo sapiens*, they also seem to contribute to the splendid isolation of the linguistic function among the other human cognitive activities. Largely because of the enormous impact in the cognitive sciences of the generative grammar theory, developed by Chomsky,[4] language is most often considered as relying on specific cognitive principles. Bickerton,[5] for instance, argues that the principles that govern language 'seem to be specifically adapted for language and have little in common with general principles of thought or other apparatuses that might be attributable to the human mind' (p. 158). The specificity of the computations involved in language processing is the main question that we would like to address in this chapter. To try to delineate which computations are specific to language and which rely on more general cognitive principles, if any, we chose to compare language with another well-organized cognitive function that, although very different in many respects, nevertheless presents interesting similarities with language: music.

We start by reviewing some of the evidence in favour of the similarities and differences between language and music, based, first, on an evolutionary perspective, and second, on a cognitive perspective. We then report a series of experiments directly aimed at comparing different aspects of language and music processing.

Similarities and differences between language and music

Evolutionary perspective

While discussions on the origin of language were banished from the *Société de Linguistique* of Paris in 1866, and although the question of the anthropological foundations of language and music certainly remains difficult, there is renewed interest in evolutionary linguistics and musicology, as can be seen, for instance, from the recent and provocative book edited by Wallin *et al.*,[6] *The Origins of Music*. The question of a common or separate origin of language and music, which was at the centre of hot debates between philosophers and scientists from the seventeenth to the nineteenth century,[7–10] is now being examined using new tools and technologies. In our opinion, one of the most promising avenues is functional brain imaging. By offering an excellent spatial and/or temporal resolution, brain imaging methods allow us to examine the brain regions that are activated by different aspects of information processing and how these processes unfold in time. Even if such methods may not help solve the problem of the common or separate origin of language and music, they provide invaluable information on the question of the similarities and differences between these two systems. Before reviewing some of the relevant brain imaging data, let us quickly consider how ideas on the origin of language and music have evolved throughout the centuries.

'The old masters'   Rousseau[9] was a strong advocate of the view that music and language share some common ancestor and that language evolved out of music for the sake of a rational organization of human societies. Darwin[7] also argued for a common origin, but considered that music evolved out of the primate's reproductive calls and that language was first. Interestingly, most of the authors who addressed this issue in the book edited by Wallin et al.[6] also seem to share the opinion of a common ancestor to language and music. The concept that the first basic function of both language and music was to express emotive meaning through variations in the intonation of the voice (intonational prosody) and rhythm also seems to be an object of consensus.[10–12] In both language and music, emotional excitement is expressed through fast, accelerating, and high-registered sound patterns. In this again they join Rousseau,[9] who considered that the first languages were sung, not spoken; they were aimed at expressing emotions, love, hate, and anger. They were passionate before being rational.

Music and culture   In Western cultures, music has evolved to become more and more isolated from other expressive forms. Moreover, most studies in music cognition are concerned with music perception, and music performance has received much less attention (but see Ref. 13). By contrast, in other cultures, in which magical thought is still alive, the bounds among music, song, dance, poetry, and rite have not been lost.[14,15]

Furthermore, ethnomusicological studies have often emphasized music as a voluntary act: music is the acoustic result of action. Kubik,[16] for instance, pointed out that African music is not just sound; action is an intrinsic part of musical performance. Motor patterns are themselves sources of aesthetic pleasure, independent from the sound that they are associated with. This strong intertwining between music and action is even reflected in language, the same word being used in several African languages to refer to music and dance.

Blacking[14] defined music as 'sound that is organized into socially accepted patterns'. Moreover, he argues that every piece of music has its own inherent logic, as the creation of an individual reared in a particular cultural background. However, his claim that patterns of sound reflect patterns of social organization seems somewhat coarse and in need of further elaboration. Still, in much the same way that a context-sensitive grammar is a more powerful analytical tool than a context-free grammar, the cognitive systems underlying different styles of music shall be better understood if music is considered in context. Different musical styles should therefore be considered not as 'sonic objects' but as humanly organized sound whose patterns are related to the social and cognitive processes of a particular society and culture.

Cognitive perspective

Structural aspects   Many definitions have been (and are still to be) proposed for language and music. The amazing point, however, is that the definition given for music will often apply to language as well, and vice versa. This is striking when we consider the comparison between language and music from both a structural and a functional perspective. Arom,[17] for instance, proposed two structural criteria to define music. One is rhythm and the temporal ratios that delineate a piece of music by the formalized segmentation of time. The other is that all cultures have divided the sound continuum into discrete pitches that form the musical scales. These two criteria may apply to language as well. Language is also composed of sequential events that unfold in time with a specific rhythm and specific segmental (phonemes) and suprasegmental (prosody) information. Moreover, the speech continuum is divided into discrete phonemes, the basic phonological unit. More generally, it is clear that both language and music are conveyed by sounds, are ubiquitous elements in all cultures, are specific to humans, and are cultural artifacts that do not correspond to natural objects.[12] They are rule-based systems composed of basic elements (phonemes, words, notes, and chords) that are combined into higher-order structures (musical phrases and sentences, themes and topics) through the rules of harmony and syntax. Therefore, there may be a musical grammar, and the experimental results to be described indeed point to the similarity of the brain's response to some specific violations of syntax in both language and music.

Functional aspects   From a functional perspective, several similarities also exist between language and music. In this respect, it is interesting to examine the following citation from Pinker[18] in his book, *The Language Instinct*: 'Language is a complex, specialized skill, which develops in the child spontaneously, without effort or formal instruction, is deployed without awareness of its underlying logic, is qualitatively the same in every individual, and is distinct from more general abilities to process information or behave intelligently' (p. 18). Except for some constraints regarding music production, we could substitute 'music' for 'language' and the characteristics would apply as well. Both language and music rely on intentionality: All music implies 'an act of creation that actualizes an intention',[17] and this is true of language as well. In other words, both language and music require a theory of mind.[19] Both develop with specific learning according to more or less standardized procedures depending on the linguistic or musical culture. Even though perception precedes production in both domains, children acquire musical and linguistic rules in a similar, effortless way. Early on, children are able to create new musical and verbal sentences by applying a rule system that they have been able to abstract without conscious intentions. Both language and music involve memory; adults can recognize and reproduce learned melodies, words, poetry, and songs.

Similarities or differences? A question of grain of analysis?   It should be noted, however, that the comparison between language and music might highlight either their similarities or their differences depending on the grain chosen for analysis. Thus, similarities at one level of processing may be interpreted as differences at another level. For example, while temporal structure and rhythmic organization play a fundamental role in both language and music, the metric structure is specific and consistent throughout a given musical piece, but the suprasegmental prosodic structure of language is less specific and more variable. Similarly, the segmentation of the sound continuum into discrete units (pitches or phonemes) is found in all music and languages. However, if we can eventually make an analogy between phonemes and intervals of a musical scale, we must also be aware of their differences. In fact, although the number of pitches by octave (degrees of the scale) is very similar across musical cultures (seven or fewer notes), the number of phonemes largely differs between languages (from 11 in Polynesian to 141 in the language of the Bushmen,[18] with 44 phonemes in English and 36 in French). Furthermore, some of the perceptual properties of the basic elements in music have no equivalent in language, as, for instance, the fact that octaves are perceived as equivalent in almost all cultures. This effect is linked with the finding that two notes separated by an octave are related by a simple frequency ratio of 2 : 1. Generally, the relationships between different pitches in a musical piece are much simpler than the relationships between different phonemes in a linguistic sentence.

As a last example, all languages are organized according to a syntactic structure that may be universal.[20,21] Indeed, verbs and nouns are always present. However, the order in which those elements are presented varies among languages: Subject–Verb–Object (French, English, etc.); Subject–Object–Verb (German, Japanese, etc.); Verb–Object–Subject (Malgache, etc.).[22] Even if it is common to refer to a musical syntax or a musical grammar, the extent to which this analogy extends beyond a simple metaphor remains to be determined. Music perception shares universal laws of auditory perception. For instance, the perception of a musical phrase is automatically influenced by factors such as the grouping of discrete notes into sequences (i.e. the melodic contour) and the feeling of closure that accompanies the playing of a cadence at the end of a phrase. Some of these factors are universally shared and others, just as verbal language, are culturally shared. However, even if there is such a thing as a musical grammar, the rules seem more flexible and ambiguous than the syntactic rules used in language. Ambiguity is a key element of the grammar and aesthetics of music.[23] There are always several ways to perceive and enjoy a musical piece. Finally, musical elements are most often played simultaneously, and each element may have its own 'syntax'. This vertical dimension of musical structure, commonly referred to as harmony, is not present in language. While different words sung at the same time may melt in a sublime combination of rhythm, melody, and harmony (as in the polyphonic madrigals of Monteverdi), different words produced at the same time by different speakers will only create an unpleasant cacophony, like that in a political debate.

Meaning and expectancy   Even if the similarities and differences between language and music depend on the level of details considered for the analysis, one fundamental difference nevertheless remains. Whereas the meaning of words is understood in relation to an extralinguistic designated space, music is considered mostly self-referential.[24-27] This does not mean that music is asymbolic. However, while the meaning of words is defined by an arbitrary convention relating sounds to meaning, notes or chords have no extramusical space in which they would acquire meaning. The internal sense of music may be conceived as something that goes beyond any objective reference structure and the possibilities of verbal language.[28] Much as Wittgenstein[29] who asked: 'Describe the coffee aroma!', music is the kingdom of the ineffable. As stated by Meyer in his wonderful book *Emotion and Meaning in Music*,[25] 'Music means itself. That is, one musical event (be it a tone, a phrase, or a whole section) has meaning because it points to and makes us expect another musical event' (p. 35). Interestingly, this statement not only highlights one of the most important differences between language and music, that is, the unsolved question of musical semantics, but also emphasizes their strongest similarity: in their own way, both systems generate strong expectancies. Just as a specific word is expected within a specific linguistic context, specific notes or chords are expected at a given moment within a musical phrase. Either these expectations are fulfilled, giving rise to resolution or satisfaction, or they are not fulfilled, giving rise to tension or surprise.

We should not believe, however, that expectation may 'bear the entire burden of deriving affect'.[30] Other factors such as tempo, volume, and nonmechanical interpretation of music certainly influence musical emotions. Still, the structure of music has intrinsic points of instability that tend to resolve, and the tension/resolution phenomenon results in affects. Moreover, tensions are perceived at different levels depending on the analysis performed. Jackendoff,[30] in analogy to language, points out that a modular and informational encapsulated parser might be at work independently from conscious memory. This independence from memory may explain why we keep enjoying a piece on repeated hearings 'in spite of the consequences of an intuitive theory of affect based on expectation'. In fact, an autonomous parser will keep analysing and recreating whatever structure is retrieved from memory. Then 'surprise will still occur within the parser'.[30]

If rather than asking ourselves what is the meaning of music, we make a more fruitful reflection on 'what can I do with sounds'? we may discover that music is, first of all, a set of choices. The flow of these choices might possibly become visible as a musical thought. Behind all this, the image of children playing appears. When the child plays with small wood blocks, we could say that the game is a way of answering the question: what can I do with my small wood blocks? Then, from the pleasure of playing we get directly into the aesthetic pleasure.

Concluding this brief and necessarily incomplete excursus, it is important to keep in mind that musical meaning is the sum of analytic approaches (musical parser), individual and/or cultural associations to the external/internal world (during some periods in the last centuries 'music was conceived as conveying precise emotional and conceptual meanings, established by codes, or at least, *repertoires*'[31]), and aesthetic reaction. The importance of the aesthetic component of music becomes evident in considering that 'the form of a work of art gains its aesthetics validity precisely in proportion to the number of different perspectives from which it can be viewed and understood'.[32]

Levels of processing   From a cognitive perspective, language and music cannot be considered as single entities. To be analysed and compared they need to be reduced to their constitutive elements. Within music, one classically differentiates the temporal (metre and rhythm), melodic (contour, pitch, and interval), and harmonic (chords) aspects. Each aspect most likely involves different types of processing, so that the processes called into play to process rhythm may differ from those involved in the processing of pitch and melodic intervals. Similarly, within language, at least four different levels of processing have been taken into consideration. The phonetic-phonological level, which comprises both segmental (phonemes) and suprasegmental (prosody) levels; the morphosyntactic level, which encompasses the combination of phonemes into morphemes and of morphemes into words; the syntactic level, which governs the relations between words; and the lexicosemantic level, with access to the meaning of words and sentences. Finally, while often ignored in psycholinguistic and neurolinguistic experiments, the pragmatic level that comprises discourse organization and contextual influences represents an essential aspect of language organization.

Insofar as we agree with the concept that language and music cannot be considered as wholes but need to be subdivided into their component operations, it becomes unrealistic, for instance, to view the linguistic function as localized in the left hemisphere and music in the right. Rather, some aspects of language processing may preferentially involve left cerebral structures, whereas others require structures on the right. The same remark applies to music as well. With this view in mind, the task of the cognitive neuroscientist is to delineate the different computations performed within one level of processing, to understand the mechanisms that underlie these computations, and to localize where in the brain these mechanisms are implemented. This task is fraught with both philosophical and method-ological problems,[19] but science is advancing rapidly, and new methods are now available to track these issues. In the second part of this presentation, we summarize the results of our research on the comparison between different levels of processing in language and music. Before going into the details of the experiments, we briefly review the position of linguistic theories on the question of the specificity of language processing.

Specificity of the computations involved in language processing?

The generative grammar theory

One of the most important claims of the generative grammar (GG) theory is that language is autonomous from other cognitive functions.[4,18,21,33,34] Language is considered a compu-tational module that entails its own functional and neural architecture.[12] Moreover, the linguistic module comprises different submodules, each responsible for different aspects of language processing, phonology, morphology, syntax, semantics, and pragmatics. Each submodule is encapsulated,[35] so that the processing of information in a module is per-formed independently of the processing of information in another submodule. Phonological processing, for instance, is realized without being influenced by the morpho-logical, syntactic, semantic, or pragmatic aspects of language processing. Thus, the compu-tations required to process language are specific to language, and the computations in one module are performed independently of those in the other modules.

Another basic claim of the GG theory is that languages are defined by their deep syntac-tic structure: syntax plays a dominant role in the structural organization of language. Moreover, from a functional perspective, syntax is first.[36] Logico-mathematic computa-tions are first performed on symbols that have no intrinsic meaning; they only acquire meaning in a second step. Therefore, the chain of computations necessary to process lan-guage is considered to be serially and hierarchically organized.

Other linguistic theories

It should be noted, however, that other linguistic theories have been developed in the last 20–30 years that advocate very different views of language structural and functional organ-ization.[22,37] Although it is beyond the scope of this presentation to go into the details of these different linguistic theories, which differ from each other in many respects (functional grammar,[38,39] cognitive grammar,[40–42] and linguistic functional typology[43–45]), the impor-tant point is that these theories call into question the two basic claims of the GG theory just summarized. First, they reject the idea that language is an autonomous function, relying on its own structural and functional architecture. By contrast, they consider that languages rely on general cognitive principles, linked with perceptual and sensorimotor motor experi-ences.[46,47] Second, they reject the syntacticocentrism of the GG theory and the idea of the autonomy of syntax relative to phonology, morphology, semantics, and pragmatics.[22]

Following Langacker,[41] for instance, semantics, morphology, and syntax form a continuum with specific meaning associated with lexicosemantic units and schematic meaning associated with grammatical units. Thus, in contrast to the GG view that grammatical units are semantically empty, all grammatical elements have meaning. Moreover, linguistic units are not static but constructed through a dynamic process influenced by the context of enunciation[48] and the interactions between individuals in a situation of communication.[49] Therefore, language should be studied not in isolation but in relation to other cognitive functions, specifically, attention and short-term and episodic memory.[45]

Success of generative grammar theory in cognitive neurosciences

Several reasons may explain the success of the GG theory in both linguistic and cognitive sciences, but two are of particular interest. First, the cognitive stakes of the GG theory have been clearly explained. It has therefore been possible to make predictions and design experiments to test these predictions.[21,47] Second, the modular organization of the functional aspects of language processing is clearly neurocompatible. The concept that language is organized in submodules, each responsible for one specific processing stage, finds strong support in the localizationist views of cerebral organization. The recent development of brain imaging methods, together with older data from the neuropsychological literature, largely contributes to the idea that specific functions are implemented in specific brain structures. A brief review of the literature shows that while this concept of the mapping of basic sensory functions into the organization of primary, sensory brain areas is probably correct, the story certainly becomes more complicated when trying to localize such higher-order cognitive abilities as language or music.

Evidence from brain imaging

Brain imaging methods are aimed at understanding the functional activity of the brain either directly through measures of the electrical activity of single neurons (intracellular recordings), or of neuronal populations (electroencephalography, EEG), or through the magnetic activity that is coupled with the electrical activity (magnetoencephalography, MEG), or indirectly through the measures of brain metabolic activity (positon emission tomography, PET, and functional magnetic resonance imaging, fMRI). Overall, direct methods have excellent temporal resolution and relatively poor spatial resolution, whereas the reverse is true for indirect methods. Elegant works have been conducted using these different methods to demonstrate, for instance, the retinotopic organization of the visual cortex using fMRI[50] and the tonotopic organization of the auditory cortex using intracellular recordings (see Chapter 9 this volume), MEG,[51] or fMRI.[52] Hence, there is strict mapping between the organization of the receptor fields at the periphery, in either the retina or the cochlea, and the functional organization of the primary visual and auditory cortex. Aside from extending to humans previous discoveries in animals, these findings validate the use of such complex methods as fMRI to study human perception and cognition.

   To address the specificity of the brain structures involved in language processing, we would need metanalysis of the results obtained across the many experiments aimed at localizing the different aspects of language processing. We would then need to do the same for music or for any other cognitive function of interest and then compare the results of these metanalyses. Although such metanalyses are being performed for some aspects of language processing, such as language production[53] or prelexical and lexical processes in language comprehension,[54] data in the neuroimaging of music are still too scarce for such an enterprise. Moreover, assuming that such metanalyses are performed for music as well, it still remains extremely difficult to compare results of experiments that were not directly designed to compare language and music processing. Indeed, leaving aside the theoretical problem of which level of processing in language is best compared with which level of processing in music, the choice of the task to be performed on the stimuli, its difficulty, as well as experimental factors, such as the mode (blocked vs mixed) and rate of stimulus presentation, stimulus repetition, and data analysis (e.g. subtraction method, correlative analyses), have been shown to exert a predominant influence on the results obtained. With these remarks in mind, it is nevertheless interesting to mention some of the results found for language and music to determine the extent to which the brain structures that are activated are similar or different.

Few experiments have been designed to directly compare language and music using brain imaging methods. Binder et al.[55] compared tones and word processing in an fMRI study. Results showed that several brain structures, including the left superior temporal sulcus, middle temporal gyrus, angular gyrus, and lateral frontal lobe, showed stronger activation for words than tones. However, both types of stimuli activated the Heschl gyrus and the superior temporal plane, including the planum temporale. The investigators concluded that whereas the planum temporale is similarly involved in the auditory processing of words and tones, other broadly distributed areas are specifically involved in word processing. Gandour et al.[56] conducted a PET study in which both Thai and English participants were required to discriminate pitch patterns and Thai lexical tones derived from accurately filtered Thai words. Results of the tone minus pitch subtraction indicated that only native Thai speakers showed activation of the left frontal operculum (BA 44/45). This finding was taken as evidence that Thai lexical tones are meaningful for native Thai speakers but not for English speakers. However, for our purposes, it is also interesting that for both Thai and English speakers, several structures, including the left anterior cingulated gyrus (BA 32), the left and right superior temporal gyrus (BA 22), and the right cerebellum, were activated in both pitch and tone tasks.

More generally, results have shown that primary auditory regions (BA 41 and BA 42) respond in similar ways to speech and music.[57] Secondary auditory regions (BA 22) are activated by hearing and understanding words[58] as well as by listening to scales,[59] auditory imagery for sounds,[60] and access to melodic representations.[61] The supramarginal gyrus (BA 40) seems involved in understanding the symbolism of language[58] and the reading of musical scores.[59] Broca's area is known to be involved in motor activity related to language and was also shown to be active when playing music[59] and when musicians were engaged in a rhythmic task.[61] The supplementary motor areas (BA 6) and the right cerebellum are also active when playing and imaging playing music.[59,62] Although this list is far from exhaustive, it nevertheless suffices to show that some of the most important language areas are clearly involved in music processing as well. Some brain structures also seem to be specifically or preferentially involved in language processing,[63] and the converse is true for

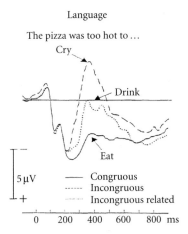

Figure 18.1 ERPs elicited by final sentence words at the central recording site (Cz) for congruous and incongruous words and for incongruous words that are semantically related to the best sentence completion. The amplitude of the negative component, peaking at 400 ms postfinal word onset (N400) is largest for incongruous words, intermediate for incongruous words related to the best sentence completion, and smallest for congruous words. In this and subsequent figures, amplitude (μV) is represented on the ordinate, with negative voltage up, and time (ms) on the abscissa. (Adapted from Ref. 66.)

music.[64] Results of metanalysis of the type just mentioned should clearly help in drawing maps of the structure–function relationships known for language and music.

Semantics, melody, and harmony

A starting point in the study of the neurophysiological basis of language processing was the discovery of the N400 component by Kutas and Hillyard.[65] This negative component of the event-related brain potentials (ERPs), peaking around 400 ms after word onset, is elicited by words that are semantically unexpected, incongruous, and within a linguistic context (e.g. 'The pizza was too hot to cry'; Figure 18.1). Further results have shown that N400 amplitude is modulated by semantic priming, so that an unexpected word related to the best sentence completion (e.g. 'drink' when the expected word is 'eat'; Figure 18.1) elicits a smaller N400 than a completely unexpected word (e.g. 'cry'[66]). These results, together with those issued from a large number of experiments, have led to the consensus that the N400 is a good index of the integration process of a word within its linguistic context.

The first experiments that we designed were aimed at finding out whether an N400 component would also be elicited when melodically and harmonically unexpected notes were presented within a melodic context.[67–69] We presented both familiar and unfamiliar monodic musical phrases to musicians and nonmusicians. The familiar melodies were chosen from the classical repertoire of Western occidental music from the eighteenth and nineteenth centuries, and the unfamiliar musical phrases were composed by a musician following the rules of tonal harmony (Figure 18.2). These melodies were ended by the congruous or most expected note, by a note out of the tonality of the musical phrase (non diatonic incongruities perceived as wrong notes), or by a note within the tonality but not

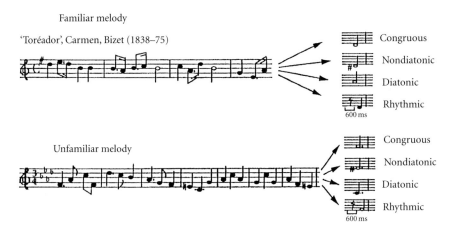

Figure 18.2 Examples of the stimuli used in the experiment. (Adapted from Ref. 69.)

the most expected ending (melodic or diatonic incongruities). Thus, we created a degree of musical incongruity from diatonic to nondiatonic.

Results clearly showed that both types of unexpected notes elicited the occurrence of late positive components, peaking around 600 ms (P600). As demonstrated for the N400 component, P600 amplitude was shown to depend on the degree of musical incongruity: it was larger for the most unexpected, nondiatonic wrong notes than for the less unexpected, diatonic incongruities. Moreover, the amplitude of the P600 was larger for familiar than for unfamiliar musical phrases and for musicians than for nonmusicians (Figure 18.3). These findings clearly demonstrate not only that specific notes are expected within a musical phrase, but also that such expectations depend on the familiarity of the musical excerpts and the expertise of the listener. Thus, an interesting similarity between language and music, just mentioned, their ability to generate strong expectancies, is supported by empirical evidence. However, our results also show that the processes that govern semantic expectancy and that are reflected by a negative component, peaking around 400 ms, the N400, are qualitatively different from those involved in musical expectancies and reflected by a positive component peaking around P600 ms, the P600. While, to our knowledge, the functional significance of positive vs negative polarities in the ERPs is not clearly established, our results, by demonstrating qualitative differences between language and music processing, nevertheless strongly argue for the specificity of the processes involved in computing the semantic aspects of language. Thus, one of the most important differences between language and music, outlined in the introduction, the fact that, in contrast to language, music has no intrinsic meaning and is a self-referential system, seems to find some support in these experimental findings.

Semantics and harmony in opera

Opera is perhaps the most complete art form, as it calls upon music, language, drama, and choreography. It originated in Italy at the end of the sixteenth century with *Dafne*, set to

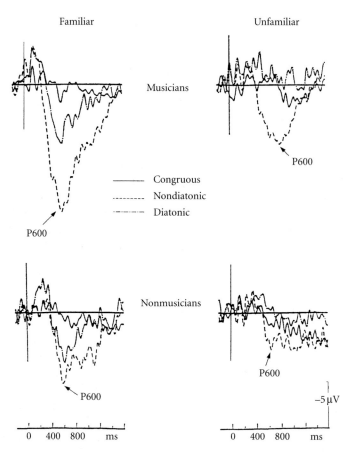

Figure 18.3 ERP results for musicians and nonmusicians are presented separately for familiar and unfamiliar musical phrases. The vertical lines mark the onset of the final note. Results are from one typical recording site, the parietal location (Pz). The amplitude of the positive component, P600, is larger for nondiatonic than for diatonic incongruity, for musicians than for nonmusicians and for familiar than for unfamiliar musical phrases. (Adapted from Ref. 69.)

music in 1594 by the Florentine composers Corsi and Peri. The first opera to survive intact is probably *Euridice*, set to music by Peri and Caccini and performed in 1600 as a wedding gift to Maria de Medici and Henri IV. Opera, as a new art form, then spread to other Italian courts with the better-known *Orfeo* of Monteverdi in 1604. Since that time, a question that has interested both music analysts and composers has been to determine which of the words or the music plays the most important role in opera. In his *Life of Rossini*, Stendhal (1783–1842) argued that music is most important: 'its function is to animate the words'. Later, ethnomusicologists, such as Levman,[70] pointed out that the lyrics are subordinate to the music in tribal songs and rituals. By contrast, Richard Wagner (1813–83) considered that both aspects are intrinsically linked: 'Words give rise to the music and music develops and reinforces the language', an opinion shared by Pierre Boulez:[71] 'The text is the centre and the absence of the musical piece'. Richard Strauss (1864–1949) even composed an opera, *Capriccio* (1940), to illustrate the complementarity of words and music.

To determine, based on scientific grounds, if the words or the music is most important when we listen to opera, we selected 200 excerpts from French operas of the nineteenth and twentieth centuries.[72] Each excerpt lasted between 8 and 20 s and was sung *a capella* by a female singer under each of four experimental conditions, that is, the final word of the excerpt was (1) semantically congruous and sung in tune, (2) semantically incongruous and sung in tune, (3) semantically congruous and sung out of tune, and (4) both semantically incongruous and sung out of tune (Figure 18.4).

Based on previous results,[65] it was of interest to determine whether semantically incongruous words will also elicit an N400 component when they are sung. Similarly, it was of interest to determine whether congruous words sung out of tune will also elicit a P600 component.[69] Of most interest was the double incongruity condition: will semantically incongruous words sung out of key elicit both an N400 and a P600 component? If language plays the most important role when we listen to opera, then results may show an N400 but not a P600. Conversely, if music is the cornerstone of opera, then results may show a P600 without an N400. Maybe both effects will be elicited, however; they may then be additive (i.e. equal to the sum of the effect associated with each type of incongruity alone) or interactive. To answer these questions, we recorded the ERPs associated with the final words of each excerpt, from 16 professional musicians from the opera company in Marseille.

To summarize, results demonstrated that sung incongruous words did elicit an N400 component, thus extending to songs results previously reported for written and spoken language[65,73] (Figure 18.5A). Moreover, words sung out of tune did elicit a P600 component, thus extending to songs results previously reported for out-of-tune notes[69,74–76] (Figure 18.5B). Most interesting are the results in the double incongruity condition. They show that incongruous words sung out of tune elicit both an N400 and a P600 component (Figure 18.5C). Interestingly, the N400 occurred earlier than the P600, which is taken as evidence that the words were processed faster than the music. Finally, effects in the double incongruity condition were not significantly different from the sum of the effects observed in each condition of simple incongruity (see Figure 18.6). This finding provides a strong argument in favour of the independence (i.e. the additivity) of the computations involved in processing the semantic aspects of language and the harmonic aspects of music. Therefore, when we listen to opera, we process both the lyrics and the tunes in an independent fashion, and language seems to be processed before music.

Influence of attention   We tracked these results further by conducting another series of experiments aimed at studying the effect of attention, again testing some professional musicians from the opera company in Marseille.[76] We hypothesized that if lyrics and tunes are processed independently, listeners should be able to focus their attention only on the lyrics or only on the tunes, depending on the instructions. Without going into the details of the results, an N400 component was elicited to sung incongruous words, and a P600 was associated with congruous words sung out of tune, thus replicating our previous findings.[72] Most interestingly, the N400 to incongruous words completely vanished when participants focused their attention on the music (Figure 18.7). Thus, musicians were able not to process the meaning of words; they did not notice whether the terminal word made sense

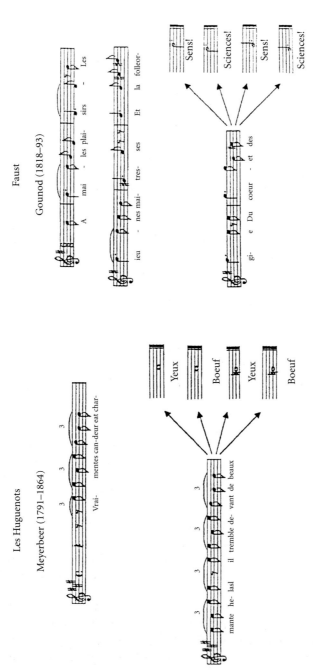

Figure 18.4 Example of the opera's excerpts used in the experiment. Approximate translation of the excerpts, from *Les Huguenots* (Meyerbeer): 'Really, his naïvity is charming. However, he trembles in front of beautiful eyes', and from *Faust* (Gounod): 'For me, the pleasures and young mistresses, the crazy orgy of the heart and the senses'. Note that in French, the final incongruous words 'boeufs' and 'sciences' rhyme with the expected completions 'yeux' and 'sens'. The final note of the excerpt is in or out of tune. (Adapted from Ref. 72.)

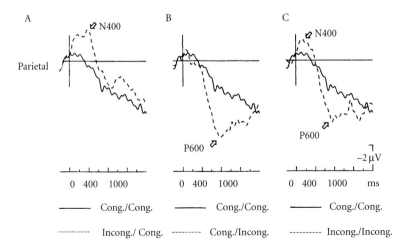

Figure 18.5 ERPs results averaged across 16 professional musicians and recorded from the parietal electrode (Pz). Terminal congruous words sung in key (Cong./Cong.) are compared to (A) semantically incongruous words sung in tune (Incong./Cong.), (B) semantically congruous words sung out of tune (Cong./Incong.), and (C) semantically incongruous words sung out of tune (Incong./Incong.). The *vertical lines* mark the onset of the final word of the excerpts. A large N400 component develops in the 50–600 ms that follow the presentation of semantically incongruous words (A). In marked contrast, a P600 develops in the 400–1200 ms that follow the presentation of words sung out of tune (B). Most importantly, both an N400 and a P600 develop in response to the double incongruity (C). (Adapted from Ref. 72.)

within the linguistic context when they only listened to the music. Conversely, P600 amplitude was significantly reduced when musicians focused attention on language, so that they did not hear that the final word was sung out of tune. Taken together these results again provide strong arguments in favour of the independence of lyrics and tunes. There is some limit to such processing independence, however. Results in the double incongruity condition showed that the presence of one type of incongruity influenced the processing of the other type. When words were both semantically incongruous and sung out of tune, musicians could not help but hear the musical incongruity, even if they were asked to focus their attention on language.

Syntax and harmony

The rules of harmony and counterpoint are often described as the grammar of tonal music. As syntax is used to extract the fundamental structure of an utterance by assigning different functions to different words, the rules of harmony allow us to specify the different elements, notes and chords, that fulfill a specific harmonic function. Results of experiments manipulating the harmonic function of target chords have shown that violations of harmonic expectancies are associated with P600 components.[76,77] Interestingly, research on syntax using ERPs has also shown that different types of syntactic violations, such as violations of gender, word order or noun-verb agreement, elicit a positive component, peaking around 600 ms.[78–80] Moreover, both components show a similar parietal

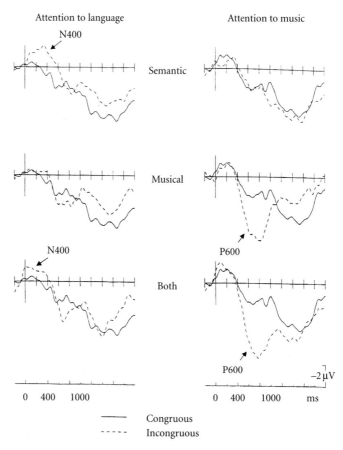

Figure 18.6 Overlapped are the ERPs to congruent and incongruent endings, recorded at the central recording site (Cz), when participants paid attention only to the language (*left column*) or only to the music (*right column*) of the opera's excerpts. A large N400 effect is generated when participants focus their attention on language. This effect completely vanishes when attention is focused on music (*top row*). Similarly, the P600 effect is much greater when participants paid attention to music than when they paid attention to language (*medium row*). Finally, when words are both semantically incongruous and sung out of tune, the N400 effect is greater when participants paid attention to the language, and the P600 effect is greater when they paid attention to the music (*bottom row*). (From Regnault and Besson, in preparation.)

distribution over the scalp, which, together with their similar polarity and latency, seems to indicate that they reflect qualitatively similar processes.

To further test this hypothesis, Patel and collaborators[81] conducted an experiment directly aimed at comparing the P600 components elicited by harmonic and syntactic violations. ERPs associated with a word within a grammatically simple, complex, or incorrect sentence were compared to those associated with the presentation of a chord that belonged to the tonality induced by the chord sequence, a nearby, or a distant tonality. Results showed that aside from early morphologic differences in the ERPs to words and chords, due to the differences in the acoustic characteristics of these two types of auditory signals, the effects associated with the

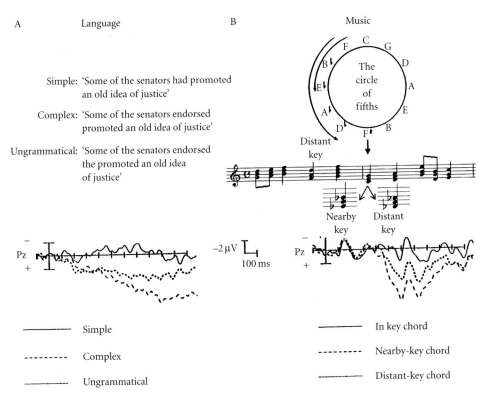

Figure 18.7 (A) Examples of the sentences presented in the auditory language experiment. Results showed increased positivity from simple to ungrammatical sentences. (B) Representation of the circle of fifths. Examples of the stimuli used in the experiment. The target chord, shown by the downward-pointing *vertical arrow*, is the congruous chord. The two *arrows* below the musical notation point to moderately incongruous (nearby key) and highly incongruous (distant key) target chords. Results also showed increased positivity from the in-key chords to the distant-key chords. (Adapted from Patel Ref. 81.)

violation of syntactic and harmonic expectancies were not significantly different (Figure 18.8). Therefore, these results raise the interesting possibility that a general cognitive process is called into play when participants are asked to process the structural aspects of an organized sequence of sounds, be it language or music. Finally, an early right anterior negativity was found at around 300–400 ms in response to a chord belonging to a distant tonality. These results paralleled those obtained in language experiments showing that an early left anterior negativity is also associated with some syntactic violations.[82] Whereas these two negative components showed a different distribution over the scalp, with a left predominance for language and a right predominance for music, they may reflect functionally similar processes.

Temporal structure

Spoken language, as music, is composed of acoustic events that unfold in time. Because of the temporal structure inherent in both language and music, specific events are expected at specific times. The main question addressed in the next series of experiments was to

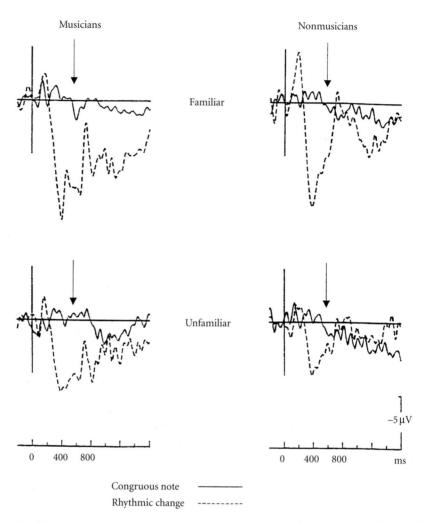

Figure 18.8 Overlapped are the ERPs to congruous notes and to the rhythmic incongruities ending familiar and unfamiliar musical phrases for musicians and nonmusicians. Recordings are from the parietal electrode (Pz). Large emitted potentials are elicited when the final note should have been presented (*vertical bar*) but was delayed by 600 ms. The *arrow* points to the moment in time when the final note was presented. (Adapted from Ref. 69.)

determine whether the processes involved in analysing temporal structures rely on general cognitive mechanisms or differ as a function of the specific characteristics of the materials to be processed. We used both the ERP and the MEG methods to analyse the time course of the effects of temporal structure violations in language and music, and fMRI to localize the cerebral structures activated by these violations. We hypothesized that if a general mechanism is responsible for processing the temporal structures in language and music, qualitatively similar effects should be revealed in the ERP and MEG recordings, and similar brain areas should be shown to be activated by temporal violations. By contrast, if processing temporal information in both systems relies on different mechanisms, qualitatively different effects and different brain areas should be found in language and music.

In previous experiments,[69] we introduced an unexpected silence between the penultimate note and the last note of a musical phrase (Figure 18.2). Results showed that a large biphasic, negative then positive, potential, the emitted potential,[83] was elicited when the final note should have been presented but was not, because it was delayed by 600 ms. The amplitude of this effect was similar in musicians and nonmusicians, but it was larger for familiar than unfamiliar melodies (Figure 18.9). These findings clearly indicate that both musicians and nonmusicians could anticipate the precise moment when the final note was to be presented and were surprised when it was not. Moreover, known melodies allowed participants to generate more precise expectancies than did unfamiliar melodies. Therefore, these results indicate that the occurrence of an emitted potential is a good index of temporal expectancy.

It was then of interest to determine whether similar results would be found for spoken language.[84] To this aim, we presented both familiar (e.g. proverbs) and unfamiliar auditory sentences to participants. In half of the sentences, final words occurred at their normal position, while in the other half, they were delayed by 600 ms. Results showed that an emitted potential, similar to the one described for temporal ruptures in music, developed when the final word should have been presented (Figure 18.9). Therefore, these ERP results indicate that qualitatively similar processes seem to be responsible for temporal processing in language and music.

To strengthen this interpretation, it was important to determine whether the same brain structures are activated by the processing of temporal ruptures in language and music. As already mentioned, fMRI allows localization of brain activation with excellent spatial resolution. Moreover, the MEG permits localization of the generators of the effects observed on the scalp more precisely than the ERP method, while offering an excellent temporal resolution. Therefore, in collaboration with Heinze and his research team, we conducted three experiments in which we presented both auditory sentences and musical phrases.[85] These experiments used a blocked design in which only sentences or musical phrases without temporal ruptures were presented within a block of trials, and only sentences or musical phrases with temporal ruptures at unpredictable positions were presented within another block of trials. The ERP method was used in the first experiment to replicate, within subjects, the results found previously with two different groups of subjects,[69,84] and the fMRI and the MEG methods were used, respectively, in the other two experiments, trying to localize the effects of interest.

Overall, the ERP results replicated, within subjects, those previously found in music and language separately (i.e. an emitted potential). However, comparison of the conditions with and without temporal violations revealed a different pattern of activation using the MEG and fMRI methods. Source localization based on MEG data revealed that the underlying generators of the biphasic potential recorded on the scalp were most likely located in the primary auditory cortex of both hemispheres. By contrast, fMRI results showed activation of the associative auditory cortex in both hemispheres as well as some parietal activation. Several factors may account for these differences,[85] but the main point is that similar brain areas were activated by temporal violations in both language and music. Therefore,

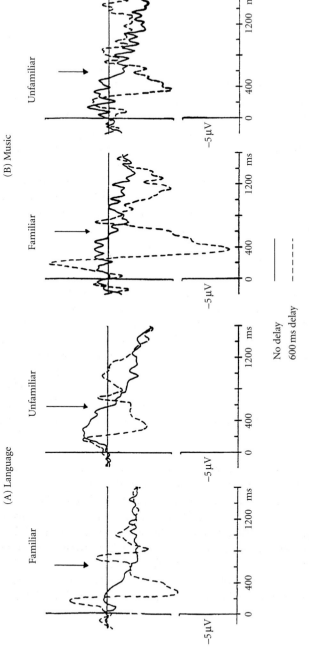

Figure 18.9 Comparison of the effects of temporal violations in (A) language and (B) music. Recordings are from the parietal electrode (Pz). (A) Overlapped are the ERPs to congruous words and to the temporal disruptions ending familiar and unfamiliar sentences. In both language and music, large emitted potentials are elicited when the final event should have been presented (*vertical bar*) but was delayed by 600 ms. Note that the amplitude of the emitted potential is greater in music than in language, but that, in both cases, its amplitude is greater for familiar than for unfamiliar materials. (Adapted from Ref. 84 (A) and Ref. 69. (B).)

taken together our results suggest that processing temporal information in both language and music relies on general cognitive mechanisms.

Conclusion

We have addressed one of the central questions of human cognition, the specificity of language processing. Is language an autonomous system, independent from other human cognitive abilities or does language rely on general cognitive principles? To address this question, we have conducted several experiments aimed at comparing some aspects of language processing with some aspects of music processing. We mainly used the ERPs method, which offers excellent temporal resolution and therefore permits study of the time course of information processing and determination of whether the processes involved in language and music are qualitatively similar or different.

Taken together, results have shown that the semantic computations required to access the meaning of words, and their integration within a linguistic context, seem to be specific to language. Indeed, whereas unexpected words within a sentence context are associated with the occurrence of an N400 component, unexpected notes or chords within musical phrases elicit a P600 component. By contrast, words that are unexpected on the basis of the syntactic structure of the sentence, and chords that are unexpected as a function of the harmonic structure of the musical sequence, elicit similar effects in both cases, namely, a P600 component. Early negative effects, that is, left and right anterior negativity, which developed between 200 and 300 ms, have also been reported in experiments manipulating syntax and harmony, respectively. Although their different scalp distributions seem to reflect involvement of different brain structures, more research is needed to further track their functional significance. Finally, violations of temporal structure within language and music also elicit similar effects, a biphasic negative–positive complex, the emitted potential. The occurrence of the emitted potential shows that in both language and music, words and notes or chords are expected at specific moments in time. Therefore, when we listen to language and music, not only do we expect words or chords with specific meaning and function, but we also expect them to be presented on time!

The question of the specificity of language processing has broad implications in our understanding of the human cognitive architecture and, even more generally, for the fundamental problem of the relationship between structures (different brain regions) and functions (e.g. language, music). Although the research reported here sheds some light on certain aspects of language processing and highlights some similarities and differences with music processing, more research is clearly needed in this fascinating research domain. Of utmost interest is the use of brain imaging methods that offer complementary information about the spatiotemporal dynamics of brain activity in order to pinpoint the networks of cerebral structures that are involved in two of the most human cognitive abilities: language and music.

References

1. Rangacharya, A. (1966) *Introduction to Bharata's Natya-Sastra*. Bombay, India: Popular Prakashan.

2. Nadel, S. (1930) The Origin of Music. *Musical Q* 16, 531–46.

3. Leroi-Gourhan, A. (1988) *Le geste et la parole. I: La mémoire et les rythmes. Sci. d'aujourd'hui*. Paris: Albin-Michel.

4. Chomsky, N. (1957) *Syntactic Structures*. The Hague, the Netherlands: Mouton and Co.

5. Bickerton, D. (2000) Can biomusicology learn from language evolution studies? In N. L. Wallin, B. Merker and S. Brown (eds) *The Origins of Music*. Cambridge, MA: MIT Press, pp. 153–64.

6. Wallin, N. L., B. Merker, and S. Brown (eds) (2000) *The Origins of Music*. Cambridge, MA: MIT Press.

7. Darwin, C. (1871) *The Descent of Man, and Selection in Relation to Sex*. London: Murray.

8. Descartes, R. (1618/1987) *Abrégé de musique. Compendium musicae. Épiméthée*. Paris: P.U.F.

9. Rousseau, J. J. (1781/1993) *Essai sur l'origine des langues*. Paris, France: Flammarion.

10. Spencer, H. (1857) The origin and function of music. *Fraser's Mag.* 56, 396–408.

11. Brown, S. (2000) The 'musilanguage' model of music evolution. In N. L. Wallin, B. Merker, and S. Brown (eds) *The Origins of Music*. Cambridge, MA: MIT Press, pp. 271–300.

12. Molino, J. (2000) Toward an evolutionary theory of music and language. In N. L. Wallin, B. Merker, and S. Brown (eds) *The Origins of Music*. Cambridge, MA: MIT Press, pp. 165–76.

13. Sloboda, J. A. (2000) Individual differences in music performance. *Trends Cognit. Sci.* 4, 397–403.

14. Blacking, J. (1973) *How Musical is Man?* Seattle: University of Washington Press.

15. Schön, A. and D. Schön (1999) Il potere del suono e della musica. *Fuga a più voci. Psiche* 1–2, 159–65.

16. Kubik, G. (1969) Composition techniques in Kiganda xylophone music. *Afr. Music J.* 4, 22–72.

17. Arom, S. (2000) Prolegomena to a biomusicology. In N. L. Wallin, B. Merker, and S. Brown (eds) *The Origins of Music*. Cambridge, MA: MIT Press, pp. 27–30.

18. Pinker, S. (1994) *The Language Instinct: How the Mind Creates Language*. New York: Harper Perennial.

19. Pacherie, E. (1999) Philosophie et sciences cognitives. In J. F. Mattéi (ed.) *Encyclopédie Philosophique Universelle*. Paris: PUF.

20. Chomsky, N. (1988) *Language and Problems of Knowledge: The Managua Lectures*. Cambridge, MA: MIT Press.

21. Chomsky, N. (1991) Linguistics and cognitive science: problems and mysteries. In A. Kasher (ed.) *The Chomskyan Turn*. Cambridge, MA: Basil Blackwell, pp. 26–53.

22. François, J. (1998) Grammaire fonctionnelle et dynamique des langues—de nouveaux modèles d'inspiration cognitive et biologique. *Verbum* XX, 233–56.

23. Aiello, R. (1994) Music and language: parallels and contrasts. In R. Aiello and J. Sloboda (eds) *Musical Percep*. New York, NY: Oxford University Press, pp. 40–63.

24. Jakobson, R. (1973) Essais de linguistique générale. II. Rapports internes et externes du langage. Editions de Minuit, Arguments. Paris.

25. Meyer, L. (1956) *Emotion and Meaning in Music*. Chicago, IL: University of Chicago Press.

26. Kivy, P. (1991) *Music Alone. Philosophical Reflection on the Purely Musical Experience*. New York: Cornell Paperbacks.

27. **Boucourechliev, A.** (1993) *Le langage musical. Collections les chemins de la musique.* Paris: Fayard.

28. **Piana, G.** (1991) *Filosofia della Musica.* Milan: Guerini e associati.

29. **Wittgenstein, L.** (1953) *Philosophical Investigations.* In G. E. M. Anscombe and R. Rhees (eds). Oxford: Blackwell, pp. 209.

30. **Jackendoff, R.** (1991) Musical parsing and musical affect. *Music Percept.* 9, 199–230.

31. **Eco, U.** (1979) *Trattato di Semiotica Generale.* Milano: Bompiani.

32. **Eco, U.** (1962) *Opera Aperta.* Milan: Bompiani.

33. **Jackendoff, R.** (1997) *The Architecture of the Lang. Faculty.* Cambridge, MA: MIT Press.

34. **Pollock, J. Y.** (1997) *Langge et cognition. Introduction au programme minimaliste de la grammaire générative.* Paris: PUF.

35. **Fodor, J.** (1983) *Modularity of Mind.* Cambridge, MA: MIT Press.

36. **Frazier, L.** (1987) Sentence processing: a tutorial review. In M. Coltheart (ed.) *Attention and Performance. XII.* Hillsdale, NJ: Erlbaum, pp. 559–86.

37. **Victorri, B.** (1999) Le sens grammatical. *Languages* 136, 85–105.

38. **Dik, S.** (1997) *The Theory of Functional Grammar.* Berlin: Mouton De Gruyter.

39. **Van Valin, R. D.** and **R. J. LaPolla** (1997) *Syntax Structure, Meaning and Function.* Cambridge: Cambridge University Press.

40. **Lakoff, G.** (1987) *Women, Fire and Dangerous Things.* Chicago, IL: University of Chicago Press.

41. **Langacker, R. W.** (1987) *Foundations of Cognitive Grammar. Vol. I: Theoretical Prerequisites.* Stanford, CA: Stanford University Press.

42. **Talmy, L.** (1988) The relation of grammar to cognition. In B. Rudzka-Ostyn (ed.) *Topics in Cognitive Linguistics.* Amsterdam: Benjamins.

43. **Croft, W.** (1995) Autonomy and functionalist linguistics. *Lang.* 71, 490–532.

44. **Greenberg, J.** (1995) The diachronic typological approach to language. In M. Shibatani and T. Bynon (eds) *Approaches to Language Typology.* Oxford: Clarenton, pp. 145–66.

45. **Givón, T.** (1995) *Functionalism and Grammar.* Amsterdam: Benjamins.

46. **Fuchs, C.** (1997) Diversité des représentations linguistiques: Quels enjeux pour la cognition? In C. Fuchs and S. Robert (eds) *Diversité des langues et représentations cognitives.* Paris: Ophrys, pp. 5–24.

47. **Robert, S.** (1997) Variation des représentations linguistiques: des unités à l'énoncé. In C. Fuchs and S. Robert (eds) *Diversité des langues et représentations cognitives.* Paris: Ophrys, pp. 25–39.

48. **Culioli, A.** (1999) *Pour une linguistique de l'énonciation.* Paris: Ophrys.

49. **Fauconnier, G.** (1997) *Mappings in Thought and Language.* Cambridge, MA: Cambridge University press.

50. **Tootell, R. B. H., N. K. Hadjkhani, J. D. Mandola,** *et al.* (1998) From retinotopy to recognition: fMRI in human visual cortex. *Trends Cognit. Sci.* 2, 174–83.

51. **Pantev, C., M. Hoke, B. Luetkenhoener,** *et al.* (1989) Tonotopic organization of the auditory cortex: pitch versus frequency representation. *Sci.* 246, 486–8.

52. **Strainer, J. C., J. L. Ulmer, F. Z. Yetkin,** *et al.* (1997) Functional magnetic resonance imaging of the primary auditory cortex: analysis of pure tone activation and tone discrimination. *Am. J. Neuroradiol.* 18, 601–10.

53. **Indefrey, P.** and **W. J. M Levelt** (2000) The neural correlates of language production. In M. S. Gazzaniga (ed.) *The New Cognitive Neurosci.* Cambridge, MA: MIT Press, pp. 845–65.

54. Norris, D. and R. Wise (2000) The study of prelexical and lexical processes in comprehension: psycholinguistics and functional neuroimaging. In M. S. Gazzaniga (ed.) *The New Cognit. Neurosci.* Cambridge, MA: MIT Press, pp. 867–80.

55. Binder, J. R, J. A. Frost, T. A. Hammeke, *et al.* (1996) Function of the left planum temporale in auditory and linguistic processing. *Brain* 119, 1239–47.

56. Gandour, J., D. Wong and G. Hutchins (1998). Pitch processing in the human brain is influenced by language experience. *Neuroreport* 9, 2215–119.

57. Zatorre, R. A., C. Evans, E. Meyer, *et al.* (1992) Lateralization of phonetic pitch discrimination in speech processing. *Sci.* 256, 846–9.

58. Falk, D. (2000) Hominid brain evolution and the origin of music. In N. L. Wallin, B. Merker, and S. Brown (eds) *The Origins of Music.* Cambridge, MA: MIT Press, pp. 197–216.

59. Sergent, J., E. Zuck, S. Terriah, *et al.* (1992) Distributed neural network underlying musical sight-reading and keyboard performance. *Sci.* 257, 106–9.

60. Zatorre, R. J., A. Halpern, D. W. Perry, *et al.* (1996) Hearing in the mind's ear: a PET investigation of musical imagery and perception. *J. Cognit. Neurosci.* 8, 29–46.

61. Platel, H., C. Price, J. C. Wise, *et al.* (1997) The structural components of music perception. *Brain* 120, 229–43.

62. Chen, W., T. Kato, X. H. Zhu, *et al.* (1996) Functionnal mapping of human brain during music imagery processing. *NeuroImage* 3, S205.

63. Grabowski, T. J. and A. R. Damasio (2000) Investigating language with functional neuroimaging. In A. W. Toga and J. C. Mazziotta (eds) *Brain Mapping: The Systems.* London: Academic Press, pp. 425–58.

64. Zatorre, J. and J. R. Binder (2000) Functional and structural imaging of the human auditory system. In A. W. Toga and J. C. Mazziotta (eds) *Brain Mapping: The Systems.* London: Academic Press, pp. 365–402.

65. Kutas, M. and S. A. Hillyard (1980) Reading sens.ess sentences: brain potentials reflect semantic incongruity. *Science* 207, 203–05.

66. Kutas, M. and S. A. Hillyard (1984) Event-related brain potentials (ERPs) elicited by novel stimuli during sentence processing. *Ann. N.Y. Acad. Sci.* 425, 236–41.

67. Besson, M. and F. Macar (1987) An event-related potential analysis of incongruity in music and other non-linguistic contexts. *Psychophysiol.* 24, 14–25.

68. Besson, M., F. Faïta, and J. Requin (1994) Brain waves associated with musical incongruity differ for musicians and non-musicians. *Neurosci. Lett.* 168, 101–5.

69. Besson, M. and F. Faïta (1995) An event-related potential (ERP) study of musical expectancy: comparison of musicians with non-musicians. *J. Exp. Psychol. Human Percept. Perform.* 21, 1278–96.

70. Levman, B. G. (1992) The genesis of music and language. *Ethnomusicology* 36, 147–70.

71. Boulez, P. (1966) Relevés d'apprenti. Editions du Seuil. Paris.

72. Besson, M., F. Faita, I. Peretz, *et al.* (1998) Singing in the brain: independence of lyrics and tunes. *Psychol. Sci.* 9, 494–8.

73. MacCallum, W. C., S. F. Farmer, and P. V. Pocock (1984) The effects of physical and semantic incongruities on auditory event-related potentials. *Electroencephal. Clin. Neurophysiol.* 59, 477–88.

74. Paller, K. A., G. McCarthy, and C. C. Wood (1992) Event-related potentials elicited by deviant endings to melodies. *Psychophysiology* 29, 202–6.

75. Verleger, R. (1990) P3-evoking wrong notes: unexpected, awaited or arousing? *Int. J. Neurosci.* 55, 171–9.

76. Regnault, P., E. Bigand, and M. Besson (2001) Different brain mechanisms mediate sensitivity to sensory consonance and harmonic context: evidence from auditory event related brain potentials. *J. Cognit. Neurosci.* 13, 1–17.

77. Janata, P. (1995) ERP measures assay the degree of expectancy violation of harmonic contexts in music. *J. Cognit. Neurosci.* 7, 153–64.

78. Hagoort, P., C. Brown, and J. Groothusen (1993) The syntactic positive shift as an ERP-measure of syntactic processing. *Lang. Cognit. Processes* 8, 439–83.

79. Osterhout, L. and P. J. Holcomb (1992) Event-related brain potentials elicited by syntactic anomaly. *J. Mem. Lang.* 31, 785–804.

80. Friederici, A. D. (1998) The neurobiology of language comprehension. In A. D. Friederici (ed.) *Lang. Comprehension: A Biological Approach.* New York: Springer, pp. 263–301.

81. Patel, A. D., E. Gibson, and J. Ratner (1998) Processing syntactic relations in language and music: an event-related potential study. *J. Cognit. Neurosci.* 10, 717–33.

82. Friederici, A. D., E. Pfeifer, and A. Hahne (1993) Event-related brain potentials during natural speech processing: effects of semantic, morphological and syntactic violations: *Cognit. Brain Res.* 1, 182–92.

83. Soutton, S., M. Braren, J. Zubin, and E. R. John (1967) Evoked potential correlates of stimulus uncertainty. *Sci.* 150, 1187–8.

84. Besson, M., F. Faïta, C. Czternasty, and M. Kutas (1997) What's in a pause: event-related potential analysis of temporal disruptions in written and spoken sentences. *Biol. Psychol.* 46, 3–23.

85. Weyert, II., M. Besson, C. Templemann, *et al.* (2001) An analysis of temporal structure in language and music using ERPs, MEG and fMRI techniques. In preparation.

CHAPTER 19

MUSICAL SOUND PROCESSING: EEG AND MEG EVIDENCE

MARI TERVANIEMI

Abstract

Even during the performance of a simultaneous task unrelated to the sounds, the human auditory cortex is able to model precisely the invariances of the acoustic environment. Data acquired in mismatch negativity (MMN) paradigm have shown that temporally and spectrally complex sounds as well as their relations are automatically represented in the human auditory cortex. Furthermore, the MMN data indicate that these neural sound representations are spatially distinct between phonetic and musical sounds within and between the cerebral hemispheres. Majority of the MMN studies were conducted in pitch dimension but also temporal aspects of sound processing are under increasing experimentation. Up to some extent, also musical expertise is reflected in sound representation accuracy as indexed by the MMN.

Introduction

Sound perception and cognition can be conceptualized as a process, in which the first stages are the least and the latest stages the most dependent on the attentional efforts of the listener.[1–3] For a long time, due to micro- and macro-level complexity of the acoustic signal, music sound encoding was assumed to require attentional effort of the listener. In the present review, some of these assumptions will be challenged.

In the majority of the studies to be reviewed below, the mismatch negativity (MMN) paradigm was utilized.[2] The MMN is evoked by an infrequently presented sound ('deviant') differing from the frequently occurring stimuli ('standard') in one or several parameters. Its presence implies that the invariant parameters of the standard sound were neurally encoded, thus producing a neural mismatch with those of the deviant sound. In other words, the MMN is an index for the neural traces of short-term auditory memory.

The MMN can be recorded even when the subject is performing a task unrelated to the stimulation under interest such as reading a book or playing a computer game. Thus it offers a direct measure for the similarity of neural sound representations, without being contaminated by differences, for instance, in attentional or motivational involvement of the subject during an experimental session or between the subject groups.

Yet, several data indicated that the MMN parameters closely correlate to the indicators of the subjects' perceptual accuracy as determined in a separate behavioural session. For instance, the MMN amplitude and latency reflect perceptual accuracy, as determined by tests of musical aptitude (for a review, see Ref. 4) and by hit rates and reaction times.[5–8] In addition, the degree of perceptual similarity between different musical instrument timbres highly correlates with the MMN amplitude.[9] This correlation between the MMN parameters and behavioural responses imply that preattentive neural functions determine the accuracy of the subsequent attentive processes.[2,3,10]

Since the MMN is elicited without attention, it received particular interest during past years among clinicians who need to evaluate the integrity of neurocognitive functions in patients unable or unwilling to participate in a neuropsychological (behavioural) testing. For instance, it was found that the MMN elicitation predicts the recovery of consciousness in comatose patients[11,12]) (for reviews, see Refs 13, 14). In addition, the deficits in MMN elicitation might help target perceptual training or rehabilitation in milder perceptual disorders. For instance, recently it was revealed that automatic discriminative functions of dyslexic adults are worse than those of control subjects.[15–18] In addition, the MMN is also correlated with the improvement of the reading performance in dyslexic children.[19]

Since differences in subjects' attention or motivation might confound studies in music psychology especially in between-group comparisons, the MMN recordings offer a promising means in determining the accuracy of neural sound representations prior to involvement of the perceptual and cognitive functions also in music studies. In the following, an overview on studies using musical sounds and sound successions to investigate the automatic neural sound processing will be given. In addition, recent studies comparing musicians and nonmusicians will be reviewed.

MMN generators for speech vs musical sounds

MMN is generated mainly in the primary auditory cortex or in its immediate vicinity. This has been indicated by several brain research methods such as magnetoencephalography (MEG),[20,21] intracranial electrode recordings,[22,23] positron emission tomography (PET),[24] and functional magnetic resonance imaging (fMRI).[25–27] In addition, this is reflected in electric recordings by polarity reversal above the Sylvian fissure from the fronto-central negative maximum to positivity in mastoids leads (when the nose reference is used) (for a review, see Ref. 28).

In late 1990s, a whole-head MEG experiment was conducted to determine whether the auditory cortex has spatially distinct areas for encoding musical vs phonetic sounds.[29] The subjects, while watching a silent movie with subtitles, were presented with frequent and infrequent phonemes (/e/ vs /o/) or chords (A major vs A minor). These phonetic and musical stimuli were matched in complexity as well as in the magnitude of the frequency change embedded in them. It was found that the source of the MMNm elicited by the deviant phoneme or chord was located posteriorly to the source of an earlier P1m component (see footnote a). In addition, the MMNm source for a phoneme change was located superiorly to that of the chord change. On the contrary, P1m sources did not differ between

---

[a] Early exogenous ERP components and their MEG equivalents are mainly determined by the physical sound characteristics, for instance, the intensity and rise time, while endogenous ERP/MEG components with longer onset latencies are modulated by cognitive and attentional factors.[2]

phonemes and chords. These data thus suggest that there are distinct cortical areas specialized in representing phonetic and musical sounds in both hemispheres. In other words, the functional specialization does not only cover stimulus complexity (as shown by Alho *et al.* comparing MMNm generator loci between single tones and chords)[30] but also the informational content (phonetic vs musical).[29] However, this specialization is not present prior to memory-related auditory processing as suggested by the dissociation between the present P1m and MMNm data.

Additionally, the data reviewed above indicated that in the right hemisphere, the MMNm was larger in amplitude for changes among chords than among phonemes. However, in the left hemisphere, no corresponding dominance for phoneme changes was found when compared with chord changes. This result was obviously discrepant with the previous results.[31,32] To solve this discrepancy, a further study was conducted with PET technique (see footnote b).

This PET study[24] used the phonetic and musical sounds developed for the MEG study described above.[29] However, the phoneme duration was prolonged from originally used 200 ms until 400 ms, since in pilot studies, presence of deviant phonemes elicited no changes in brain metabolism with phonemes of 200 ms duration. The subjects were concentrating on classifying the gender of visually presented words while they were presented with sound sequences consisting of (1) both deviant and standard sounds or (2) standard sounds only (phonemes and chords in separate sequences). The data, obtained after subtracting the activity elicited by the standard sounds only from that elicited by both deviant and standard sounds when intermixed, showed that the change from vowel /e/ to /o/ was processed in the left auditory cortex, more specifically, in the middle and supratemporal gyri. In a mirror-like manner, the change from A major to A minor chord was processed in the right auditory cortex, in the supratemporal gyrus. These data thus indicate that hemispheric specialization for phonetic vs musical processing, previously seen in dichotic-listening studies and brain-imaging studies using an active task, may be present even during the performance of a task unrelated to the sound stimulation. However, this phenomenon is very vulnerable to changes in stimulus parameters as indexed by the importance of an adequate sound duration[24,29] (see also Refs 36–38 for recent evidence about the effects of acoustic noise on lateralization of phonetic processing).

Sound complexity and perceptual accuracy

All natural speech and instrumental sounds consist of several parallel harmonic partials, which, despite their wide frequency range, produce a percept of one single sound. The presence of harmonic partials is known to facilitate pitch naming in the possessors of absolute pitch (for a review on absolute pitch, see Ref. 39) as well as the tuning of music instruments.[40] Only recently it was systematically investigated whether harmonic partials facilitate pitch discrimination in ignore and attend conditions in nonmusicians.

---

[b] Localizing the active neural population with MEG (and EEG) necessarily involves inverse modelling of the active neural source. Accuracy of this operation depends from the adequacy of the head model available.[33] This source of uncertainty can be avoided by using brain-imaging techniques such as PET and fMRI. Those methods detect directly the locus of activation change in brain metabolism, presumably caused by increased neural activity.[34,35]

In the first study, the subjects were presented with pitch changes of 2.5, 5, and 10 per cent at 500 Hz sounds, first, during reading a book and, second, during a target-detection task.[41] It was found that they detected more accurately the sounds which consisted of three lowest partials than pure sinusoidal tones. Correspondingly, the frequency-MMN amplitude was larger and latency shorter in spectrally rich tones than in pure tones. This result suggests that pitch discrimination, under attentional control as well as prior to that, is facilitated by the presence of the harmonic partials.

Subsequently it was determined whether adding harmonic partials or prolonging the sound would further facilitate pitch discrimination.[42] To this aim, the frequency-MMN was recorded to a 2.5 per cent pitch change in pure tones with only one sinusoidal frequency component (500 Hz) and in spectrally rich tones with three (500...1500 Hz) and five (500...2500 Hz harmonic partials. Stimuli were 100 and 250 ms in duration (in separate blocks). During these recordings, subjects concentrated on watching a silent movie. The data show that the MMN amplitude was enhanced with spectrally rich sounds when compared with pure tones, with no difference between spectrally rich tones having three or five partials. Moreover, the prolonged sound duration did not significantly enhance the MMN. This suggests, first of all, that relatively few harmonic partials (at least when they

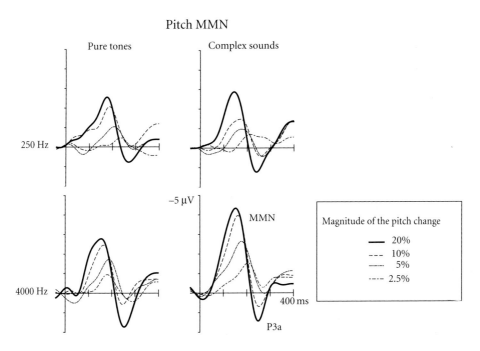

Figure 19.1 The MMN elicited by 2.5, 5, 10, and 20 per cent pitch changes in pure sinusoidal tones (left) and in spectrally rich sounds (right) at 250 Hz (top) and 4000 Hz (bottom). The lines denote difference waves in which the event-related potential elicited by the standard tone has been subtracted from the deviant-tone ERP. The MMN was consistently larger when the pitch change was presented among spectrally rich sounds. Its amplitude also systematically reflected the magnitude of the pitch change. Adapted from Ref. 43.

fall inside the dominance region of pitch perception) are sufficient to sharpen the neural representations underlying pitch discrimination. Second, prolonging sound duration does not further facilitate pitch discrimination with spectrally rich sounds, at least when duration of 100 ms is exceeded.

Most recently, the neural and behavioural accuracy of frequency discrimination across different frequency ranges (250–4000 Hz) with pure sinusoidal vs spectrally rich sounds was compared.[43] Also magnitude of the frequency change (2.5, 5, 10, 20 per cent) was varied in both MMN and behavioural paradigms. The data showed that, in general, the spectrally rich sounds elicited larger MMN across the whole frequency range. Additionally, the changes at the middle frequencies elicited larger MMN, which, in parallel, had a shorter latency than at the lowest and highest frequencies. Replicating earlier findings, the MMN amplitude and latency reflected the magnitude of the frequency change.[5] These neural indices were mirrored in behavioural performance as well, the hit rate being the most accurate and the reaction time fastest at the middle frequency range, with the widest deviants, and with harmonically rich sounds. To summarize, the facilitation in pitch discrimination caused by the spectrally rich sound structure exceeds relatively broad frequency range.

Sequential stimulation

Behavioural evidence shows that, in addition to spectral complexity, also temporal proximity of adjacent sounds may facilitate pitch encoding in its several forms. For instance Dewar et al.[44] presented subjects with standard tonal or atonal sequences followed by two comparison tones in the no-context condition or by two comparison sequences in the full-context condition. The listeners recognized the target tone more accurately under the full-context condition than under the no-context condition. In addition, they performed more accurately when the target tone was embedded in tonal rather than atonal sequences and musicians outperformed nonmusicians in all recognition tasks. This and related findings inspired us to investigate if the presence of Western, familiar sound context facilitates pitch processing even at the preattentive level and, further, whether it might be enhanced by musical expertise.[45]

To this end, 10 musicians and 10 nonmusicians were presented with a 144-Hz frequency change in three contexts. First, the frequency change was among single sounds (554 vs 698 Hz). Second, it was embedded among sound sequences in which the subsequent sounds belonged to the Western musical scale (440–493–**554**–587–659 vs 440–493–**698**–587–659 Hz). Third, the change was presented within sound sequences, which were composed of arithmetically determined intervals, compromising between Western semitones and whole-tone steps (446–467–**499**–547–622 vs 446–467–**643**–547–622 Hz). During the recordings, the subjects were (once again) reading a book of their own choice.

The MMN data indicate that, first of all, MMN amplitude was larger when the frequency change occurred among temporally complex sound sequence with the familiar scale than when it occurred among the unfamiliar scale and, further, larger in unfamiliar scale than among single tones (see Figure 19.2). This suggests that musical context facilitates pitch discrimination most effectively when it is familiar to the subjects. Second, with both familiar and unfamiliar complex sound sequences, the musicians had a generalized facilitation of the MMN in terms of a shorter MMN latency when compared to that by nonmusicians.

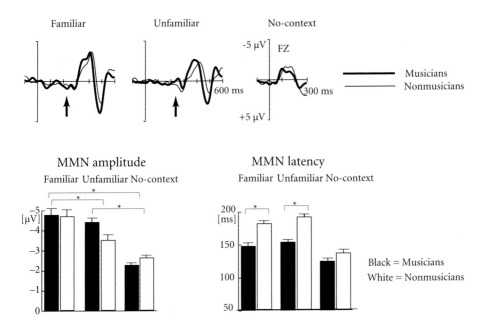

Figure 19.2 Upper panel: The MMN elicited by a pitch change within familiar (tonal) pattern (left), Unfamiliar (atonal) pattern (middle) and in pure sinusoidal tones (right) in musicians (thick line) and nonmusicians (thin line) at Fz electrode. The arrows denote the onset of the pitch change in deviant patterns. The lines denote difference waves in which the event-related potential elicited by the standard tone has been subtracted from the deviant-tone ERP. Bottom panel: the MMN mean amplitude (left) and latency (right) these conditions in musicians (black) and nonmusicians (white) (s.e.m. at the top of each bar). The values were averaged across 10 fronto-central electrodes.

In both subject groups, the MMN amplitude was larger in familiar than in unfamiliar condition and, further, smallest in no-context condition. In addition, in musicians, the MMN latency was shorter in musicians than in nonmusicians. Adapted from Ref. 45.

This suggests that the musicians can adopt the unfamiliar sound environment more readily than nonmusicians.

Abstractions and expectations

Despite the emphasis given in above-described ERP studies on sound processing accuracy at the sensory level in audition, music perception and cognition cannot be reduced merely to a successful sensory-level processes. For instance, despite transpositions and modulations within a musical piece, the 'core' of the melody can be easily remembered and recognized, in other words, abstract sound and melody features are implicitly extrapolated from the continuously changing acoustic input. Consequently, it was questioned whether abstract sound relations and primitive concepts such as 'ascending' or 'descending' interval, pitch continuum, or chord cadences could also be neurally encoded during a performance of a parallel task.

Abstractions

The first studies investigated the interval perception using tone pairs with a whole-tone frequency change within a tone pair.[46,47] To determine whether the direction of a sound change within a pair is encoded by the auditory cortex irrespectively of the absolute sound frequency, the pitch of the standard tone pairs was randomly varied between five different frequency levels (AB, CD, BC, ... , EF, DE, AB, ...).[47] Deviant pairs had either reversed frequency change (BA, ... , FE) or a frequency repetition (AA, BB, ... , EE), also at five different frequency levels. It was found that despite this complexity in stimulation and the parallel reading task given to the subjects, the deviant sound pairs elicited MMN, indicating that the change in the direction of the interval was discriminated in the auditory cortex. This line of research has been continued by Paavilainen and his colleagues.[48] They found that in addition to the direction of the tone interval, also the interval size is automatically encoded in the auditory cortex. This was evidenced by the MMN elicitation by smaller or larger intervals among minor seventh standard intervals (all intervals were randomly presented at 10 frequency levels). Furthermore, the cortical interval representation may also be formed on the basis of converging information from both ears as indicated by the MMN elicitation when the two successive sounds of an interval are delivered to separate ears.[49]

In sum, the present results show that the human auditory cortex can automatically encode highly complex and abstract auditory information (see Ref. 50 for a review).

Expectations

In the two studies to be summarized below, the regularity of the sound change itself created a rule about the sound continuum, in other words, an expectation for the next sound of the sequence either in terms of pitch or sound location. An MMN elicitation by abrupt changes in such sound continuums would strengthen the above-documented conclusions about the 'intelligence' of automatically formed neural sound representations in extracting invariant rules from the continuously varying sound information.

Tervaniemi *et al.* presented reading subjects with regularly spaced sound sequences consisting of regular pitch decrease of one semitone as the standard event.[51] In two conditions, the sounds were Shepard sounds and in two conditions they were pure sinusoidal tones. Randomly, a pitch repetition or an ascending pitch interrupted this line of regularly descending pitch. The MMN was elicited by ascending sounds, be them Shepard or sinusoidal sounds, and by pitch repetition when they were Shepard sounds. These data suggested the existence of primitive expectation formation even without conscious attention being directed to the sounds.

To confirm and expand the previous data obtained by using sound sequences based on regular pitch change, the follow-up experiment was conducted in which the regularity was created by virtual sound movement.[52] To create a subjective feeling of sound movement, sounds were presented via nine loudspeakers extending in a horizontal symmetrical arc in front of the subject. Short noise bursts were presented about three times a second, continuously moving back and forth between the two extreme loudspeakers. Occasionally the regular virtual sound movement was broken by the sound skipping two loudspeakers, which is experienced as a jump in the movement. ERPs recorded from reading subjects showed that 'jumps' elicited a large centrally negative response resembling the MMN. This suggests that expectation about the source location of the next sound was automatically formed (for related data about automatic sound source discrimination, see Refs 53–55).

Chord cadences

How syntactic rules of major-minor tonal music are represented in the brain has been addressed by a chord-cadence paradigm.[56] Cadences of five chords (first four chords 600 ms, fifth chord 1200 ms in duration) were continuously presented at several randomly varying frequency levels. The majority of the chords were presented with synthesized piano timbre, the task of the subject being to detect the chords presented with a different timbre (e.g. celesta, marimba). The study was conducted to reveal whether chords violating musical regularities would elicit differential ERPs compared to 'music-syntactically' appropriate chords, although the subject's attention was directed away from these regularity-violating chords.

The ERPs, recorded from subjects without any formal training in music, were found to differ at two latencies between harmonically appropriate chords and Neapolitan chords violating the context established by the previous chords. The first difference was labelled as the early right anterior negativity (ERAN) according to its relatively early peak latency at around 200 ms, right preponderant distribution, and negative polarity (its linguistic counterpart being termed as the left anterior negativity, ELAN[57]). (See also Ref. 58 for previous related data in music neurocognition.) The second difference was called the N5 (negative polarity and peak latency at around 500 ms; without hemispheric dominance in distribution). The authors concluded that musically untrained subjects may have several neural mechanisms activated for extrapolating the tonal harmony and musical regularities of musical sequences, and, further, that this may occur despite the direction of their conscious attention. In fact, the second argument was confirmed in a subsequent experiment. There, the subjects were reading a book during the stimulation (Reading condition) or listening to the cadences and indicating the presence of a Neapolitan chord (Attend condition).[59] The ERAN did not differ between these two conditions. MEG evidence suggests that the ERAN is generated in the inferior fronto-lateral cortex (in the left hemisphere known as Broca's area), suggesting the involvement of the language areas in music-syntactic processing.[60]

Taken together, the auditory system appears to be able to encode automatically regularity of the sound environment. For this regularity extraction, acoustic repetitiveness of the sound material is not necessary; instead, also more abstract sound relations (direction of the sound change, interval size, chord progression) are encoded.

Musical expertise

Pitch encoding

Musical expertise is reflected in early auditory ERPs even 100 ms after the sound onset, at least when the attention of the subject is not directed away from the sounds.[61] Likewise, it is reflected in the cognitive late-latency ERPs such as P3 and LPC when the subjects are required to attend to the sound stimulation.[62–64] Recently it was also investigated whether musical expertise may be reflected in the auditory ERPs during a performance of a parallel task in another modality. The first set of these studies addressed the accuracy of the violin players' and, more generally, the musicians' auditory system to process slight pitch changes. In the first study, 3-part major chords with a perfect major were used as the standard stimulus.[65] The deviant stimulus was the same chord as the standard stimulus, except that the middle tone of the chord was marginally mistuned (<1 per cent), leading the chord towards a minor chord. This stimulation was presented to subjects while they were reading a book (the first and third blocks of the experiment; reading condition) and while they were asked to detect the deviant chords (the second block; discrimination condition). In the reading condition, the deviants elicited the MMN only in musicians. In the discrimination condition, nonmusicians detected about 10 per cent and musicians about 80 per cent of the deviant chords. In this condition, the parallel ERP recordings showed a significant MMN followed by N2b and P3b deflections in musicians. This N2b–P3 complex reflects higher cognitive processes concerned with the conscious detection and evaluation of deviants. Nonmusicians had a small (but statistically significant) MMN without a subsequently elicited N2b or P3. The third block was presented to see whether the intermediate attentive task facilitated subjects' automatic pitch processing. This, however, was not the case. Musicians showed a MMN that did not differ from that elicited in the first block while nonmusicians showed no MMN. These results suggest that professional violin players automatically are able to detect tiny pitch changes in auditory information, which were undetectable for nonmusicians and, further, that these automatic functions could not be modified by attentional manipulations. Interestingly, the MMN evoked by a small (<1 per cent) or large (10 per cent) pitch change in pure sinusoidal tones did not differentiate violinists and nonmusicians. This suggests that the superior pitch processing accuracy of the violinists was activated only when the pitch change was presented among musical sounds.

In the subsequent experiment the superiority of musicians in automatic and attentive pitch discrimination, originally observed in violin players,[65] was further investigated.[66] Thirteen professional musicians (guitarists, pianists, and wind instrument players) and 13 nonmusicians were presented with harmonically rich sounds of 300 ms in duration. Standard sounds were of 528 Hz in fundamental frequency while deviant sounds were 0.7, 2, or 4 per cent higher. It was found that in the discrimination condition, the musicians detected the pitch changes faster and more accurately than the nonmusicians. This was reflected also in their P3b component, which was significantly larger in musicians than in nonmusicians. However, the event-related brain responses recorded during the reading condition showed a different data pattern—the MMN or P3a amplitude or latency did not differ between the musicians and nonmusicians.

To summarize, the data reviewed above on pitch discrimination in violin players suggest that musical expertise is reflected at preattentive cortical auditory processing especially when the sound structure is musically relevant and when the stimulus change is of musically relevant magnitude. However, in musicians with other instrumental training, despite their superiority in pitch discrimination during attentional listening, preattentive neural mechanisms were not enhanced when compared with those of nonmusicians. This implies that automated neural functions in pitch discrimination are most sensitive in musicians who most consistently need such ability. In other musicians, such a sensitivity to pitch changes exists but is activated only during attentive listening. Whether we here evidence an effect of differential training on brain plasticity or a result of appropriately chosen musical instrument, remains unresolved on the basis of the present evidence. However, recent evidence obtained by using both structural and functional methods of cognitive neuroscience promotes the importance of training in reorganizing the brain functions.[61,67,68]

Temporal encoding

Very recently, also temporal domain of sound processing has attracted attention in musician–nonmusician comparisons in MMN paradigm. This is valuable especially if the temporal accuracy of the event-related potentials is taken into account—it allows one to track the processing of very minute changes also in temporally complex sound sequences.

The first study investigated the accuracy of musicians vs nonmusicians to preattentively encode regularity in relatively fast sound presentation rate and to react to infrequent sound omissions in that sound stream.[69] In separate conditions, the sinusoidal sounds of 50 ms were delivered every 100, 120, 180, and 220 ms to the subjects who concentrated on a reading task. 15 musicians and 15 subjects without any formal training in music were employed. Sound omissions occurred with the probability of 3 per cent. It was found that while the sound omissions evoked the MMN in musicians in all conditions, in nonmusicians the MMN was present only with two shortest stimulation rates. This suggests that musicians have a prolonged window of sound integration.[70] Furthermore, the results of the second experiment of these authors suggest that the temporal processing of musicians within this window is also more accurate than in nonmusicians. In that study, musicians and nonmusicians were presented with tone pairs. In the standard pair, the sound onsets were separated by 150 ms whereas in the deviant pairs, they were separated by 100 or 120 ms. It was found that the MMN was elicited in musicians by both deviant pairs but in nonmusicians only by 100 ms pair.

The second set of related experiments investigated the accuracy and efficacy of musicians vs nonmusicians to preattentively encode sound sequences up to 1.5 s and to detect violations in the regularities established by the sequences.[71] In the first of these experiments, the sound sequences were either 750 ms or 1.5 s in duration (in separate conditions). Four tones, ascending in pitch, were presented in a looped manner. The deviant sequence consisted of five tones, thus being one tone longer than the standard sequence. The MMN elicitation implied that musicians were able to encode the length and frequency content of such a subsequence with both sequence durations. In contrast, in nonmusicians, no MMN was elicited. In the second experiment, the standard sound sequences were also either 750 ms or 1.5 s in duration but were made very simple in their pitch structure: they consisted of four repetitions of the same pitch. After four tones, the pitch of all of them was changed. Also here, the deviant sequences were one tone longer. It was found that the MMN was elicited by the tone sequence lengthening in both subject groups with 750 ms sequences and in musicians also with 1.5 s sequences. These data suggest that grouping of sequential sounds can take place on a preattentive processing level irrespective of musical skill with moderate sequence durations, but that professional musicians have more advanced preattentive ability to group sequential sounds than nonmusicians when sequences are lengthy. In other words, in its simple forms, auditory grouping does not differ between subjects with different levels of expertise. However, with more complicated

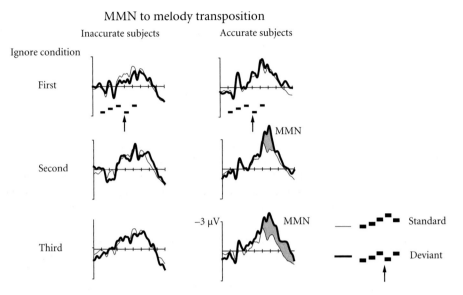

Figure 19.3 Event-related potentials elicited by the standard (90 per cent; thin line) and the deviant (10 per cent; thick line) melodic patterns. In the accurate subjects, an MMN was elicited during the second and third Ignore conditions following the first attend condition (right column). In the inaccurate subjects, no MMN was observed at any phase of the experiment despite intermediate attend conditions (left column). Adapted from Ref. 72.

pitch information or longer sound sequences, the musicians have more advanced encoding ability even during a performance of a parallel task.

Recently it was also studied whether musicians and nonmusicians may encode melodic transpositions without attentional effort.[72] The subjects were presented with short melodic patterns of 0.5 s at 12 different frequency levels within one octave. In alternating order, the experimental session consisted of three Ignore conditions (during which the subjects watched a silent video with subtitles) and three Attentive conditions (during which they detected a target with a different melody contour). The data indicated that especially musicians who perform music mainly without a score easily learn to detect contour changes in the pitch transposed melodic patterns (see Figure 19.3). However, even those musicians had no MMN during the first Ignore condition, in other words, also they needed some conscious, explicit effort to learn to extract the melodic contour from the constantly varying sound material. After learning, their auditory cortex detected violations from the standard melodic contour even when their attention was directed away from the sounds. Interestingly, all non-musicians and the 'score-dependent musicians' were not assisted by the presence of the active task.

Conclusions

The data reviewed above was acquired by electromagnetic and hemodynamic recordings on healthy adult subjects. In majority of those studies, an experimental paradigm was employed in which the subject performed a parallel task outside the auditory modality during the stimulation and brain recordings. Thus, these findings offer fundamental insight to the brains's ability to encode and differentiate acoustically complex sounds despite the focus of the listener's attention.

The results indicated, first, that the cortical networks are able to automatically encode temporally and spectrally complex musical sounds as well as their abstract relations. Moreover, it was shown that pitch changes among spectrally complex sounds and temporally complex sound patterns are more readily discriminated than equivalent pitch changes among pure single sinusoidal sounds. These findings might rephrase our views on the ability of the human brain to represent the continuously changing sound environment beyond the 'listener's' attentional focus. In other words, although music and music sounds are acoustically and cognitively demanding entities, majority of relevant sound information is neurally encoded even if we are not consciously aware of it.

Second, the loci of the cortical sound representations were found to differ between musical and phonetic sounds both within and between the cerebral hemispheres. This suggests that the auditory cortex is able to represent not only the acoustical but also the informational sound content. Further, the data reviewed above imply that the tonality processing as probed by neurocognition of chord cadences involves also the brain regions primarily devoted to language, that is, the Broca's area. These two lines of research may first seem to be in conflict. However, the level of auditory material and thus the level of processing is not comparable. While isolated sounds represent one fragment of an auditory scene, a chord cadence is actually already an auditory scene of its own. In future, it will hopefully be possible to further illuminate the degree and timing of the neurocognitive modularity of music and language processing.

Third, in several experimental paradigms, musical expertise was reflected in automatically elicited brain responses to violations in pitch and temporal sound features as a response enhancement and/or latency decrease. It was also indicated that musical expertise does not guarantee facilitated neuronal processing of music sounds or sound sequences. Based on the above reviewed findings (see also Ref. 73), it might be argued that the commonly used differentiation between 'musicians' when contrasted with 'nonmusicians' does not necessarily provide a researcher with an accurate enough categorization. Preferably, we should identify and subdivide musicians more accurately on the basis of their major instruments (e.g. whether just or fixed tuning is used); the importance of pitch vs timing cues in the genre and instrument, and their relationship to musical score. Also the quantity and quality of the musical activities the 'nonmusical' subjects have, for instance, in terms of dance, sports, or music listening, should be taken into account. Hopefully, by optimizing the contrasts between the subject groups in their relationship to music in its broadest meaning, the purest forms of neurocognitive expertise in musicians could be more readily unveiled.

To summarize, during past decade, plenitude of electromagnetic evidence together with increasing number of hemodynamic data underlined the importance of the automatically activated neural networks in the auditory cortex also in musically relevant forms of cognition. In future, our task is to further illuminate the degree of modularity in audition for music vs speech sounds and also the role of automatically activated sound representations in musical expertise.

Acknowledgements

The author thanks the Academy of Finland, University of Helsinki, and the Marie Curie Fellowship of the European Commission. Special thanks to Elvira Brattico, M.A., for her comments on an earlier version of the manuscript.

References

1. Shiffrin, R. M. and W. Schneider (1977) Controlled and automatic human information processing: II. Perceptual learning, automatic attending and a general theory. *Psychol. Rev.* 84, 127–90.

2. Näätänen, R. (1992) *Attention and Brain Function.* Hillsdale: Lawrence Erlbaum Associates.

3. Näätänen, R. and I. Winkler (1999) The concept of auditory stimulus representation in cognitive neuroscience. *Psychol. Bull.* 125, 826–59.

4. Tervaniemi, M. (1999) Pre-attentive processing of musical information in the human brain. *J. New Music Res.* 28, 237–45.

5. Tiitinen, H., P. May, K. Reinikainen, *et al.* (1994) Attentive novelty detection in humans is governed by pre-attentive sensory memory. *Nature* 372, 90–2.

6. Kraus, N., T. McGee, T. D. Carrell, *et al.* (1996) Auditory neurophysiologic responses and discrimination deficits in children with learning problems. *Science* 273, 971–3.

7. Tremblay, K., N. Kraus, and T. McGee (1998) The time course of auditory perceptual learning: neurophysiological changes during speech-sound training. *Neuroreport* 9, 3557–60

8. Amenedo, E. and C. Escera. (2000) The accuracy of sound duration representation in the human brain determines the accuracy of behavioural perception. *Euro. J. Neurosci.* 12, 2570–4.

9. Toiviainen, P., M. Tervaniemi, J. Louhivuori, *et al.* (1998) Timbre similarity: convergence of neural, behavioral, and computational approaches. *Music Percept.* 16, 223–41.

10. Novak, G. P., W. Ritter, H.G. Vaughan Jr, *et al.* (1990) Differentiation of negative event-related potentials in an auditory discrimination task. *Electroencephal. Clin. Neurophysiol.* 75, 255–75.

11. Kane, N. M., S. H. Curry, C.A Rowlands, *et al.* (1996) Event-related potentials—neurophysiological tools for predicting emergence and early outcome from traumatic coma. *Intensive Care Med.* 22, 39–46.

12. Fischer, C., D. Morlet, P. Bouchet, *et al.* (1999) Mismatch negativity and late auditory evoked potentials in comatose patients. *Clin. Neurophysiol.* 110, 1601–10.

13. Gene-Cos, N., H. A. Ring, R. C. Pottinger, *et al.* (1999) Possible roles for mismatch negativity in neuropsychiatry. *Neuropsychiatry, Neuropsychol. Behav. Neurol.* 12, 17–27.

14. Näätänen, R. and M. Hoke (eds) (2000) Special issue on mismatch negativity and its clinical applications. *Audiol. Neuro-Otol.* 5, 101–246.

15. Schulte-Korne, G., W. Deimel, J. Bartling, *et al.* (1998) Auditory processing and dyslexia: evidence for a specific speech processing deficit. *Neuroreport* 9, 337–40.

16. Schulte-Korne G., W. Deimel, J. Bartling, *et al.* (1999) Pre-attentive processing of auditory patterns in dyslexic human subjects. *Neurosci. Lett.* 276, 41–4.

17. Baldeweg, T., A. Richardson, S. Watkins, *et al.* (1999) Impaired auditory frequency discrimination in dyslexia detected with mismatch evoked potentials. *Ann. Neurol.* 45, 495–503.

18. Kujala, T., K. Myllyviita, M. Tervaniemi, *et al.* (2000) Basic auditory dysfunction in dyslexia as pinpointed by brain-activity measurements. *Psychophysiology* 37, 262–6.

19. Kujala, T., K. Karma, R. Ceponiene, *et al.* (2001) Plastic neural changes and reading improvement caused by audio–visual training in reading-impaired children. *PNAS* 98, 10509–14.

20. Sussman, E., I. Winkler, and M. Huotilainen (2002) Top–down effects on stimulus-driven auditory organization. *Cogn. Brain Res.* 13, 393–405.

21. Tiitinen, H., K. Alho, M. Huotilainen, *et al.* (1993) Tonotopic auditory cortex and the magnetoencephalographic (MEG) equivalent of the mismatch negativity. *Psychophysiology* 30, 537–40.

22. Kropotov, J. D., R. Näätänen, A.V. Sevostianov, *et al.* (1995). Mismatch negativity to auditory stimulus change recorded directly from the human temporal cortex. *Psychophysiology* 32, 418–22.

23. Halgren, E., K. Marinkovic, and P. Chauvel (1997) Generators of the late cognitive potentials in auditory and visual oddball tasks. *Electroencephal Clin. Neurophysiol.* 106, 156–64.

24. Tervaniemi, M., S. V. Medvedev, K. Alho, *et al.* (2000) Lateralized automatic auditory processing of phonetic versus musical information: a PET study. *Hum. Brain Map.* 10, 74–9.

25. Opitz, B., A. Mecklinger, D. Y. von Cramon, *et al.* (1999) Combining electrophysiological and hemodynamic measures of the auditory oddball. *Psychophysiology* 36, 142–7.

26. Opitz, B., A. Mecklinger, A. D. Friederici, *et al.* (1999) The functional neuroanatomy of novelty processing: integrating ERP and fMRI results. *Cerebr. Cortex* 9, 379–91.

27. Opitz, B., T. Rinne, A. Mecklinger, *et al.* (2002) Differential contribution of frontal and temporal cortices to auditory change detection: fMRI and ERP results. *Neuroimage* 15, 167–74.

28. Alho, K. (1995) Cerebral generators of mismatch negativity (MMN) and its magnetic counterpart (MMNm) elicited by sound changes. *Ear Hear* 16, 3–50.

29. Tervaniemi, M., A. Kujala, K. Alho, *et al.* (1999) Functional specialization of the human auditory cortex in processing phonetic and musical sounds: a magnetoencephalographic study. *Neuroimage* 9, 330–6.

30. Alho, K., M. Tervaniemi, M. Huotilainen, *et al.* (1996) Processing of complex sounds in the human auditory cortex as revealed by magnetic brain responses. *Psychophysiology* 33, 369–75.

31. Näätänen, R., A. Lehtokoski, M. Lennes, *et al.* (1997) Language-specific phoneme representations revealed by the electric and magnetic brain responses. *Nature* 385, 432–4.

32. Rinne, T., K. Alho, P. Alku *et al.* (1999) Hemispheric asymmetry of cortical activation as reflected by the mismatch negativity reveals when a sound is processed as speech. *Neuroreport* 10, 1113–17.

33. Hämäläinen, M., R. Hari, R. J. Ilmoniemi, *et al.* (1993) Magnetoencephalography—theory, instrumentation, and applications to noninvasive studies of the working human brain. *Rev. Mod. Phys.* 65, 413–97.

34. Tervaniemi, M. and T. L. van Zuijen (1999) Methodologies of brain research in cognitive musicology. *J. New Music Res.* 28, 200–8.

35. Rugg, M. D. (1999) Functional neuroimaging in cognitive neuroscience. In C. M. Brown and P. Hagoort (eds) *The Neurocognition of Language*. Oxford: Oxford University Press, pp. 15–36.

36. Shtyrov, Y., T. Kujala, J. Ahveninen, *et al.* (1998) Noise-induced shift in hemispheric lateralization of speech processing. *Neurosci. Lett.* 251, 141–4.

37. Shtyrov, Y., T. Kujala, R. J. Ilmoniemi, *et al.* (1999) Noise affects speech-signal processing differently in the cerebral hemispheres. *Neuroreport* 10, 2189–92.

38. Herrmann, C. S., U. Oertel, Y. Wang, *et al.* (2000) Noise affects auditory and linguistic processing differently: an MEG study. *Neuroreport* 11, 227–9.

39. Takeuchi, A. H. and S. H. Hulse (1993) Absolute pitch. *Psychol. Bull.* 113, 345–61.

40. Sundberg, J. (1991) *The Science of Musical Sounds.* San Diego: Academic Press.

41. Tervaniemi, M., T. Ilvonen, J. Sinkkonen, *et al.* (2000) Harmonic partials facilitate pitch discrimination in humans: electrophysiological and behavioral evidence. *Neurosci. Lett.* 279, 29–32.

42. Tervaniemi, M., E. Schröger, M. Saher, *et al.* (2000) Effects of spectral complexity and sound duration in complex-sound pitch processing in humans—a mismatch negativity study. *Neurosci. Lett.* 290, 66–70.

43. Tervaniemi, M., N. Novitski, M. Huotilainen, *et al.* (2002) Frequency discrimination at different frequency levels as reflected by electrophysiological and behavioral indices. Submitted.

44. Dewar, K., L. L. Cuddy, and D. J. K. Mewhort (1977) Recognition memory for single tones with and without context. *J. Exp. Psychol.* 3, 60–7.

45. Brattico, E., R. Näätänen, and M. Tervaniemi (2002) Context effects on pitch perception in musicians and non-musicians: evidence from ERP recordings. *Music Percept.* 19, 199–222.

46. Tervaniemi, M., J. Saarinen, P. Paavilainen, *et al.* (1994) Temporal integration of auditory information in sensory memory as reflected by the mismatch negativity. *Biol. Psychol.* 38, 157–67.

47. Saarinen, J., P. Paavilainen, E. Schröger, *et al.* (1992) Representation of abstract stimulus attributes in human brain. *Neuroreport* 3, 1149–51.

48. Paavilainen, P., M. Jaramillo, R. Näätänen, *et al.* (1999) Neuronal populations in the human brain extracting invariant relationships from acoustics variance. *Neurosci. Lett.* 265, 179–82.

49. Paavilainen, P., M. Jaramillo, and R. Näätänen. (1998) Binaural information can converge in abstract memory traces. *Psychophysiology* 35, 483–7.

50. Näätänen, R., M. Tervaniemi, E. Sussman, *et al.* (2001) 'Primitive intelligence' in the auditory cortex. *Trends Neurosci.* 24, 283–8.

51. Tervaniemi, M., S. Maury, and R. Näätänen (1994) Neural representations of abstract features in the human brain as reflected by the mismatch negativity. *Neuroreport* 5, 844–6.

52. Winkler, I., W. Teder, M. Tervaniemi, *et al.* (2002) Event-related potential (ERP) correlates of unexpected jumps of a continuously moving auditory stimulus. In preparation.

53. Paavilainen, P., M. L. Karlsson, K. Reinikainen, *et al.* (1989) Mismatch negativity to changes in the spatial location of an auditory stimulus. *Int. J. Psychophysiol.* 7, 342–3.

54. Schröger, E. and C. Wolff (1996) Mismatch response of the human brain to changes in sound location. *Neuroreport* 7, 3005–8.

55. Winkler, I., M. Tervaniemi, E. Schröger, *et al.* (1998) Processing of spatial cues used for auditory lateralization as revealed by the mismatch negativity. *Neurosci. Lett.* 242, 49–52.

56. Koelsch, S., T. C. Gunter, A. D. Friederici, *et al.* (2000) Brain indices of music processing: 'non-musicians' are musical. *J. Cogn. Neurosci.* 12, 520–41.

57. Hahne, A. and A.D. Friederici (1999) Electrophysiological evidence for two steps in syntactic analysis: early automatic and late controlled processes. *J. Cogn. Neurosci.* 11, 194–205.

58. Patel, A. D., E. Gibson, J. Ratner, *et al.* (1998) Processing syntactic relations in language and music: an event-related potential study. *J. Cogn. Neurosci.* 10, 717–33.

59. Maess, B., S. Koelsch, T. C. Gunter, *et al.* (2001) Musical syntax is processed in Broca's area: an MEG study. *Nature Neurosci.* 4, 541–5.

60. S. Koelsch, E. Schröger, and T. C. Gunter (2002) Music matters: preattentive musicality of the human brain. *Psychophysiology* 39, 38–48.

61. Pantev, C., R. Oostenveld, A. Engelien, *et al.* (1998) Increased auditory cortical representation in musicians. *Nature* 392, 811–14.

62. Verleger, R. (1990) P3-evoking wrong notes: unexpected, awaited, or arousing? *Int. J. Neurosci.* 55, 171–9.

63. Besson, M., F. Faïta, and J. Requin (1994) Brain waves associated with musical incongruities differ for musicians and non-musicians. *Neurosci. Lett.* 168, 101–5.

64. Crummer, G. C., J. P. Walton, J. W. Wayman, *et al.* (1994) Neural processing of musical timbre by musicians, nonmusicians, and musicians possessing absolute pitch. *J. Acoust. Soc. Am.* 95, 2720–7.

65. Koelsch, S., E. Schröger, and M. Tervaniemi (1999) Superior attentive and pre-attentive auditory processing in musicians. *Neuroreport* 10, 1309–13.

66. Tervaniemi, M., V. Just, S. Koelsch, *et al.* (2002) Pitch-discrimination accuracy in musicians vs. non-musiciansan event-related potential and behavioral study. In preparation.

67. Schmithorst, V. J. and M. Wilke (2002) Differences in white matter architecture between musicians and non-musicians: a diffusion tensor imaging study. *Neurosci. Lett.* 321, 57–60.

68. Pantev, C., L. E. Roberts, M. Schulz, *et al.* (2001) Timbre-specific enhancement of auditory cortical representations in musicians. *Neuroreport* 12, 1–6.

69. Rüsseler, J., E. Altenmüller, W. Nager, *et al.* (2001) Event-related brain potentials differ in musicians and non-musicians. *Neurosci. Lett.* 308, 33–6.

70. Yabe, H., M. Tervaniemi, J. Sinkkonen, *et al.* (1998) The temporal window of integration of auditory information in the human brain. *Psychophysiology* 35, 615–19.

71. van Zuijen, T., I. Winkler, E. Sussman, *et al.* (2002) Pre-attentive grouping of sequential sounds-an event-related potential study comparing musicians and non-musicians. Submitted.

72. Tervaniemi, M., M. Rytkönen, E. Schröger, *et al.* (2001) Superior formation of cortical memory traces for melodic patterns in musicians. *Learning Mem.* 8, 295–300.

73. Kishon-Rabin, L., O. Amir, Y. Vexler, *et al.* (2001) Pitch discrimination: are professional musicians better than non-musicians? *J. Basic Clin. Physiol. Pharmacol.* 12, 125–43.

CHAPTER 20

PROCESSING EMOTIONS INDUCED BY MUSIC

L. J. TRAINOR AND L. A. SCHMIDT

Abstract

Can music induce emotions directly and, if so, are these emotions experienced similarly to emotions arising in other contexts? We explore these questions from the perspective of neuroscience. Emotional processing has a deep evolutionary history because it is essential for self-regulation and social approach vs withdrawal. In humans, emotional processing involves autonomic, subcortical, and cortical structures. Despite the fact that music does not appear to have an obvious survival value for modern adults, research indicates that listening to music does activate autonomic, subcortical, and cortical systems in a manner similar to other emotional stimuli. We propose that music may be so intimately connected with emotional systems because caregivers use music to communicate emotionally with their infants before they are able to understand language.

Introduction

Music is often referred to as the language of emotions, but there is considerable controversy as to whether music actually induces emotions directly in listeners and, if so, whether these musically induced emotions are the same as other emotional experiences. In this chapter, we examine evidence from neuroscience to explore these questions.

The question of meaning in music has been a subject of philosophical debate for a very long time.[1] Music is peculiar because in large part it appears to be a closed system, with musical meaning defined only in terms of music itself. Music can be referential in the sense of having an intended outside meaning (e.g. it can be about a thunderstorm, a war, or a love story), but this specific reference to events or things in the world is usually far from transparent to the listener. Music can also come to have meaning, in terms of convention (e.g. particular turns of phrase in Baroque music may be meaningful for listeners familiar with these conventions; particular *rags* may signal particular moods or moral qualities in Indian listeners educated in this tradition) or through association with events in the world (e.g. a particular song can signal bedtime for a child; lovers may associate a particular song with their courtship). However, conventional and associational referential meanings do not seem to account for the majority of meaningful responses to music. Rather, meaning appears to arise largely through the unfolding of sounds over time in relation to musical expectations.[2] In other words, to a large extent the meaning appears to be simply in the musical relations themselves.

Empirical psychomusicological research suggests that both adults and young children readily discriminate musical emotions.[3,4] The acoustic cues that differentiate emotions cover virtually all aspects of musical structure and include both structural (what is given by the composer) and performance characteristics.[5–8] For example, *sadness* is conveyed by quiet, slow, legato articulation and large deviations from metrical timing, whereas *happiness* or *joy* is conveyed by high-pitched, fast, staccato features and small variations from metrical timing.[9] However, music appears to express some emotions more precisely than others. Listeners generally agree on whether music is happy or sad, but there is less agreement when it comes to other emotions.[3,10] Acoustically, the differences between, for example, tenderness and sadness are rather subtle. According to Juslin,[9] both are quiet, have slow tempos, legato articulation, and large timing variations. Although they may differ in other subtle features, it does not appear that musical structure is set up to differentiate these emotions robustly. The notion that music may express readily only certain emotions must lead us to further question the nature of musical emotions, and how they relate to emotions in general.

It is likely surprising to psychologists to learn that some philosophers have argued that music does not express emotion, given the empirical data showing substantial agreement between listeners as to the emotion expressed in particular pieces of music. For example, a century and a half ago, Hanslick[11] proposed that music appreciation had nothing to do with emotion. Half a century ago, Langer[12] proposed that music bears some relation to emotion in that the rise and fall of tension in music, the interplay between uncertainty and resolution, mimics the time course of emotional experience. In this view, music does not express emotion, but we understand music through its similarity to emotional dynamics. On the other hand, Meyer[2] has argued that music does express emotions. According to his argument, musical emotions are induced through musical uncertainty, expectation for what will follow, and the way in which this uncertainty is resolved, similarly to how emotions are induced by other stimuli and events in the world.

Emotions can be classified in a number of ways. One approach is to extract the underlying dimensions of emotion, and to situate each specific emotion in this multi-dimensional space. Such analyses reveal two main dimensions of emotion: valence (negative to positive) and intensity (low to high).[13] Positive emotions are associated with approach behaviours and negative emotions with withdrawal behaviours. The ventromedial prefrontal cortex is thought to play a role in approach/withdrawal evaluations.[14] Although emotional processing in general tends to be more lateralized to the right than to the left,[15] there is also evidence that lateralization follows valence, with left prefrontal areas specialized for positive emotions and right prefrontal areas for negative emotions.[16–19] Despite the common view that 'music is the language of emotions', these models were developed without reference to musical stimuli. Music is an interesting stimulus in this regard, because in most cases it does not lead to overt approach or withdrawal behaviour. In fact, people often 'approach' sad music, in that they find it beautiful. Because music does not seem to be directly connected with approach/withdrawal behaviour, it is possible that music is *about* emotion, that music *communicates* emotional information, but that music does not directly *induce* emotions. One interesting question, then, is whether musical stimuli generate activity in the prefrontal cortex, and whether differential activation can be seen for music expressing different emotions.

There is currently much debate among psychologists and neuroscientists as to the nature of emotional experience in general and its relation to cognition, behaviour, consciousness, and the sense of self. According to one view, cognitive evaluation must take place first, and the emotional response is generated subsequent to this.[20] An opposite view posits that emotions correspond to unconscious activity in the autonomic nervous system, and that our conscious feelings are interpretations of this activity.[21,22] According to Damasio,[23] emotions are induced in a relatively small number of brain sites, most of which are below the cerebral cortex. These comprise various components of the limbic system that have long been implicated in emotion,[24] including the amygdala (particularly the central nucleus), the hypothalamus, and the basal forebrain. In this view, emotion evolved through mechanisms of evolutionary adaptation, and performs an essential role in life regulation.[25] An animal needs to know when to approach a stimulus or situation and when to avoid a stimulus or situation, and it is through innate emotional biases and learned emotional associations that the animal does this. Thus, according to Damasio,[26] all experiences are emotionally tagged and influence emotional reactions in future situations, even though the person or animal may no longer have conscious access to the original experience. For example, an early unpleasant experience with a dog may induce a fear response to dogs, even though the person may not remember the origin of the association.

Although it has been argued that music may be an evolutionary adaptation serving social group cohesion (e.g. Chapter 5, this volume), it has also been argued that music does not have any survival function at all.[27,28] However, if music engages both phylogenetically old and newer emotional systems, this would suggest that music evolved alongside emotion in humans. In this chapter, we will first explore whether music engages the autonomic nervous system, sub-cortical emotion networks, and cortical areas involved in the emotional processing of other types of stimuli. Second, we will consider whether emotional reactions to music are simply cultural conventions by asking whether and how infants process musical emotions.

Physiological responses to music

The subcortical emotion-processing parts of the brain affect the rest of the body through two basic mechanisms: the release of chemical molecules into the blood that act on various parts of the body; and the spread of neural activation to various brain centres and muscles. Through these mechanisms, the experience of an emotion is connected with a myriad of physiological responses, from muscle contractions, to changes in breathing and heart rate, to changes in blood flow in various parts of the body, to sweating. If music is simply about emotion, but does not induce emotion, one would not expect listening to music to activate the autonomic system, and physiological changes should not be evident. However, studies using both self-report[29] and direct measures of autonomic function[30,31] have now shown that listening to music does indeed produce autonomic changes associated with emotional processing. For example, adults report shivers down the spine, laughter, tears, and 'lump in the throat' as some physiological responses to music.[29]

Nyklicek et al.[31] presented listeners with musical excerpts expressing happiness, sadness, serenity, or agitation. These four emotions cover the extremes of an intensity/valence matrix: happiness and agitation are intense, whereas sadness and serenity are not; happiness and serenity are positively valenced, whereas sadness and agitation are negatively valenced. They found that changes in respiration clearly followed the intensity dimension. Respiration rate was higher, and inspiration and expiration times shorter, for the happy and agitated excerpts than for the sad and serene excerpts. This is consistent with the findings of Krumhansl,[30] who found respiration rate to be higher during fear and happy excerpts than during sad excerpts. The valence dimension, however, is less clearly seen in the autonomic measures. Using discriminant analysis, Nyklicek et al.[31] found that an arousal dimension accounted for 63 percent of the variance across a number of physiological variables related to respiration and cardiac function, whereas a dimension related to valence accounted for only 10 percent of the variance. Krumhansl[30] did find that respiration depth decreased more during happy excerpts than sad or fear excerpts, and that finger temperature decreased less for happy excerpts than for sad or fear excerpts. However, as a low-intensity, positive-valence emotion was not present in this study, it is difficult to determine definitively whether these measures reflect valence *per se*. It is clear, then, that music induces physiological changes consistent with the processing of emotional intensity, and perhaps also with emotional valence.

One approach to determining the relation between emotions induced by music and those induced through other means is to consider whether excerpts of music conveying different emotions produce distinctive autonomic signatures, and whether these signatures are consistent with emotions induced in other ways. However, there are inconsistencies in the autonomic signatures of specific emotions across studies using varying stimuli such as static visual stimuli, films, and directed facial action tasks. Thus, the idea that specific emotions are uniquely represented by specific autonomic patterns is still controversial.[22] Distinctive autonomic patterns for specific emotions are found when the directed facial action task is used.[32,33] However, there is little correspondence between these autonomic signatures and those found by Krumhansl[30] and Nyklicek et al.[31] For example, heart rate tends to be higher for sad than for happy facial actions and finger temperature does not differ, whereas heart rate tends to be slower for musically-induced sadness than for musically induced happiness, and finger temperature is higher for happy than for sad musical emotions. Facial action studies have been criticized as perhaps reflecting the difficulty of producing the facial expression rather than the emotion expressed.[34] In fact, many factors may influence the specific autonomic responses observed. Emotion is complex (e.g. there are many different kinds of happiness and fear) and differential effects may arise when overt responses are made or blocked.[35] Interestingly, musically induced autonomic responses are most consistent with those measured in studies employing manipulations that extend over time, such as watching a film or listening to a radio play.[30]

One difference between musical emotion and emotion arising in other domains is that overt action is not normally required in response to musical emotion. With development, people learn to control the overt expression of emotion to some extent. They may be able to stop themselves from uttering hurtful or angry words, but controlling their autonomic responses is more difficult. In the case of musical performers, however, feeling the music too much, and allowing autonomic responses free rein, could lead to an inability to perform. A singer with a tight throat will not have optimal sound control, and a violin player with sweaty, shaking fingers will not be able to play well. Damasio[23] gives a wonderful example of a pianist, Maria Joao, who claimed that she could cut off the flow of emotion to her body at will. Damasio's skepticism turned out to be unfounded, as laboratory tests confirmed that she could allow or block physiological responses during music listening. This leads to the interesting question of whether musical emotions are somehow more subject to cognitive control than other emotions, or whether all emotional autonomic responses can be controlled through learning.

In summary, music does induce emotion directly. However, more research is needed before we can answer the question of whether musical emotions have the same autonomic signatures as emotions induced in other situations. Similarly, we can only speculate at present as to whether musical emotions are more under cognitive control than emotions induced through other means.

Central nervous system responses to emotion in music

Music stimulates wide networks of bilateral activity across the brain, and specific areas within these networks appear to be specialized for the perception of various aspects of music such as melody, rhythm, and timbre (see Chapter 17, this volume). In particular, auditory cortex and frontal regions appear to be essential for musical processing.[36,37] Changes in pitch intervals and pitch contour are processed in auditory cortex even in the absence of attention,[38] and right frontal areas are activated during tasks involving pitch memory.[37] While right-hemisphere dominance is often found for pitch-based musical tasks (e.g. Chapter 16, this volume), laterality can be moved around by instruction (analytic vs holistic) and degree of musical training.[39,40] In contrast to the *perception* of music, much less is known about the networks for processing *emotional* aspects of music.

It is generally agreed that emotional processing of all types involves wide networks of central nervous system activity, including limbic and sensory areas as well as those related to cognition and consciousness.[41] However, consensus on the specific brain regions that are activated for each specific emotion is far from achieved.[22] This is likely due in part to the employment of different methodologies (e.g. PET, fMRI, EEG) across studies. However, it is also likely due to large effects on neural activity of the *contents* of emotional experience (e.g. which sensory systems are involved; the specific stimulus triggering the feelings), the salience of an emotion or extent to which the emotion is felt, different shadings of emotion within one category such as 'happiness', and, very importantly, differences between the induction of emotion, the feeling of emotion, and the conscious memory or discrimination of emotions. For example, the amygdala is strongly implicated in the induction and learning of fear responses,[41] but does not appear to be involved when fear states are recalled.[25]

Does emotion induced by music activate the same cortical structures as emotion induced by other stimuli? How is the processing of musical emotion affected by the contents of the stimulus? Given that research into the neural processing of emotion in music is just beginning, and given the lack of consensus on a model of emotional processing in general, definitive answers to these questions cannot be given. However, a few very interesting studies are providing a starting point. We will review here three approaches that have been taken. First, lesion cases involving impairment of musical ability can give a hint as to the brain regions involved. Second, PET imaging studies in normal adults who listen to music varying in its emotional content can also suggest the brain regions involved. Third, EEG studies examining general patterns of regional activation can be compared across conditions of musical and nonmusical induction of emotion.

Peretz et al.[42] presented a case study of a patient, IR, who showed a dissociation between perceptual and emotional processing of music, a dissociation that appears to parallel that found between the identification of faces and the processing of emotional expression in faces.[43] IR suffered bilateral damage to her auditory cortices, such that in the left hemisphere Heschl's gyrus and the anterior portion of the planum temporale are completely destroyed, the superior temporal gyrus is infracted, and the damage extends to adjoining regions. On the right, Heschl's gyrus and the planum temporale are spared, but the anterior and superior portions of the superior temporal gyrus are damaged, and there is a large frontal lesion that includes the precentral and inferior frontal gyri and part of the orbitofrontal gyri. Despite the left hemisphere damage, IR's language is normal. However, her musical perception abilities are severely damaged, and she is unable to recognize or discriminate melodies. Despite these perceptual deficits, IR is able to tell whether musical excerpts are happy or sad.[44] Furthermore, she can do this based only on the mode and tempo of the excerpts. Thus, at least in this one case, not only are music and language dissociated, but perceptual and emotional aspects of music are as well. Further research is needed, however, to determine whether IR uses modality-general emotional processing areas for determining musical emotion.

As an initial step into examining musical emotions, Blood et al.[45] used PET imaging to identify regions whose activity correlated with changes in musical stimuli along the consonance/dissonance dimension. This dimension is defined such that tones sounding pleasant or smooth together are said to be consonant whereas those sounding unpleasant or rough together are said to be dissonant.[46] Dissonance is interesting as it relies on the peripheral structure of the auditory system: the critical band structure of the basilar membrane[46,47] and the firing patterns in the auditory nerve (see Chapter 9, this volume). In brief, tones with harmonics that are close enough in frequency to be difficult to resolve along the tonotopic organization of the basilar membrane are perceived to be dissonant. Likely because of its peripheral origins, infants as young as two months of age are sensitive to this dimension, preferring to listen to simultaneous tones in consonant relations over those in dissonant relations.[48,49] This dimension is also critical to musical structure, as virtually all musical systems rely on dissonance to generate tension, and consonance to resolve that tension.

Blood et al.[45] found that some regions involved in affective processing from previous nonmusic studies were also activated with changes in consonance and dissonance, including right parahippocampal gyrus, right precuneus, bilateral orbitofrontal, medial subcallosal singulate, and right frontal polar regions. Furthermore, the degree of activation of certain areas differed across consonance and dissonance presentation, suggesting that music conveying positive and negative valence may have distinct cortical signatures. While interesting and suggestive, a caveat is necessary before making strong conclusions about musical emotional processing on the basis of this study. Although pleasant/unpleasant ratings correlated with activity in right parahippocampal gyrus, these dimensions did not correlate with ratings of happy/sad. Thus, while this study appears to capture something about the processing of musical valence, simply varying the amount of dissonance across a musical phrase is not the equivalent to inducing happiness or sadness. Dissonance without resolution likely corresponds more to irritation, which is a high-arousal negative emotion, rather than sadness, which is a low-arousal negative emotion. Furthermore, there is evidence for the cortical separation of consonance and dissonance from happiness and sadness. IR, described above, is unable to discriminate consonance and dissonance although she can discriminate happy from sad music.[50] In any case, this study suggests that musically induced emotions are processed in brain regions overlapping those involved in general emotional processing.

In a second study, Blood and Zatorre[51] explored intense positive emotional reactions to music by having each subject choose an except that gave them 'chills', and listen to it while PET responses were recorded. Compared to control conditions, the music induced increased cerebral blood flow in the left ventral striatum, dorsomedial midbrain areas, and paralimbic regions, areas that have been associated with euphoria, pleasant emotion, and cocaine administration in other studies. In addition, music listening was associated with decreases in blood flow to the amygdala, hippocampus, and ventral medial prefrontal cortex, which is also consistent with the experience of intense emotions in other contexts. In sum, these PET studies suggest that the experience of positive emotional responses to music activate the same brain circuits as positive emotions induced in other contexts.

There are two related lines of EEG research on emotion that may shed light on how musical emotion is processed in the brain. One line concerns the pattern of EEG activity that is observed in anterior regions during the processing of emotion. For example, a number of EEG studies have found evidence that frontal activation patterns differ across emotions.[16,17,52,53] A second line of research concerns the pattern of resting frontal EEG activity recorded during baseline or neutral states and its relation to individual differences in affective style or personality. In the personality literature, current thinking is that different personality styles emerge from how emotions are regulated.[16,17,52] For example, depression is thought to be characterized and maintained by an inability to experience positive affect; shyness and anxiety are thought to be characterized by an inability to regulate fear; sociability and extraversion are thought to be characterized and maintained by the experience of positive affect and the ability to control negative affect.

Interestingly, the pattern of resting frontal EEG activity has been shown to discriminate these various profiles, suggesting that the resting frontal EEG metric is indexing the predisposition to experience different affect states. This in turn suggests that the neural correlates of transient emotion may be similar to those shown for different personality types. One model has associated the intensity of emotion with overall amount of frontal activation.[54–56] For example, infants separated from their mothers show an increase in frontal activation.[57] A second model posits that emotions with positive valence, such as joy, interest, and happiness, show greater left than right activation whereas those with negative valence, such as fear, disgust, and sadness show greater right than left activation.[16,17,52,54,58] (It should also be noted that Blood et al.[45] also found that the positively valenced consonance excerpts tended to activate left frontal areas more than the negatively valenced dissonant excerpts.) Evidence for the frontal activation/emotion valence model has been found across a number of stimulus modalities including pictures, films, and taste[16,17,52] and in infants as well as in adults.[52] Furthermore, baseline or neutral EEG asymmetries have been linked to personality types, with outgoing individuals tending to exhibit greater relative left activation and shy individuals greater relative right activation.

Because the frontal activation/emotion valence model is based on the idea of a dichotomy between approach and withdraw behaviours with a deep evolutionary history, it is not clear a priori whether it would apply to music. However, we[56] found clear evidence that it holds for music as well. We presented listeners with music expressing emotions at the extremes of the intensity/valence matrix. Specifically, we used orchestral excerpts expressing joy (high intensity, positive valence), happiness (low intensity, positive valence), fear (high intensity, negative valence), and sadness (low intensity, negative valence) that had been rated by adults along the valence and intensity dimensions. Evidence was found supporting both the intensity and the frontal activation/emotion valence models. The measure of activation was the inverse of alpha band activity (8–13 Hz), as energy in this band decreases with increased activation.[58] The amount of frontal activation was correlated with adults' ratings of the intensity of their emotional response to the excerpts (from least to most intense: sad, happy, joy, fear), supporting the intensity model (Figure 20.1). Both joy and happiness showed greater relative left frontal activation whereas both fear and sadness showed greater relative right activation (Figure 20.1), supporting the frontal activation/emotion valence model. Thus, we[56] found evidence that emotion induced by music activates frontal circuits in the brain similar to those activated by other emotional stimuli.

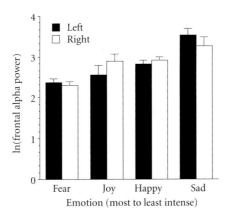

Figure 20.1 Differences among fear, joy, happy, and sad left and right frontal EEG alpha power. Note that EEG power is thought to be inversely related to activity, thus lower power reflects more activity. Overall activation is related to intensity, and positive emotions show greater relative left activation whereas negative emotions show greater relative right activation. Error bars represent the standard error of the mean. Reprinted with permission from Schmidt and Trainor.[56]

In summary, although there are rather few studies to date addressing how musical emotion is processed in the brain, the preliminary evidence suggests that, despite the fact that music has questionable evolutionary advantages, and despite the fact that music normally does not motivate approach or withdraw behaviours, music does appear to activate the same emotional circuits as other stimuli.

Development of emotional responses to music

The strongest argument that music is an important evolutionary adaptation arguably comes from the developmental perspective. Caregivers around the world sing to infants, and young infants are responsive to such music.[59] Singing directed at infants is rendered in a style that is distinct from other types of singing,[60,61] and infants prefer to listen to infant-directed over non-infant-directed renditions of the same song. The function of infant-directed singing remains somewhat elusive. However, one of the main theories is that caregivers use infant-directed singing to express emotional information, and to regulate their infant's state.[59-61] Young infants are, of course, not good at state regulation, and require intervention in order to calm down when upset. Mothers sing in two distinct styles, a lullaby style and a playsong style.[61-63] Adults can discriminate playsong and lullaby styles easily, and they rate playsongs as more rhythmic, brilliant, clipped, and smiling in character, and less soothing and airy than lullabies.[63] Furthermore, infants react differently when exposed to lullabies and playsongs, focussing their attention inward during the former and outward during the latter.[63] Thus, music has the power to affect an infant's state.

On the basis of the evidence that music is universally used in caretaking contexts for emotional expression and state regulation, and that infants react differently to different musical styles, it is possible that singing to infants serves an important adaptive function in development. Specifically, music may provide one route into learning about social interaction and self-regulation before infants understand any language.

Children are also able to distinguish different emotions in music. Cunningham and Sterling[64] showed that 4- to 6-year-olds could discriminate happy, sad, angry, and fearful musical excerpts. Trainor and Trehub[4] found that children as young as 4 years could reliably associate excerpts from Prokofiev's Peter and the Wolf and Saint Saens' Carnival of the Animals with pictures of the animals, giving emotion-laden justifications for their responses such as that the wolf excerpt sounded 'scary'.

The bases for early emotional reactions to music have not been investigated widely, but they likely involve interpretations based on pitch, tempo, and timbre characteristics of the music. One aspect of pitch structure has been investigated. As discussed previously, consonant intervals are associated with positive emotion and dissonant intervals with negative emotion. Using a visual looking paradigm in which infants control how long they listen to consonant vs dissonant chords by how long they fixate on a visual target, Trainor and colleagues[48,49] have demonstrated that infants as young as two months prefer to listen to consonant over dissonant musical intervals. These results complement previous findings that older infants also prefer consonance over dissonance.[65-67]

Given the behavioural evidence that young infants respond to the emotional content of music, the same question that we addressed previously with adults arises with infants: Does musical emotion stimulate the same brain circuits as other emotional experiences in infants? A number of EEG studies of nonmusical emotional processing in infants support the presence of frontal asymmetries related to valence.[52] For example, infants tend to show greater relative right frontal EEG activation during the processing of negatively valenced stimuli (i.e. faces displaying distress or fear, tastes that are sour) and greater relative left frontal EEG activation during the processing of positively valenced stimuli (i.e. faces displaying joy, smiling, and sweet tastes). As well, infants who show greater right than left resting frontal EEG activation tend to show heightened distress to novel events and maternal separation.

In order to test whether infants' EEG responses would show the same asymmetry effects for emotion induced by music, we[68] recently recorded EEG and ECG as 3-, 6-, 9-, and 12-month old infants listened to the joy, fear, and sad orchestral excerpts used in Ref. 56. Infant alpha band activity (4–8 Hz) was recorded, and activation was taken as the inverse of this measure. There were interesting changes across age (Figure 20.2). Compared to baseline, the presence of music significantly increased brain activity at 3 months of age, had little effect at 6 and 9 months of age, and significantly attenuated brain activity at 12 months of age (Figure 20.2),

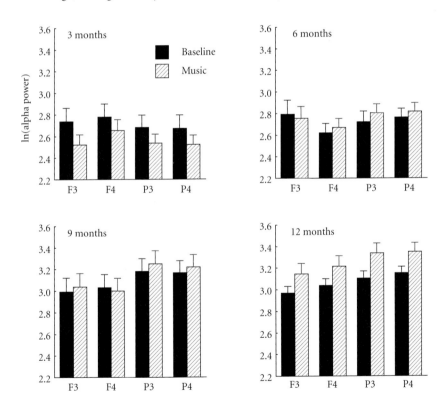

Figure 20.2 Infant alpha power for frontal (F3, F4) and parietal (P3, P4) regions and left (F3, P3) and right (F4, P4) hemispheres. Note that music has opposite effects compared to baseline at 3 and 12 months of age. Error bars represent the standard error of the mean. Reprinted with permission from Schmidt, Trainor, and Santesso.[68]

suggesting that music is having a calming effect by 12 months as infants are increasingly able to regulate their sensory input. However, no left/right asymmetries were found in any condition.

There are a number of possible reasons for the lack of asymmetric responses to musical emotion in infants. It is possible that musical emotion is processed differently than other emotions in infancy, but this would be surprising given the behavioural evidence for a central role of musical emotion in everyday infant caregiving activities. Another possibility is that the orchestral musical excerpts used were simply too complex for infants. While it is advantageous to use the same musical excerpts with infants and adults, this music is certainly not very similar to typical infant-directed singing. Still another explanation is that sufficient frontal lobe maturation for the cognitive appraisal of musical stimuli is not yet developed in the first year of life.

To address these possibilities, studies are underway to measure infant EEG with more ecologically valid stimuli. In particular, we are using vocal singing, infant-directed speech, and infant-directed singing conveying various emotions. At this point it is not possible to answer the questions of whether infants process musical emotions with similar brain circuits to those used for other emotions, or whether infants and adults use similar brain circuits to process musical emotion. However, methodologies now exist to ask these questions, and hopefully more data will be forthcoming.

Conclusions

The popular notion that music elicits powerful emotions appears to be close to the truth. That music is not only about emotion, but that it elicits emotion directly, can be seen clearly from the physiological responses it induces. The changes in heart rate, respiration rate, blood flow, and skin conductance are clear indications that music activates the phylogenetically old parts of the nervous system, and that music elicits a cascade of subconscious activity. Music also appears to activate the cortical systems associated with emotion, including circuits in the frontal lobes. Further research is needed, however, to address the questions of how discrete emotions are processed, and how various dimensions of emotion such as valence and intensity are encoded in the brain. There are many unanswered questions with respect to music, such as why happiness and sadness are so easily expressed in musical structure whereas emotions such as anger are so much more difficult to express.

Despite the fact that, for adults in the modern world, music does not command the same approach/withdrawal reactions as other emotion-laden stimuli, much evidence suggests that music does activate the same cortical, subcortical, and autonomic circuits as other emotions. Perhaps the answer to the puzzle of why music appears to activate the essential survival circuits of the nervous system—when music does not appear to serve any obvious survival function—lies in the evolution of development and child care. Human infants are particularly helpless for an extended period of time, and are reliant on their caregivers for survival. An emotional bond and the communication of positive and prohibitory emotional information is essential for survival. Perhaps music evolved in order to further emotional communication between infants and caregivers. And perhaps infant-directed singing and infant-directed 'musical' speech[69] are intimately connected with approach and withdrawal behaviour on the part of the infant. Taking this one step further, as children develop other means of communication such as language, and as they learn to keep overt expressions of emotion under control, music may go 'underground'. Music still elicits emotion, but more direct and precise methods of emotional communication can occur with language. Perhaps, however, music retains a survival role in adults in that it allows the 'practice' of feeling emotions without having to risk the consequences of acting on these emotions. Thus, we are free to laugh and cry to music, to feel our heart race, to feel chills, and to hold our breath, and perhaps once again to feel like the infant who is exquisitely tuned to the emotion in its mother's voice.

Acknowledgements

This work was supported by grants from the Canadian Institutes of Health Research and the National Science and Engineering Research Council of Canada. We thank Joanne Leuzzi for technical support, and Terri Lewis and Judy Plantinga for comments on an earlier draft.

References

1. **Juslin, P. N.** and **J. A. Sloboda** (eds) (2001) *Music and Emotion: Theory and Research*. Oxford: Oxford University Press.
2. **Meyer, L. B.** (1956) *Emotion and Meaning in Music*. Chicago: University of Chicago Press.
3. **Terwogt, M. M.** and **F. Van Grinsven** (1991) Musical expression of moodstates. *Psychol. Music* 19, 99–109.
4. **Trainor, L. J.** and **S. E. Trehub** (1992) The development of referential meaning in music. *Music Percept.* 9, 455–70.
5. **Gabrielsson, A.** and **E. Lindstrom** (2001) The influence of musical structure on emotional expression. In P. N. Juslin and J. A. Sloboda (eds) *Music and Emotion*. Oxford: Oxford University Press.
6. **Hevner, K.** (1935) The affective character of the major and minor modes in music. *Am. J. Psychol.* 47, 103–18.
7. **Hevner, K.** (1936) Experimental studies of the elements of expression in music. *Am. J. Psychol.* 48, 246–68.
8. **Balkwill, L. L.** and **W. F. Thompson** (1999) A cross-cultural investigation of the perception of emotion in music: psychophysical and cultural cues. *Music Percept.* 17, 43–64.
9. **Juslin, P. N.** (2001) Communicating emotion in music performance: a review and a theoretical framework. In P. N. Juslin and J. A. Sloboda (eds) *Music and Emotion*. Oxford: Oxford University Press, pp. 309–37.
10. **Gabrielsson, A.** and **P. N. Juslin** (1996) Emotional expression in music performance: between the performer's intention and the listener's experience. *Psychol. Music* 24, 68–91.
11. **Hanslick, E.** (1957) (originally published in 1854). *The Beautiful in Music*. New York: Liberal Arts Press.
12. **Langer, S.** (1942) *Philosophy in a New Key: A Study in the Symbolism of Reason, Rite, and Art*. Cambridge, MA: Harvard University Press.

13. Watson, D. and A. Tellegen (1985) Toward a consensual structure of mood. *Psychonomic Bulletin* 98, 219–35.

14. Davidson, R. J., K. R. Scherer, and H. H. Goldsmith (2003) *Handbook of Affective Sciences.* New York: Oxford Unversity Press.

15. Bryden, M. P. and R. G. Ley (1983) Right-hemispheric involvement in the perception and expression of emotion in normal humans. In K. M. Heilman and P. Satz (eds) *Neuropsychology of Human Emotion.* New York: Guilford Press.

16. Davidson, R. J. (2000) Affective style, psychopathology, and resilience: brain mechanisms and plasticity. *American Psychologist* 55, 1196–214.

17. Davidson, R. J. (1993) The neuropsychology of emotion and affective style. In M. Lewis and J. M. Haviland (eds) *Handbook of Emotion.* New York: The Guilford Press, pp. 143–54.

18. Fox, N. A. (1994) Dynamic cerebral processes underlying emotion regulation. *Monographs of the Society for Research in Child Development* 59, 152–66, 250–83.

19. Silberman, E. K. and H. Weingartner (1986) Hemispheric lateralization of functions related to emotion. *Brain and Cognition* 5, 322–53.

20. Lazarus, R. S. (1991) Progress on a cognitive-motivational-relational theory of emotion. *American Psychologist* 46, 819–34.

21. James, W. (1950) (originally published in 1890). *The Principles of Psychology* vol. 2. New York: Dover Publications.

22. Zajonc, R. B. and D. N. McIntosh (1992) Emotions research: some promising questions and some questionable promises. *Psychol. Sci.* 3, 70–4.

23. Damasio, A. (1999) *The Feeling of What Happens: Body and Emotion in the Making of Consciousness.* San Diego, CA: Harcourt Inc.

24. Papez, J. W. (1937) A proposed mechanism of emotion. *Archives of Neurology and Psychiatry* 38, 725–43.

25. Damasio, A. R., T. J. Grabowski, A. Bechara, *et al.* (2000) Subcortical and cortical brain activity during the feeling of self-generated emotions. *Nat. Neurosci.* 3, 1049–56.

26. Damasio, A. R. (1994) *Descartes' Error: Emotion, Reason, and the Human Brain.* New York: Putnam.

27. Pinker, S. (1997) *How the Mind Works.* New York: William Morrow.

28. Pinker, S. (1994) *The Language Instinct.* New York: William Morrow.

29. Sloboda, J. A. (1991) Music structure and emotional response: some empirical findings. *Psychol. Music* 19, 110–20.

30. Krumhansl, C. L. (1997) An exploratory study of musical emotion and psychophysiology. *Canadian J. Exp. Psychol.* 51, 336–52.

31. Nyklicek, I., J. F. Thayer and L. J. P. Van Doornen. (1997) Cardiorespiratory differentiation of musically-induced emotions. *J. Psychophysiol.* 11, 304–21.

32. Levenson, R. W., P. Ekman and W. V. Friesen (1990) Voluntary facial action generates emotion-specific autonomic nervous system activity. *Psychophysiol.* 27, 363–84.

33. Levenson, R. W. (1992) Autonomic nervous system differences among emotions. *Psychol. Sci.* 3, 23–7.

34. Boiten, F. (1996) Autonomic response patterns during voluntary facial action. *Psychophysiology* 33, 123–31.

35. Gross, J. J. and R. W. Levenson (1993) Emotional suppression: physiology, self-report, and expressive behavior. *J. Pers. Soc. Psychol.* 64, 970–86.

36. **Zatorre, R. J.** and **S. Samson** (1991) Role of the right temporal neocortex in retention of pitch in auditory short-term memory. *Brain* 114, 2403–17.

37. **Zatorre, R. J., A. C. Evans**, and **E. Meyer** (1994) Neural mechanisms underlying melodic perception and memory for pitch. *J. Neurosci.* 14, 1908–19.

38. **Trainor, L. J., K. L. McDonald**, and **C. Alain** (2002) Automatic and controlled processing of melodic contour and interval information measured by electrical brain activity. *J. Cog. Neurosci.* 14, 430–42.

39. **Peretz, I.** and **J. Morais** (1987) Analytic processing in the classification of melodies as same or different. *Neuropsychologia* 25, 645–52.

40. **Peretz, I., J. Morais**, and **P. Bertelson** (1987) Shifting ear differences in melody recognition through strategy inducement. *Brain and Cognition* 6, 202–15.

41. **LeDoux, J. E.** (1996) *The Emotional Brain: The Mysterious Underpinnings of Emotional Life.* New York: Simon and Schuster.

42. **Peretz, I.** and **L. Gagnon** (1999) Dissociation between recognition and emotional judgements for melodies. *Neurocase* 5, 21–30.

43. **Peretz, I.** (2001) Listen to the brain: a biological perspective on musical emotions. In P. N. Juslin and J. A. Sloboda (eds) *Music and Emotion.* Oxford: Oxford University Press.

44. **Peretz, I., L. Gagnon**, and **B. Bouchard** (1998) Music and emotion, perceptual determinants, immediacy, and isolation after brain damage. *Cognition* 68, 111–41.

45. **Blood, A. J., R. J. Zatorre, P. Bermudez**, and **A. C. Evans** (1999) Emotional responses to pleasant and unpleasant music correlate with activity in paralimbic brain regions. *Nat. Neurosci.* 2, 382–7.

46. **Plomp, R.** and **W. J. Levelt** (1965) Tonal consonance and critical bandwidth. *J. Acoust. Soc. Am.* 38, 548–60.

47. **Schellenberg, E. G.** and **L. J. Trainor** (1996) Sensory consonance and the perceptual similarity of complex-tone harmonic intervals: tests of adult and infant listeners. *J. Acoust. Soc. Am.* 100, 3321–8.

48. **Trainor, L. J.** and **C. D. Tsang** (2000) Paper presented at the International Conference on Infant Studies. England: Brighton.

49. **Trainor, L. J., C. D. Tsang**, and **V. H. W. Cheung** (2002) Preference for musical consonance in 2-month-old infants. *Music Perception*, 20, 185–92.

50. **Peretz, I., A. J. Blood, V. Penhune**, and **R. Zatorre** (2001) Cortical deafness to dissonance. *Brain* 124, 928–40.

51. **Blood, A. J.** and **R. Zatorre** (2001) Intensely pleasurable responses to music correlate with activity in brain regions implicated in reward and emotion. *Proc. Natl. Acad. Sci.* 98, 11818–23.

52. **Fox, N. A.** (1991) If it's not left, it's right: electroencephalogram asymmetry and the development of emotion. *American Psychologist* 46, 863–72.

53. **Canli, T.** (1999) Hemispheric asymmetry in the experience of emotion: A perspective from functional imaging. *The Neuroscientist* 5, 201–7.

54. **Dawson, G.** (1994) Frontal electroencephalographic correlates of individual differences in emotional expression in infants. *Monographs of the Society for Research in Child Development* 135–51.

55. **Schmidt, L. A.** and **N. A. Fox** (1999) Conceptual, biological, and behavioural distinctions among different types of shy children. In L. A. Schmidt and J. Schulkin (eds) *Extreme Fear, Shyness and Social Phobia: Origins, Biological Mechanisms, and Clinical Outcomes.* New York: Oxford University Press, pp. 27–46.

56. **Schmidt, L. A.** and **L. J. Trainor** (2001) Frontal brain electrical activity (EEG) distinguishes valence and intensity of musical emotions. *Cognit. Emotion* 15, 487–500.

57. **Dawson, G. W., L. Grofer-Klinger., H. Panagiotides, D. Hill,** and **S. Spieker** (1992) Frontal lobe activity and affective behavior of infants of mothers with depressive symptoms. *Child Dev.* 63, 725–37.

58. **Davidson, R. J.** and **A. J. Tomarken** (1989) Laterality and emotion: an electrophysiological approach. In F. Boller and J. Grafman (eds) *Handbook of Neuropsychology.* Amsterdam: Elsevier Science.

59. **Trehub, S. E.** and **L. J. Trainor** (1998) Singing to infants: lullabies and play songs. In C. Rovee-Collier, L. P. Lipsitt, and H. Hayne (eds) *Advances in Infancy Research.* Stamford, Connecticut: Ablex Publishing Corporation, pp. 43–77.

60. **Trehub, S. E., A. M. Unyk,** and **L. J. Trainor** (1993) Maternal singing in cross-cultural perspective. *Infant Behav. Dev.* 16, 285–95.

61. **Trainor, L. J.** (1996) Infant preferences for infant-directed versus noninfant-directed playsongs and lullabies. *Infant Behav. Dev.* 19, 83–92.

62. **Trainor, L. J., E. D. Clark, A. Huntley,** and **B. A. Adams.** (1997) The acoustic basis of preferences for infant-directed singing. *Infant Behav. Dev.* 20, 383–96.

63. **Rock, A. M. L., L. J. Trainor,** and **T. L. Addison** (1999) Distinctive messages in infant-directed lullabies and play songs. *Developmental Psychol.* 35, 527–34.

64. **Cunningham, J. G.** and **R. S. Sterling** (1988) Developmental change in the understanding of affective meaning in music. *Motivation and Emotion* 12, 399–413.

65. **Trainor, L. J.** and **B. J. Heinmiller** (1998) The development of evaluative responses to music: infants prefer to listen to consonance over dissonance. *Infant Behav. Dev.* 21, 77–88.

66. **Zentner, M. R.** and **J. Kagan** (1998) Infants' perception of consonance and dissonance in music. *Infant Behav. Dev.* 21, 483–92.

67. **Crowder, R. G., J. S. Reznick,** and **S. L. Rosenkrantz** (1991) Perception of the major/minor distinction: V. Preferences among infants. *Bull. Psychon. Soc.* 29, 187–8.

68. **Schmidt, L. A., L. J. Trainor,** and **D. L. Santesso** Development of electroencephalogram (EEG) and autonomic (ECG) responses to affective musical stimuli during the first 12 months of postnatal life. *Brain and Cognit.* (in press).

69. **Fernald, A.** (1992) Meaningful melodies in mothers' speech to infants. In H. Papousek and U. Jurgens (eds) *Nonverbal Vocal Communication.* Cambridge, UK: Cambridge University Press, pp. 262–82.

CHAPTER 21

A NEW APPROACH TO THE COGNITIVE NEUROSCIENCE OF MELODY

ANIRUDDH D. PATEL

Introduction

What is a musical melody? At the physical level, it is simply an organized succession of individual tones. At the perceptual level, however, it is much more. One perceptually oriented definition of melody has been suggested by the ethnomusicologist Simon Shaheen: a melody is 'a group of notes that are in love with each other'.[1] A related definition, which I hope to illustrate in this chapter, is that a musical melody is a tone sequence in which the individual tones are processed in terms of multiple structured relationships.[a] This definition emphasizes the active role of the mind in melody perception. That is, a melody (like a spoken sentence) depends on a listener's perceptual system to convert a 'mere sequence of sounds' into a meaningful mental experience.

This chapter has two goals. The first is to illustrate the cognitive richness of melody perception. The second is to introduce a new method for the neural study of melody. To illustrate melody perception I have chosen one particular melody from the Western European tradition, a children's song indexed as K0016 in the Essen database of Bohemian folk melodies.[2,3,b] Figure 21.1 shows the melody in Western music notation and in 'piano-roll' notation with each tone's pitch plotted as a function of time (this melody and all sound examples in this chapter can be heard at www.nsi.edu/users/patel/sound_examples/pz_chapter). The reasons for choosing this melody are threefold. First, it is historically recent yet likely to be unfamiliar to readers of this chapter: thus it follows familiar musical conventions while being free of specific memory associations. Second, as a folksong this melody has been through a period of preservation and transmission by ear rather than by music notation, so that it has survived a certain amount of natural testing for its perceptual coherence. Third, as a children's song the melody is short and illustrates basic structural relations in relatively simple form. Beyond these constraints, there is nothing special about K0016, and any number of melodies would have served the same purpose.

---

[a] Throughout this chapter the term 'melody' refers to monophonic melody, that is, melody without accompaniment.
[b] The database is available from the Center for Computer Assisted Research in the Humanities (Stanford University) and at www.esac-data.org (K0016 is in the kinder0 file of this database).

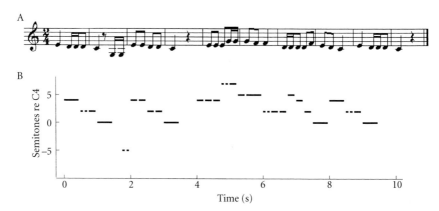

Figure 21.1   A children's melody from the ESAC database (K0016). The melody has been transposed to the key of C. (A) Western music notation. (B) Piano roll notation, with each tone's fundamental frequency (in semitones from C4 or 261.63 Hz) plotted as a function of time. A semitone is a ratio of ~1.06 in fundamental frequency, and corresponds to the distance between a neighbouring white and black piano key. K0016 ranges over 12 semitones (one octave, a doubling in fundamental frequency), that is, −5 semitones below C4 to 7 semitones above it.

Thirteen ways of hearing a melody

One way to appreciate the cognitive richness of melody perception is to enumerate the different things a listener hears during melodic processing. The following list is based on perception of a simple melody by a listener familiar with Western European tonal music. The list is not exhaustive, but merely touches on some of the more obvious features of melodic perception. Readers who wish to delve deeper into the structure of melody may consult Leonard Meyer's *Explaining Music*[4] and Eugene Narmour's two volumes on the analysis and cognition of melodies.[5,6]

Instrument identity

An immediate and salient aspect of melody perception is recognition of the instrument producing the tones (e.g. piano vs violin). Instrument recognition takes place very rapidly (instruments can often be recognized from single tones), and relies heavily on timbre or 'sound quality', which is a complex feature relying on the spectral and temporal shape of sound.[7]

Grouping

Grouping refers to the segmentation of a melody into units larger than single tones.[8] This can be illustrated with K0016, which consists of 33 separate tones. These tones define 33 minimal 'pitch-time units', each defined by a particular pitch and duration. In listening to this melody, there is a clear sense of larger pitch-time units between the levels of the individual pitches and the entire melody. For example, the melody is perceived as divided into phrases, schematically marked in Figure 21.2. The boundaries of the first two phrases are

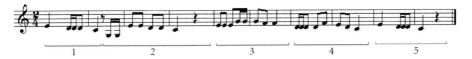

Figure 21.2   K0016 segmented into melodic phrases.

marked by silences (musical rests). Of greater interest are the boundaries at the end of the third and fourth phrases, which are not marked by any physical discontinuity in the tone sequence. Instead, these boundaries are marked by local durational lengthening and lowering of pitch, cues which also serve a boundary-marking role in speech.[9]

Beat and metre

A beat refers to 'a psychological, more-or-less isochronous, pulse train—that provides the stimulus for synchronization'.[10] K0016 readily evokes a beat: if asked to tap the beat of this melody, listeners are likely to tap at the positions marked in Figure 21.3 by the dots at the level labelled '1x'.[c] Note that three of these taps occur during silent intervals, showing that the beat is not a simple marking of physically accented events. Indeed, in the sound examples all tones in K0016 have the same amplitude: there are no accents based on the intensity of tones. Instead, the beat is inferred from the pattern of durations and pitches.[11]

When beats are grouped into larger repeating units the result is metre, that is, periodicity at multiple time scales.[12] In K0016 the beats are organized into higher-level groups of two (as indicated by the time signature) and four (examination of Figures 21.2 and 21.3 shows that each phrase has four beats).[d] Melodic sequences frequently exhibit these sorts of multiple periodicities, which can be demonstrated by asking listeners to tap at different rates on successive listenings to a piece. Musically experienced listeners can tap at different rates related by simple integer ratios (e.g. 1/2 or 2× the basic beat), suggesting that the rate at which one spontaneously taps the beat is simply one level (the 'tactus') in a hierarchy of beats, as shown in Figure 21.3.[8,13]

Scale structure

The numerical ratios between the fundamental frequencies of successive musical tones define the set of pitch intervals used in a melody. The intervals used in any given melody typically adhere to culture-specific schemata, for example, the scales of Western tonal music.[14,15] The intervals of K0016 are drawn from the major (Ionian) scale, characterized by a particular pattern of frequency steps between adjacent tones within an octave (in semitones, step sizes are: 2 2 1 2 2 2 1; a semitone is a ratio of approximately 1.06 in fundamental frequency). Listeners are sensitive to the structure of pitch intervals relative to the schemata of one's

---

[c] The tempo of K0016 has been set to 120 beats per minute (bpm) in the sound examples, that is, one beat every 500 ms. Any tempo between between ~75 and 150 bpm would likely be acceptable.

[d] This helps explain why the music notation for this melody includes a rest in the final position, rather than simply ending with the final note: this rest occurs on a beat. The psychological reality of this rest can be demonstrated by memorizing K0016 and singing it twice in immediate succession. There will be a natural tendency to pause after the final sung note before beginning again.

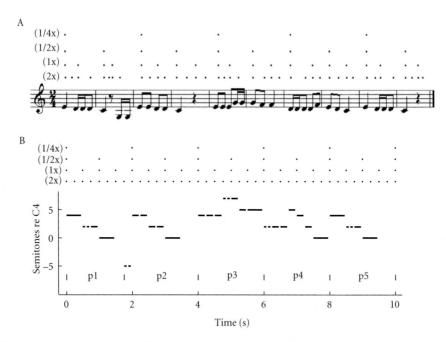

Figure 21.3 Metrical structure of K0016, indicated as a hierarchy of beats above (A) Western music notation. (B) Piano roll notation. To help orient the reader, phrase boundaries are marked below the pitch sequence in (B), and phrases are labelled as p1, p2, etc. (cf. Figure 21.2).

culture.[14] Violations of these schemata are quite salient (sound example 2). In fact, insensitivity to such violations is diagnostic of true 'tune deafness' (congenital amusia).[16]

Contour

The overall pattern of ups and downs created by a sequence of pitch intervals, regardless of precise interval size, defines a pitch contour. A pitch contour and its temporal pattern together define a melodic contour,[15] a perceptually salient aspect of melodies, which plays an important role in memory for unfamiliar melodies.[17] Sensitivity to melodic contour emerges early in infancy[18] and is likely to be related to the importance of intonation in speech perception.[19]

Parallelism

Parallelism refers to motivic/thematic similarity between different parts of a melody. For example, the first and last phrase of K0016 are identical, which helps to provide this melody with a sense of closure. Parallelism need not be so literal: for example, it can be based on similar melodic contours. The study of parallelism is based on the measurement of structural and perceptual similarity. Since similarity is a matter of degree, and is influenced by many factors, the study of parallelism has lagged behind other aspects of music which have more discrete and easily measurable characteristics (e.g. grouping, metre, and interval/tonal relations (see below)). Thus despite its fundamental role in melodic perception, parallelism and its perception is only beginning to be investigated in a quantitative framework.[20]

Intervallic implications

Listeners are sensitive to the patterning of successive pitch intervals in a melody. One source of evidence for this is that if a melody is stopped midstream, listeners typically have well-defined expectations of how it will continue.[21] Interval-based expectancies are the focus of Narmour's 'implication-realization' (IR) model.[5,6] A flavour for the model's principles can be gleaned from Schellenberg,[22] who investigated melodic expectancy in British and Chinese melodies using American and Chinese listeners. Two principles emerged as important factors cross-culturally: 'pitch proximity' (an overall expectancy for small intervals) and 'pitch reversal' (an expectation that after a large interval, the pitch direction will change). The source of these bottom-up principles may be auditory Gestalt principles[23] or experience with the intonation contours of speech.

Tension vs resolution

A remarkable aspect of melody perception is an unfolding sense of tension vs resolution over the course of the entire melody. That is, at each point a listener has some sense of whether the melody must continue or could naturally come to a halt. Bigand[24] has empirically measured this aspect of melody by having participants listen to increasingly long fragments of a melody and judge the stability of each fragment's end.[e] His results confirm that perceived tension varies widely during the course of a single melody. This is easily illustrated with K0016: consider two fragments which stop at the ends of phrase 3 and 4, respectively (sound examples 3 and 4). These differ dramatically in the degree of tension experienced at the final tone, even though both fragments stop at the ends of phrases.

Two factors that contribute to the degree of perceived tension are 'tonal weight' and tone duration.[24] The latter is simple (longer tone = less tension), but the former requires a brief explanation. In 'tonal' music of the Western European tradition different pitches take on distinct structural roles in the fabric of the music. Consider Figure 21.4, in which each note of K0016 has been marked with a number representing each tone's position (or 'scale degree') in the scale from which the melody is built (e.g. tone 1 is do, 2 is re, 3 is mi, etc.). Music perception research shows that once a melody is perceived as being in a particular key, certain scale degrees act as perceptual reference points,[25] especially scale degree 1 (also known as the 'tonic'). K0016, for example, is in the key of C, and the central role of the C note (scale degree 1) is marked in several ways. It is the final tone of phrases 1, 2, 4, and 5, and thus serves as a resting point within the melody and at the melody's end. Furthermore, it always occurs on a beat and is always long in duration. Thus scale degree 1 acts as a perceptual 'centre of gravity' for the entire melody, a role which can be contrasted with that of another tone in the melody (D), marked by the numeral 2 in Figure 21.4. Tone 2 is far more

---

[e] Bigand[24] (p. 811) defined high stability at the end of a fragment as 'the feeling that the melody could naturally stop at this point ... [while] low stability [is] the feeling that there must be a continuation of the melody'. Listeners rated stability on a scale of 1–7. My use of 'tension' is equivalent to Bigand's 'low stability'. Bigand[24] reported stability profiles, which can easily be converted to tension profiles by taking their inverse.

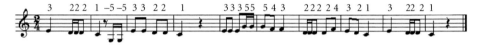

Figure 21.4 Scale degree of each tone in K0016. 1 = do, 2 = re, 3 = mi, etc. (−5 = so in the octave below).

common than tone 1 in the melody (13 vs 4 occurrences), yet tone 2 never serves as a resting point: instead, it almost always leads back to tone 1. Furthermore, it is never long in duration, and frequently occurs off the beat. Thus scale degrees 1 and 2, though neighbours in frequency, play very different structural roles in the melody.

Bigand's 'tonal weight' is simply the degree of structural stability or centrality of each tone in a key, as quantified in perception experiments by Krumhansl.[25] Krumhansl has demonstrated an empirical hierarchy of stability for the notes in a particular key, with scale degree 1 being the most stable, followed by scale degrees 5 and 3 (G and E in the key of C) while degrees 2, 4, 6, and 7 have lower stability (D, F, A, & B in the key of C).

Ornamentation

The concept that some pitches serve to elaborate or ornament others is central to Western European music theory (e.g. the theories of Schenker,[26] Meyer,[4] and Lerdahl & Jackendoff;[8] cf. Cook[27]), and is also found in the music theory of many non-Western cultures, including China and India. For example, in one Chinese folk tradition musicians speak of ornamenting a melodic skeleton in terms of 'adding flowers' to a melody.[28] The ability to distinguish structural from ornamental pitches is thought to play an important role in melody perception, for example, in a listener's ability to recognize one passage as an elaborated version of another.[8] An important issue for the study of melodic ornamentation is understanding the basis upon which pitches are perceived as structural vs ornamental. One relevant study in this regard is that of Bharucha,[29] who used a memory experiment to show that the salience of a tonally unstable note was influenced by its serial position relative to the following note. Specifically, Bharucha demonstrated that an unstable note which is immediately followed by a tonally stable pitch neighbour (e.g. B–C in a C major context) is less prominent/detectable than an unstable note which is not 'anchored' in this way. It is as if the stable tone subordinates the preceding tone as a local ornament and makes it less conspicuous than if the same preceding tone were inserted randomly into the sequence. This suggests that the tonal hierarchy is involved in perceived elaboration relations in music.

Implicit harmony

While melodies present tones one at a time (i.e. 'horizontally'), chords present tones in combination (i.e. 'vertically'). The organization of chords in musical sequences is the domain of harmony. As with the tones of a melody, different chords play distinct structural roles in the fabric of the music, reflecting some of the same relationships which applied to the roles of individual tones. For example, different chords are associated with different degrees of stability, with one chord acting as a point of greatest structural stability: the triadic chord built on the first degree of the scale. This 'tonic chord', together with the chords built on the fourth and fifth scale degrees (the 'subdominant' and 'dominant' chords,

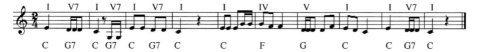

Figure 21.5 Harmonization of K0016. The letters below the staff give the chords in the key of C major, while the Roman numerals above the staff indicate chord functions (e.g. I = tonic, IV = subdominant, V = dominant).

respectively), form a structural core of chords in any key.[25] Although unaccompanied melodies do not have explicit harmony, they can have a strong implicit harmony based on the principle of 'broken chords', whereby chord tones occur successively (often with other intervening pitches) rather than simultaneously.[30] Thus K0016 has a strong underlying dominant-tonic harmonic organization (Figure 21.5), which can easily be perceived by harmonizing this melody with additional tones (sound example 5).

Expression

'Mechanical' performances of a melody (as in sound example 1, which was produced by a computer) involve strict adherence to the relative time values of notes as indicated by the musical score, and lack any amplitude variation. Human performances are never mechanical in this sense, but feature systematic variations in timing and amplitude, which help communicate the structure of the music and the performer's artistic and emotional interpretation of it.[31–33] In addition, there are fluctuations in timing and amplitude due to the limits of sensorimotor control. Listeners are quite sensitive to expressive variations. They can easily distinguish an expressive performance from a mechanical one, and can grasp an emotional valence intended by a performer.

Complexity

In listening to a melody a listener has intuitions concerning its structural complexity. K0016, for example, is relatively simple (informally evidenced by the fact that it can be learned by heart after one or two hearings). Recently, Eerola and North have proposed a computational model of perceived melodic complexity, which successfully predicts data from complexity-rating experiments[34] (Eerola and North, submitted). Their model suggests that perceived complexity is related to the degree to which tonally stable pitches are emphasized and to the strength of a beat, among other factors.[f]

Meta-relations

In processing a melody a listener hears basic perceptual relations (such as grouping and metre) as well as relations between these relations, that is, meta-relations.[4,37] For example, the slight misalignment of grouping and beat at the onset of phrase 2 in K0016 adds rhythmic energy to the melody (the presence of a note or notes before the first beat of a phrase

---

[f] It is worth noting that perceived complexity has also been computationally modelled in sentence processing.[35,36] Sentence complexity appears to be related to the number and distance of dependent syntactic heads in a sentence. It would be instructive to contrast computational theories of complexity in the melodic and linguistic domains.

is termed anacrusis or upbeat). Another meta-relation illustrated by K0016 is the relation between contour and beat. Consider phrase 4, where the highest tone (F) does *not* occur on a beat: thus this tone is melodically prominent (as a contour peak) but rhythmically weak. This creates a syncopation (i.e. accent on an off-beat tone), which adds rhythmic interest to the melody. As suggested by these two examples, beat is an important player in forming meta-relations with other aspects of melody.

Summary: 'relational richness' in musical melody

This brief review illustrates that musical melodies are a prime example of 'rich relations arising from modest means',[38] and as such are of considerable interest for aesthetic theory as well as for cognitive science. One way to appreciate this relational richness is to compare musical melody to speech intonation. Speech intonation is often referred to as 'speech melody' by linguists and phoneticians.[39] This is reasonable because voice pitch in speech is used in an orderly fashion to convey a variety of information, including semantic focus, pragmatic category (e.g. marking statements vs questions), emotional valence, and even lexical identity (in tone languages). Thus melody is not unique to music. Musical melody is quite different from speech melody, however, as evidenced by the fact that people rarely hum or whistle intonation contours (i.e. these contours seldom attract independent interest).[g] In other words, speech melodies rarely draw attention to themselves and away from the semantic message being conveyed. Indeed, one might think of speech melodies as pitch sequences designed to carry out certain quotidian functions without themselves being memorable auditory patterns. In contrast, musical melodies are designed to attract the attention and interest of listeners, and as a result can remain in memory for decades. This difference between musical and linguistic melodies arises from the nature of the perceptual relations between the basic elements of pitch sequences. These relations are far more intricate in musical melody. If a musical melody is 'a group of tones in love with one another', then a speech melody is a loose affiliation of tones (or pitch movements) that work together to get a job done.[h]

The cognitive neuroscience of melody

The many-faceted nature of melody means that even simple tunes (such as K0016) engage a rich set of mental operations, which serve to structure the relations between tones. Furthermore, these operations occur quite rapidly. For example, K0016 is approximately 10 s long, yet during this time at least 13 aspects of this melody are processed in parallel by a listener. Clearly, then, one desideratum for the cognitive neuroscience of melody is the ability to 'tap into the moment-to-moment history of mental involvement with the music'.[43] In this section I briefly review different approaches to the neural study of melody

---

[g] The Czech composer Leos Janáček (1854–1928) is an interesting exception. He notated speech intonation contours in music notation and incorporated 'musicalized' versions of these contours into his compositions.[40]

[h] I am referring to speech melody in non-tonal languages such as English. In languages with elaborate tone systems (such as many African languages),[41,42] the organization of tones can be quite complex, though I would argue that they still do not attain the relational richness of musical melodies.

and then introduce a new technique for measuring cortical activity during the perception of melodies.[44]

Existing approaches to the neuroscience of melody

The study of melody and the brain has relied primarily on three approaches. The first is the neuropsychological approach. This approach focuses on melodic perception deficits in individuals with localized brain damage (e.g. from stroke or surgery), in order to determine if the affected brain regions are involved in aspects of melody perception.[45,46] For example, such studies have suggested that left superior temporal cortex is involved in the processing of pitch interval information, while analogous regions in the right hemisphere have similar capacities but also play a special role in the perception of melodic contour.[19,47]

The second method for studying the neuroscience of melody is the evoked potential or ERP (event-related potential) approach. This approach is based on extracting stimulus-locked population-level neural activity from the EEG or electroencephalogram.[48–50] ERPs provide excellent time resolution—on the order of 10s to 100s of milliseconds—but due to the spatial spreading of bioelectric currents by the skull and scalp it is extremely difficult to localize the brain sources of ERPs. Thus ERPs are not used for localization, but to examine the neural response to individual tones in melodies in fine temporal detail. Initially it might seem that ERPs are ideally suited to studies of melodic processing, since they can resolve the details of neural responses to single tones. However, the low signal-to-noise ratio of evoked potentials means that they must be extracted from the EEG by averaging, that is, by repeating a similar stimulus many (e.g. 30–60) times and averaging the brain's response time-locked to stimulus onset. Thus ERP studies have not been used to study the brain's response to successive tones in a single melody, but have focused instead on responses to a particular tone in multiple repetitions of similar melodies (e.g. an out-of-key note at the end of a melody).[i] Despite this limitation, ERPs have proved a valuable tool: for example, they have demonstrated the influence of musical training on the brain's processing of tonality relations.[51]

The third approach to melody and the brain is the haemodynamic approach, based on techniques such as positron emission tomography (PET) and functional magnetic resonance imaging (fMRI). These methods provide indirect measures of neural activity via the measurement of metabolism and/or blood flow in different regions of the brain. In contrast to the ERP method, these techniques provide excellent spatial resolution, and can identify specific brain regions whose activity is modulated by particular types of perceptual processes. For example, research by Zatorre and colleagues points to regions in the right inferior frontal gyrus and the right superior temporal gyrus, which are involved in the maintenance of a tone in memory during the perception of a melodic sequence.[52] Unfortunately, both PET and fMRI have relatively poor temporal resolution since blood

---

[i] Theoretically, there is no reason why the responses to each tone in a repeated melody could not be examined. However, this would require a listener to hear the same melody dozens of times in an experimental session. This could lead to perceptual/neural responses which are quite different from those occurring in natural listening situations.

flow and metabolism are sluggish signals, which grow and decay over many seconds in response to the physiological demands of the underlying neural tissue. These techniques thus do not operate at the rapid time-scale of melody perception.

Each of the approaches outlined above continues to provide valuable information about melody and the brain, yet none of them fulfils the desideratum mentioned at the beginning of this section. That is, none of them follows brain activity as perception unfolds in time over the course of individual melodies. The ERP method, for example, 'zooms in' to examine the temporal details of neural responses to individual tones, while PET and fMRI 'zoom out' to examine the overall response of various brain regions to entire tone sequences. Melodic processing in the brain, however, is more than the sum of responses to single tones, and more than an average response to an entire sequence. It is a dynamic process of building mental relations between tones during the course of individual melodies. For this reason, techniques are needed that measure patterns of neural activity as perception unfolds within individual sequences. The study described below is one attempt in this direction.

A new approach for the neural study of melody: the dynamic aSSR (auditory steady-state response) method

Background   Patel & Balaban[44] set out to examine the temporal evolution of stimulus-related brain activity during perception of tone sequences. To accomplish this, we used a brain signal known as the aSSR.[53] The aSSR is a sinusoidal neural oscillation produced in primary auditory cortex in response to an acoustic stimulus with constant amplitude modulation (AM). aSSR frequency equals the acoustic AM rate, and it is strongest when the AM is in the 40 Hz range.[54,55] Figure 21.6A shows an acoustic signal with constant carrier frequency (400 Hz) and constant AM (40 Hz), and Figure 21.6B shows the power spectrum of a brain signal recorded with an MEG (magnetoencephalography, see later) sensor over auditory cortex while an individual listened to this tone for 1 min. A clear energy peak is visible at 40 Hz. When the same tone is presented without AM, no peak at 40 Hz is visible in the power spectrum (Figure 21.6C). Thus the aSSR is a frequency-specific, stimulus-related brain response with a high signal-to-noise ratio. Unlike an evoked potential, the aSSR represents continuous cortical activity, that is, the oscillation is present as long as the stimulus is on.

How can this seemingly esoteric brain signal be of use to the cognitive neuroscience of melody? The answer to this question has two parts. The first is an empirical observation, namely that the frequency specificity of the aSSR is preserved even when the carrier frequency of a tone changes in a step-wise fashion over the course of two octaves, as long as the AM rate stays constant.[44] Thus one can impose a constant AM on a melody and extract stimulus-related neural activity from the brain by measuring activity at the AM rate. Second, while aSSR frequency does not vary in response to changes in carrier frequency, the amplitude and phase (relative to the stimulus AM) of this oscillation *do* change dynamically over time during the perception of musical sequences.[56] It is these latter variables (the 'dynamic' aspect of the aSSR) which are of primary interest. In particular, the key question is whether aSSR amplitude and phase are sensitive to cognitively relevant processes during melody perception, such as expectancy. If aSSR dynamics are sensitive to cognitive

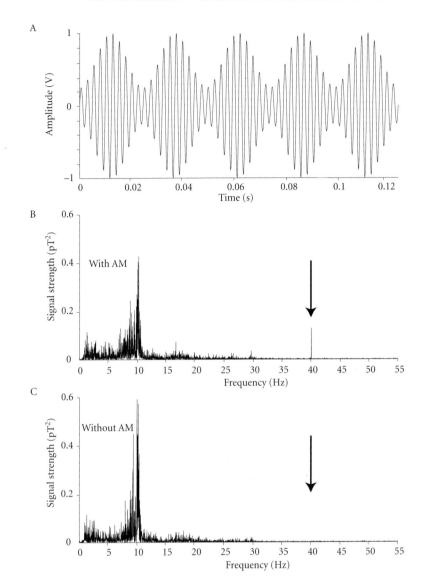

Figure 21.6 The aSSR. Panel (A) shows a 400 Hz pure tone with 40 Hz AM. Panel (B) shows the power spectrum of the neural response to the tone, recorded from an MEG sensor located over auditory cortex in an adult human listener. Note the strong peak at 40 Hz (arrow) marking the aSSR and indicating the presence of stimulus-related cortical activity. Panel (C) shows a power spectrum of the brain signal when the listener hears a 400 Hz tone without 40 Hz AM. Stimulus-related activity can no longer be distinguished.

processes, it is presumably because cognitive processes influence the state of auditory cortex (e.g. its balance of excitatory and inhibitory activity), which in turn influences how the cortex responds to the AM oscillation. Thus the aSSR may serve as an ongoing probe of cortical function, that is, an indirect measure of cognitive processes over time.

Details of the tone sequences employed   To explore brain dynamics during tone sequence perception, we used statistically generated tone sequences. This allowed us to generate novel stimuli which lay on a spectrum from random to deterministic in structure. We elected to use statistical tone sequences rather than precomposed melodies so that the sequences would be unfamiliar to participants, easily generated in quantity, and mathematically well characterized. The latter two points were of particular importance because we were employing a novel brain imaging technique and wanted to have good control over the stimuli.

All tone sequences were approximately 1 min long, consisting of ~150 pure tones (415 ms each) with no temporal gaps. Sequences were diatonic, and ranged between A3 (220 Hz) and A5 (880 Hz) in pitch. Four structural categories of sequences were employed: random, deterministic (musical scales), and two intermediate 'fractal' categories of constrained variation more reminiscent of musical melody. These categories were given mathematical names in accordance with the technique used to generate them:[j] $1/f$ ('one over f') and $1/f^2$ ('one over f squared').[57]

A qualitative understanding of these categories is possible without delving into the underlying mathematics. In random sequences each successive pitch is chosen independently of the previous one, and there are no long-term pitch trends. Deterministic sequences represent the opposite case: they consist entirely of long-term pitch trends (predictable stair-like patterns) with no short-term unpredictability. The fractal sequences are intermediate. $1/f$ sequences have a hint of long-term pitch trends but still have much unpredictable variation from one pitch to the next. $1/f^2$ sequences are strong in long-term pitch trends, but retain a small amount of unpredictability in the behavior of successive tones (Figure 21.7, sound examples 6–9).

Perceptual task and brain recordings   Participants ($n = 5$ right-handed males, 2 with musical training) were familiarized with the different stimulus categories in a training session where examples of each category were presented along with an arbitrary category label (the numbers 1–4). Participants quickly learned to identify the different categories, and during the experiment, classified novel sequences by their category with little difficulty. The experiment consisted of 28 such sequences (7 per category) presented in random order. Stimuli in each category were equally distributed among seven Western diatonic modes (ionian, dorian, phrygian, lydian, mixolydian, aeolian, and locrian). Each participant heard a unique set of stimuli for the random, $1/f$, and $1/f^2$ conditions (all heard the same set of scales).

During stimulus presentation, neural data were recorded using 148-channel whole head MEG. MEG measures magnetic fields produced by electrical activity in the brain, providing a signal with similar time resolution to EEG but with certain advantages relating to source localization and independence of signals recorded from different parts of the sensor array.[58]

aSSR measurements   We used the aSSR to detect stimulus-related neural activity. Each sequence was given a constant rate of AM (41.5 Hz). This AM gave the tone sequences a slightly warbly quality, without disrupting their perceived pitch pattern: listeners heard them as sequences of pitches at the underlying pure tone frequencies (sound examples

---

[j] Inverse Fourier transforms of power spectra with different slopes. See Patel and Balaban[44] for details.

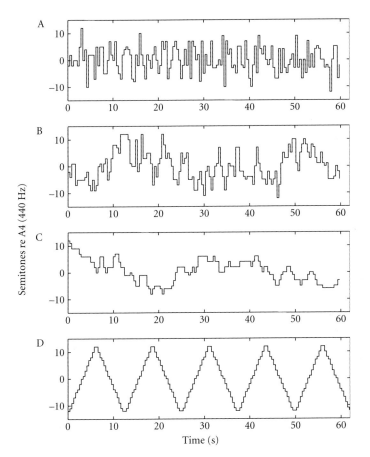

Figure 21.7   Examples of pitch contours from the different conditions used by Patel and Balaban[44] (A) Random sequence, (B) $1/f$ sequence, (C) $1/f^2$ sequence, (D) scales. All sequences had ~150 tones of 415 ms each, with no pauses between tones. The sequences in this figure can be heard in sound examples 6–9.

10–13). For each sequence heard by a subject we studied the amplitude and phase (relative to the acoustic AM) of the aSSR in contiguous 2-s epochs from each channel.[k] That is, one amplitude and phase value of the aSSR was obtained from each successive 2-s epoch of the channel's brain signal via a Fourier transform, yielding approximately 30 amplitude and phase values ×148 channels per sequence.

Since a good deal of our analysis concerns phase information, it is worth giving a brief conceptual explanation of phase. By amplitude modulating our tone sequences at 41.5 Hz, we are introducing an oscillatory signal into the brain at that same frequency. This causes an oscillatory response (the aSSR) at that frequency in certain brain regions. The relative

---

[k] Two-second epochs were chosen on the basis of pilot analysis suggesting that this was the shortest epoch we could study and still maintain a desired signal to noise ratio.

degree of lag between the time-referenced input signal and the oscillatory brain response is measured by the phase of the aSSR.

Results I: phase tracking   Our first finding was that the phase of the measured brain signal varied with the pitch of the tone sequence. As pitch increased, phase advanced (corresponding to a *decreased* lag between stimulus and brain response), and vice-versa. This relationship between aSSR phase and carrier frequency was suggested by early work,[53] and has been confirmed by recent studies,[55,59] but had not previously been studied in a dynamic fashion. The underlying mechanism for this phenomenon likely involves the tonotopic layout of the basilar membrane in the cochlea of the human ear, where higher frequencies are closer to the oval window and hence are stimulated earlier than lower frequencies. However, the degree of phase change observed in the aSSR cannot be solely explained by peripheral neural mechanisms (Patel and Balaban, in preparation).

In our study, variation of phase with stimulus carrier frequency manifested itself in 'phase tracking', that is, in a correlation between the shape of the phase-time contour and the stimulus carrier frequency-time contour (Figure 21.8). As just mentioned, this tracking may be largely driven by peripheral neural mechanisms, and we make no claim that phase tracking has a causal relationship to tone sequence processing (indeed, it is only present because of the AM we have imposed on the tone sequences). Rather, the interesting question is whether phase tracking is modulated by perceptual aspects of the stimulus. We found evidence that this may be the case, in that phase tracking improved as sequences became more predictable in structure. Examples of phase-time contours (solid lines) overlaid on their corresponding pitch-time contours (dashed lines) are shown in Figure 21.8A–D, showing how tracking improves across the stimulus conditions. The best tracking occurred for musical scales, which have a completely predictable structure.

Each subject showed a number of sensor locations where this 'phase tracking' of pitch was observed. Across participants, these locations tended to be in fronto-temporal regions, with a slight right-hemisphere bias. A similar set of locations was identified when we looked for sensors where the amplitude of the aSSR was strong. However, we found no evidence that the amplitude time series of the aSSR correlated with the heard pitch contour (see Patel and Balaban[44] for details).

Results II: phase coherence   Knowing that the phase of the brain response reflected stimulus properties (i.e. pitch contour), we then turned to looking at patterns of phase coherence between different brain regions. Phase coherence does not measure the lag between an oscillatory signal and brain response but rather the stability of the phase *difference* between oscillatory activity in different brain areas. Thus phase coherence measures the degree of temporally correlated activity in distinct brain regions. If two brain areas show greater phase coherence during certain conditions, this is suggestive of a greater degree of functional coupling between regions under those conditions.[60,1]

---

[1] In studying phase coherence at the aSSR frequency, we are not assuming that the aSSR is itself part of the causal chain of melodic processing, but rather that its dynamics are influenced by ongoing brain processes which *are* involved in melody perception. Thus aSSR coherence serves as a proxy for coherent brain activity, which is related to melodic processing. (It should be noted that the idea that phase coherence between brain regions has some functional significance is a topic of active research in modern neuroscience, which enjoys increasing evidence but which has yet to be conclusively proved.)

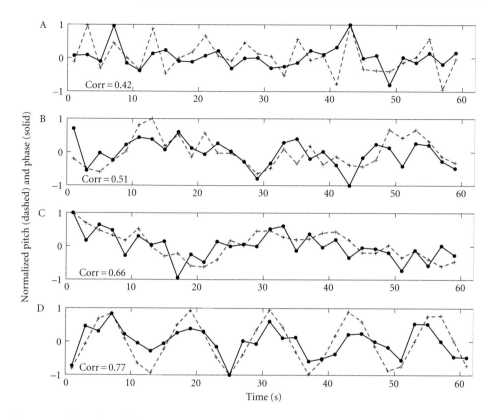

Figure 21.8   Examples of phase-time contours (solid lines) extracted from brain signals recorded with MEG sensors over auditory cortical regions. Each phase-time contour is overlaid on its associated pitch-time contour (dashed lines: these contours have been down sampled to show the average pitch during each 2-s epoch in which aSSR phase was measured). These contours represent single channel, single-trial data recorded from one listener. Correlations between each phase-time contour and its associated down-sampled pitch-time contour are shown in the inset to each graph. Full details of correlation between phase and pitch across sensors, conditions, and subjects is given in Patel and Balaban.[44]

We found that across participants, the different conditions were characterized by differing degrees of phase coherence. Random sequences generated less phase coherence than all other categories, and among the structured categories, scales (which showed the best phase tracking) did *not* generate the highest coherence. Rather, $1/f^2$ sequences were associated with the greatest degree of phase coherence (Figure 21.9A). Interestingly, statistical research on Western music suggests that melodies have approximately $1/f^2$ statistics,[61,62] suggesting that melody-like sequences generated more brain interactions than sequences which were either overly random or overly deterministic.

To better understand the nature of these interactions, we examined topographic patterns of phase coherence, subdividing the brain into four quadrants (anterior and posterior left and right). We found that the greater phase coherence of $1/f^2$ sequences was driven by interactions between the left posterior hemisphere and the rest of the brain, including the

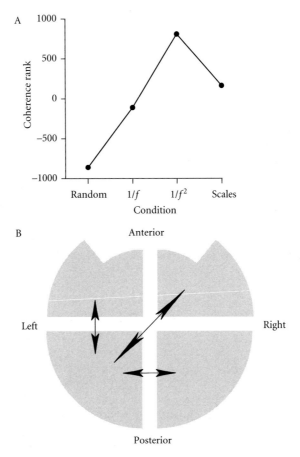

Figure 21.9 Results of phase coherence analysis conducted in order to study the interaction of brain regions during the perception of different sequence types. Panel (A) shows that coherence is lowest for random sequences, and that among the structured sequences, is greatest in the $1/f^2$ sequences (which most closely resemble real musical melodies in their statistical structure). Panel (B) shows the regional interactions underlying this result. The relatively higher coherence in $1/f^2$ sequences results from interactions between the left posterior brain quadrant and other brain quadrants. The coupling between left posterior and right anterior and posterior brain regions may represent a dynamic neural correlate of the integration of pitch interval and pitch contour perception, that is, local and global pitch processing (see text and Patel and Balaban[44] for details).

two right hemisphere quadrants (Figure 21.9B). This is of interest because neuropsychological studies of brain-damaged patients suggests that left superior temporal regions are involved with the discrimination of precise interval sizes, while right fronto-temporal circuits have an additional role in the perception of more global contour patterns.[19,47] Thus the observed pattern of coherence may reflect the dynamic integration of local and global pitch perception, and suggests that this integration is greatest when tone sequences resemble musical melodies.

Conclusions

The study of melody perception provides both a challenge and an opportunity for cognitive neuroscience. Melodies, like sentences, are complex structures, and unraveling the neural mechanisms by which they are understood is a project which is still in its infancy. However, melodies do afford some attractive properties to the cognitive neuroscientist. Their raw materials can be extremely simple (e.g. pure tones instead of phonemes), and their complexity can be systematically varied using quantitative principles.[34] Thus they provide a valuable tool with which to study basic issues in cognitive neuroscience, such as the interaction of bottom-up and top-down processes in sequence perception. Indeed, it is possible that neural principles learned from using melodies may prove useful in understanding brain processing of other types of complex sequences, such as sentences.

This chapter has described a new approach to the neuroscience of melody, based on a method which monitors stimulus-related cortical activity over time during the perception of individual tone sequences.[44,m] Using the aSSR, we have demonstrated that it is possible to extract a signal from the human cerebral cortex which reflects the pitch contour an individual is hearing. The accuracy with which this signal reflects the pitch contour improves as the pitch sequence becomes more predictable. Thus there may be top-down influences of musical expectancy which influence this brain signal, suggesting that future studies may be able to use aSSR dynamics to monitor how expectancy is structured in time.

The basis of aSSR phase tracking is *temporal* information in cortical activity. When the *amount* of activity was examined, no relationship with pitch contour was observed. This suggests that dynamic imaging techniques have an important role to play in the study of music perception, complementing techniques sensitive to the amount of neural activity but insensitive to the fine temporal structure of that activity (e.g. PET & fMRI).

Dynamic imaging techniques also offer the opportunity to study how brain areas interact during perception. It is clear from decades of neural research that the brain is divided into different regions, each of which has a special role to play in perception and cognition. Yet it is also clear that these brain areas must interact to form coherent and unified percepts. Complex patterns such as music and speech engage multiple brain regions, and sequences with different perceptual properties may be distinguished by the pattern of brain interactions they engender rather than by the particular brain regions which respond to them. Using phase coherence, we examined brain interactions as a function of stimulus structure and found that sequences with melody-like statistics were associated with the greatest degree of neural interactions. In particular, we found evidence for strong functional coupling between left posterior hemisphere and right hemisphere regions during the perception of melody-like sequences. This may reflect the perceptual integration of local and global pitch patterns, and suggests that one neural signature of melody is the dynamic integration of brain areas which process structure at different time scales.

Two obvious directions to pursue with the dynamic aSSR approach are the examination of tonality's influence on brain dynamics and the dynamic neural correlates of rhythm perception. The dynamic aSSR approach may also provide a way to examine brain interactions

---

[m] For a related approach based on the visual steady-state response, see Harris and Silberstein.[63]

as a function of stimulus structure in real melodies. This may allow an objective quantification of perceptual coherence of melodies in individuals who cannot easily give details of their perception, such as young children and infants. Without question, future studies of melody and the brain will benefit from the integration of existing approaches (e.g. neuropsychology, ERPs, fMRI, and dynamic aSSR), as well as the development of new approaches. No matter what the approach, the goal is the same: to understand how the mind converts 'mere sequences of tones' into meaningful cognitive and aesthetic experiences, which can reside in memory for a lifetime.

Acknowledgements

This work was supported by Neurosciences Research Foundation as part of its program on music and the brain at The Neurosciences Institute, where A.D. Patel is the Esther J. Burnham fellow. I thank Joseph Daniele and John Iversen for technical assistance with figures and sound examples, and W. Jay Dowling, John Iversen, and Bruo Repp for comments which improved the manuscript.

References

1. **Hast, D. E., J. R. Cowdery,** and **S. Scott** (eds) (1999) *Exploring the World of Music.* Dubuque: Kendall Hunt. (Quote from interview with Simon Shaheen in video program #6: Melody.)
2. **Schaffrath, H.** (1995) In D. Huron (ed.) *The Essen Folksong Collection in the Humdrum Kern Format.* Menlo Park, CA: Center for Computer Assisted Research in the Humanities.
3. **Selfridge-Feld, E.** (1995) *The Essen Musical Data Package.* CCARH (Center for Computer Assisted Research in the Humanities) Technical Report No. 1. Menlo Park, CA: CCARCH.
4. **Meyer, L. B.** (1973) *Explaining Music: Essays and Explorations.* Berkeley: University of California Press.
5. **Narmour, E.** (1990) *The Analysis and Cognition of Basic Melodic Structures: The Implication-realization Model.* Chicago: University of Chicago Press.
6. **Narmour, E.** (1992) *The Analysis and Cognition of Melodic Complexity: The Implication-realization Model.* Chicago: University of Chicago Press.
7. **Hajda, J. M., R. A. Kendall, E. C. Carterette,** and **M. L. Harshberger** (1997) Methodological issues in timbre research. In I. Deliège and J. Sloboda (eds) *Perception and Cognition of Music.* Hove, UK: Psychology Press, pp. 253–306.
8. **Lerdahl, F.** and **R. Jackendoff** (1983) *A Generative Theory of Tonal Music.* Cambridge, MA: MIT Press.
9. **Jusczyk, R.** and **C. Krumhansl** (1993) Pitch and rhythmic patterns affecting infants' sensitivity to musical phrase structure. *J. Exp. Psychol.: Hum. Percept. Perform.* 19(3), 627–40.
10. **Large, E.** (2000) On synchronizing movements to music. *Hum. Movement Sci.* 19, 527–66.
11. **Snyder, J.** and **C. L. Krumhansl** (2001) Tapping to ragtime: cues to pulse finding. *Music Percept.* 18(4), 455–89.
12. **Cooper, G. W.** and **L. B. Meyer** (1960) *The Rhythmic Structure of Music.* Chicago: University of Chicago Press.

13. **Drake, C., M. R. Jones,** and **C. Baruch** (2000) The development of rhythmic attending in auditory sequences: attunement, referent period, focal attending. *Cognition* 77, 251–88.

14. **Dowling, W. J.** (1978) Scale and contour: two components of a theory of memory for melodies. *Psychol. Rev.* 85(4), 341–54.

15. **Dowling, W. J.** (2001) Perception of music. In E. B. Goldstein (ed.) *Blackwell Handbook of Perception.* Malden, MA: Blackwell.

16. **Ayotte, J., I. Peretz,** and **K. Hyde** (2002) Congenital amusia: A group study of adults afflicted with a music-specific disorder. *Brain* 125, 238–51.

17. **Dowling, W. J., S. Kwak,** and **M. Andrews** (1995) The time course of recognition of novel melodies. *Percept. Psychophys.* 57(2), 136–49.

18. **Trehub, S. E., D. Bull,** and **L. A. Thorpe** (1984) Infant's perception of melodies: the role of melodic contour. *Child Dev.* 55, 821–30.

19. **Patel, A. D., I. Peretz, M. Tramo,** and **R. Labrecque** (1998) Processing prosodic and musical patterns: a neuropsychological investigation. *Brain Lang.* 61, 123–44.

20. **Schmuckler, M. A.** (1999) Testing models of melodic contour similarity. *Music Percept.* 16, 295–326.

21. **Krumhansl, C. L., J. Louhivuori, P. Toiviainen, T. Järvinen,** and **T. Eerola** (1999) Melodic expectancy in Finnish folk hymns: convergence of behavioral, statistical, and computational approaches. *Music Percept.* 17, 151–96.

22. **Schellenberg, G.** (1996) Expectancy in melody: Tests of the Implication-realization Model. *Cognition* 58, 75–125.

23. **Bregman, A.** (1990) *Auditory Scene Analysis: The Perceptual Organization of Sound.* Cambridge, MA: MIT Press.

24. **Bigand, E.** (1997) Perceiving musical stability: The effect of tonal structure, rhythm and musical expertise. *J. Exp. Psychol.: Hum. Percept. Perform.* 23, 808–12.

25. **Krumhansl, C. L.** (1990) *Cognitive Foundations of Musical Pitch.* New York: Oxford University Press.

26. **Schenker, H.** (1969) *Five Graphic Music Analyses.* New York: Dover.

27. **Cook, N.** (1987) *A Guide to Musical Analysis.* Oxford: Oxford University Press.

28. **Jones, S.** (1995) *Folk Music of China.* NY: Oxford University Press.

29. **Bharucha, J. J.** (1984) Event hierarchies, tonal hierarchies, and assimilation: a reply to Deutsch and Dowling. *J. Exp. Psychol.: Gen.* 113(3), 421–5.

30. **Povel, D.-J.** and **E. Jansen** (2001) Perceptual mechanisms in music processing. *Music Percept.* 19(2), 169–97.

31. **Repp, Bruno H.** (1995) Expressive timing in Schumann's 'Traeumerei': an analysis of performances by graduate student pianists. *J. Acoust. Soc. Am.* 98(5, Pt 1), 2413–27.

32. **Palmer, C.** (1997) Music performance. *Ann. Rev. Psychol.* 48, 115–38.

33. **Juslin, Patrik N.** (2000) Cue utilization in communication of emotion in music performance: relating performance to perception. *J. Exp. Psychol.: Hum. Percept. Perform.* 26(6), 1797–813.

34. **Eerola, T.** and **A. North** (2000) Expectancy-based model of melodic complexity. In C. Woods, G. Luck, R. Brochard, F. Seddon, and J. A. Sloboda (eds) *Proceedings of the 6th International Conference on Music Perception and Cognition.* Keele, UK: Keele University Department of Psychology.

35. **Gibson, E.** (1998) Linguistic complexity: locality of syntactic dependencies. *Cognition* 68(1), 1–76.

36. **Gibson, E.** (2000) The dependency locality theory: a distance-based theory of linguistic complexity. In Y. Miyashita *et al.* (eds) *Image, Language, Brain.* Cambridge, MA: MIT Press, pp. 95–126.

37. **Jones, M. R.** and **P. Q. Pfordresher** (1997) Tracking musical patterns using Joint Accent Structure. *Can. J. Exp. Psychol.* 51(4), 271–90.

38. **Meyer, L. B.** (2000) *The Spheres of Music: A Gathering of Essays.* Chicago: University of Chicago Press.

39. **'t Hart, J., R. Collier,** and **A. Cohen** (1990) *A Perceptual Study of Intonation: An Experimental-Phonetic Approach to Speech Melody.* Cambridge: Cambridge University Press.

40. **Wingfield, P.** (ed) (1999) *Janáček Studies.* Cambridge: Cambridge University Press.

41. **Connell, B.** (2000) The perception of lexical tone in Mambila. *Lang. Speech* 43(2), 163–82.

42. **Hyman, L.** (2001) Tone systems. In M. Haspelmath (ed.) *Language typology and language universals: an international handbook.* Berlin: W. de Gruyter.

43. **Sloboda, J.** (1985) *The Musical Mind: The Cognitive Psychology of Music.* Oxford: Oxford University Press.

44. **Patel, A. D.** and **E. Balaban** (2000) Temporal patterns of human cortical activity reflect tone sequence structure. *Nature* 404, 80–4.

45. **Peretz, I.** (1990) Processing of local and global musical information in unilateral brain-damaged patients. *Brain* 113, 1185–205.

46. **Steinke, W. R., L. L. Cuddy,** and **L. S. Jakobson** (2001) Dissociations among functional subsystems governing melody recognition after right hemisphere damage. *Cognit. Neuropsychol.* 18, 411–37.

47. **Liégeois-Chauvel, C., I. Peretz, M. Babaï, V. Laguitton,** and **P. Chauvel** (1998) Contribution of different cortical areas in the temporal lobes to music processing. *Brain* 121, 1853–67.

48. **Besson, M.** (1997) Electrophysiological studies of music processing. In I. Deliège and J. Sloboda (eds) *Perception and Cognition of Music.* Hove, UK: Psychology Press, pp. 217–50.

49. **Tervaniemi, M.** *et al.* (2001) Superior formation of cortical memory traces for melodic patterns in musicians. *Learning Memory* 8, 295–300.

50. **Trainor, L. J., K. L. McDonald,** and **C. Alain** (2002) Automatic and controlled processing of melodic contour and interval information measured by electrical brain activity. *J. Cognit. Neurosci.* 14(3), 430–42.

51. **Besson, M.** and **F. Faïta** (1995) An event-related potential (ERP) study of musical expectancy: comparison of musicians with non-musicians. *J. Exp. Psychol.: Hum. Percept. Perform.* 21, 1278–96.

52. **Zatorre, R. J., A. C. Evans,** and **E. Meyer** (1994) Neural mechanisms underlying melodic perception and memory for pitch. *J. Neurosci.* 14, 1908–19.

53. **Galambos, R., S. Makeig,** and **P. J. Talmachoff** (1981) A 40-Hz auditory potential recorded from the human scalp. *Proc. Natl. Acad. Sci. USA* 78, 2463–647.

54. **Gutschalk, A.** *et al.* (1999) Deconvolution of 40 Hz steady-state fields reveals two overlapping source activities of the human auditory cortex. *Clin. Neurophys.* 110, 856–68.

55. **Ross, B., C. Borgmann, R. Draganova, L. Roberts,** and **C. Pantev** (2000) A high-precision magnetoencephalographic study of human auditory steady-state responses to amplitude-modulated tones. *J. Acoust. Soc. Am.* 108, 679–91.

56. **Galambos, R.** and **S. Makeig** (1988) Dynamic changes in steady-state responses. In E. Başar (ed.) *Dynamics of Sensory and Cognitive Processing by the Brain.* Berlin: Springer-Verlag, pp. 103–22.

57. Schmuckler, M. A. and D. L. Gilden (1993) Auditory perception of fractal contours. *J. Exp. Psychol. Hum. Percept. Perform.* 19, 641–60.

58. Lewine, J. D. and W. W. Orrison (1995) Magnetoencephalography and magnetic source imaging. In W. W. Orrison *et al.* (ed.) *Functional Brain Imaging.* St Louis: Mosby, pp. 369–417.

59. John, M. S. and T. W. Picton (2000) Human auditory steady-state responses to amplitude modulated tones: phase and latency measurements. *Hearing Res.* 14, 57–79.

60. Bressler, S. (1995) Large-scale cortical networks and cognition. *Brain Res.: Brain Res. Rev.* 20(3), 288–304.

61. Nettheim, N. (1992) On the spectral analysis of melody. *Interface* 21, 135–48.

62. Boon, J. P. and O. Decroly (1995) Dynamical systems theory for music dynamics. *Chaos* 5, 501–8.

63. Harris, P. and R. Silberstein (1999) Steady-state visual evoked potential (SSVEP) responses correlate with musically trained participants' encoding and retention phases of musical working memory task performance. *Aust. J. Psychol.* 51(3), 140–6.

CHAPTER 22

HOW MANY MUSIC CENTRES ARE IN THE BRAIN?

ECKART O. ALTENMÜLLER

Abstract

When reviewing the literature on brain substrates of music processing, a puzzling variety of findings can be stated. The traditional view of a left–right dichotomy of brain organization—assuming that in contrast to language, music is primarily processed in the right hemisphere—was challenged 20 years ago, when the influence of music education on brain lateralization was demonstrated. Modern concepts emphasize the modular organization of music cognition. According to this viewpoint, different aspects of music are processed in different, although partly overlapping neuronal networks of both hemispheres. However, even when isolating a single 'module', such as, for example, the perception of contours, the interindividual variance of brain substrates is enormous. To clarify the factors contributing to this variability, we conducted a longitudinal experiment comparing the effects of procedural vs explicit music teaching on brain networks. We demonstrated that cortical activation during music processing reflects the auditory 'learning biography', the personal experiences accumulated over time. Listening to music, learning to play an instrument, formal instruction, and professional training result in multiple, in many instances multisensory, representations of music, which seem to be partly interchangeable and rapidly adaptive. In summary, as soon as we consider 'real music' apart from laboratory experiments, we have to expect individually formed and quickly adaptive brain substrates, including widely distributed neuronal networks in both hemispheres.

Keywords: Music; Brain; Neuromusicology; Music centres

Changing concepts in neuromusicology

During the past two decades, the concepts of brain substrates underlying music processing have changed. Although never unequivocally supported by classical lesion studies,[1,2] traditional theories proposed a simple right-vs-left–hemisphere dichotomy, with music being processed in the right brain, language in the left. This simple viewpoint—still represented in many textbooks—could not be held any longer, when in 1974 Bever and Chiarello[3] were able to demonstrate the influence of professional training on hemispheric lateralization during music processing, nonmusicians exhibiting right, professionals left hemispheric preponderance. In the following years, results of several brain imaging studies supported this idea. In our laboratory, for example, brain activation patterns were investigated during demanding harmonic and melodic discrimination tasks in a large group of nonmusicians, amateurs, and professional musicians. Professional musicians processed these tasks primarily in the left frontotemporal lobes, whereas amateurs as well as nonmusicians bilaterally activated the frontal lobes and the right temporal lobe.[4] It was assumed that professional musicians had access to different cognitive strategies ascompared to amateurs and nonmusicians. The left hemisphere activation in professionals was attributed to covert inner speech, since trained musicians—as a consequence of hundreds of lessons of ear training and solfège—reported that they named the intervals and harmonies more or less automatically during processing of the task. In other words and speaking more generally, access to 'auxiliary' representations of music acquired during training was discussed as accounting in part for the variability in brain activation patterns during music listening. Consequently, brain substrates of music processing were supposed to reflect the *way of listening and processing* rather than more-or-less fixed 'music centres'.

Listening to music: concepts of perceptive modules and hierarchies

Before considering brain substrates of music processing, we have to clarify what we term 'music' in this context. To our understanding, music is not a mere acoustic structure in time, or a stimulus created in a laboratory to fit a well-controlled experimental design, but a phenomenon of subjective human experience. Such an experience is not based on a uniform mental capacity but on a complex set of perceptive and cognitive operations represented in the central nervous system. These operations act interdependently in some parts, independently in others. They are integrated in time and linked to previous experiences with the aid of memory systems, thus enabling us to perceive, or better, to 'feel' a sort of meaning while listening. Neuromusicology has been profoundly influenced by the idea of the *modularity of musical functions*.[5,6] According to Fodor,[5] a module corresponds to a specialized computational device that is devoted to the execution of some biologically important function. Applied to music, this concept has been put forward by the groups of Isabelle Peretz and Robert Zatorre, demonstrating convincingly the neuropsychological fractionation of different musical subfunctions in patients following brain lesions.[7–12] Taking together the results of these studies, we see that a complex pattern of distinct dissociation syndromes with isolated loss of cognitive subunits of music processing following a lesion emerges. For example, there is evidence that separate modules are processing time or pitch structures of complex musical stimuli. Generally speaking, time structures seem to be processed to a greater extent in the left temporal lobe, whereas pitch structures may be processed primarily in right temporal lobe networks. According to recent results, a predominance of the posterior portions of the right supratemporal lobe for processing of pitch structures may exist.[13]

Such a modular organization concerning processing of segregated physical (temporal or pitch) properties of musical structures could account for the involvement of separated, in part, overlapping, neuronal substrates. However, the situation becomes more complex when one considers that perception of music may occur on different hierarchical levels. With respect to temporal structures, for example, two levels of organization may be distinguished: metre and rhythm. Rhythm is defined as the serial relation of durations between different acoustical events in a train of sounds—that is, rhythm represents a serial durational pattern—whereas metre involves a temporal invariance in terms of the regular recurrence of pulses or beats marking off equal durational units, which can be organized as measures. Metre therefore represents a more complex acoustical 'gestalt', since its perception and production require information on sound intensity (accented and unaccented events) and on periodicity of rhythmical events, the latter based on integration of information over longer time periods. Again, by means of neuropsychological fractionation of perceptive subfunctions in patients with brain lesions, it was possible to isolate neuronal networks processing metre and rhythm, demonstrating spared metric judgement but disrupted rhythmic discrimination.[7] It is beyond the scope of the present contribution to discuss the complex issue of local vs global gestalt processing in the auditory domain. Whereas in the visual modality, a dissociation of neuronal substrates concerned with local (left parietal) or global (right parietal) processing can clearly be demonstrated,[14] in the auditory modality such a clear-cut neuroanatomical distinction is still under debate. This may be related to the methodological problem of fractionating time structures in appropriate perceptive units allowing for a clear and interindividually consistent discrimination between local or global processing units. In fact, most experimental designs have not been very convincing in excluding variable time fractionation based on rapidly changing individual auditory habits.

'Music centres' in the brain reflecting the auditory biography

Although lesion studies conducted in larger groups of patients suffering from well-defined lesions support the idea of modularity and hierarchy and yield relatively clear results, it still remains a scientific challenge to further clarify the nature and function of these hypothesized modules and hierarchies and to delineate their degree of autonomy and specificity to music. Another, in our opinion, even more urgent problem arises when taking a look at the individual data. In a recently published study,[15] where procedures were performed on patients suffering from small unilateral ischemic lesions of the temporal, parietal, or frontal lobe, respectively, a surprising heterogeneity of the patterns of impairment with respect to modular subfunctions of auditory processing emerged. Whereas none of the patients had a deficit in basic auditory perception as, for example, in pitch discrimination, in some individuals right hemispheric lesions produced deficits in more complex temporal or pitch organization tasks, including in all instances, however, a combined deficit of local as well as global processing stages. Following left hemispheric stroke, surprisingly dissociated impairments of rhythm, metre, interval, or contour processing occurred, irrespective of whether the lesion was localized anterior or posterior to the central sulcus. In summary, it emerged that individually variable varieties of brain regions were necessary to ensure complex auditory functions, including parts of the posterior parietal lobes and the frontal lobes. It therefore becomes evident that not only the temporal lobes, as suggested in the comprehensive study of Liégois-Chauvel and co-workers,[13] but widespread and individually developed neuronal networks may underlie music processing. Without going into methodological details, it should be mentioned in this context that our patients were investigated relatively early—7–14 days following the ischemic stroke—before profound plastic changes compensating for impaired functions had reached their full extent. The discrepancies with earlier studies applying similar test batteries can in part be explained by the early timing of the investigation.

When considering individual factors as possible sources of variability in brain substrates of music processing, the next step is to further delineate the nature of these factors. In order to clarify whether the *way of learning music* plays an important role, we investigated the impact of music education on brain activation patterns in a group of 13- to 15-year-old students[16] in close cooperation with the music educator Wilfried Gruhn. The hypotheses were that (1) learning music and acquiring a new mental representation of music changes brain activation patterns while listening to music, and that (2) different ways of music learning may cause various mental representations that are reflected in different cortical activation patterns.

The task was to judge formal aspects of symmetrically structured phrases, so-called musical periods that consist of corresponding parts, 'antecedent' and 'consequent'. Students had to distinguish between correct and incorrect (balanced or unbalanced) phrases. Whereas the antecedent phrase ends in a weak cadence on the dominant, suspending the expected tonic (half cadence), the consequent phrase leads to a stable ending on the tonic (perfect cadence). This different quality of cadences and the balance of the two melodic parts can easily be recognized merely by an internal feeling of musical balance and the tension of the cadence. For training, subjects were divided into three subgroups: (1) a 'declarative' learner group that received traditional instructions about the antecedent and consequent and their tonal relationship with respect to the closing on a complete or incomplete cadence (the instructions included verbal explanations, visual aids, notations, verbal rules, and some musical examples that were played for the subjects, but never sung or performed); (2) a 'procedural' learner group that participated in musical experiences for establishing genuine musical representations by singing and playing, improvising with corresponding rhythmic and tonal elements, or performing examples from the music literature; and (3) a control group of nonlearners who did not receive any instruction about or in music. Low-frequency DC shifts of the electroencephalogram (EEG) were measured prior to learning and after a five-week training period.

In Figure 22.1, the main results of the study are summarized. After learning, in the verbally trained 'declarative' group, music processing produced an increased activation of the left frontotemporal brain regions, which probably reflects inner speech and analytical, step-by-step processing. By contrast, the musically trained 'procedural' group showed increased activation of the right frontal and of bilateral parietooccipital lobes, which may be ascribed to a more global way of processing and to visuospatial associations. These results demonstrate for the first time directly that musical expertise influences auditory brain activation patterns and that changes in these activation patterns depend on the teaching strategies applied. In other words, *brain substrates of music processing reflect the auditory learning 'biography', the personal experiences accumulated over time.* Listening to music, learning to play an instrument, formal instruction, and professional training result in multiple, in many instances multisensory, representations of music, which seem to be partly interchangeable and rapidly adaptive.

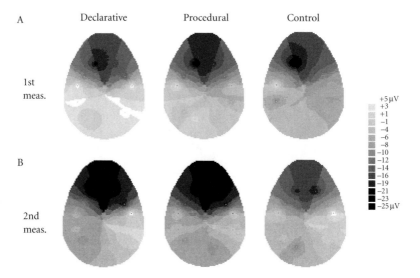

Figure 22.1 Brain maps demonstrating cortical activation patterns (A) before and (B) after learning in the 'Declarative' learning group, in the 'Procedural' learning group, and in the 'Control' group. Group averages are displayed. Activation is *dark*, inactivation is *white* (see microvolt scale on the *right*). The brain diagrams are displayed as *top views*, frontal regions up, left hemisphere on the *left*, right hemisphere on the *right*. As can be recognized, declarative, mainly verbally mediated training leads to an increase in brain activity over the left frontal areas, whereas procedural, genuinely musical training produces an increase in activity over right frontal and bilateral parietooccipital regions. In controls, overall activity decreased slightly. (Modified from Ref. 16.)

A tentative model on brain substrates of music processing

It is not a particularly fruitful approach to look at brain substrates of music processing from such a solipsistic viewpoint, stating that presently around six billion different auditory biographies may produce the same number of different 'music centres' in the brain. Many aspects of auditory processing in general and music processing in particular are necessarily bound to fixed neuronal substrates common to all humans and mainly located in the superior temporal gyrus. As a sort of division of labour, hemispheric specialization may take place at a very early stage of auditory processing: the left superior temporal gyrus seems to be specialized for very rapid processes requiring high temporal resolution such as the identification of different phonemes, whereas the right superior temporal lobe is specialized for spectral analyses of sound.[17] Even at such an early stage, however, the brain substrates underlying auditory processing remain adaptive and subject to plastic changes as a consequence of conditioning or training.[18,19]

In Figure 22.2, a tentative model illustrating the interrelationship between the complexity of neuronal networks involved in music processing (*y*-axis) and the complexity of auditory processing (*x*-axis) is outlined. An additional dimension can be added on the *z*-axis, accounting for effects of acculturation. The complexity of neuronal networks increases

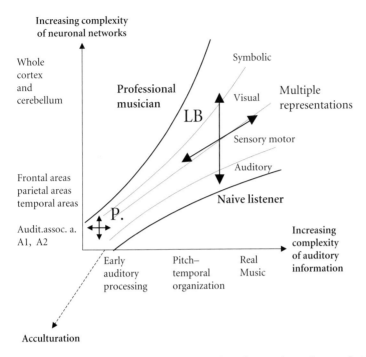

Figure 22.2 A simplified model demonstrating the interdependency between increasing complexity of auditory information processing (*x*-axis) and increasing complexity of neuronal networks (*y*-axis). *P.* = plasticity, *L.B.* = learning biography. *A1, A2,* and *audit. assoc. a* stand for primary auditory cortex, secondary auditory cortex, and auditory association cortices. For further explanation, see text.

with the complexity of processing demands. Training and practice add additional mental representations of music that rely on different brain substrates. Therefore, professionals presumably use larger and more complex neuronal networks during music processing than do nonprofessionals. The actual network engaged in a defined processing task is not fixed, but is subject to short- and long-term plastic changes, allowing at early processing stages for adaptations and compensations in case of damage to certain brain substrates. For example, a bilateral lesion of the primary auditory cortices with complete cortical deafness may be compensated for.[20] The vertical axis of the small cross 'P'. (for plasticity) on the left symbolizes such a reciprocal replacement of brain functions by other brain structures. The horizontal axis relates to the fact that listeners may add or reduce complexity of auditory processing by adapting their listening strategies. When entering more advanced processing stages, including many neuropsychological laboratory experiments, the learning biography, determining the multiplicity of different auditory representations may influence the actual network used for music processing. According to actual demands or as a reaction to brain lesions, processing strategies may lead to a simplified or to a more complex way to listen to the stimuli or music, respectively. Learning biography (*LB*) and auditory strategies are symbolized by the larger cross on the right in the diagram. For the sake of clarity, other variables influencing brain activation patterns during music processing have been omitted: guidance of attention, emotions, working memory, procedural and explicit short- and long-term memory systems, and effects of acculturation play an important role, rendering the brain substrates of music processing still more complex.

In summary, as soon as we consider 'real music' apart from laboratory experiments, we have to expect individually formed and quickly adaptive brain substrates, including widely distributed neuronal networks in both hemispheres. In our laboratories, we are just beginning to face the enormous challenges linked to the clarification of rules determining this puzzling variety of findings, determining the complexity and transitoriness of neuronal interactions during music processing. Two hundred years ago, the German poet Johann Wolfgang von Goethe recognized and expressed this problem in a masterful way in the 'scene in the laboratory':

> *Homunculus*: That is the way that things are apt to take:
> The cosmos scarce will compass nature's kind
> But man's creations need to be confined. (Johann Wolfgang von Goethe, *Faust*, Part II, Act II. Scene in the Laboratory. Translated by Philip Wayne)

References

1. Henschen, S. E. (1920) Über Amusie. In *Klinische und anatomische Beiträge zur Pathologie des Gehirns*, vol. 5. Stockholm: Nordiska Bokhandeln, pp. 137–213.

2. Uvstedt, H. J. (1937) The method of examination in amusia. *Acta Psychiatr. Neurol.* 12, 447–55.

3. Bever, T. G. and R. I. Chiarello (1974) Cerebral dominance in musicians and non-musicians. *Science* 185, 537–40.

4. Altenmüller, E. (1989) Cortical DC-potentials as electrophysiological correlates of hemispheric dominance of higher cognitive functions. *Int. J. Neurosci.* 47, 1–14.

5. Fodor, G. A. (1983) *The Modularity of Mind*. Cambridge, MA: MIT Press.

6. Gardner, H. (1983) *Frames of Mind. The Theory of Multiple Intelligences*. New York: Basic Books.

7. Peretz, I. (1990) Processing of local and global musical information by unilateral brain-damaged patients. *Brain* 113, 1185–205.

8. Peretz, I. (1993) Auditory agnosia: a functional analysis. In S. McAdams and E. Bigand (eds) *Thinking in Sound: The Cognitive Psychology of Human Audition*. Oxford: Clarendon Press, pp. 199–230.

9. Peretz, I., R. Kolinsky, M. Tram, *et al.* (1994) Functional dissociations following bilateral lesions of auditory cortex. *Brain* 117, 1283–301.

10. Peretz, I. and L. Gagnon (1999) Dissociation between recognition and emotional judgements for melodies. *Neurocase* 5, 21–30.

11. Zatorre, R. J. and S. Samson (1991) Role of right temporal neocortex in retention of pitch in auditory short-term memory. *Brain* 114, 2403–17.

12. Zatorre, R. J., A. C. Evans, and E. Meyer (1994) Neural mechanisms underlying melodic perception and memory for pitch. *J. Neurosci.* 14, 1908–19.

13. Liégeois-Chauvel, C., I. Peretz, M. Babaï, *et al.* (1998) Contribution of different cortical areas in the temporal lobes to music processing. *Brain* 121, 1853–67.

14. Heinze, H. J., G. R. Mangun, W. Burchert, *et al.* (1994) Combined spatial and temporal imaging of brain activity during visual selective attention in humans. *Nature* 372, 543–6.

15. Schuppert, M., T. F. Münte, B. M. Wieringa, *et al.* (2000) Receptive amusia: evidence for cross-hemispheric neural networks underlying music processing strategies. *Brain* 123, 546–59.

16. Altenmüller, E., W. Gruhn, D. Parlitz, *et al.* (1997) Music learning produces changes in brain activation patterns: a longitudinal DC-EEG-study. *Int. J. Arts Med.* 5, 28–34.

17. Zatorre, R. J. (2001) Neural specialization for tonal processing. In R. Zatorre and I. Peretz (eds) *The biological foundations of music*. Annals of the New York Academy of Sciences, Vol. 290, pp. 193–210.

18. Pantev, C., A. Wollbrink, L. E. Roberts, *et al.* (1999) Short-term plasticity of the human auditory cortex. *Brain Res.* 842, 192–9.

19. Weinberger, N. M. and J. S. Bakin (1998) Learning-induced physiological memory in adult primary auditory cortex: receptive field plasticity, model and mechanisms. *Audiol. Neuro-Otol.* 3, 145–67.

20. Tramo, M. J., J. J. Bharucha, and F. Musiek (1989) Music perception and cognition following bilateral lesions of auditory cortex. *J. Cognit. Neurosci.* 2, 195–212.

PART V

MUSICAL EXPERTISE/BRAIN PLASTICITY

CHAPTER 23

FUNCTIONAL ORGANIZATION AND PLASTICITY OF AUDITORY CORTEX

JOSEF P. RAUSCHECKER

Remarkable as our cerebral cortex is in many respects, its ability to self-organize in response to extrinsic stimuli is perhaps the most astonishing property of all. The three chapters in this section are all impressive testimony to this ability. The effects of musical experience can be found on various levels: in the gross-anatomical differences between professional musicians with absolute pitch[1] (Chapter 24, this volume) to the subtle functional differences after musical training found with magnetoencephalography[2] (Chapter 25, this volume) or transcranial magnetic stimulation[3] (Chapter 26, this volume). Of course, even the ability to learn and memorize a simple tune is an expression of the brain's ability to change with musical experience. In this case, the changes would have to be sought in even finer modifications of synaptic strength in distributed cortical networks.

Basic principles of cortical plasticity

The tenet that learning and memory is based on changes of synaptic efficacy was propagated, among others, by Hebb.[4] More specifically, he postulated that the conjunction of pre- and postsynaptic activity contributes to a strengthening of synaptic connections. Hebb's ideas were applied to many different areas of neuroplasticity, but perhaps most prominently so in the field of visual cortical plasticity. Developing visual cortex became a model system for the study of neural plasticity when Wiesel and Hubel had established many of the fundamental facts, such as ocular dominance plasticity after monocular lid closure.[5] The development of orientation selectivity was also proposed early on as an example of experience-dependent plasticity at the single-neuron level[6] and was later shown to follow Hebbian rules.[7,8]

Improved auditory abilities in the blind

Deprivation in one sensory modality, such as vision, can also lead to dramatic reorganization in other modalities, such as hearing or touch.[9] The mechanisms of cross-modal plasticity of

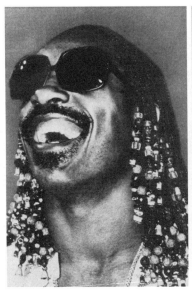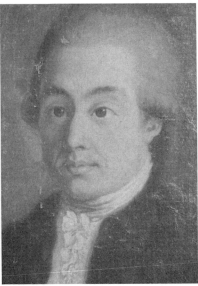

Figure 23.1 Anecdotal evidence reports superior musical abilities in blind individuals. *Left*: Stevie Wonder. From: *The Rolling Stone. Illustrated History of Rock and Roll.* A. DeCurtis, J. Henke, H. George-Warren (eds) New York: Random House, p. 294. *Right*: Wolfgang Amadeus Mozart, though not blind, possibly suffered from strabismic amblyopta, reducing vision in one or both eyes by an unknown amount. Portrait attributed to Kymli of Mannheim, Germany, 1783 (held in a private collection). (See Plate 17 in colour section.)

the auditory cortex appear to be the same as those of visual cortical plasticity.[10] Compensatory improvement of auditory abilities in the blind had long been postulated, claiming, among other things, improved musical abilities (Figure 23.1).

While it is often difficult to quantitatively assess musical abilities, other auditory perceptual capacities can be tested more easily. An ability of blind people to localize sounds with greater precision has been found in a number of recent studies.[11,12] These studies followed on the footsteps of work in visually deprived cats[13] and ferrets[14] that had also demonstrated improved sound localization abilities in these animals. Animal studies can additionally be used to find the neural bases of these behavioural improvements. In blind cats, visually deprived by binocular lid suture from birth, an area in the parietal cortex (the anterior ectosylvian visual area [AEV]) that is normally innervated by visual fibres originating in extrastriate cortex and visual pulvinar[15] is completely taken over by auditory and somatosensory inputs.[16] At the single unit level, auditory cortical neurons show greater selectivity for the position of sounds in space.[17] Taken together, these findings suggest a greater sampling density of auditory space in the cerebral cortex as the basis for the greater precision in sound localization of blind individuals.[9] Furthermore, the expansion of auditory territory in the cerebral cortex would appear to enable other refinements of auditory perception as well.

Modern neuroimaging techniques, such as positron emission tomography (PET), can be used to look for such crossmodal map changes directly in blind humans. During localization

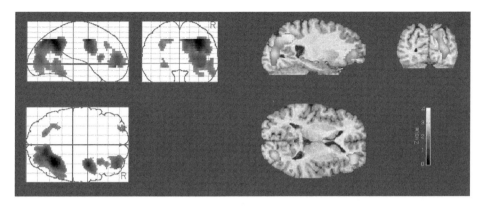

Figure 23.2 Results of PET scanning in congenitally blind subjects during localization of sounds presented via headphones in virtual auditory space (data from Ref. 19). Areas in the occipital cortex that are driven by visual stimuli in sighted individuals are now activated during sound localization. Note that the right hemisphere seems to profit more from the expansion of auditory into visual territory. The 'rewiring' seems to be mediated by the parietal cortex, consistent with studies on visually deprived animals.[9] (See Plate 18 in colour section.)

of sounds in virtual auditory space via headphones, sighted humans normally activate parts of their posterior parietal cortex in an area separate from known visual areas involved in spatial analysis.[18] Blind humans, in addition to activating a much more extended area in the same region, also activate large parts of the occipital lobe, which is normally used for seeing[19] (Figure 23.2). The results of cross-correlating activities in different brain regions suggest that the auditory input to the occipital cortex is relayed via posterior parietal cortex, but a sustenance or strengthening of direct connections from auditory to visual cortex, as they occur especially in young animals,[20–22] cannot be excluded. These surprising results warrant further testing in animals with neurophysiological and neuroanatomical techniques.

'What' and 'where' in auditory cortex

Another fundamental tenet of Hebbian models of long-term memory is that information gets stored in the same places where it is processed. We are far from understanding how lengthy sequences of musical melodies or even more complex pieces of music are stored in our brains, although it is clear that music is a powerful stimulus that activates large parts of auditory cortex in both hemispheres (Figure 23.3). What we are slowly beginning to understand is that complex sounds are first broken down into their frequency components in the periphery of the auditory system and in primary auditory cortex. Then, at later stages of cortical processing this tonal information is integrated into more complex response properties,[23,24] and single units respond to more and more complex contents. The hierarchical processing of such 'what' information seems to take place in more antero-lateral portions of the superior temporal gyrus (STG),[25–28] all the way to the temporal pole. By

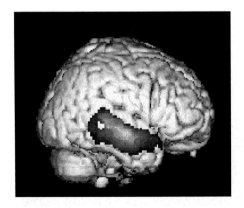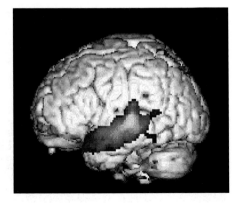

Figure 23.3 Auditory cortical activation while listening to music. Averaged group results of functional magnetic resonance imaging are shown. While the processing of music by the right cerebral hemisphere has often been emphasized[32] (as opposed to language, which is thought to be processed primarily on the left), it is now generally accepted that different aspects of music are processed by *both* hemispheres.[33] (See Plate 19 in colour section.)

contrast, location and movement of sounds are determined in more posterior aspects of the STG.[27,29,30] The latter regions project to the posterior parietal cortex,[31] also known to be involved in auditory spatial processing, as mentioned above.[18,34,35] Anterior STG projects to orbitofrontal cortex, which plays a role in working memory for objects,[36] whereas the caudal STG projects to dorsolateral prefrontal cortex, directly and via parietal cortex, again highly consistent with its role in spatial processing.[37]

Musical learning and auditory imagery

If the anterior STG and orbito-frontal cortex are responsible for the processing of complex auditory 'images', patterns, or objects, they should also be the storage houses of musical memories. Indeed, when we try to imagine music, we activate parts of the auditory cortex that is anterior to Heschl's region (primary auditory cortex) plus areas in frontal cortex.[38] Even when we simply anticipate familiar music, inferior frontal cortex lights up.[39] This may correspond to the involvement of left frontal regions in the retrieval of complex memories, as predicted in a model put forward by Tulving and coworkers.[40] Other brain regions, such as the cerebellum and the anterior cingulate cortex, are also active during anticipatory imagery of music (Figure 23.4). This justifies the idea that mental rehearsal, by activating some of the same brain regions as during a real performance, helps to practice and memorize music, even though we do not actually play the instrument at that time. It is also well known that professional conductors are not only able to conduct hundreds of pieces from memory but also rehearse them mentally, stressing again the partial equivalence of brain activation through attention and mental exercise.

'What' and 'where' information in music come together for conductors of large orchestras. In these situations, the content of what is being played is of utmost importance, but

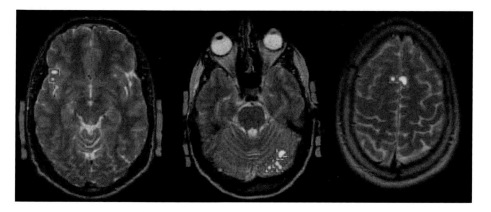

Figure 23.4 Results of functional magnetic resonance imaging during anticipatory imagery of music. The axial sections from individual subjects are displayed in radiological coordinates showing the left side of the brain on the right and vice versa. Imagery leads to activation of anterior regions of auditory cortex in the right hemisphere (in conjunction with right inferior frontal regions; panel on the left of the figure). This emphasizes the role of sensory cortices in mental imagery. However, brain regions outside auditory cortex, such as the cerebellum (left cerebellar hemisphere; middle panel) and the anterior cingulate bilaterally (right panel), are also activated, demonstrating their role in cognitive processing. (See Plate 20 in colour section.)

the location of a particular instrument on the stage helps the conductor to pinpoint the source of errors. Training this ability obviously helps, as has been found in a recent study with event-related brain potentials.[41] Conductors show greater differentiation between positions in peripheral auditory space than nonmusicians or pianists. As attention has been shown to increase brain activation in nonprimary auditory cortex,[42] attentional modulation during rehearsal would be expected to sharpen conductors' skills by modulating the activity of brain regions encoding auditory space. This situation is not unlike that of blind individuals focusing completely on nonvisual events, although in this situation attention only provides the initial vehicle that leads to permanent change. At the single-neuron level, cells have been found in area CL of the monkey's nonprimary auditory cortex that are selective to both the content and the location of complex sounds.[29] Such cells could well provide the neural substrate for the above effects.

Sensitive periods of auditory cortical plasticity

Auditory cortical plasticity can be demonstrated in everyday processes as musical learning, and it becomes even more overtly obvious in the reorganization of auditory cortex across areal borders after early blindness. Age certainly plays an important role in these plastic changes, as the age of onset of musical training as well as the age of onset of blindness have both been shown to be critical for the extent of reorganization. Learning a musical instrument is easier during childhood not only because our motor abilities are more malleable during these early phases, but also because our auditory cortex has sensitive periods for self-organization. This does not mean that we cannot acquire these abilities any longer later in life, but an equivalent outcome will require greater effort. Similar sensitive periods apply to language learning: Learning a second language after the age of eight is definitely still possible, but a foreign accent will usually remain.[43] Again, this effect may have its ultimate cause in a decreasing malleability with age of recipient auditory cortical structures for auditory perception and discrimination.[44]

Conclusions

The connection between brain activation and musical perception is becoming clearer as more and more refined techniques become available to image neural activity. Brain imaging can be performed while subjects are listening to music or imagining it. One can measure the immediate correlates of music as well as its effects on brain development and later brain organization. And, although animals do not have music (just as, in a strict sense, they do not speak), one can still get a grasp of the exact neural mechanisms of music perception by measuring the responses of single neurons in animal studies to various types of complex sounds. An analysis, for instance, of how sound sequences are processed and stored by neural networks would go a long way towards understanding the neural basis of music perception. Other aspects, such as timbre and rhythm perception, could equally be tackled by simpler paradigms in animal models.

Cortical plasticity has to be considered in at least two ways in the context of studies on music and the brain. First, early experience with the world of sound will inevitably shape our brain in an indelible fashion. Enhanced experience with sound, as it occurs with musical training and, inevitably, in blind individuals, can profoundly alter the circuitry of the part of the brain that processes complex sounds in general and music in particular. As we experience these brain changes resulting from cortical plasticity from studies in both humans and animals, we learn to appreciate how expanded areas of the brain lead to enhanced perceptual abilities in the corresponding senses.

Acknowledgements

Supported in part by a grant from the National Institute of Deafness and Other Communication Disorders (R01-DC03489).

References

1. Schlaug, G., L. Jäncke, Y. Huang, and H. Steinmetz (1995) In vivo evidence of structural brain asymmetry in musicians. *Science* 267, 699–701.

2. Pantev, C., R. Oostenveld, A. Engelien, B. Ross, L. E. Roberts, and M. Hoke (1998) Increased auditory cortical representation in musicians. *Nature* 392, 811–14.

3. Pascual-Leone, A., D. Bartres-Faz, and J. P. Keenan (1999) Transcranial magnetic stimulation: studying the brain-behaviour relationship by induction of 'virtual lesions'. *Philos. Trans. Roy. Soc. Lond. B. Biol. Sci.* 354, 1229–38.

4. Hebb, D. O. (1949) *The Organization of Behavior.* New York: Wiley.

5. Wiesel, T. N. and D. H. Hubel (1963) single-cell responses in striate cortex of kittens deprived of vision in one eye. *J. Neurophysiol.* 26, 1003–17.

6. Blakemore, C. and G. F. Cooper (1970) Development of the brain depends on the visual environment. *Nature* 228, 477–8.

7. Rauschecker, J. P. (1991) Mechanisms of visual plasticity: hebb synapses, NMDA receptors and beyond. *Physiol. Rev.* 71, 587–615.

8. Singer, W. (1995) Development and plasticity of cortical processing architectures. *Science* 270, 758–64.

9. Rauschecker, J. P. (1995) Compensatory plasticity and sensory substitution in the cerebral cortex. *Trends in Neurosci.* 18, 36–43.

10. Rauschecker, J. P. (1999) Auditory cortical plasticity: a comparison with other sensory systems. *Trends in Neurosci.* 22, 74–80.

11. Lessard, N., M. Pare, F. Lepore, and M. Lassonde (1998) Early-blind human subjects localize sound sources better than sighted subjects. *Nature* 395, 278–80.

12. Röder, B., W. A. S. Teder-Salejärvi, F. Rösler, S. A. Hillyard, and H. J. Neville (1999) Improved auditory spatial tuning in blind humans. *Nature* 400, 162–6.

13. Rauschecker, J. P. and U. Kniepert (1994) Auditory localization behaviour in visually deprived cats. *Eur. J. Neurosci.* 6, 149–60.

14. King, A. J. and C. Parsons (1999) Improved auditory spatial acuity in visually deprived ferrets. *Eur. J. Neurosci.* 11, 3945–56.

15. Norita, M., L. Mucke, G. Benedek, B. Albowitz, Y. Katoh, and O. D. Creutzfeldt (1986) Connections of the anterior ectosylvian visual area (AEV). *Exp. Brain Res.* 62, 225–40.

16. Rauschecker, J. P. and M. Korte (1993) Auditory compensation for early blindness in cat cerebral cortex. *J. Neurosci.* 13, 4538–48.

17. Korte, M. and J. P. Rauschecker (1993) Auditory spatial tuning of cortical neurons is sharpened in cats with early blindness. *J. Neurophysiol.* 70, 1717–21.

18. Bushara, K. O., R. A. Weeks, K. Ishii, M.-J. Catalan, B. Tian, J. P. Rauschecker, and M. Hallett (1999) Modality-specific frontal and parietal areas for auditory and visual spatial localization in humans. *Nat. Neurosci.* 2, 759–66.

19. Weeks, R., B. Horwitz, A. Aziz-Sultan, B. Tian, C. M. Wessinger, L. Cohen, M. Hallett, and J. P. Rauschecker (2000) A positron emission tomographic study of auditory localization in the congenially blind. *J. Neurosci.* 20, 2664–72.

20. Clarke, S. and G. M. Innocenti (1990) Auditory neurons with transitory axons to visual areas form short permanent projections. *Eur. J. Neurosci.* 2, 227–42.

21. Falchier, A., L. Renaud, P. Barone, and H. Kennedy (2001) Extensive projections from the primary auditory cortex and polysensory area STP to peripheral area V1 in the macaque. *Soc. for Neurosci. Abstracts* 31, 511.21.

22. Rockland, K. S. and Ojima (2001) Calcarine area V1 as a multimodal convergence area. *Soc. for Neurosci. Abstracts* 31, 511.20.

23. Rauschecker, J. P. (1998) Cortical processing of complex sounds. *Curr. Opin. Neurobiol.* 8, 516–21.

24. Wessinger, C. M., J. Van Meter, B. Tian, J. Van Lare, J. Pekar, and J. P. Rauschecker (2001) Hierarchical organization of human auditory cortex revealed by functional magnetic resonance imaging. *J. Cognitive Neurosci.* 13, 1–7.

25. Belin, P., R. J. Zatorre, P. Lafaille, P. Ahad, and B. Pike (2000) Voice-selective areas in human auditory cortex. *Nature* 403, 309–12.

26. Binder, J. R., J. A. Frost, T. A. Hammeke, P. S. Bellgowan, J. A. Springer, J. N. Kaufman, and E. T. Possing (2000) Human temporal lobe activation by speech and nonspeech sounds. *Cereb. Cortex* 10, 512–28.

27. Rauschecker, J. P. and B. Tian (2000) Mechanisms and streams for processing of "what" and "where" in auditory cortex. *PNAS* 97, 11800–6.

28. Scott, S. K., C. C. Blank, S. Rosen, and R. J. Wise (2000) Identification of a pathway for intelligible speech in the left temporal lobe. *Brain* 123 (12), 2400–6.

29. Tian, B., D. Reser, A. Durham, A. Kustov, and J. P. Rauschecker (2001) Functional specialization in rhesus monkey auditory cortex. *Science* 292, 290–3.

30. Zatorre, R. J., A. C. Evans, and E. Meyer (1994) Neural mechanisms underlying melodic perception and memory for pitch. *J. Neurosci.* 14, 1908–19.

31. Peretz, I. (1990) Processing of local and global musical information in unilateral brain damaged patients. *Brain* 13, 1185–205.

32. Warren, J. D., B. A. Zielinski, G. G. Green, J. P. Rauschecker, and T. D. Griffiths (2002) Perception of sound-source motion by the human brain. *Neuron* 34, 139–48.

33. Lewis, J. W. and D. C. Van Essen (2000) Corticocortical connections of visual, sensorimotor, and multimodal processing areas in the parietal lobe of the macaque monkey. *J. Comp. Neurol.* 428, 112–37.

34. Griffiths, T. D., G. Rees, A. Rees, G. G. Green, C. Witton, D. Rowe, C. Buchel, R. Turner, and R. S. Frackowiak (1998) Right parietal cortex is involved in the perception of sound movement in humans. *Nat. Neurosci.* 1, 74–9.

35. Weeks, R. A., A. Aziz-Sultan, K. O. Bushara, B. Tian, C. M. Wessinger, N. Dang, J. P. Rauschecker, and M. Hallett (1999) A PET study of human auditory spatial processing. *Neurosci. Lett.* 262, 155–8.

36. Goldman-Rakic, P. S. (1996) The prefrontal landscape: implications of functional architecture for understanding human mentation and the central executive. *Philos. Trans. R. Soc. Lond. B. Biol. Sci.* 351, 1445–53.

37. Romanski, L. M., B. Tian, J. Fritz, M. Mishkin, P. S. Goldman-Rakic, and J. P. Rauschecker (1999) Dual streams of auditory afferents target multiple domains in the primate prefrontal cortex. *Nat. Neurosci.* 2, 1131–6.

38. Halpern, A. R. and R. J. Zatorre (1999) When that tune runs through your head: a PET investigation of auditory imagery for familiar melodies. *Cereb. Cortex* 9, 697–704.

39. Van Lare, J. E., B. A. Zielinski, and J. P. Rauschecker (1999) Anticipatory musical imagery: functional MRI studies of the human brain. In *Intl. Soc. for Sys. and Comparative Musicol.* Norway: Oslo.

40. Tulving, E., S. Kapur, F. I. Craik, M. Moscovitch, and S. Houle (1994) Hemispheric encoding/retrieval asymmetry in episodic memory: positron emission tomography findings. *Proc. Natl. Acad. Sci. USA* 91, 2016–20.

41. Münte, T. F., C. Kohlmetz, W. Nager, and E. Altenmüller (2001) Superior auditory spatial tuning in conductors. *Nature* 409, 580.

42. Grady, C. L., J. W. VanMeter, J. M. Maisog, P. Pietrini, J. Krasuski, and J. P. Rauschecker (1997) Attention-related modulation of activity in primary and secondary auditory cortex activation. *Neuroreport* 8, 2511–6.

43. Newport, E. L. (1990) *Cognitive Sci.* 14, 11–28.

44. Kuhl, P. K., J. E. Andruski, I. A. Chistovich, L. A. Chistovich, E. V. Kozhevnikova, V. L. Ryskina, E. I. Stolyarova, U. Sundberg, and F. Lacerda (1997) Cross-language analysis of phonetic units in language addressed to infants. *Science* 277, 684–6.

CHAPTER 24

THE BRAIN OF MUSICIANS

GOTTFRIED SCHLAUG

Introduction

Musicians perform complex physical and mental operations such as translating musical symbols into complex motor operations, performing independent movements of fingers and hands, remembering long musical phrases, improvising music, and identifying tones absolutely without a reference tone. The neural correlates of most of these musical operations are not fully understood yet.[1] Several studies have shown that musicians differ from nonmusicians in certain aspects of brain function and structure,[2-14] but questions remain as to whether 'musical' skills and functions are related to these functional and structural differences. The commencement of motor and auditory training for students of music starts at a time when the brain and its components are in a critical period of development. This early commencement combined with long-term training makes musicians ideal subjects in which to investigate whether the almost daily practice of auditory and motor skills over many years leads to functional and/or structural cerebral adaptations. On the one hand, the brain may be highly plastic, capable not only of changes in functional brain networks,[15,16] but also in structural components as a response to increased use.[17-19] On the other hand, the brains of musicians may be 'atypical' prior to training, both anatomically and functionally, and hence a special anatomy or brain function would be a prerequisite for musical skill acquisition rather than its consequence.

Several animal studies have shown that microstructural changes such as increases in number of synapses, glial cells number and volume, and capillary density occur after long-term motor exercises and motor learning in rats within the cerebellum and primary motor cortex.[20-23] More recently, studies have also shown evidence for neurogenesis, mainly in the hippocampus, in rats reared in a complex environment[24] or as a result of long-term motor activity (i.e. running in a running wheel) which was associated with behavioural advantages.[25] It is unknown whether the sum of these microstructural changes could amount to structural differences detectable on a macrostructural level. Only a few studies examined the results of presumed structural plasticity in the human brain.[26,27] The only study in humans besides our own studies on musicians that suggested plastic structural changes in response to environmental demands is a study by Maguire and colleagues.[27] In this study a larger posterior hippocampal volume was found in experienced taxi drivers who are under intense visual-spatial demands of driving a taxi in a large metropolitan region.

Functional reorganization of adult mammalian sensory and motor cortical representations after peripheral or central stimulation or as an adjustment after injury has been found in many different experimental animal models of brain plasticity.[28-31,19] Similar adaptive changes in the cortical organization after skill learning and as an adjustment after injury have been found in humans using electrophysiological or neuroimaging methods.[32–40] These findings have advanced the understanding that functional properties of central nervous system neurons as well as the neural circuitry either within the same or different brain areas, are malleable and retain a significant degree of functional plasticity which could lead to microstructural changes. The term plasticity is a broad term that can mean an adjustment or adaptation of a sensory or motor system to environmental stimuli or performance requirements or a compensation of some cerebral structures for others that are impaired due to injury or deafferentiation.[15–17]

Three human studies are particularly relevant to our studies on structural adaptation which show differences in the sensorimotor representation maps as a response to skill learning and acquisition of new skills. Pascual-Leone et al.[35] showed that as subjects learned a five-finger exercise on the piano over the course of 5 days, the cortical representation area targeting the long finger flexor and extensor muscles enlarged. Karni et al.[38] showed that a few minutes of daily practice of a sequential finger opposition task induced large, incremental performance gains over a few weeks of training, which was associated with changes in cortical movement representation within the primary motor cortex. These authors argued that the changes in the primary motor cortex reflected the setting up of a task-specific motor processing routine while the subsequent changes indicated the consolidation of a motor program. Although several reports have stressed the rapid reversal of representational changes, other studies have found persistent representational changes in response to the early acquisition of fine sensorimotor skills such as having a larger sensory finger representation in the left hand of string players.[7]

Structural brain differences between musicians and nonmusicians

In the search for a morphological substrate of musicianship, several cross-sectional studies comparing adult musicians with nonmusicians were done. A priori defined anatomical regions were selected based on the relevance for musical functions and on data derived from human developmental studies as well as animal experimental studies suggesting a high degree of plasticity.

Subjects, neuroimaging methods, and analysis

All of our study participants were either righthanded, classically trained professional musicians or nonmusicians. A professional musician was defined as someone who was either enrolled as a student in a full time music program in music school or music conservatory or someone who was a graduate of a music program and had his or her main income derived from a professional career in music. The majority of musicians in our studies were keyboard players. We also had a subgroup of string players who were mostly keyboard players as well. For our studies, we contrasted different groups of musicians with groups of nonmusicians who were matched for age, gender, and handedness. A non-musician was defined as someone who did not have any formal training in music and never played a musical instrument for any reasonable period of time. Hand preferences was typically assessed with the 12-item Annett questionnaire.[41] Consistent right-handedness corresponded to performance of all 12 tasks with the right hand with up to two 'either hand' preferences being acceptable.[8,42] In addition to hand preference, we also assessed distal hand motor skills using an index finger tapping test.[43] A laterality coefficient was calculated according to the following formula $(R-L)/(R+L)$, where L (left) and R (right) were the number of finger taps with either hand within 20 s. A subgroup of our subjects also underwent a battery of behavioural and cognitive tests including subsets taken from the Wechsler Adult Intelligence Scale tests (WAIS-R, Ref. 44) as well as other test of verbal intelligence (Shipley-Hartford Scale) and visual-spatial tests such as a mental rotation task and the block design test from the WAIS-R inventory as well as other memory tests and tests of attention.

Neuroimaging studies were performed using a whole-body Siemens 1.5 T MR machine acquiring volumetric T1-weighted brain images with a typical voxel resolution of 1^3 mm. Functional MR imaging studies were done using a T2*-weighted MR sequence that was sensitive to changes in the local concentrations of oxy- and deoxyhemoglobin. Changes in the relative concentrations of oxy-/deoxyhemoglobin are indirect markers of regional blood flow changes that again are indirect markers of changes in regional neuronal synaptic activity. Analysis of fMRI data was done using SPM99, AFNI, and other custom made software. All morphometric analyses were done using custom made software running on HP workstations and mostly implemented in the Advanced Visual System (AVS) image analysis package. Morphometric studies were typically done by two independent investigators who were blinded to the identity as well as to the hemisphere of each brain. Interobserver correlations for the anatomical measurements were usually higher than 0.9.

Corpus callosum

There is evidence that the functional and possibly structural maturation of the corpus callosum extends into late childhood and early adolescence and coincides with the termination of its myelination cycle.[45,46] In comparing 30 professional musicians and 30 age-, sex-, and handedness-matched non-musician controls, we found that the anterior half of the corpus callosum was significantly larger in musicians (Figure 24.1; Table 24.1), particularly in musicians who started training early (<7 years old) compared to those who started late

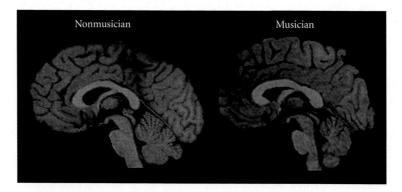

Figure 24.1 *Two MR images showing the mid-sagittal area of the corpus callosum in a musician and a nonmusician. The anterior part of the corpus callosum was significantly larger in musicians compared to nonmusicians.

Table 24.1   Midsagittal area of the corpus callosum

Group	Size of corpus callosum (mm² (mean + SD))	Anterior part	Posterior part
Musicians (n = 30)	687 (85)	371 (46)*	314 (43)
≤ 7 years (n = 21)	709 (81)	384 (42)+	321 (44)
> 7 years (n = 9)	637 (77)	340 (43)	297 (38)
Nonmusicians (n = 30)	649 (88)	344 (48)*+	305 (43)

The anterior part of the corpus callosum differs insignificantly between musicians and nonmusicians (*). This difference was mainly due to musicians who started before 7 years of age with their musical training (+).

(>7 years old).[8] The differences in callosal size might be due to more fibres crossing through the corpus callosum, a larger proportion of thicker myelinated fibres with faster interhemispheric transfer, or fibres with thicker axons or more axon collaterals. The anterior part of the corpus callosum contains mainly fibres from frontal motor related regions and prefrontal regions,[47] and the anterior corpus callosum matures the latest of all callosal subregions. The anatomical difference in the mid-sagittal area of the anterior corpus callosum has to be seen in the context of a requirement for increased inter-hemispheric communication subserving complex bimanual motor sequences in musicians. This structural difference could have been triggered by performing and continuously practicing complicated and independent bimanual finger movements.

Motor cortex

The exact histological extents of the primary motor cortex cannot be defined on current MR images. Therefore, we used a gross anatomical marker of the motor cortex, the intrasulcal length of the posterior bank of the precentral gyrus (ILPG). This marker corresponds roughly with the histological extent of the primary motor cortex.[48] All brains were spatially oriented and normalized to the coordinate system of Talairach and Tournoux. The ILPG was measured in horizontal slices (parallel to the AC–PC plane) from the deepest point of the central sulcus following the contour line of the posterior bank of the precentral gyrus to a lateral surface tangent which connected the crests of the pre- and postcentral gyrus. Results revealed a greater symmetry of the ILPG in the musician group in a dorsal subregion of the motor cortex (Talairach coordinates $z = 69$ to $z = 55$; Figure 24.2).

In addition to the greater symmetry, both left and right hemispheric measures were larger in musicians in this region. The greater symmetry was due primarily to a much larger size of the ILPG in the right hemisphere controlling the nondominant left hand. In addition, we found strong correlations (Figure 24.3) between the age of commencement of musical training and the mean right as well as left ILPG size.[10]

Cerebellum

Several animal studies have provided compelling evidence that the cerebellum shows microstructural changes (e.g. increased number and density of synapses, glial cells, and

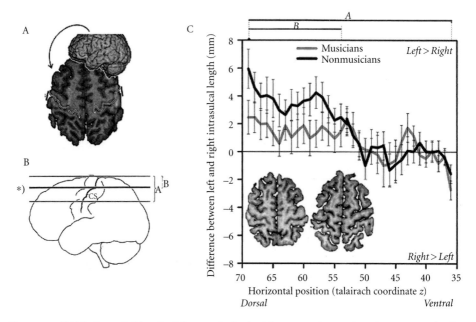

Figure 24.2 (A) The intrasulcal length of the posterior bank of the precentral gyrus (ILPG) was measured in horizontal slices (parallel to the AC–PC plane) from the deepest point of the central sulcus following the contour line of the precentral gyrus to a lateral surface tangent that connected the crests of the pre- and postcentral gyrus. (B and C) We differentiated a dorsal and a ventral subregion. The dorsal subregion roughly corresponds to the location of the functional hand motor area. We found prominent differences in the intrasulcal length of the precentral gyrus in the dorsal subregion between musicians and nonmusicians. Musicians had more symmetrical lengths which was due to a disproportional increase in length of the nondominant hemisphere. (See Plate 21 in colour section.)

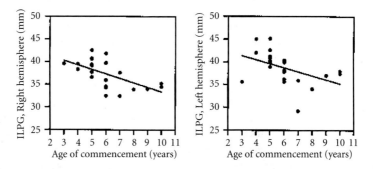

Figure 24.3 Significant correlations between age of commencement of musical training and the intrasulcal length of the right and left precentral gyrus which was chosen as a marker of primary motor hand area.

capillaries) after long-term motor activity and motor skill acquisition. These findings combined with the role of the cerebellum in movement coordination, timing of sequential movements, and possibly other cognitive functions,[49] lead us to examine whether the cerebellum of adult musicians differs structurally from those of nonmusicians.[12] From a

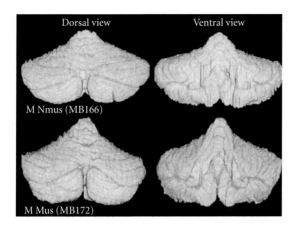

Figure 24.4 Dorsal and ventral views of the cerebellum. Cerebellar volume was normalized to whole brain volume to reduce intersubject variability. The relative cerebellar volume of male musicians was about 5 per cent larger than that of matched nonmusicians. There was a discrete positive correlation between cerebellar volume and intensity of musical training.

Table 24.2   Absolute brain volume and absolute and relative cerebellar volume in musicians and nonmusicians. There was a significant difference in relative cerebellar volume comparing male musicians to male nonmusicians ($p < 0.05$), but no difference in relative cerebellar volume comparing female musicians to female nonmusicians. Female musicians showed a trend for total brain volume differences ($p = 0.08$)

Group	Brain volume (cc)	Rel. cerebellar volume (%)	Abs. cerebellar volume (cc)
Musicians (males; $n = 30$)	1412.0 (84.5)	10.4 (0.7)*	146.2 (9.3)
Nonmusicians (males; $n = 30$)	1405.2 (120.0)	9.9 (0.7)*	139.9 (14.4)
Musicians (females; $n = 26$)	1308.4 (92.3)	10.5 (0.6)+	136.7 (9.6)
Nonmusicians (females; $n = 26$)	1266.6 (76.7)	10.6 (0.7)+	134.8 (11.4)

prospective databank of anatomical MR images of musicians and nonmusicians, we selected MRIs of 56 classically trained, professional musicians matched by gender, age, and handedness to a control group of nonmusicians. In order to compensate for the high intersubject variability in cerebellar volume, absolute cerebellar volume was normalized as a percentage of total brain volume. We found a significant gender effect with female subjects having a higher relative cerebellar volume although males showed a trend for a higher mean absolute cerebellar volume and total brain volume. Male musicians had a significantly higher mean relative cerebellar volume (10.4 vs 9.9 per cent; Figure 24.4; Table 24.2) compared to male nonmusicians. This was not due to a difference in total brain volume since male musicians and male nonmusicians did not show any significant difference in total brain volume. No significant difference in relative cerebellar size was found when female musicians were compared with their nonmusician counterparts. However, female musicians had a trend towards a higher absolute brain volume (Table 24.2).

The results in the male subgroup may suggest microstructural adaptations in the human cerebellum in response to early commencement and continual practice of complicated bimanual finger sequences, similar to findings in animal experiments.[50,20,22] The absence of an observable effect in the cerebellum in the female subgroup may be due to several reasons. First, females seem to reach adult cerebellar size much earlier than males during development.[51] Second, the relative cerebellar volume of females is larger than that of males, possibly indicating that a ceiling effect might have been reached. Third, synaptic up-and-down regulation during the female menstrual cycle has been described and could have diminished a group difference.[52] Fourth, there was a trend for a difference in total brain volume between female musicians and nonmusicians indicating that other brain regions outside the cerebellum might show structural differences. This could indicate gender related differences in presumed structural plasticity.

Regional differences in gray matter volume

A voxel-by-voxel morphometric technique was used to detect local differences in gray matter volume and concentration between musicians and nonmusicians across the entire brain space (SPM99, Functional Imaging Laboratory, Institute of Neurology, London). This method involves spatial normalization of all images to the same anatomical space, extracting the gray matter from the normalized images, and analysing group differences in local concentration of gray matter on a voxel-by-voxel basis.[53] Professional musicians showed higher gray matter concentrations (Figure 24.5) compared to nonmusicians in the perirolandic region, the premotor region, the posterior superior parietal region, the posterior mesial perisylvian region bilaterally, and the cerebellum.[54]

This study replicates and significantly expands upon our previous studies using more traditional morphometric techniques describing size and volume differences in the motor

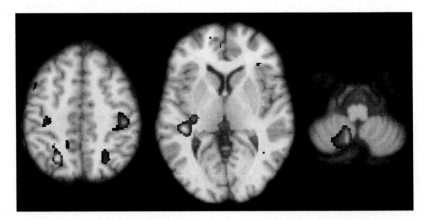

Figure 24.5 Preliminary findings of a voxel-by-voxel morphometric study comparing a group of 15 male musicians with 15 male nonmusicians. Three axial slices show significant differences ($p < 0.05$ corrected) between musicians and nonmusicians superimposed on corresponding T1-weighted structural images. Yellow and red voxels indicate more graymatter concentration in the musicians, blue voxels indicate more gray matter concentration in the nonmusicians. (See Plate 22 in colour section.)

cortex, the cerebellum and the posterior perisylvian regions. In addition, this study showed differences in gray matter concentrations in regions not expected to show differences, such as the posterior superior parietal cortex. The superior parietal cortex does play an important role in music performance, since it may serve as an integrator of visual and auditory information with motor planning activities. Its importance in musical sight-reading has already been shown.[55]

Functional brain differences between musicians and nonmusicians

Most pronounced functional differences between musicians and nonmusicians have been found in perisylvian brain regions with various perceptual tasks ranging from listening to musical pieces, pitch discrimination and memory, harmony, melody, and rhythm tasks.[4–6,11,56,57] It appears from these studies that musicians and nonmusicians process music in a different way, leading to more left hemispheric activation with increased musical sophistication. The reason for this is unclear and the historic explanation of a more emotional or holistic approach to music by the nonmusician vs a more analytic approach to music by the trained musician is an oversimplification of the underlying processes. However, music is certainly not just a right or left hemisphere issue. There may be aspects of music that will be processed more on the right hemisphere by both musicians and non-musicians (e.g. melodic contour tasks) while there are others that will be more processed on the left by both groups (e.g. rhythmic tasks). Of interest are of course those aspects of music that may be processed differently. One example for this may be the processing of pitch information.

A region that seems to play an important role in the processing of musical stimuli is the posterior perisylvian region. This region is known to be very asymmetric in normal right-handers. The planum temporale has long been used as a marker of this asymmetry and in general as a marker of cerebral dominance, at least for language and handedness.[58] It has been found that the majority of right-handers have a leftward planum temporale asymmetry whereas the majority of left-handers have either a symmetric planum temporale or show a rightward asymmetry. The planum temporale is not only a structural marker of left-hemispheric dominance for language, it is also involved in auditory processing and as such is of great interest for studies investigating laterality effects of auditory processing. Recent studies have found associations between PT surface area and functional dominance when listening to stories[59] and the PT has been found to be activated in various musical tasks.[60–64,57]

In an anatomical MRI study designed to test the hypothesis that musicians might have a different degree of hemispheric dominance than nonmusicians, we found that musicians differed significantly from nonmusicians by having an increased leftsided asymmetry of the planum temporale (Figure 24.6). The surprising finding was that a subgroup of musicians, those with absolute pitch, explained all the difference between the musician and nonmusician group. The absolute pitch musician subgroup showed an increased leftsided asymmetry of the planum temporale.[9] Absolute pitch is the ability to identify a tone in the absence of a reference tone. The incidence varies between different studies, but is presumed to be between 5 and 20 per cent among musicians. In a subsequent study, Keenan et al.[13] compared

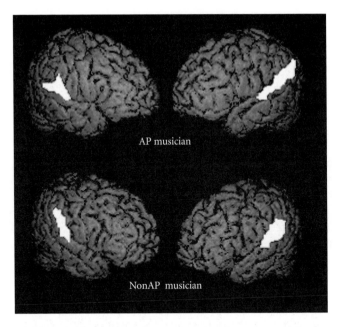

Figure 24.6 Two representative brain renderings. The PT is highlighted in each brain. The AP musician has a pronounced leftward asymmetry that is not seen in the nonAP subject.

subgroups of AP and nonAP musicians with a similar early commencement of music training. Only the AP musicians showed extreme leftward PT asymmetry. Furthermore, Keenan *et al.*[13] found that a decrease of the right PT rather than an increase in the left PT determined the leftward asymmetry of the PT. From these and other studies[65,66] it appears that two factors are of importance in acquiring AP: age of commencement of musical training and an extreme PT asymmetry. In our sample and in other large samples, it is extremely seldom that someone developed absolute pitch if they did not start musical training or were exposed to music before the age of seven.

Although the functional significance of the increased leftsided PT asymmetry in AP musicians is not clear, it has to be examined in the context of their ability to assign any pitch to a pitch class or category in the absence of a reference tone.[67] Siegel[68] demonstrated the influence of possession of verbal labels on recognition memory for pitch. In her study, AP subjects were able to assign different verbal labels to tones that belonged to different pitch classes resulting in a better performance than nonAP subjects. Comparing different tones that belonged to the same pitch class did not result in a performance difference between AP and nonAP subjects since both groups were supposedly using a sensory coding strategy. These results could be taken as evidence for the categorical nature of absolute pitch.[68] We designed a functional MRI experiment that aimed to investigate the functional significance of the increased left-sided PT asymmetry in AP by contrasting two conditions with each other, a tone and a phoneme memory task. In the tone condition, subjects heard a string of sine wave tones (each tone was 500 ms long). A two-alternative forced choice

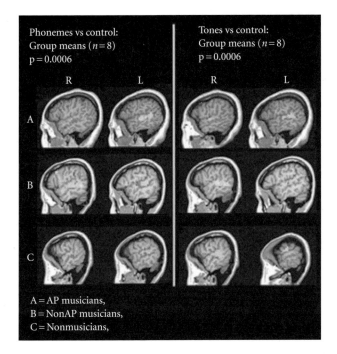

Figure 24.7 Results of a fMRI experiment aimed to investigate the functional significance of the increased leftsided anatomical PT asymmetry in AP musicians. Three groups of subjects were examined: AP musicians, nonAP musicians, and nonmusicians. A phoneme memory task and a tone memory task were contrasted with a rest condition. Suprathreshold voxels showing significant task related activity changes were superimposed on a representative sagittal anatomical image of right and left hemisphere. AP musicians showed prominent left superior temporal lobe activation during the tone memory task that was not seen in the other two groups. The cerebral activation pattern of the phoneme memory task was similar between the three groups. (See Plate 23 in colour section.)

paradigm was used requiring the subjects to indicate whether each new tone was 'same' or 'different' compared to two tones ago. In the phoneme task five different consonant-vowel syllables were presented in the same way as in the tone memory task. AP musicians, nonAP musicians and nonmusicians showed pronounced left-sided temporal lobe activation in the phonemes vs control task comparison. Similar activations were seen in the tone memory condition for the AP musicians. However, the nonAP musicians as well as the nonmusicians showed either symmetric or right-sided activation of the superior temporal lobe in the tone memory task (Figure 24.7). It appeared that in AP musicians, the perception of phonemes and tones is mediated by the same superior temporal lobe structures on the left hemisphere. Nonabsolute pitch control subjects showed a differential involvement of the superior temporal lobe depending on the stimuli. The left superior temporal lobe may be a mediator of a specialized perception that enables the categorization of auditory stimuli.[57]

Recently, Ohnishi et al.[64] were able to demonstrate the preferential involvement of the PT in music perception in trained musicians, with particularly strong activation of the left PT in AP musicians. Zatorre et al.[61] did find left hemisphere activation when contrasting pitch perception in musicians with and without absolute pitch, however, in the critical comparison, only a dorsal posterior frontal region became significant.

Pantev et al.[11] found evidence for an increased auditory cortical representation of piano tones in highly skilled musicians which was not seen for pure tones. There was a correlation between the enhanced representation of tones in the auditory cortex and age of commencement of musical training. No significant difference was seen between musicians with and without absolute pitch. This may have been due to the fact that mainly the N1 which occurs up to 100 ms after tone onset was examined. In a subsequent report, a functional difference was found between musicians with and without absolute pitch. AP musicians showed a distinct activity more posterior in the left superior temporal lobe than the nonmusicians.[69]

Implicit musical ability of the human brain

Although there are differences in the way that musical stimuli are processed between musicians and nonmusicians, it has also become clear over the last years that nonmusicians possess some implicit ability to process musical stimuli. This then leads to the question whether the differences between musicians and nonmusicians observed in neurophysiological studies are either due to training and experience in processing complex auditory stimuli or are due to innate anatomical or functional differences.

Although enhanced cortical responses in the N1[11] as well as in the transient N1/P2 complex have been seen comparing musicians with nonmusicians, there have been other studies showing that early cortical responses to musical stimuli (such as contour violations, etc.) may be processed similarly between musicians and nonmusicians.[70] Koelsch and colleagues[63] examined early brain potentials in subjects listening to violations of musical syntax. The mapping of these changes indicated that neural activity covaried with these events in regions of the brain that were previously thought to play an important role in language processing.[71] Furthermore, these results were obtained in naïve subjects without explicit musical knowledge. On the contrary, Ruesseler et al.[72] showed that professional musicians exhibited a mismatch negativity (MMN), a frontal negative wave in the event-related potential (ERP), for tones anticipated by as little as 20 ms within a series of regularly spaced tones while nonmusicians did not.

Thus, there is evidence for an implicit ability of the human brain to process musical stimuli. It will need to be determined in future studies how training and experience changes the neural elements subserving the perceptual processing of musical stimuli and subserving the planning and execution of highly complex motor action requiring the integration of multimodal sensory information and precise monitoring and feedback.

Summary

Musicians are an ideal human model to investigate possible functional and structural neural changes due to the acquisition and continuous practice of complex perceptions and actions. Experimental animal studies strongly support the existence of microstructural plasticity. Many studies have provided evidence for functional and structural differences comparing musicians with nonmusicians. Although self-selection for musicianship by individuals with innate functional and structural brain differences cannot be completely ruled out, there is now more and more evidence to support the notion that musical training will lead to changes in brain function and structure.

Acknowledgements

I would like to thank all the subjects, musicians and nonmusicians, who participated in our studies and allowed us to learn more about the brain that makes music. I like to acknowledge the enormous contributions that have been made during various parts of these ongoing studies by my former mentor Helmuth Steinmetz as well as by my friends, colleagues and coworkers Lutz Jaencke, Katrin Amunts, Ben Martin Bly, Andrea Halpern, Michael Charness, Ven Thangaraj, Julian Keenan, Siobhan Hutchinson, Yi Chen, and Christian Gaser. Furthermore, this work would have not been possible without the invaluable help, dedication, and efforts of my students Leslie Lee, Maria Picone, Katrin Schulze, Eileen Lüders, and Nadine Gaab. I am also very thankful to my wife, Lisa Jones, for her constant support and her many invaluable contributions to this work.

References

1. Tramo, M. J. (2001) Music of the hemispheres. *Science* 291, 54–6.

2. Bever, T. G. and R. J. Chiarello (1974) Cerebral dominance in musicians and nonmusicians. *Science* 185, 537–9.

3. Meyer, A. (1977) The search for a morphological substrate in the brains of eminent persons including musicians: a historical review. In M. Critchley and R. A. Henson (ed.) *Music and the Brain.* London: W. Heinemann, pp. 255–97.

4. Mazziotta, J. C., M. E. Phelps, R. E. Carson, and D. E. Kuhl (1982) Tomographic mapping of human cerebral metabolism: auditory stimulation. *Neurology* 32, 921–37.

5. Altenmueller, E. (1986) Electrophysiological correlates of music processing in the human brain. *Euro. Archives Psychiatry Neurol. Sci.* 235, 342–54.

6. Besson, M., F. Faita, and J. Requin (1994) Brain waves associated with musical incongruities differ for musicians and non-musicians. *Neurosci. Lett.* 168, 101–5.

7. Elbert, T., C. Pantev, C. Wienbruch, B. Rockstroh, and E. Taub (1995) Increased cortical representation of the fingers of the left hand in string players. *Science* 270, 305–6.

8. Schlaug, G., L. Jaencke, Y. Huang, and H. Steinmetz (1995) In vivo evidence of structural brain asymmetry in musicians. *Science* 267, 699–701.

9. Schlaug, G., L. Jaencke, Y. Huang, and H. Steinmetz (1995) Increased corpus callosum size in musicians. *Neuropsychologia* 33, 1047–55.

10. Amunts, K., G. Schlaug, L. Jaencke, A. Dabringhaus, H. Steinmetz, A. Schleicher, and K. Zilles (1997) Motor cortex and hand motor skills: structural compliance in the human brain. *Hum. Brain Map.* 5, 206–15.

11. **Pantev, C., R. Oostenveld, A. Engelien, B. Ross, L. E. Roberts**, and **M. Hoke** (1998) Increased auditory cortical representation in musicians. *Nature* 392, 811–14.

12. **Schlaug, G.** (2001) The brain of musicians: a model for functional and structural adaptation. In R. J. Zatorre and I. Peretz (ed.) *The Biological Foundations of Music*, vol. 930, New York: Annals of the New York Academy of Sciences, pp. 281–99.

13. **Keenan, J. P., V. Thangaraj, A. Halpern**, and **G. Schlaug** (2001) Planum temporale and absolute pitch. *Neuroimage* 14, 1402–8.

14. **Hutchinson, S., L. H. L. Lee, N. Gaab**, and **G. Schlaug** (2003) Cerebellar volume in musicians. *Cerebral Cortex*, in press.

15. **Rauschecker, J. P.** (1995) Compensatory plasticity and sensory substitution in the cerebral cortex. *Trends Neurosci.* 18, 36–45.

16. **Hallett, M.** (1995) The plastic brain. *Ann. Neurol.* 38, 4–5.

17. **Zilles, K.** (1992) Neuronal plasticity as an adaptive property of the central nervous system. *Annals of Anatomy* 174, 383–91.

18. **Zheng, D.** and **D. Purves** (1995) Effects of increased neural activity on brain growth. *Proc. Natl. Acad. Sci. USA* 92, 1802–6.

19. **Nudo, R. J., G. W. Milliken, W. M. Jenkins**, and **M. M. Merzenich** (1996) Use-dependent alterations of movement representations in primary motor cortex of adult squirrel monkeys. *J. Neurosci.* 16, 785–807.

20. **Black, J. E., K. R. Isaacs, B. J. Anderson, A. A. Alcantara**, and **W. T. Greenough** (1990) Learning causes synaptogenesis whereas motor activity cause angiogenesis, in cerebellar cortex of adult rats. *Proc. Natl. Acad. of Sci. USA* 87, 5568–72.

21. **Isaacs, K. R., B. J. Anderson, A. A. Alcantara, J. E. Black**, and **W. T. Greenough** (1992) Exercise and the brain: angiogenesis in the adult rat cerebellum after vigorous physical activity and motor skill learning. *J. Cerebr. Blood Flow and Metabolism* 12, 110–19.

22. **Anderson, B. J., X. Li, A. Alcantara, K. R. Isaacs, J. E. Black**, and **W. T. Greenough** (1994) Glial hypertrophy is associated with synaptogenesis following motor-skill learning, but not with angiogenesis following exercise. *Glia* 11, 73–80.

23. **Kleim, J. A., E. Lussnig, E. R. Schwarz, T. A. Comery**, and **W. T. Greenough** (1996) Synaptogenesis and FOS expression in the motor cortex of the adult rat after motor skill learning. *J. Neurosci.* 16, 4529–35.

24. **Kempermann, G., H. G. Kuhn**, and **F. H. Gage** (1997) More hippocampal neurons in adult mice living in an enriched environment. *Nature* 386, 493–5.

25. **Praag, H., B. R. Christie, T. J. Sejnowski**, and **F. H. Gage** (1999) Running enhances neurogenesis, learning and long-term potentiation in mice. *Proc. Natl. Acad. Sci. USA* 96, 13427–31.

26. **Dettmers, C., J. Liepert, T. Adler**, *et al.* (1999) Abnormal motor cortex organization contralateral to early upper limb amputation in humans. *Neurosci. Lett.* 263, 41–4.

27. **Maguire, E. A., D. G. Gadian, I. S. Johnsrude**, *et al.* (2000) Navigation-related structural change in the hippocampi of taxi drivers. *Proc. Natl. Acad. Sci. USA* 97, 4398–403.

28. **Merzenich, M. M., G. Recanzone, W. M. Jenkins**, *et al.* (1988) Cortical representational plasticity. In P. Rakic and W. Singer (ed.) *Neurobiology of Neocortex*. New York: John Wiley Sons Limited, pp. 41–7.

29. **Recanzone, G. H., T. T. Allard, W. M. Jenkins**, *et al.* (1990) Receptive-field changes induced by peripheral nerve stimulation in S1 of adult cats. *J. Neurophysiol.* 63, 1213–25.

30. Jacobs, K. M. and J. P. Donoghue (1991) Reshaping the cortical motor map by unmasking latent intracortical connections. *Science* 251, 944–7.

31. Wang, X., M. M. Merzenich, K. Sameshima, *et al.* (1995) Remodeling of hand representation in adult cortex determined by timing of tactile stimulation. *Nature* 378, 71–5.

32. Cohen, L. G., S. Bandinelli, T. W. Findeley, *et al.* (1991) Motor reorganization after upper limb amputation in man. *Brain* 114, 615–27.

33. Jenkins, I. H., D. J. Brooks, P. D. Nixon, *et al.* (1994) Functional reorganization of primary somatosensory cortex in adult owl monkeys after behaviorally controlled tactile stimulation. *J. Neurosci.* 14, 3775–90.

34. Pascual-Leone, A., J. Grafman, and M. Hallett (1994) Modulation of cortical motor output maps during development of implicit and explicit knowledge. *Science* 263, 1287–9.

35. Pascual-Leone, A., N. Dang, L. G. Cohen, *et al.* (1995) Modulation of muscle responses evoked by transcranial magnetic stimulation during the acquisition of new fine motor skills. *J. Neurophysiol.* 74, 1037–44.

36. Pascual-Leone, A., E. M. Wassermann, N. Sadato, *et al.* (1995) The role of reading activity on the modulation of motor cortical outputs to the reading hand in Braille readers. *Ann. Neurol.* 38, 910–15.

37. Schlaug, G., U. Knorr, and R. J. Seitz (1994) Inter-subject variability of cerebral activations in acquiring a motor skill: a study with positron emission tomography. *Exp. Brain Res.* 98, 523–34.

38. Karni, A., G. Meyer, P. Jezzard, M. M. Adams, R. Turner, and L. G. Ungerleider, (1995) FMRI evidence for adult motor cortex plasticity during motor skill learning. *Nature* 377, 155–8.

39. Hund-Georgiadis, M. and Y. von Cramon (1999) Motor-learning-related changes in piano players and non-musicians revealed by functional magnetic-resonance signals. *Exp. Brain Res.* 125, 417–25.

40. Charness, M. and G. Schlaug (2000) Cortical activation during finger movements in concert pianists, dystonic pianists, and non-musicians. *Neurology* 54, A221

41. Annett, M. (1970) A classification of hand preference by association analysis. British *J. Psychol.* 61, 303–21.

42. Jancke, L., G. Schlaug, and H. Steinmetz (1997) Hand skill asymmetry in professional musicians. *Brain and Cognit.* 34, 424–32.

43. Peters, M. and B. M. Durding (1978) Handedness measured by finger tapping: a continuos variable. *Canadian J. Psychol.* 32, 257–61.

44. Wechsler, D. (1981) Wechsler Adult Intelligence Scale – revised. New York: The Psychological Corporation.

45. Yakovlev, P. I. and A. R. Lecours (1994) The myelogentic cycles of regional maturation of the brain. In A. Minkowski (ed.) *Regional Development of the Brain in Early Life.* Oxford: Blackwell, pp. 3–70.

46. Pujol, J., P. Vendrell, C. Jungue, *et al.* (1993) When does human brain development end? Evidence of corpus callosum growth up to adulthood. *Ann. Neurol.* 34, 71–5.

47. Pandya, D. N. and B. Seltzer, (1986) The topography of commissural fibers. In F. Lepore, M. Ptito, and H. H. Jasper (ed.) *Two Hemispheres – One Brain. Functions of the Corpus Callosum,* New York: Alan R Liss, pp. 47–73.

48. Amunts, K., G. Schlaug, A. Schleicher, H. Steinmetz, A. Dabringhaus, P. E. Roland, and K. Zilles (1996) Asymmetry in the human motor cortex and handedness. *Neuroimage* 4, 216–22.

49. **Schmahmann, J. D.** and **J. C. Sherman** (1998) The cerebellar cognitive affective syndrome. *Brain* 121, 561–79.

50. **Psych, J. J.** and **G. M. Weiss,** (1979) Exercise during development induces an increase in purkinje cell dendritic tree size. *Science* 206, 230–1.

51. **Caviness, V. S., D. N. Kennedy, C. Richelme, J. Rademacher,** and **P. A. Filipek** (1996) The human brain age 7–11 years: a volumetric analysis based on magnetic resonance images. *Cerebr. Cortex* 6, 726–36.

52. **Woolley, C. S.** and **B. S. McEwen** (1992) Estradiol mediates fluctuation in hippocampal synapse density during the estrous cycle in the adult rat. *J. Neurosci.* 12, 2549–54.

53. **Ashburner, J.** and **K. J. Friston** (2000) Voxel-based morphometry – the methods. *Neuroimage* 11, 805–21.

54. **Gaser, C.** and **G. Schlaug** (2001) Brain structures differ between musicians and non-musicians. *Neuroimage* 13, S1168.

55. **Sergent, J., E. Zuck, S. Terriah,** and **B. MacDonald** (1992) Distributed neural network underlying musical sight-reading and keyboard performance. *Science* 257, 106–9.

57. **Bly, B. M., C. Gaser,** and **G. Schlaug** The functional anatomy of pitch perception, submitted.

58. **Steinmetz, H., J. Volkmann, L. Jäncke,** and **H. J. Freund** (1991) Anatomical left-right asymmetry of language-related temporal cortex is different in left- and right-handers. *Ann. Neurol.* 29, 315–19.

59. **Tzourio, N., B. Nkanga-Ngila,** and **B. Mazoyer** (1998) Left planum temporale surface correlates with functional dominance during story listening. *Neuroreport* 9, 829–33.

60. **Zatorre, R. J., A. C. Evans,** and **E. Meyer** (1994) Neural mechanisms underlying melodic perception and memory for pitch. *J. Neurosci.* 14, 1908–19.

61. **Zatorre, R. J., D. W. Perry, C. A. Beckett, C. F. Westbury,** and **A. C. Evans** (1998) Functional anatomy of musical processing in listeners with absolute pitch and relative pitch. *Proc. Natl. Acad. Sci. USA* 95, 3172–7.

62. **Rauschecker, J. P., B. Tian,** and **M. Hauser** (1995) Processing of complex sounds in the macaque non-primary auditory cortex. *Science* 268, 111–14.

63. **Koelsch, S., T. Gunter,** and **A. D. Friederici** (2000) Brain indices of music processing: 'nonmusicians' are musical. *J. Cognitive Neurosci.* 12, 520–41.

64. **Ohnishi, T., H. Matsuda, T. Asada,** *et al.* (2001) Functional anatomy of musical perception in musicians. *Cerebr. Cortex* 11, 754–60.

65. **Sergeant, D.** (1969) Experimental investigation of absolute pitch. *Journal of Research in Music Education* 17, 135–43.

66. **Baharloo, S., P. A. Johnston, S. K. Service, J. Gitschier,** and **N. B. Freimer** (1998) Absolute pitch: an approach for identification of genetic and nongenetic components. *Am. J. Hum. Genetics* 62, 224–31.

67. **Takeuchi, A. H.** and **S. H. Hulse** (1993) Absolute pitch. *Psychological Bulletin* 113, 345–61.

68. **Siegel, J. A.** (1974) Sensory and verbal coding strategies in subjects with absolute pitch. *J. Exp. Psychol.* 103, 37–44.

69. **Hirata, Y., S. Kuriki,** and **C. Pantev** (1999) Musicians with absolute pitch show distinct neural activities in the auditory cortex. *Neuroreport* 10, 999–1002.

70. Trainor, L. J., R. N. Desjardins, and C. Rockel (1999) A comparison of contour and interval processing in musicians and non-musicians using event-related potentials. *Australian Journal of Psychology* 51, 147–53.

71. Maess, B., S. Koelsch, T. C. Gunter, and A. D. Friederici (2001) Musical syntax is processed in Broca's area: an MEG study. *Nature Neurosci.* 4, 540–5.

72. Ruesseler, J. E., W. Altenmuller, C. Nager, T. F. Kohlmetz, and T. F. Munte (2001) Event-related brain potentials to sound omissions differ in musicians and non-musicians. *Neurosci. Lett.* 308, 33–6.

CHAPTER 25

REPRESENTATIONAL CORTEX IN MUSICIANS

C. PANTEV, A. ENGELIEN, V. CANDIA, AND T. ELBERT

Abstract

The lifelong ability to adapt to environmental needs is based on the capacity of the central nervous system for plastic alterations. In a series of neurophysiological experiments, we studied the impact of music and musical training in musicians on the specific functional organization in auditory and somatosensory representational cortex. In one such study, subjects listened to music from which one specific spectral frequency was removed. This led to rapid and reversible adaptation of neuronal responses in auditory cortex. Further experimental evidence demonstrated that long years of practice and training by professional musicians to enable them to reach their capacity is associated with enlarged cortical representations in the somatosensory and auditory domains. This tuning of neuronal representations was specifically observed for musical tones and was absent when pure sinusoidal tones were used as stimuli. In the somatosensory cortex, plastic changes proved to be specific for the fingers frequently used and stimulated. These changes were not detected in the fingers of the hand that were not involved in playing the particular instrument. Neuroplastic alterations also may be driven into a domain where they may become maladaptive. The clinical syndrome of focal hand dystonia that may occur in musicians who engage in forceful practice may be one such consequence. We will discuss the possibilities of reversing maladaptive responses leading to the successful treatment of focal hand dystonia, which relies on basic research about cortical reorganization. This example elucidates how neuroscientific progress can guide the development of practice guidelines and therapeutic measures for the benefit of professional musicians.

Introduction

The structural and functional organization of the human brain becomes increasingly differentiated during child development. In higher mammals, including humans, neurons are formed prenatally as are some of their interconnections into neural networks. For many years the prevailing opinion suggested that network connections between neurons are built primarily during cerebral maturation processes in childhood, with the exception of only those structures that were directly involved in memory. It was thought that this network pattern, almost like a connection diagram, would not change later. However, humans respond with considerable flexibility to new challenges throughout their entire life. Since the early 1980s, increasing experimental evidence demonstrated that the connectivity of the adult brain is in fact only partially determined by genetics and early development, and may be substantially modified through sensory experiences, even during adulthood.

Practising and performing music entails intense auditory and somatosensory peripheral sensory excitations, which are transmitted via specific receptors and fibre systems to the corresponding specialized regions of the cerebral cortex. Because the functional organization of representational cortex has been intensely studied, the examination of sensory cortical areas in the somatosensory and auditory systems provides an excellent model for studying the plastic changes that are associated with being a musician. The sensory cortex of both systems has a known topographical order of neuronal representations: a homuncular mapping of the body surface on somatosensory cortex[1-3] and a tonotopic mapping of acoustic frequency in auditory cortex.[4-7] Thus, modifications of representations can be specifically assessed. For example, different fingers of a given hand may not be equally used (and thus not equally stimulated) when playing certain musical instruments.

Based on W. James's suggestion at the end of the nineteenth century that learning may alter synaptic connectivity, the prominent Canadian neuropsychologist Donald Hebb formulated an important and innovative theory to view the brain not as a static but as a dynamic system. Hebb's rule asserts that effective connections between neurons are formed depending on synchronous activation: 'Cells that fire together, wire together'.[8] The development of new scientific methods for recording neuronal activity has made it possible to prove the hypothesis of plasticity in functional neuronal networks. The electrical activity of single neurons can only be recorded invasively in animals, but derived potentials that reflect the activity of a group of neurons can be recorded noninvasively on the scalp surface by means of electroencephalography (EEG). The magnetic counterpart of the EEG is the magnetoencephalography (MEG), which has become an established method for non-invasive study of the activity of the human cortex.[9] The main sources of cortical evoked magnetic fields are the pyramidal cells, which produce currents flowing tangentially to the surface of the head. Although MEG measurements provide only a macroscopic view of the function of the brain, the spatial resolution achieved with this technique is sufficient to give indications of functional organization and reorganizational plasticity of the human cortex by localizing the sources of evoked magnetic fields, which are elicited by defined and standardized peripheral excitation.

The first studies to clearly demonstrate reorganizational plasticity of the adult cortex were performed in the 1980s in 'deafferentation' experiments. Typically, in these studies the afferent information influx specific to certain cortical areas was eliminated.[10-15] One mechanism of change observed was that neurons that had lost their regular input were recruited by neighbouring regions. For example, neurons that were specialized for processing information from the fifth digit (little finger) may process information coming in on the second digit after the fifth digit was amputated. Similarly, neurons that were specific to a certain acoustic frequency may respond to neighbouring spared frequencies after the part of the cochlea transmitting their originally preferred input was destroyed.

Experimental studies in monkeys have demonstrated that intensive sensory stimulation may lead to an expansion of the corresponding cortical area.[16,17] Here we briefly review the experimental paradigm for one such study in the somatosensory modality concerning finger representation in adult monkeys. The animals were trained to touch a rotating disk with the tip of their index and middle fingers for 15 s. The surface of that disk was an irregular grid, so that it caused a sensation (and somatosensory excitation) specifically for those two fingertips. Anytime the monkeys touched the disk for 15 s, they received a reward (chips with banana taste). After about 600 stimulation periods, the representation of the hand in the somatosensory cortex was measured. The representation for the two stimulated fingers had become enlarged. Recanzone *et al.* trained owl monkeys for 60–80 daily sessions to make fine-pitch discriminations in selected regions of the auditory frequency spectrum (these regions differing among animals).[17] Tonotopic mapping carried out invasively afterward showed that the cortical area tuned to the trained frequencies was enlarged by a factor of 2–3 compared to untrained monkeys or to animals that experienced the same acoustic stimuli passively while being trained on a somatosensory discrimination task. Thus, the organization of the brain seems capable of significant change to adapt to the changing demands of the organism's environment. Synchronized sensory stimulation may be of particular importance for such changes. The common observation captured in the German proverb *Übung macht den Meister* [practice makes perfect] could therefore have its neurobiological correlate in an augmented simultaneous stimulation of neurons, which entrains a reorganization of the functional neuronal network.

Musicians practise and train for many years before they achieve their professional skills. Coordination and synchronization of somatosensory and motor control on the one hand, and audition on the other hand, are crucial when playing a musical instrument. We therefore hypothesized that musical aptitude and the training to fulfill it may be associated with plastic changes of neuronal representations in the cortical organization. We will describe below a series of experiments that support this hypothesis for the somastosensory and auditory domains.[18–20]

Neuronal representations in the given cortical field of interest were determined by measuring evoked magnetic fields contralateral to the stimulated side with a 37-channel BTi Magnes system. For the somatosensory modality, a brief pneumatic stimulation was applied to the fingertips; for the auditory modality, a variety of different auditory stimuli were delivered to the right ear. The following sections describe some experimental examples in more detail.

Short-term plasticity effect of the auditory cortex induced by notched music

Most studies of deafferentation-induced cortical reorganization have investigated cortical reorganization on a timescale of days to weeks, or longer. However, other more recent studies have documented rapid changes in cortical dynamics following deafferentation. These studies have shown that neurons broaden and shift their receptive fields to sensory surfaces near or beyond the edge of the lesioned zone within minutes of deafferentation in the somatosensory[21] and visual systems,[22] and within hours in the auditory one.[23] Rapid retuning of sensory neurons has also been observed following reversible 'functional' deafferentation in which sensory input from the environment is altered by procedures such as artificial scotomota[24] or digit ligation[25] rather than by permanent lesions of the receptor organs.

A study of 'functional deafferentation' was carried out to determine whether plastic changes of frequency representation occur on a short timescale of a few hours when the adult human auditory cortex is deprived of sensory input. Ten normal test subjects were asked to provide three favourite CDs from their CD collection. The music was manipulated in such a way that a notch between 0.7 and 1.3 kHz, centred around 1 kHz, was produced using a band rejection filter (Bessel, 96 dB/oct) in the broad-band spectrum of the music (cf. Figure 25.1a). Although this manipulation initially produced a clearly noticeable change in perception, subjects reported that they quickly adapted to the modified sound and that their appreciation of the music during the listening time was unchanged. The subjects were asked to listen attentively to the music for a continuous period of 3 h. Due to the notch filtering during this period, any afferent input to cortical neurons tuned to frequencies around 1 kHz was abolished. In order to measure the effect of notching of the music on the neuronal representation of 1 kHz, MEG recordings to the test stimulus (band-passed noise bursts centred at 1 kHz) were compared to MEG recordings to the control stimulus (band-passed noise bursts centred at 0.5 kHz; cf. Figure 25.1a). The experiment was repeated three times in each subject on consecutive days in order to address the time course and the reversibility of cortical remodelling induced by this procedure. These repetitions served to investigate the dynamics of cortical reorganization over a period of 24 h. The auditory evoked fields (AEF, channels 12 and 35, depicting the maximum and minimum of the AEF, respectively) obtained for test and control stimuli before and after listening to notched music are shown for one representative subject in Figure 25.1b. Whereas the AEF amplitudes measured before and after listening to notched music are almost the same for the control stimulus, the AEF amplitude for the test stimulus is about 10 per cent smaller after listening to notched music than before. Figure 25.1c demonstrates the differences of the strength of the cortical sources before and after listening to the notched music for the test and for the control stimulus, averaged over all subjects and days. Whereas the strength of the cortical source decreased significantly after the listening to the notched music for the test stimulus ($p < 0.01$), this value did not change appreciably for the control stimulus. In order to provide information on the reversibility of the notching effect within the time period of 24 h, the measurements taken before listening to notched music on each day were compared. Between days, no significant differences between the strength of the cortical sources were observed for these measures, a result that proves the reversibility of the short-term plasticity effect provided by the 'functional deafferentation' with respect to listening to the notched music.

Taken together, our results suggest that reorganization of cortical representations can occur within time periods as short as a few hours following functional deafferentation of the adult human auditory cortex. The temporal properties of the notching effect are consistent with animal studies that have shown that cortical neurons deafferented by cochlear lesions display elevated response thresholds initially and then shift their tuning preferences away from the lesioned area to frequencies near the edge of the deafferented region over a period of 1–3 h or longer.[23] Several interrelated mechanisms appear to contribute to cortical remodelling induced by deafferentation, including (1) changes in the efficacy of existing excitatory synapses unmasked by lesioning,[26] (2) modification of synaptic efficacy by transcription of immediate early genes,[27] and (3) the sprouting of new connections.[28] Of these mechanisms the first and second appear to be probable candidates to account for our findings. Synaptogenesis may occur within hours,[29] but axonal sprouting and dendritic growth may require more time and hence would be less likely to be involved.

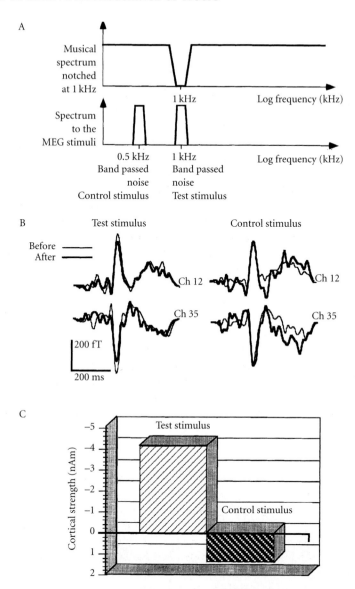

Figure 25.1 Short-term plasticity effect of the auditory cortex induced by notched music. (A) Music spectrum notched at 1 kHz (*top*) and spectral characteristics of the test and control stimuli for MEG recording (*bottom*). (B) Auditory evoked fields (AEF) of a single subject recorded for test stimulus (1 kHz, *left panel*) and control stimulus (0.5 kHz, *right panel*) before and after listening to notched music. (C) Change in cortical representation or respectively in the strength of the cortical source produced by listening to the notched music and calculated as the moment (Q, nAm) of the equivalent current dipole fitted to the Nlm component of the AEF for test and control stimuli averaged over subjects and days. (Modified from Ref. 20.)

Cortical plasticity and musical training

Somatosensory representations

Two groups of subjects were examined. The first group consisted of nine musicians who played string instruments: six violinists, two violoncellists, and one guitarist. The subjects' average age was 24 ± 3 years. They had started to play their instruments 12 years earlier on average, ranging between 7 and 17 years. They practised on their instruments for an average of 9–10 h per week. The second group consisted of six control subjects who had never played a musical instrument and did not frequently carry out tasks that involved a systematic and rhythmic finger stimulation such as typing (on a typewriter or computer). All subjects were right-handed. The fingers D1 (the thumb) and D5 (the little finger) of both hands were consecutively excited with a brief, nonpainful standardized pneumatic pressure.

After excitation of the left-hand fingers D1 and D5, the strength of the cortical sources as determined with MEG were stronger in musicians than the corresponding sources in control subjects (Figure 25.2). Thus, the cerebral representation was increased representing the excitation of those fingers that are intensively used in string instrument musicians. This effect was particularly pronounced for the fifth digit (D5). The cortical representation of the left thumb was also enhanced, but not as strongly as the one for left D5. Cortical representations obtained for right-hand stimulation did not differ between control subjects and musicians.

The amount of increase in somatosensory cortical representations of left-hand fingers in musicians depended on the age at which the musicians had started to play their instrument (Figure 25.3). The cortical response for stimulation of D5 was greater in those musicians who had begun to play their instrument earlier. Among the musicians who started to play violin or violoncello later (after the age of 13 years), the cortical representations for D5

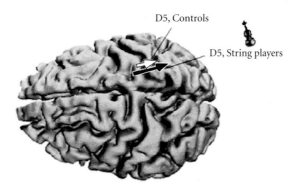

D5, Controls

D5, String players

Figure 25.2 Equivalent current dipoles (ECD) elicited by stimulation of the digit 5 (D5) of the left hand of control subjects and string players, superimposed onto an MRI-reconstruction of the cerebral cortex of a control subject, selected to provide anatomical landmarks for the interpretation of the MEG-based localization. The arrows represent the location and orientation of the ECD vector for D5 averaged across musicians (*black arrow*) and control subjects (*white arrow*). The length of the arrows represents the mean magnitude of the dipole moment for D5 in each group. The dipole moment is larger for the musicians' D5 as indicated by the greater magnitude of the black arrow. (Modified from Ref. 39.)

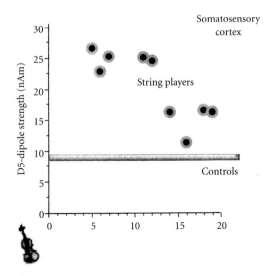

Figure 25.3 The magnitude of the D5 cortical strength as a function of the age of inception of musical practice: string players (*circles*), mean value for control subjects (*line*). Note the larger dipole moment for individuals beginning musical practice before the age of 12. (Modified from Ref. 39.)

were somewhat smaller, but still larger than those observed in the control subjects who had never played an instrument.

Auditory representation

Three groups of subjects were examined. The first group consisted of musicians with absolute pitch ($n = 9$), the second group of musicians with relative pitch ($n = 11$), and the third group of subjects were controls who had never played a musical instrument ($n = 13$). In the first group, the mean number of years the musicians had played their instruments was 21 ± 6, in the second group 15 ± 3 years. The musicians were recruited from the conservatory in Münster. The musicians with absolute pitch reported practising their instruments for 27 ± 14 h per week, and the musicians with relative pitch 23 ± 12 h per week, during the 5 years preceding participation in the study. The musicians who claimed to have absolute pitch were subjected to a testing procedure that was developed according to criteria established in the musical psychological literature.[30–34] A random sequence of 35 piano tones from H2 to C7 was presented to the musicians. For our study, in order to be considered a musician with absolute pitch, correct recognition of at least 90 per cent of the tones was required. Musicians with relative pitch were either self-identified ($n = 9$) or were subjects who failed the test for absolute pitch ($n = 2$). The mean age in the three groups was 29 ± 6 years for musicians with absolute pitch, 26 ± 5 years for musicians with relative pitch, and 26 ± 4 years for control subjects. All participants were right-handed, as established by the Edinburgh handedness questionnaire[35] and did not have recent or past audiology, otology, or neurology medical history. Audiological status was normal at the time the study was performed for each subject.

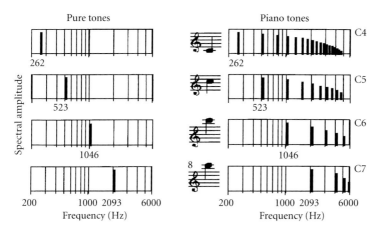

Figure 25.4 Spectra of piano tones C4–C7 (American notation, having fundamental frequency at 262, 523, 1046, and 2093 Hz, respectively) and four pure tones of the same fundamental frequencies. (Modified from Ref. 19.)

The acoustic stimulation consisted of a pseudorandom sequence of four piano tones (C4–C7; with the fundamental frequencies of 262, 523, 1046, and 2093 Hz), and four pure (sinusoidal) tones matching the fundamental frequencies (Figure 25.4). Each stimulus was presented 128 times to determine the location and strength of the electrical source in the auditory cortex.

In all musicians larger neuronal excitation was noted for piano tones as compared to pure tones. Our measure for the cortical neuronal representation, the strength of the electrical dipole moment in both musician groups, was significantly 25 per cent stronger for the piano tones as compared to the one for the pure tones ($p < 0.001$). By contrast, in the control subjects, who never played an instrument, no such difference was noted (Figure 25.5).

This finding demonstrates an increase in neuronal representation specific for the processing of the tones of the musical scale in musicians. Similar to the described enhancement of somatosensory representation, the degree of this increase was also dependent on the age at which the musicians had started to play their instruments. The earlier the initiation of musical practice, the stronger the neuronal response to the piano tones. In this study a marked difference was found between those who had begun practising music before and after 9 years of age.

The cortical representations for processing information from the fingers and the ears of musicians give an impressive demonstration that not only deafferentation, but also intensive training, can trigger a functional adaptation of the cortical organization. In general, this suggests that training can induce plastic changes of the adult human brain. In the musicians proficient in playing stringed instruments, the representation of the frequently used left-hand fingers is enlarged relative to control subjects. The more a given finger is stimulated, the larger the expansion of the cortical response. The representation for the thumb, which is not as frequently used as the other fingers, is not increased as much. However, the amount of practice is not the only factor that influences the organization of the somatosensory cortex. The plastic change of cortical representation is not directly

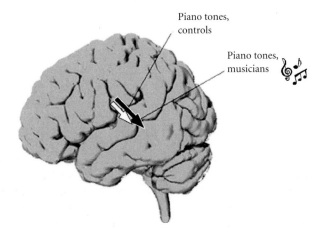

Figure 25.5 Mean values of the strength of cortical activation during the auditory N1 evoked field for piano tones as compared to pure tones in control subjects and musicians with absolute or relative pitch. (Modified from Ref. 19.)

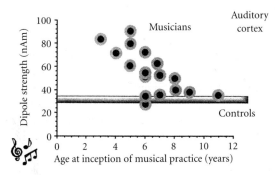

Figure 25.6 Mean strength of cortical activation for the different piano tones as a function of the age at which musical training began in musicians with absolute or relative pitch. The line denotes mean dipole moment in control subjects who never played a musical instrument. (Modified from Ref. 19.)

correlated to the number of hours played per week, but rather to the age at which the training was started in childhood.

For the auditory system, the representation of pure tones, which are not part of our natural acoustic environment and also not encountered in musical training and practice, does not differ between musicians and control subjects. By contrast, the representation of piano tones, which in control subjects is of the same strength as the one for pure tones, is specifically enhanced in musicians. The analysis of reports of these musicians revealed that neither the passive exposure to music as a child nor the amount of time spent listening to music passively as an adult significantly influences functional cortical organization. It seems that active practice is necessary to induce plastic alterations. This reorganization of the auditory system also exhibits a trend towards more pronounced brain plasticity with a younger age of starting to play the musical instrument (Figure 25.6). The musicians who started playing before they were 9 years old demonstrated the largest cortical representations.

The fact that the degree of expansion of the neuronal representations depends on the age training is started suggests that the enormous capacity of plasticity in the adult brain is, however, more limited than the plasticity of the infant brain. This corresponds to the pre-scientific observation that it is more difficult for adults to learn to play a musical instrument. To achieve an equivalent musical aptitude, adults can still adapt their cortical organization but they have to work harder to do so.

The dark side of neuroplasticity in musicians

As mentioned above, neuronal networks are thought to be particularly plastic during 'sensitive periods' in the development of cortical structures. However, they maintain the ability to alter their architecture and function to afferent input throughout life. Perceptual and behavioural correlates of this reorganization indicate that neuroplasticity can be adaptive, as illustrated previously. Another type of reorganization includes the smearing of representational zones. An example has been described in blind multifinger Braille readers where overlap of digit representation may aid the ability to process different types of digital input simultaneously, thus enabling more rapid reading.[36] However, cortical reorganization can also be maladaptive, as is indicated by its association with phantom limb pain,[37] tinnitus,[38] and focal hand dystonia.[39,40] Intense training, as found in professional musicians, employs mechanisms of cortical plasticity with the inherent danger that maladaptive processes may also occur. Evidence from several laboratories suggests that one such danger is focal hand dystonia. Focal dystonia of the hand falls into a class often termed occupational hand cramp.[41,42] It involves manual discoordination occurring in individuals engaging in extensive or forceful use of the fingers. The disorder involves a disorganization of control of the digits such that the movements of some fingers on a hand become involuntarily linked to those of others, something particularly incapacitating to professional instrumental musicians.

Repetitive and behaviourally relevant stimulation to several digits performed with healthy subjects results in a fusion and in a disordered arrangement of the representation of individual digits.[36,43] At the same time subjects in these experiments consistently mislocalize light pressure stimuli applied to the fingertips. Consistent with earlier work in animals, source imaging in humans demonstrates that synchronous stimulation of the digits may create a fusion of cortical representational zones, whereas asynchronous stimulation leads to separation. Could such a process of cortical reorganization become maladaptive and thus contribute to focal dystonia? By means of magnetic and neuroelectric source imaging, an overlap or smearing of the homuncular organization of the representation of the digits in the primary somatosensory and the motor cortex was indeed observed (Figure 25.7).[39,44,45]

Work by N. Byl, M. Merzenich, and colleagues in New World monkeys has indicated that lack of digital motor coordination resulting from digital overuse is associated with an induced disorder in the representation of the digits in the somatosensory cortex.[42,46] These findings suggest that overuse-dependent central nervous system (CNS) plasticity is the basis of the focal hand dystonia. Therefore, because evidence suggests that behavioural usage and a CNS plastic response to this usage could be the cause of both the cortical

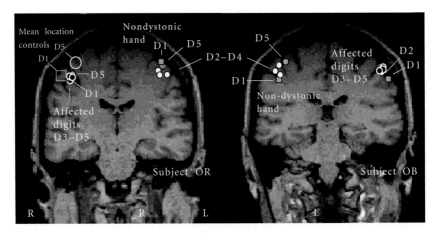

Figure 25.7   A coronal MRI section is shown through the somatosensory cortices of an organ player (*left*) and an oboist (*right*), both suffering from focal hand dystonia. The symbols indicate cortical representations (dipole locations) of digits 1–5 (D1–D5) resulting from contralateral stimulation of the finger tips. The large *open symbols* in the right hemisphere of subject O.R. indicate the mean location of dipoles for D1 and D5 in normal control subjects. (Modified from Ref. 39.)

disorder and the involuntary lack of movement coordination, it was thought that a behavioural intervention focusing on movement could be of value in reducing or eliminating these conditions. Any such treatment approach should include practice in a behaviourally relevant setting. A number of studies have shown that the behavioural relevance of the stimulation is the critical factor for reorganization to occur, whereas simple passive stimulation seems to be ineffective in altering cortical connectivity.[17] For example, Kilgard et al. suggested that the cholinergic nucleus basalis might play an important role in labelling stimuli as behaviourally relevant because nucleus basalis activation facilitated cortical plasticity induced by correlated stimulation in the periphery.[47] Further evidence points to the additional involvement of dopaminergic pathways. It seems possible that blockade of dopamine, released by a potentially rewarding condition, for example, through neuroleptics, will not allow cortical reorganization to occur.

On the basis of these considerations, Candia et al. have developed a successful therapy for focal hand dystonia.[40] Professional musicians (pianists, guitarists, and wind players), with long-standing symptoms, who had previously received a variety of treatments, practised their instrument according to rules derived from insights into the mechanisms of cortical reorganization. The therapy involved immobilization by splints of one or more of the digits other than the focal dystonic finger. The focal dystonic finger was required to carry out repetitive exercises in coordination with one or more of the other digits for 1.5–2.5 h a day over an intended period of eight consecutive days under supervision of a therapist. The patients were instructed to continue the exercises using the splint at home for 1 h every day for 1 year posttreatment. The wind players, who, in effect, constituted placebo controls, did not improve substantially. However, each of the pianists and guitarists showed marked and significant improvement in spontaneous repertoire performance without the splint at the end of treatment, up into the normal range. Neuroimaging results obtained in successfully treated subjects indicated normalization of the cortical representational maps, highlighting again the continued role of plasticity in the adult human brain for successful adaptation. The outcome demonstrates that learning-induced alterations in the functional architecture of the brain can be maladaptive, and that the resulting pathology can be treated using behavioural techniques that are based on learning principles that take into account recent research on neuroplasticity.

Conclusions

By use of MEG, it was shown that it is possible to noninvasively study mechanisms of cerebral organization and reorganization in humans. Listening to music attentively for as little as 3 h can have a temporary influence on auditory cortical representation, as was shown in our study with music notched at a specific frequency. It was further shown that musical education and training is reflected in the organization of auditory and somatosensory representational cortex in musicians. From the results obtained, the following questions arise: Can we draw conclusions on the behavioural plasticity after knowing about the neuronal one? How do alterations in functional cortical organization affect musical accomplishment? Do the best virtuosos have the most atypical cortical organization?

The results of the studies presented here do not allow final conclusions. However, as shown in the case of focal dystonia, current research can lead to recommendations about musical practice and help design methods of treatment. The observed correlation between the age of initiation of musical practice and the amount of cortical change should not be overinterpreted from a music-pedagogical perspective. The complex relationships between genetic and familial, as well as educational pedagogical factors, would have to be studied by an interdisciplinary team of scientists. Such a team should comprise neuroscientists, as well as musicians and experts in music psychology, because it would be necessary to evaluate subtle differences in musical achievement to address these questions and establish causal links.

Acknowledgements

This research was supported by the Deutsche Forschungsgemeinschaft. The work presented here was made possible through multiple collaborations with Drs Larry Roberts, Brigitte Rockstroh, Bernhard Ross, Edward Taub, and Christian Wienbruch. We wish to thank Deborah Urdang and Dr Harvey Salomon for comments on the manuscript.

References

1. Clark, S. A., *et al.* (1988) Receptive fields in the body-surface map in adult cortex defined by temporally correlated inputs. *Nature* 332, 444–5.

2. Narici, L., *et al.* (1991) Neuromagnetic somatosensory homunculus: a non-invasive approach in humans. *Neurosci. Lett.* 121, 51–4.

3. **Elbert, T.**, *et al.* (1995) The separation of overlapping neuromagnetic sources in first and second somatosensory cortices. *Brain Topogr.* 7, 275–82.

4. **Merzenich, M. M., P. L. Knight**, and **G. L. Roth** (1975) Representation of cochlea within primary auditory cortex in the cat. *J. Neurophysiol.* 38, 231–49.

5. **Pantev, C.**, *et al.* (1988) Tonotopic organization of the human auditory cortex revealed by transient auditory evoked magnetic fields. *EEG Clin. Neurophysiol.* 69, 160–70.

6. **Pantev, C.**, *et al.* (1989) Tonotopic organization of the auditory cortex: pitch versus frequency representation. *Science* 246, 486–8.

7. **Pantev, C.**, *et al.* (1995) Specific tonotopic organizations of different areas of the human auditory cortex revealed by simultaneous magnetic and electric recordings. *EEG Clin. Neurophysiol.* 94, 26–40.

8. **Hebb, D. O.** (1949) *The Organization of Behavior*. Chichester, UK: John Wiley and Sons.

9. **Hari, R.** (1990) Magnetic evoked fields of the human brain: basic principles and applications. *EEG Clin. Neurophysiol.* 41 (Suppl.), 3–12.

10. **Merzenich, M. M.**, *et al.* (1984) Somatosensory cortical map changes following digit amputation in adult monkeys. *J. Comp. Neurol.* 224, 591–605.

11. **Merzenich, M. M.**, *et al.* (1983) Topographic reorganization or somatosensory cortical areas 3b and 1 in adult monkeys following restricted deafferentation. *Neuroscience* 8, 33–55.

12. **Elbert, T.**, *et al.* (1994) Extensive reorganization of the somatosensory cortex in adult humans after nervous system injury. *Neuroreport* 5, 2593–7.

13. **Elbert, T.**, *et al.* (1997) Input-increase and input-decrease types of cortical reorganization after upper extremity amputation in humans. *Exp. Brain Res.* 117, 161–4.

14. **Rajan, R.**, *et al.* (1993) Effect of unilateral partial cochlear lesions in adult cats on the representation of lesioned and unlesioned cochleas in primary auditory cortex. *J. Comp. Neurol.* 338, 17–49.

15. **Irvine, D. R. F.** and **R. Rajan** (1995) In G. A. Manley *et al.* (eds) *Advances in Hearing Research*. Singapore: World Scientific Publishing Co. pp. 3–23.

16. **Jenkins, W. M.**, *et al.* (1990) Functional reorganization of primary somatosensory cortex in adult owl monkeys after behaviorally controlled tactile stimulation. *J. Neurophysiol.* 63, 82–104.

17. **Recanzone, G. H., C. E. Schreiner**, and **M. M. Merzenich** (1993) Plasticity in the frequency representation of primary auditory cortex following discrimination training in adult owl monkeys. *J. Neurosci.* 13, 87–103.

18. **Elbert, T.**, *et al.* (1995) Increased cortical representation of the fingers of the left hand in string players. *Science* 270, 305–7.

19. **Pantev, C.**, *et al.* (1998) Increased auditory cortical representation in musicians. *Nature* 392, 811–14.

20. **Pantev, C.**, *et al.* (1999) Short-term plasticity of the human auditory cortex. *Brain Res.* 842, 192–9.

21. **Doetsch, G. S.**, *et al.* (1996) Short-term plasticity in primary somatosensory cortex of the rat: rapid changes in magnitudes and latencies of neuronal responses following digit denervation. *Exp. Brain Res.* 112, 505–12.

22. **Gilbert, C. D.** (1997) Cortical dynamics. *Acta Paediatr. Suppl.* 422, 34–7.

23. **Robertson, D.** and **D. R. Irvine** (1989) Plasticity of frequency organization in auditory cortex of guinea pigs with partial unilateral deafness. *J. Comp. Neurol.* 282, 456–71.

24. **Gilbert, C. D.**, *et al.* (1996) Spatial integration and cortical dynamics. *Proc. Natl. Acad. Sci. USA* 93, 615–22.

25. **Rossini, P. M.**, *et al.* (1994) Short-term brain 'plasticity' in humans: transient finger representation changes in sensory cortex somatotopy following ischemic anesthesia. *Brain Res.* 642, 169–77.

26. **Ziemann, U., M. Hallet**, and **L. G. Cohen** (1998) Mechanisms of deafferentation-induced plasticity in human motor cortex. *J. Neurosci.* 18, 7000–7.

27. **Kaczmarek, L.** and **A. Chaudhuri** (1997) Sensory regulation of immediate-early gene expression in mammalian visual cortex: implications for functional mapping and neural plasticity. *Brain Res. Brain Res. Rev.* 23, 237–56.

28. **Florence, S. L., H. B. Taub**, and **J. H. Kaas** (1998) Large-scale sprouting of cortical connections after peripheral injury in adult macaque monkeys. *Science* 282, 1117–21.

29. **Engert, F.** and **T. Bonhoeffer** (1999) Dendritic spine changes associated with hippo-campal long-term synaptic plasticity. *Nature* 399, 66–70.

30. **Bachem, A.** (1937) Various types of absolute pitch. *J. Acoust. Soc. Am.* 9, 146–51.

31. **Miyazaki, K.** (1988) Musical pitch identification by absolute pitch possessors. *Percept. Psychophys.* 44, 501–12.

32. **Neu, D. M.** (1947) A critical review on the literature on 'absolute pitch'. *Psychol. Bull.* 44, 249–66.

33. **Takeuchi, A.** and **S. H. Hulse** (1993) Absolute pitch. *Psychol. Bull.* 113, 345–61.

34. **Ward, W. D.** (1998) In D. Deutsch (ed.) *The Psychology of Music.* San Diego, CA: Academic Press.

35. **Oldfield, R. C.** (1971) The assessment and analysis of handedness: the Edinburgh inventory. *Neurophysiologia* 9, 97–113.

36. **Sterr, A.**, *et al.* (1998) Perceptual correlates of changes in cortical representation of fingers in blind multifinger Braille readers. *J. Neurosci.* 18, 4417–23.

37. **Flor, H.**, *et al.* (1995) Phantom limb pain as a perceptual correlate of massive cortical reorganization in upper limp amputees. *Nature* 375, 482–4.

38. **Muhlnickel, W.**, *et al.* (1998) Reorganization of auditory cortex in tinnitus. *Proc. Natl. Acad. Sci. USA* 95, 10340–3.

39. **Elbert, T.**, *et al.* (1998) Alteration of digital representations in somatosensory cortex in focal hand dystonia. *Neuroreport* 9, 3571–5.

40. **Candia, V.**, *et al.* (1999) Constraint-induced movement therapy for focal hand dystonia in musicians. *Lancet* 353, 42.

41. **Lederman, R. G.** (1988) Occupational cramp in instrumental musicians. *Med. Probl. Perform. Art* 3, 45–51.

42. **Byl, N. N., M. M. Merzenich**, and **W. M. Jenkins** (1996) A primate genesis model of focal dystonia and repetitive strain injury: I. Learning-induced dedifferentiation of the representation of the hand in the primary somatosensory cortex in adult monkeys. *Neurology* 47, 508–20.

43. **Braun, C.**, *et al.* (2000) Differential activation in somatosensory cortex for different discrimination tasks. *J. Neurosci.* 20, 446–50

44. **Elbert, T.** and **A. Keil** (2000) Imaging in the fourth dimension. *Nature* 404, 29–31.

45. **Bara-Jimenez, W.**, *et al.* (1998) Abnormal somatosensory homunculus in dystonia of the hand. *Ann. Neurol.* 44, 828–31.

46. **Byl, N. N.**, *et al.* (1997) A primate model for studying focal dystonia and repetitive strain injury: effects on the primary somatosensory cortex. *Phys. Ther.* 77, 269–84.

47. **Kilgard, M. P.** and **M. M. Merzenich** (1998) Cortical map reorganization enabled by nucleus basalis activity. *Science* 279, 1714–18.

CHAPTER 26

THE BRAIN THAT MAKES MUSIC AND IS CHANGED BY IT

ALVARO PASCUAL-LEONE

Abstract

Playing a musical instrument demands extensive procedural and motor learning that results in plastic reorganization of the human brain. These plastic changes seem to include the rapid unmasking of existing connections and the establishment of new ones. Therefore, both functional and structural changes take place in the brain of instrumentalists as they learn to cope with the demands of their activity. Neuroimaging techniques allow documentation of these plastic changes in the human brain. These plastic changes are fundamental to the accomplishment of skilful playing, but they pose a risk for the development of motor control dysfunctions that may give rise to overuse syndromes and focal, task-specific dystonia.

Keywords: Brain plasticity; Musical training

Introduction

The most intricately and perfectly coordinated of all voluntary movements in the animal kingdom are those of the human hand and fingers, and perhaps in no other human activity do memory, complex integration, and muscular coordination surpass the achievements of the skilled pianist.

Homer W. Smith, *From Fish to Philosopher*

Playing a musical instrument requires more than factual knowledge about the musical instrument and the mechanics of how it is played. For example, given complete information about hand position, finger motions, and sequence of keys to push for how long and with what force, I would still be unable to play even the simplest piano sonata. The central nervous system has to acquire and implement a 'translation mechanism' to convert knowledge into action. These translation capabilities constitute the skill that enables the pianist to act on memory systems, select the relevant facts, choose the proper response goals, activate the necessary sensorimotor structures, and execute the sonata successfully. We generally think of such a skill as being acquired with practice. The pianist confronted with a new composition, after understanding the task and its demands, develops a cognitive representation of it and initiates a first, centrally guided response that results in sensorimotor feedback and movement correction. It seems certain that both sensory and motor aspects have to be exquisitely coordinated. At the beginning, the limbs move slowly, with fluctuating accuracy and speed, and success requires visual, proprioceptive, and auditory feedback. Eventually, each single movement is refined, the different movements chained into the proper sequence with the desired timing, a high probability of stability in the ordered sequence attained, and a fluency of all movement developed. Only then can the pianist shift his or her attentional focus away from the mechanical details of the performance towards the emotional content of the task. We can think of the acquisition of such a skill as the conversion of declarative knowledge (facts) into procedural knowledge (actions, skills).[1–3]

Learning and memory might be considered integral parts of all the operations of any neural circuit, a concept for which Fuster[4] recently made an eloquent and convincing argument. In this view, 'perception and action are phenomena of memory and, conversely, memory is an integral part of perceptual and motor processing' (Ref. 4, p. 21). The nervous system comes to be viewed as a dynamic, dialectic organization in which plasticity is an intrinsic property that relates to the acquisition of new memories and skills as an obligatory consequence of perceptions and motor actions. To play an instrument, the nervous system is modified as a consequence of practice to yield the necessary changes in ability. We refer to this experience-dependent modification in neural structure as plasticity. These changes take place both in sensory and motor systems as well as in their interface. The consequence of this notion is that these changes do not necessarily represent behavioural benefits to the subject but might in fact be misguided and functionally deleterious. The development of noninvasive imaging and neurophysiologic techniques enables us to pursue the study of such changes in humans.

Learning to play the piano changes your brain

> ... the work of a pianist ... is inaccessible for the untrained human, as the acquisition of new abilities requires many years of mental and physical practice. In order to fully understand this complicated phenomenon it is necessary to admit, in addition to the strengthening of pre-established organic pathways, the establishment of new ones, through ramification and progressive growth of dendritic arborizations and nervous terminals. ... Such a development takes place in response to exercise, while it stops and may be reversed in brain spheres that are not cultivated.
>
> Santiago Ramón y Cajal, *Textura del Sistema Nervioso del Hombre y de los Vertebrados*

Normal subjects were taught to perform with one hand a five-finger exercise on a piano keyboard connected by a MIDI interface to a computer.[5] Subjects did not play any musical instrument, did not know how to typewrite using all fingers, and held jobs not demanding skillful hand and finger activities. The exercise required pressing a piano key sequentially with thumb (C), index finger (D), middle finger (E), ring finger (F), little finger (G), ring finger (F), middle finger (E), index finger (D), thumb (C), index finger (D), and so forth. The subjects were instructed to attempt to perform the sequence of finger movements fluently, without pauses and without skipping any key, while paying particular attention to keep the interval between the individual key presses constant and the duration of each key press the same. A metronome gave a tempo of 60 beats per minute, which the subjects were asked to aim for. Subjects performed the exercise under auditory feedback. They were studied on five

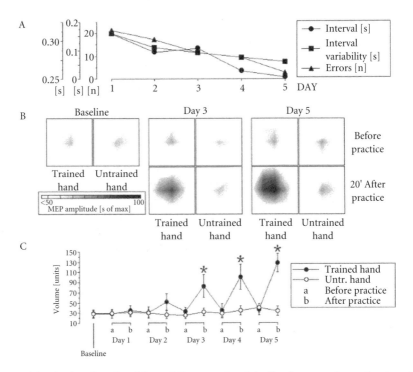

Figure 26.1 (A) Behavioural results of the week-long practice of the five-finger exercise on the piano. Interval between key presses, variability of these intervals, and number of errors in 20 repetitions of the exercise all show a highly significant decrease. This documents learning for all subjects studied. (B) Cortical output maps for the finger flexors of the trained and untrained hands of a representative subject. (See text and Ref. 5 for details on mapping method.) Note the marked changes of the output maps for the trained hand and the lack of changes for the untrained hand and the maps obtained for either hand before the daily practice sessions. (C) Graphic display of mean (± SD) volumes of the cortical output maps for all subjects studied. Note the significant (*star*) changes in cortical output maps for the trained hands after practice sessions on days 3–5.

consecutive days, and each day they had a two-hour practice session followed by a test. The test consisted of the execution of 20 repetitions of the five-finger exercise and was eventually analysed with the computer for the exact sequence of key presses, the interval between keys, and the duration and velocity of each key press. Following each test the subjects were given feedback about their performance and tips about how to improve. Figure 26.1 illustrates the great improvement in the subjects' playing skill over the course of the five study days. The number of sequence errors and the duration and variability of the intervals between key presses (as marked by the metronome beats) all decreased significantly.

The aim of the experiment was to correlate skill acquisition with changes in motor cortical output. Therefore, before the first practice session on the first day of the experiment, we used focal transcranial magnetic stimulation (TMS) to map the motor cortical areas targeting long finger flexor and extensor muscles bilaterally. Thereafter, this mapping was repeated daily. The baseline maps can be compared with those obtained during the five days. As the subjects' performance improved, the threshold for TMS activation of the finger flexor and extensor muscles decreased steadily; even taking into account this change in threshold, the size of the cortical representation for both muscle groups increased significantly (Figure 26.1).[5] However, this increase could be demonstrated only when the cortical mapping studies were conducted following a 20- to 30-minute rest after the practice (and test) session. No such modulation in the cortical output maps was noted when maps were obtained before each daily practice session (Figure 26.1).[6]

When a near-perfect level of performance was reached at the end of a week of daily practice, subjects were randomized into two groups (Figure 26.2). Group 1 continued daily practice of the same piano exercise during the following four weeks. Group 2 stopped practising. During the four weeks of follow-up, cortical output maps for finger flexor and extensor muscles were obtained in all subjects on Mondays (before the first practice session of that week in group 1) and on Fridays (at the end of the last practice session for the week in group 1). In the group that continued practising (group 1), the cortical output maps obtained on Fridays showed an initial plateau and eventually a slow decrease in size despite continued performance improvement (Figure 26.2). On the other hand, maps obtained on Mondays before the practice session and after the weekend rest showed a small change from baseline with a tendency to increase in size over the course of the study (Figure 26.2). In group 2, who stopped practising after one week, the maps returned to baseline after the first week of follow-up and remained stable thereafter.

This experiment reveals that acquisition of the necessary motor skills to perform a five-finger movement exercise correctly is associated with reorganization in the cortical motor outputs to the muscles involved in the task. There are two main mechanisms to explain this reorganization: establishment of new connections, or sprouting, and unmasking of previously existing connections. The rapid time course in the initial modulation of the motor outputs, by which a certain region of motor cortex can reversibly increase its influence on a motoneuron pool, is most compatible with the unmasking of previously existing connections.[7–10] Supporting this notion, the initial changes are transient, demonstrable after practice, but return to baseline after a weekend of rest. We suggest that such flexible, short-term modulation represents a first and necessary step, leading to longer-term structural changes in the intracortical and subcortical networks as the skill becomes overlearned and automatic.

It is important to realize that our TMS mapping technique demonstrates a trace or memory of the activation of the motor cortical outputs that took place during the performance of the task rather than the activation during the task itself, as would be the case with neuroimaging studies. Long-term potentiation has been demonstrated in the motor cortex,[11,12] and our results might reveal a similar phenomenon. During the learning of the task, the cortical output maps obtained after task performance show a progressive increase in size, suggesting that skill acquisition is associated with a change in the pattern of activation of the executive structures. These changes are not demonstrable before the task performance, and we might hypothesize that 'learning' to activate the cortical outputs appropriately (in this case, activating a progressively larger cortical output map) constitutes the neurophysiological correlate of performance improvement.

As the task becomes overlearned over the course of five weeks, the pattern of cortical activation for optimal task performance might change as other neural structures take a

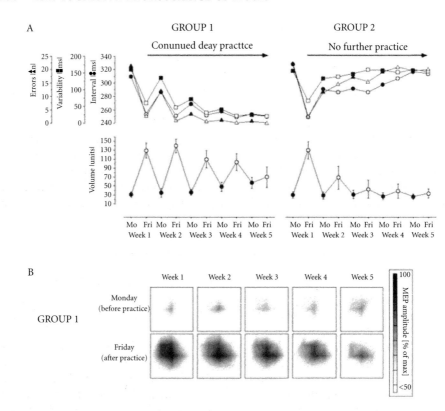

Figure 26.2 (A) Behavioural results for subjects in groups 1 (continued practice after 1 week) and 2 (practice limited to 1 week) learning the five-finger exercise on the piano. Interval between key presses, variability of these intervals, and number of errors in 20 repetitions of the exercise are shown. Data from Monday and Friday of each week are shown. (B) Cortical output maps for the finger flexors of the trained hand of a representative subject. (See text and Ref. 5 for details on mapping method.) Note the marked changes in the output maps. There appear to be two parallel processes in action, one accounting for the rapid modulation of the maps from Monday to Friday and the other responsible for the slow and more discrete changes in Monday maps over time.[5,6]

more leading role in task performance. This might result in the decreasing size of the cortical output maps after practice and the increasing size before practice. For example, if basal ganglia play a more important role in driving task performance, the changed activity in the basal ganglia motor circuit might enhance thalamocortical connections. This may account for changes in the cortical motor representation, which would be more stable than that observed during the initial acquisition of a skill. Greenough *et al.*[13] showed that motor training is associated with changes in the dendritic branching patterns of motor and sensory cortical cells involved in the performance of a task. Sprouting may account for plastic changes in such situations, as likely occurred in monkeys deafferented for 10 years,[14] and represent the correlate of long-standing 'memories'. Neuroimaging studies suggest a similar phenomenon.[15–22] Related changes in the pattern of cortical activation and the resulting modulation of cortical outputs might be induced by changes in the subject's strategy as explicit learning mechanisms are engaged.[23]

Our findings stress the role of the primary motor cortex (M1) in skill acquisition. It is not unreasonable to expect plastic changes in M1 during motor skill learning, because M1 is clearly involved in movement, and its cells have complex patterns of connectivity, including variable influences on multiple muscles within a body part.[24,25] Recent animal studies also illustrate the importance of the M1 in skill learning. For example, increases in excitability of primary motor cortex neurons have been found during conditioning,[26,27] and repeated activation of somatosensory inputs into the motor cortex results in long-term potentiation of motor neurons.[11,12] Even so, at the low stimulus intensities used in our mapping studies, TMS activates cortical cells largely transsynaptically.[28,29] Therefore, the demonstrated modulation in motor cortical outputs might be conditioned by changes in premotor areas projecting to M1, rather than by changes in M1 itself.

If you cannot do it, at least think about it: mental practice

In the quote reproduced above, Cajal talks about rapid and slower plastic changes in the brain in the context of practice. Our results confirm his intuitions. Furthermore, Cajal writes about physical and *mental* practice. Might the latter result in plastic brain changes similar to those induced by the former?

Mental practice is the imagined rehearsal of a motor act with the specific intent of learning or improving it, without overt movement output. Mental practice can be viewed as a virtual simulation of behaviour by which the subject develops and 'internally' rehearses a cognitive representation of the motor act. When confronted with a new motor task, the subject must develop a cognitive representation of it and initiate a centrally guided response, which secondarily can be improved using sensorimotor feedback. Mental practice may accelerate the acquisition of a new motor skill by providing a well-suited cognitive model of the demanded motor act in advance of any physical practice.[30,31]

Mental practice has found wide acceptance in the training of athletes.[32] Musicians also have long recognized the benefit of mental rehearsal. Harold Schoenberg, in his fascinating books on virtuoso intrumentalists,[33,34] provides ample information on this topic. For example, Horowitz is supposed to have practised mentally before concerts to avoid disturbing his motor skills by the feedback of pianos other than his own Steinway. Rubinstein, eager to enjoy life to its fullest and dedicate as little time to practise as possible, found mental rehearsal the best way to minimize the number of hours spent sitting in front of the piano while maintaining his skill.

Using the same experimental design as described above for the five-finger exercise, we studied subjects who, instead of practising at the keyboard 2 h daily for five days spent time at the keyboard visualizing, rather than executing, the movements.[5] They were told to repeat the movement mentally, as if they were playing, but without moving their fingers. They could rest their fingers on the piano keyboard, but the lack of voluntary movements was monitored using electromyography and video. Such mental practice resulted in a reorganization of the motor outputs to finger flexor and extensor muscles similar to the one observed in the group of subjects who physically practised the movements and led to

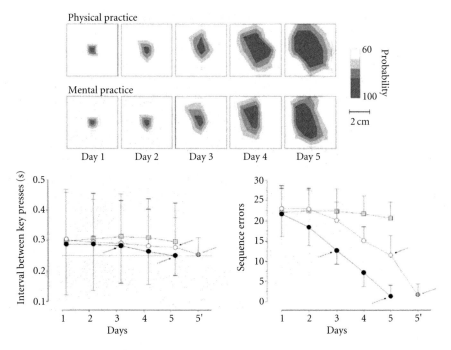

Figure 26.3 (A) Cortical output maps for the finger flexors of the trained hand in a representative subject with physical *vs* mental practice alone. Modified from Ref. 5; see also text for details. Note the parity of changes with either form of practice. (B) Graphic representation of behavioural data in a group of control subjects (no practice, *squares*) and a group of test subjects performing mental practice (*open circles*) vs physical practice (*filled circles*). Note the behavioural advantage of the physical practice group, but the significant improvement of the mental practice group as compared with controls. The last data point (5′) represents the performance achieved by the mental practice group after 5 min of physical practice at the end of day 5. Note the apparent advantage of mental practice, because subjects go from a performance equivalent to day 3 of the physical practice group to matching their day 5 performance with only 5 min of practice. Modified from Ref. 5.

similar improvement in their ability to perform the five-finger movement exercise (Figure 26.3).

Studies of regional cerebral blood flow (rCBF) suggest that the prefrontal and supplementary motor areas, basal ganglia, and cerebellum are part of the network involved in the mental simulation of motor acts.[35–38] Therefore, mental simulation of movements activates some of the same central neural structures required for the performance of the actual movements. In so doing, mental practice alone seems to be sufficient to promote the modulation of neural circuits involved in the early stages of motor skill learning. This modulation not only results in marked improvement in performance, but also seems to place the subjects at an advantage for further skill learning with minimal physical practice.[5,6] The combination of mental and physical practice leads to greater performance improvement than does physical practice alone, a phenomenon for which our findings provide a physiological explanation.

The risk of the change: sensorimotor mismatch and task-induced dystonia

As we have seen, skill acquisition requires plastic changes in the brain. This plastic reorganization is driven by efferent demand and afferent input. However, a system capable of such flexible reorganization harbours the risk of unwanted change. Increased demand of sensorimotor integration poses such a risk. We can postulate that faulty practice may result in unwanted cortical rearrangement and set the stage for motor control problems such as overuse syndrome and focal, task-specific dystonias. The style of piano playing—for example, the Russian vs the German school—seems to play a critical role in the risk of development of motor control problems. Forceful playing with the fingers bent and executing hammer-like movements is more frequently associated with overuse syndrome and dystonia than is softer playing with extended fingers 'caressing' the keys. This stresses the importance of proper, well-guided practice and illustrates the need for greater understanding of the neurobiology underlying music playing to define what proper practice actually is.

Focal hand dystonia in musicians is a strongly task-related movement disorder that can end an instrumentalist's career. Typically, symptoms become manifest only when players execute specific overpracticed skilled exercises on their instrument. Suddenly, a finger moves involuntarily, voluntary motor control is lost, the muscles tense up excessively, and pain develops. Playing is disturbed. For years, focal, task-specific dystonias were thought to be psychiatric in nature. It seemed too bizarre that involuntary muscle contraction might occur when playing a certain passage but not with any other activity or when playing on a certain instrument (organ) but not another (pianoforte). We now know that dystonias are neurologic involuntary movements due to disturbances in motor programs.[39] What, however, is their underlying pathophysiology?

We examined five guitarists with functional magnetic resonance imaging (fMRI) during dystonic symptom provocation by means of an adapted guitar inside the magnet.[40] As reference, we used the activation pattern obtained in the same subjects during other hand movements and in matched guitar players without dystonia during execution of the same guitar playing exercises. A 1.5-Tesla system equipped with echo-speed gradients and single-shot echoplanar imaging (EPI) software was used. Data acquisition was centred on the cortical motor system encompassed in eight contiguous slices.

Dystonic musicians compared in both control situations showed significantly greater activation of the contralateral primary sensorimotor cortex, which contrasted with conspicuous bilateral underactivation of premotor areas (Figure 26.4). Our results agree with studies of other types of dystonia in that they show abnormal recruitment of cortical areas involved in the control of voluntary movement. They do suggest, however, that rather than being hypoactive in idiopathic dystonic patients, the primary sensorimotor cortex may be overactive when tested during full expression of the task-induced movement disorder.

Although the primary manifestation of dystonia is abnormal motor function, evidence is increasing for a dysfunction of sensory processing that may be an associated or contributing factor.[39,41–43,46,47] In fact, dedifferentiation of the normally independent sensory representations of multiple digits may be a causative element in the etiology of dystonia.[44,45] For example, in musicians, extensive practice of co-ordinated hand postures in which

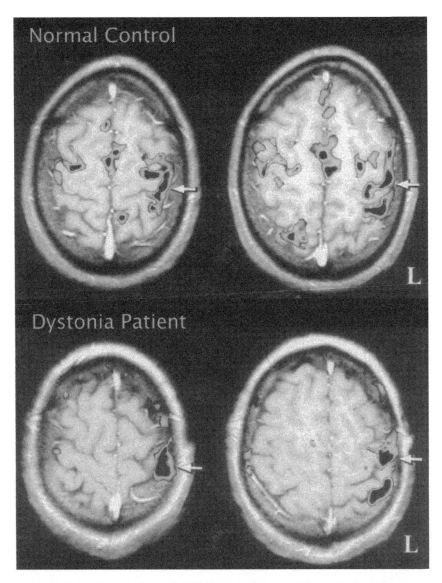

Figure 26.4 The bold fMRI images of a normal and dystonic guitar player executing right hand arpeggios in the scanner are displayed. Note the greater activation of the sensorimotor cortex (*arrows*) and the lack of activation of premotor and supplementary motor cortices in the dystonic patient. Modified from Ref. 40. (See Plate 24 in colour section.)

various digits function as a unit, such as arpeggios, could eventually induce changes in the sensory representation of the hand with blurring of the segregation of different digits. This might be the case particularly when small repeated traumas are added, as in forceful, 'hammer-finger' piano playing. Disorganization and consequent confusion of sensory

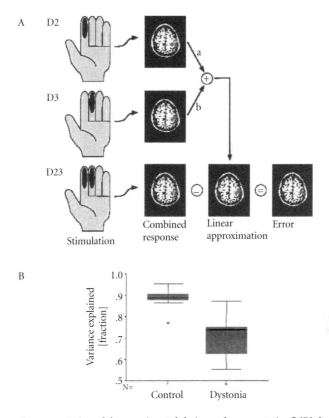

Figure 26.5 (A) Schematic representation of the experimental design and representative fMRI data in one subject. Sensory stimulation was applied to the index (D2) or middle (D3) finger alone or to both fingers at the same time (D23) while the fMRI bold signal was recorded. A linear approximation of the fMRI signal associated with combined stimulation of D2 and D3 was calculated and substracted from the measured signal, giving rise to the 'error' of 'variance'. (B) Variance results in graphic form for all control subjects and patients with dystonia. Modified from Refs 46 and 47. (See Plate 25 in colour section.)

inputs could potentially lead to poorly differentiated control of motor representations and be the mechanisms underlying the risk of faulty motor control in some instrumentalists.

Sanger *et al.*[46,47] investigated whether evidence from fMRI supports abnormal receptive fields in primary somatosensory cortex that span more than a single finger surface. We developed a new technique for investigating overlap of sensory cortical receptive fields (Figure 26.5) and hypothesized that the combined metabolic demands of two spatially separated populations of cells, when activated simultaneously, would be approximated by the sum of the metabolic demands of each population individually. Therefore, if the populations of cells activated by the second and third digits in normal subjects are distinct, we expect that the task-related component of the blood oxygenation level–dependent (BOLD) signal obtained by simultaneous activation of the two digits will be a linear combination of the task-related BOLD signals when each finger is activated individually. Conversely, if there is overlap of the receptive fields so that the same sensory populations respond to two different fingers, we do not necessarily expect linearity, because the metabolic demands of a single population stimulated by two different fingers may be determined by a complex function of the stimulus strength.

BOLD contrast was measured with fMRI during tactile stimulation of the index finger, the middle finger, or both simultaneously in five patients with focal dystonia and seven control subjects. In the control subjects, a linear combination of activation patterns for individual finger stimulation predicts an average of 88 per cent of the variance in the pattern of activity for combined stimulation. In patients with dystonia, the linear combination predicted only 70 per cent of the combined stimulation pattern ($p = 0.008$; Figure 26.6). Therefore, our results suggest that in patients with dystonia, the same region of sensory cortex may respond to tactile stimuli on more than one finger. Disorganization of sensory representations appears to be part of the pathophysiology of focal dystonia and may contribute to motor abnormalities. Hence, emphasis needs to be placed in the sensory as well as on the motor aspects of skill acquisition and practice in musicians. Perhaps all instrumentalists should learn Braille to enhance the functional segregation of individual fingers and minimize the risk of dystonia.

Conclusion

Tools are now available to study the neurophysiological correlates of skill learning in humans. The motor cortex plays an important role in motor skill learning, but so does the sensory cortex. The sensorimotor cortex changes as a consequence of skill acquisition. These plastic changes, which probably include functional and structural components, place the subjects at great advantage for skillful task performance, but harbour the risk of the development of motor control disorders. The results of our studies may be useful in understanding not only the physiology of skill acquisitions, but also the pathophysiology of movement disorders in skilled performers. Further work along these lines may lead to helpful insight into the appropriate teaching/learning technique for fine motor skills.

Acknowledgements

Part of the work summarized in this chapter was done in collaboration with Mark Hallett, Nguyet Dang, Leonardo Cohen, José María Tormos, Josep Valls-Solé, Terrance Sanger, Gottfried Schlaug, Daniel Tarsy, Jesus Pujol, and Jaume Roset-Llobet. This work was supported in part by the General Clinical Research Center at Beth Israel Deaconess Medical Center (National Center for Research Resources MO1 RR01032) and grants from the National Institute of Mental Health (MH57980 and MH60734) and the National Eye Institute (EY12091).

References

1. **Critchley, M.** and **R. A. E. Henson** (1977) *Music and the Brain: Studies in the Neurology of Music.* Southampton: The Camelot Press.

2. **Holding, D. H. E.** (1989) *Human Skills*, 2nd ed. Chichester, New York: John Wiley & Sons.

3. **Wilson, F. R.** (1989) Acquisition and loss of skilled movement in musicians. *Sem. Neurol.* 9, 146–51.

4. **Fuster, J. M.** (1995) *Memory in the Cerebral Cortex. An Empirical Approach to Neural Networks in the Human and Nonhuman Primate.* Cambridge, MA: The MIT Press.

5. **Pascual-Leone, A., D. Nguyet, L. G. Cohen,** *et al.* (1995) Modulation of muscle responses evoked by transcranial magnetic stimulation during the acquisition of new fine motor skills. *J. Neurophysiol.* 74, 1037–45.

6. **Pascual-Leone, A., F. Tarazona,** and **M. D. Catala** (1999) Applications of transcranial magnetic stimulation in studies on motor learning. *Electroencephalogr. Clin. Neurophysiol. Suppl.* 51, 157–61.

7. **Jacobs, K. M.** and **J. P. Donoghue** (1991) Reshaping the cortical motor map by unmasking latent intracortical connections. *Science* 251, 944–7.

8. **Sanes, J. N., J. Wang,** and **J. P. Donoghue** (1992) Immediate and delayed changes of rat motor cortical output representation with new forelimb configurations. *Cerebr. Cortex* 2, 141–52.

9. **Brasil-Neto, J. P., A. Pascual-Leone, J. Valls-Solé,** *et al.* (1992) Focal transcranial magnetic stimulation and response bias in a forced-choice task. *J. Neurol. Neurosurg. Psychiatry* 55, 964–6.

10. **Brasil-Neto, J. P., J. Valls-Solé, A. Pascual-Leone,** *et al.* (1993) Rapid modulation of human cortical motor outputs following ischaemic nerve block. *Brain* 116, 511–25.

11. **Iriki, A., C. Pavlides A. Keller,** and **H. Asanuma** (1989) Long-term potentiation in the motor cortex. *Science* 245, 1385–7.

12. **Iriki, A., C. Pavlides, A. Keller,** and **H. Asanuma** (1991) Long-term potentiation of thalamic input to the motor cortex induced by coactivation of thalamocortical and corticocortical afferents. *J. Neurophysiol.* 65, 1435–1.

13. **Greenough, W. T.** (1984) Structural correlates of information storage in the mammalian brain: a review and hypothesis. *Trends Neurosci.* 7, 229–33.

14. **Pons, T. P., P. E. Garraghty, A. K. Ommaya,** and **J. H. Kaas** (1991) Massive cortical reorganization after sensory deafferentation in adult macaques. *Science* 252, 1857–60.

15. **Seitz, R. J., E. Roland, C. Bohm,** *et al.* (1990) Motor learning in man: a positron emission tomographic study. *Neuroreport* 1, 57–60.

16. **Grafton, S. T., J. C. Mazziotta, S. Presty,** *et al.* (1992) Functional anatomy of human procedural learning determined with regional cerebral blood flow and PET. *J. Neurosci.* 12, 2542–8.

17. **Grafton, S. T., R. P. Woods,** and **J. M. Tyszka** (1994) Functional imaging of procedural motor learning: relating cerebral blood flow with individual subject performance. *Human Brain Mapping* 1, 221–34.

18. **Grafton, S. T., E. Hazeltine,** and **R. Ivry** (1995) Functional mapping of sequence learning in normal humans. *J. Cognit. Neurosci.* 7, 497–510.

19. **Jenkins, I. H., D. J. Brooks, P. D. Nixon,** *et al.* (1994) Motor sequence learning: a study with positron emission tomography. *J. Neurosci.* 14, 3775–90.

20. **Karni, A., G. Meyer, P. Jezzard,** *et al.* (1994) Where practice makes perfect: an fMRI study of long-term motor cortex plasticity associated with the acquisition of a motor skill (abstr). *Soc. Neurosci. Abstr.* 20, 1291.

21. **Karni, A., G. Meyer, P. Jezzard,** *et al.* (1995) Functional MRI evidence for adult motor cortex plasticity during motor skill learning. *Nature* 377, 155–8.

22. Karni, A., G. Meyer, C. Rey-Hipolito, *et al.* (1998) The acquisition of skilled motor performance: fast and slow experience-driven changes in primary motor cortex. *Proc. Natl. Acad. Sci. USA* 95, 861–8.

23. Pascual-Leone, A., J. Grafman, and M. Hallett (1994) Explicit and implicit learning and maps of cortical motor output. *Science* 265, 1600–1.

24. Schieber, M. H. (1990) How might the motor cortex individuate movements. *Trends Neurosci.* 13, 440–5.

25. Schieber, M. H. and L. S. Hibbard (1993) How somatotopic is the motor cortex hand area? *Science* 261, 489–92.

26. AOu, S. A., C. D. Woody, and D. Birt (1992) Increases in excitability of neurons of the motor cortex of cats after rapid acquisition of eye blink conditioning. *J. Neurophysiol.* 12, 560–9.

27. Woody, C. D. (1986) Understanding the cellular basis for learning and memory. *Annu. Rev. Psychol.* 37, 433–93.

28. Pascual-Leone, A., J. M. Tormos, J. Keenan, *et al.* (1998) Study and modulation of human cortical excitability with transcranial magnetic stimulation. *J. Clin. Neurophysiol.* 15, 333–43.

29. Pascual-Leone, A., D. Bartres-Faz, and J. P. Keenan (1999) Transcranial magnetic stimulation: studying the brain-behaviour relationship by induction of 'virtual lesions'. *Philos. Trans. R. Soc. Lond. B Biol. Sci.* 354, 1229–38.

30. Mendoza, D. W. and H. Wichman (1978) 'Inner' darts: effects of mental practice on performance of dart throwing. *Percept. Motor Skills* 47, 1195–9.

31. McBride, E. R. and A. L. Rothstein (1979) Mental and physical practice and the learning and retention of open and closed skills. *Percept. Motor Skills* 49, 359–65.

32. Dennis, M. Visual imagery and the use of mental practice in the development of motor skills. *Can. J. Appl. Sport Sci.* 10, 4S–16S.

33. Schonberg, H. (1987) *Great Pianists.* St. Louis, MO: Fireside Books.

34. Schonberg, H. (1988) *The Virtuosi.* New York: Vintage-Random House.

35. Ingvar, D. H. and L. Philipson (1977) Distribution of the cerebral blood flow in the dominant hemisphere during motor ideation and motor performance. *Ann. Neurol.* 2, 230–7.

36. Roland, P. E., L. Eriksson, S. Stone-Elander, and L. Widen (1987) Does mental activity change the oxidative metabolism of the brain? *J. Neurosci.* 7, 2373–89.

37. Decety, J. and D. H. Ingvar (1990) Brain structures participating in mental simulation of motor behavior: a neuropsychological interpretation. *Acta Psychol. (Amst.)* 73, 13–34.

38. Decety, J., D. Perani, M. Jeannerod, *et al.* (1994) Mapping motor representations with positron emission tomography. *Nature* 371, 600–2.

39. Hallett, M. (1998) The neurophysiology of dystonia. *Arch. Neurol.* 55, 601–603.

40. Pujol, J., J. Roset-Llobet, D. Rosines-Cubells, *et al.* (2000) Brain cortical activation during guitar-induced hand dystonia studied by functional MRI. *Neuroimage* 12, 257–67.

41. Hallett, M. (1995) Is dystonia a sensory disorder? *Ann. Neurol.* 38, 139–40.

42. Bara-Jimenez, W., M. J. Catalan, M. Hallett, and C. Gerloff (1998) Abnormal somatosensory homunculus in dystonia of the hand. *Ann. Neurol.* 44, 828–31.

43. Elbert, T., V. Candia, E. Altenmuller, *et al.* (1998) Alteration of digital representations in somatosensory cortex in focal hand dystonia. *Neuroreport* 9, 3571–75.

44. Byl, N. N. and M. Merzenich (1997) The neural consequences of repetition: clinical implications of a learning hypothesis. *J. Hand Ther.* 10, 160–74.

45. **Byl, N. N., M. M. Merzenich**, and **W. M. Jenkins** (1996) A primate genesis model of focal dystonia and repetitive strain injury. I. Learning-induced dedifferentiation of the representation of the hand in the primary somatosensory cortex in adult monkeys. *Neurology* 47, 508–20.

46. **Sanger, T., A. Pascual-Leone, D. Tarsy**, and **G. Schlaug** (2001) Non-linear sensory cortex response to simultaneous tactile stimuli in writer's cramp. *Movement Dis.* In Press

47. **Sanger, T., D. Tarsy**, and **A. Pascual-Leone** (2001) Abnormalties of spatial and temporal sensory discrimination in writer's cramp. *Movement Dis.* In press.

PART VI

RELATION OF MUSIC TO OTHER COGNITIVE DOMAINS

CHAPTER 27

THE SOUNDS OF POETRY VIEWED AS MUSIC

FRED LERDAHL

Abstract

An extended parallel is developed between musical and prosodic structures, using the author's cognitively oriented music theory and recent work in generative phonology. As illustration, the sounds of a short poem by Robert Frost are treated entirely in musical terms. The poem is assigned a phonological stress grid and then musical grouping and meter. These structures enable a durational realization. Phonological stress also helps assign the poem's normative melodic contour. Finally, the similarities and differences in sound repetition are given hierarchical structure by means of musical prolongational theory. These formal parallels suggest a corresponding realization in brain localization and function. Evidence from the neuropsychological literature is cited in support of this view. The picture emerges that grouping, metre, duration, contour, and timbral similarity are mind/brain systems shared by music and language, whereas linguistic syntax and semantics and musical pitch relations are systems not shared by the two domains.

Keywords: Poetry and music; Music and poetry; Phonology, generative; Frost, Robert

Introduction

Comparisons between music and language have traditionally been couched in terms of syntax or rhetoric.[1] The more substantive parallels, however, are between musical structures on the one hand and phonological and prosodic structures on the other, and they derive from the fact that music and language both consist of sounds organized in time. Here I explore these parallels by developing a representational and partly computational account of the sounds of a poem treated entirely as music. This approach builds on work from previous collaborations and consultations.[2–5] As I hope to show, the analysis is suggestive for the neurobiology of music.

A musical-poetic analysis

Consider in some detail the first two lines Robert Frost's short lyric 'Nothing Gold Can Stay', given in its entirety in Figure 27.1. Grouping structure, a fundamental component in music theory, segments a musical surface hierarchically into motives, phrases, and sections. Phonologists have developed a comparable concept, the prosodic hierarchy.[6] Hence linguistics now offers a second kind of tree structure, a prosodic as well as a syntactic one.

Nature's first green is gold,
Her hardest hue to hold.
Her early leaf's a flower;
But only so an hour.
Then leaf subsides to leaf.
So Eden sank to grief.
So dawn goes down to day.
Nothing gold can stay.

Figure 27.1 'Nothing Gold Can Stay', by Robert Frost.

[C Nature's] [C first] [C green] [C is gold] [C Her hardest] [C hue] [C to hold]
[P Nature's] [P first green] [P is gold] [P Her hardest hue] [P to hold]
[I Nature's first green is gold] [I Her hardest hue to hold]
[U Nature's first green is gold Her hardest hue to hold]

Figure 27.2 Bracketed, stratified representation of the prosodic analysis of the first couplet. C = clitic group, P = phonological phrase, I = intonational phrase, and U = utterance.

Even where the two coincide in their segmentations, their meanings differ. Syntactic trees represent parts of speech and syntactic phrases; phonological trees represent groupings of spoken sound.

At the lowest levels of the prosodic hierarchy are the syllable and the word. Words categorize as either content words, which carry major semantic content, or function words, which mainly fill a syntactic role. For example, in the first line of the poem, 'Nature's first green is gold', all the words are content words except 'is'. At the level above the word is the clitic group, which coincides either with a content word or combines content and function words that, together, sound as if they were one word. In the latter case, the stressed syllable of the content word is the clitic host, the sound to which the others are drawn. In 'Nature's first green is gold', 'is gold' sounds as one word, with 'gold' as clitic host. Likewise in the second line, 'Her hardest hue to hold', the content words are 'hardest', 'hue', and 'hold'; 'Her hardest' and 'to hold' are clitic groups, with 'hard-' and 'hold' as clitic hosts. Above the clitic group is a grouping of words called the phonological phrase, for example, 'first green'. Above that is the intonational phrase, which conveys the melody of speech. The entire line, 'Nature's first green is gold', is an intonational phrase. Finally, there is the utterance, which usually corresponds to a sentence. 'Nature's first green is gold,/Her hardest hue to hold' is an utterance.

Figure 27.2 displays the grouping analysis of the first two lines of the poem. The syllable and word levels are omitted for convenience. The bracketing categories are indicated in boldface. A category can repeat from one level to the next. This representation abstractly resembles a parsing of a musical phrase into subgroups and motives. As in music, pauses are more likely to occur between, rather than within, these segments, with greater pauses between superordinate boundaries.

Now consider linguistic stress, whose musical equivalent is phenomenal accent.[2] In both, the perception, whether of a syllable or of a pitch event, is one of relative sonic prominence within its immediate context. Linguists have proposed a so-called metrical grid to represent linguistic stress in words and phrases.[7] From a musical perspective, this designation is misleading; it acts as a stress grid, for its purpose is to represent not hierarchical periodicities but hierarchical patterns of stress. Within a polysyllabic word, such a pattern is given lexically, as in the first word of the poem, 'Náture's' (in English, one would not say 'Natúre's'). Within a phrase, the stress pattern obeys the nuclear stress rule, which, after the categorization of words into content and function words, assigns global stress to the strongest syllable of the last content word of a prosodic unit.[8] Thus, we say 'first gréen', rather than 'first green', because 'green' is the last stressed syllable of its phonological phrase. This principle can be overridden by the rhythm rule, which ameliorates clashes in stress between adjacent or nearby syllables. According to nuclear stress, one says 'hardest húe', but we might prefer to adjust it to 'hárdest hue', so that the nearby words 'hue' and 'hold' are not comparably stressed. The rhythm rule implicitly invokes metrical periodicity: strong beats should be more or less evenly spaced. At this level, then, the choice is between 'Her hardest húe to hóld', which obeys nuclear stress but challenges periodicity, and 'Her hárdest hue to hold', which violates nuclear stress in order to distribute the stresses. Finally, nuclear stress can be overridden by nonnormative focus on a particular word, to bring out a semantic nuance. Hence if we say 'Nature's first green is gold', the implication is that nature's second green is not gold. Generally, however, nuclear stress holds.

Setting the rhythm rule and focus to one side, a stress grid is constructed by cyclic generation of stresses from level to level in the prosodic hierarchy, observing nuclear stress starting at the phonological grouping level. As illustrated in Figure 27.3a, the procedure is first to assign an x to every syllable, second to assign an x in the next row to a lexically relatively stressed syllable in a polysyllabic word or to the host of a clitic group. For the third row, shown in Figure 27.3b, an x for the nuclear stress is added at the level of the phonological phrase. Finally, in Figure 27.3c, an x for the nuclear stress is assigned at the level of

```
A    x          x        x         x          x        x          x

     x  x       x        x         x  x       x  x  x    x        x  x

   [C Nature's] [C first] [C green] [C is gold] [C Her hardest][C hue][C to hold]


B    x                   x         x                     x          x

     x          x        x         x          x          x          x

     x  x       x        x         x  x       x  x  x    x        x  x

   [P  Nature's] [P first    green] [P is gold] [P Her hardest    hue] [P to hold]


                                   x                               x

C    x                   x         x                     x          x

     x          x        x         x          x          x          x

     x  x       x        x         x  x       x  x  x    x        x  x

   [I  Nature's    first    green    is gold] [I Her hardest    hue    to hold]
```

Figure 27.3 Assignment of the stress grid in conjunction with the prosodic hierarchy.

level d:	[Na]	[ture's]	[first]	[green]	[is]	[gold] [Her]	[hard]	[est]	[hue] [to]	[hold]
level c:	[Na-	]	[first]	[green] [		gold] [	hard-		[hue] [	hold]
level b:	[Na-	] [		green] [		gold] [			hue] [	hold]
level a:	[					gold] [				hold]

Figure 27.4 The stress pattern in Figure 27.3 put in reductional format.

the intonational phrase. There is little point in continuing to yet another level, for, as in music, distinctions in linguistic stress attenuate over long spans.

Figure 27.4 recasts the stress pattern in Figure 27.3c into an equivalent music-reductional format. Level *d* brackets the syllables and corresponds in content to the bottom row of the stress grid in Figure 27.3c. Level *c* reduces out the syllables and monosyllabic words that in Figure 27.3c are assigned only one *x*. Similarly, levels *b* and *a* keep only those units that carry three and four *x*s, respectively. This is the same layout as in musical time-span reduction, which selects relatively important pitch events at successively larger levels of rhythmic segmentation.[2] These relationships could alternatively be displayed by a tree representation with right and left branching, again as in the corresponding music theory.

Turn now to metre. In both music and poetry, metrical structure consists of hierarchic-ally related periodicities inferred from the signal. It might be objected that periodicities in language, unlike those in music, do not really exist because syllabic and phrasal durations are so variable. Yet it would be misleading to say that musical durations are invariable. Expressive musical performance depends on deviations from isochrony. Like metre itself, temporal precision is a mental construct. While it is true that durations in verse are usually more variable than in music, many poetic idioms, from nursery rhymes to sophisticated traditions, demonstrate considerable regularity.[9] As in music, these verbal idioms approach periodicity as a framework against which expressive deviations take place.

Once periodicity is understood as a relative matter, poetic and musical meter may be regarded as formally and cognitively equivalent. This has, in essence, long been recognized by music theorists in their occasional borrowing of prosodic foot notation for the rep-resention of musical metre. Now, however, it is more usual in music theory to employ a grid notation, which represents the metrical hierarchy directly and does not confuse features of metre with those of grouping.[2] A similar consensus has emerged in phonological theory.

A poetic or musical metre exists when the perceiver infers conceptually regular levels of beats from the signal, such that a beat that is strong at one level is also a beat at the next larger level. The perceptually most prominent metrical level is called the tactus; it occurs at a moderate tempo, is usually at an intermediate level within a grid, and is often more restricted in regularity than are smaller or larger levels. Beats at a given level are two or three beats apart at the next smaller level. (Even pentametre lines have intermediate strong beats, resulting in patterns of two and three.) Some poetic or musical idioms, while allow-ing a mixture of two or three beats apart across levels, discourage the mixture of two or three strong beats apart within a level. Thus, European classical tonal music uses compounds of two and three across levels as in Figure 27.5a and b, but it regards as atypical the grid in Figure 27.5c, which alternates two and three beats within a single level. Other musical cul-tures, as in the Balkan countries, would take Figure 27.5c as normative. The important point

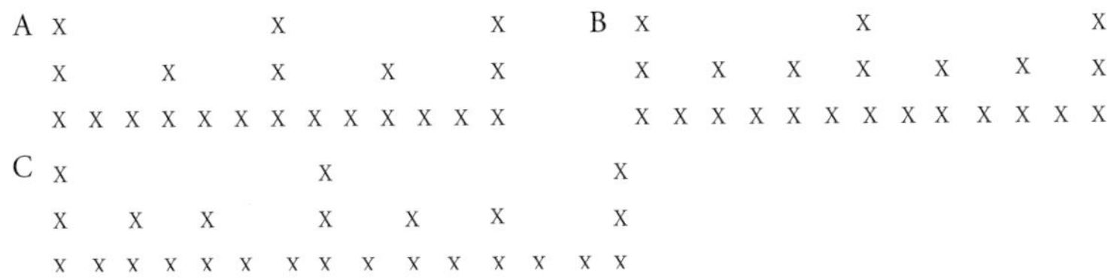

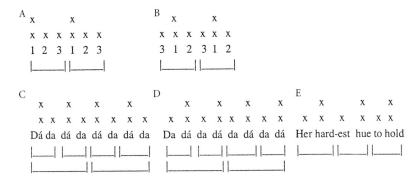

Figure 27.5 Three metrical grids: (A) 6/8 metre; (B) 3/4 metre; (C) 7/8 metre (2 + 2 + 3).

Figure 27.6 Interaction of grouping and metre: (A) 3/4 metre with afterbeats; (B) 3/4 metre with an upbeat and an afterbeat; (C) trochaic tetrametre; (D) iambic tetrametre; (E) conflict between word and foot boundaries at 'hardest'.

is not that different cultures prefer different metrical grids, but that the possible combinations of two and three, across or within levels, are very small. Cultural variation on poetic and musical metres is intrinsically limited.

In constructing a metrical grid, the perceiver seeks an optimal fit between the stresses provided by the acoustic signal and the culturally available repertory of metrical grids. To hear a musical phrase in 3/4 time or a poetic line in pentametre is to select that particular grid because, within the repertory, that grid gives the minimal number of conflicts between stress and beat. Where the fit is imperfect, the effect is one of syncopation or, to use terms from traditional scansion, of inversion, substitution, or truncation. If the fit is seriously imperfect, the perceiver switches to another available grid or perhaps abandons metrical understanding altogether.

The interaction of grouping and metre causes intuitions of upbeat and afterbeat in relation to a downbeat. The metre is 3/4 in Figure 27.6a and b, but the two differ in that Figure 27.6a has afterbeats while Figure 27.6b has an upbeat and an afterbeat. The terminology of traditional scansion recognizes this upbeat-afterbeat distinction. In current notation, Figure 27.6c and d represents the contrasting groupings of trochaic and iambic tetrametre, respectively. Traditional foot scansion becomes troublesome, however, in cases where the presumed foot contradicts the prosodic hierarchy. Supposing our lyric to be in iambic trimetre, in the line, 'Her hardest hue to hold', the foot-grouping of '-est' is not with its own word stem, 'hard-', but counterintuitively with 'hue', as shown in Figure 27.6e. It is unclear in such cases what function the poetic foot serves. In the present view, iambs, trochees, dactyls, and so on, arise not from a predetermined schema but directly from the prosodic groupings of beats. Moreover, the concept of the foot lacks a musical counterpart. While recognizing its historical practice, let us ignore the foot as an independent unit of rhythmic analysis.

Having set to one side the iambic dimension of our poem, I would now suggest that it is not in trimetre either. The punctuated pauses at the end of each line and, more elusively, the historical style that it evokes, suggest that it is in truncated tetrametre. Many short lyrics, such as those of Emily Dickinson, employ so-called common metre, comprising couplets in a four-plus-three beat pattern with an implied silent final beat: da-dá, da-dá, da-dá, da-dá; da-dá, da-dá, da-dá, —. Common metre is a variant of standard tetrameter, the final silent beat reinforcing the grouping structure. Our poem is in turn a variant of common metre. Frost uses it here because of the ineluctable decline that is the poem's theme. Every line falls into silence.

Given this paradigmatic metre, the first two lines of the poem receive the structural description in Figure 27.7. Above the lines appears the stress grid, taken from Figure 27.3c. Beneath, in boldface and inverted for visual convenience, is the metrical grid for the tactus and larger levels, showing four basic beats per line and their relative metrical strengths. The tactus is represented by upper-case Xs. To clarify the grid notation, the beats are numbered as two 4/4 measures, grouped into two intonational phrases. Only stresses of three or four xs count for the establishment of the tactus. Since the greatest stresses occur on 'gold' and 'hold', these syllables are assigned the strongest beats. The periodicity of the metrical grid requires that 'Na-' and 'hard-' receive the next strongest metrical position, with 'green', 'hue', and the silent beats getting the weaker beats. This treatment creates a slight syncopation at 'hue'. Observe that the strongest metrical beats take place at the end of each line, creating an out-of-phase relationship between the grouping boundaries and the spans between the strongest beats. This is a consequence of nuclear stress and is characteristic of poetry in English. In classical tonal music, by contrast, the strongest beat usually comes at or near the beginning of a phrase. For its ending rhythmic articulation, tonal music relies instead on the cadence, for which there is no linguistic counterpart. (In Balinese gamelan the strongest beat usually arrives at the end of a phrase.[10])

					x			x	
	x		x	x			x	x	
Stress	x	x	x	x		x	x	x	
grid:	x x	x	x	x x		x	x x	x x	
	Nature's	first	green	is	gold,	Her	hardest	hue	to hold.

Metrical	**X**		**X**	**X**	**X**	**X**	**X**	**X**	
grid:	x			x		x		x	
				x				x	
Beats in 4/4:	3		4	1	2	3	4	1	2
Phrase boundaries:	|_____||_____|							

Figure 27.7 Stress and metrical analysis for the first two lines of the Frost poem.

This analysis indicates conceptually equal durations between tactus beats. To derive subtactus levels, the two requisite principles are to seek the best possible fit (1) between stress and beat, and (2) between duration and the prosodic hierarchy. Condition 1 has already been discussed; it is a matter of matching the metrical with the stress grid, starting with the tactus level. Condition 2 invokes the Gestalt principle that proximate objects tend to group together. It follows that grouping boundaries tend to exist between objects in a string that are relatively nonproximate. The prosodic hierarchy is meant to reflect perceptual groupings of sound. Therefore, contextually longer durations—or, more precisely, distances between attack points—should occur between, rather than within, the constituents of the prosodic hierarchy. Once these subtactus levels are established, the metrical positions of all the syllables of the couplet can be translated into standard musical notation.

Let us apply these two conditions to the first three words of the poem, 'Nature's first 'green', and derive their durations. Figure 27.8a fully satisfies condition 1: 'Na-' and 'green' provide the tactus frame, and in both grids '-ture's' receives a single x and 'First' receives two x's. Translated into metrical durations, the result is a duple division with two sixteenth notes plus an eighth note. But this solution does not satisfy condition 2: the greater distance is between 'first' and 'green', weakening the perception of the phonological group 'first green'. The alternative in Figure 27.8b, an eighth plus two sixteenths, is more problematic still, for it both violates condition 1 and breaks up the word 'Nature's' with the longer duration. Figure 27.8c effects the preferable solution by smoothing out the durations in a triple-beat realization. Condition 1 is almost met, and there is no implication of an unwanted grouping boundary.

On the assumption that triple metre continues at the eighth-note level, Figure 27.9 completes the subtactus level for Figure 27.7 and realizes the rhythm for the two lines. The match between stress and beat is complete, and the durations reflect the constituents of the prosodic hierarchy: 'is gold', 'Her hardest', and 'to hold' are all clitic groups, grouped musically by temporal proximity and surrounded on either side by longer distances between attack points.

If this derivational procedure is carried out for the entire poem, the rhythmic derivation is as in Figure 27.10, cast in 12/8 metre with two-beat anacruses for each line. Minor adjustments with duple divisions appear in the second, third, and fourth lines. The first three of these have to do with syllable length. For example, in Figure 27.9 'hard-' receives an eighth note and '-est' a quarter note, even though 'hard-' is a longer syllable than '-est'. To reverse the values, however, so that 'hard-' is assigned a quarter note and '-est' an eighth note,

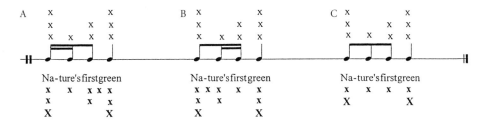

Figure 27.8 Duple and triple subtactus metrical realizations for the beginning of the first line.

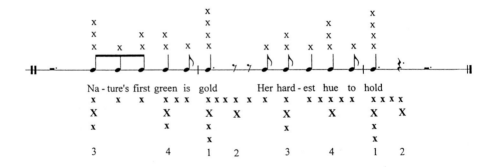

Figure 27.9 Addition of the subtactus level to Figure 27.7, with translation into musical durations.

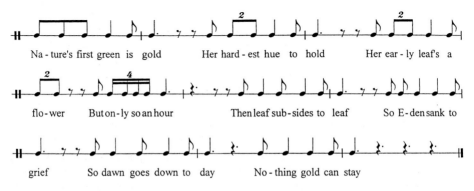

Figure 27.10 Durational reading of the poem.

would violate condition 2, weakening the word boundary. A compromise is effected in Figure 27.10 by a duple realization—two equal eighth notes—for 'hard-est'. The rhythm of 'But only so an hour' is caused by a different factor: the only content words are 'only' and 'hour', so that the monosyllabic words 'so' and 'an' are cliticized. The absence of any stress between 'on-' and 'hour' permits a quick setting. 'Hour' arrives a beat earlier than it otherwise would, and consequently there is a longer pause between the two quatrains than between the lines internal to each quatrain. These changes in lines two, three, and four induce considerable rhythmic variety in the first quatrain. This variety in turn sets up the second quatrain's rhythmic monotony, a reflection of its sense of futility.

We turn now by way of stress to contour. Three acoustic variables contribute to stress: intensity (or loudness), pitch height, and duration.[11] While duration is an independent variable, intensity and pitch height covary, for the muscles that enable greater intensity also tend to raise pitch. Even when pitch height is artifically isolated, relative height induces the perception of relative stress. Thus, pitch height is a strong projector of stress. Since pitch height is a matter of contour, stress patterns can provide a basis for the derivation of speech melody. There are many acceptable contours, however, for an intonational phrase or utterance, each having its own nuance. If our concern were grammaticality, in keeping with

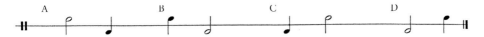

Figure 27.11 Four normative contour frameworks.

much generative linguistics, well-formedness constraints would underdetermine the options for contour realizations. A different goal, and one congenial with a musical perspective, is to ask whether a grammatical contour is normative or not. One need then derive only normative contours from stress grids, letting the other grammatical contours be seen as nuanced variants.

To pursue this question, let us initially restrict contour features to a binary classification of high and low, and apply it to the two most stressed syllables in an intonational phrase. Contour theory in linguistics has represented this classification by 'H' and 'L', with accompanying diacritics to indicate hierarchical function.[12,13] However, it is in the spirit of the approach taken here to employ musical notation, which after all is designed to show pitch height. As is common in musical reduction theory, hierarchy can be represented by note values that stand not for durations but for relative structural importance. In Figure 27.11a the first syllable is high and the second low, with the half-note first syllable acting as superordinate to the quarter-note second syllable. The high–low pattern continues in Figure 27.11b but with a superordinate low syllable. Figure 27.11c and d reverses the high–low pattern. These four cases exhaust the possibilities. The prototypical declarative contour is that in Figure 27.11a and b, a rise and fall whose musical analogue is the tensing–relaxing pattern of a standard tonal phrase. The difference between the two is whether the high or the low syllable dominates. In Figure 27.11c and d, the high syllable is to the right of the low one; this is the typical shape of an interrogative.

The claim that a higher pitch causes stress would seem to disqualify Figure 27.11b and d as normative, since in these cases the low syllable dominates. As a consequence of nuclear stress, however, a superordinate low syllable can indeed function in the position of the last clitic host of an intonational phrase. In other words, this syllable's location at the close of a major phrase boundary compensates for its lower pitch. Hence Figure 27.11b is normative. By the same token, Figure 27.11d is not normative, because in this case the dominating low syllable is not in a location to benefit from major nuclear stress. As there are no interrogatives in our poem, we can also ignore Figure 27.11c. This leaves Figure 27.11a and b as the remaining options. This very restricted repertory will provide the framework for mapping stress importance onto contour peaks and valleys.

In this presentation we take for granted but do not notate that there is sliding from one pitch level to another (in musical terms, there is a glissando from one pitch to another). We also posit that a given syllable has a single pitch level, ignoring cases in which a syllable slides between two pitch levels, especially at a phrase boundary. For example, in the utterance 'He has gone!', 'gone' normally begins high because it is stressed but ends low in order to convey its declarative status. In 'He has gone?', however, 'gone' begins low but ends high in order to convey its interrogative status. Finally, we bypass the possibility that an extended sequence of highs and lows can gradually ramp up or (more commonly) down, so that the

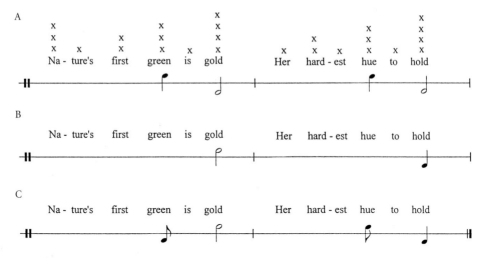

Figure 27.12 Global contour assignments for the first couplet.

pitch levels do not stay absolute but are relative. In short, our contour model is highly idealized. Even so, it generates plausible shapes derived from musical principles.

The stress analysis in Figure 27.3b and c assigns three *x*s for the most stressed syllable in each phonological phrase and four *x*s for the most stressed syllable in each intonational phrase, the latter occurring at the end of the line. Hence, as shown in Figure 27.12a, the intonational contours for the first two lines of the poem fall in the pattern of Figure 27.11b. The two lines together, however, form an utterance, leading to the assignment in Figure 27.12b of high and low to four *x*s at this level, at 'gold' and 'hold', respectively. The assignment for 'gold' is thereby reversed from low in Figure 27.12a, to high in Figure 27.12b. This step does not yet determine whether 'gold' or 'hold' dominates; for reasons beyond the present purview, 'gold' is chosen. The next step is to combine the shapes at the utterance and intonational levels. In Figure 27.12a, 'green' was realized as high, an assignment that is no longer preferred because it would conflict with the high 'gold' in Figure 27.12b. Therefore 'green' receives a low position within its intonational phrase, as shown in Figure 27.12c; the eighth-note value signifies its subordinate status. In the next line, 'hue' remains high, for it combines at the intonational level with the superordinate low 'hold', although it too receives a subordinate eighth-note value. This is the scaffolding within which more local contour shapes take place.

A two-place categorization of high and low does not provide enough distinctions as more syllables come into play. Four levels appear to be optimal: three do not afford sufficient variety, and more than four would be fussy in view of the limited ability to categorize degrees of stress. In the musical notation, there are now two lines with spaces above and below, so that the highest position is placed above the top line, the second highest on the top line, the second lowest between the lines, and the lowest on the bottom line. On the basis of the salience of registral extremes, the two most prominent syllables, again represented by half and quarter notes, are placed in the top and bottom positions.

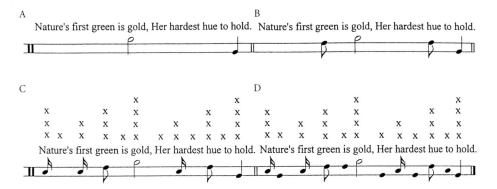

Figure 27.13 Assignment of pitch levels to the first couplet: (A,B) from the analysis in Figure 27.12; (C) for unassigned syllables with three two *x*'s; (D) for syllables with one *x*.

Figure 27.13a performs this step for the first couplet. Figure 27.13b appends pitch heights for the syllables in the third hierarchical position, again represented by eighth notes, and places them one slot lower than their adjacent superordinate high syllable. These locations preserve the rising–falling shape of the contour schema in Figure 27.11a and b. Except where a superordinate low syllable occurs at the right edge of an intonational phrase, the contour reflects the shape of the stress grid, with its peaks and valleys of *x*s. Thus, in Figure 27.13c the syllables with three and two *x*s, notated by sixteenth notes, appear one slot below the positions of the syllables that were already given three *x*s in Figure 27.13b. Then in Figure 27.13d come the syllables with one *x*, represented by unstemmed noteheads. These syllables are cliticized and are typically spoken as schwas (the default neutral vowel for an unstressed syllable). They are placed one step below their clitic hosts, except when the latter are in the lowest slot, in which case they are located one step above the clitic host. Hence '-ure's' is one step below 'Na-' in 'Nature's', and 'is' one step below 'gold', but 'to' is one step above 'hold', since the latter is in the bottom slot.

This derivation of contour is musical not only in its attention to normative shapes but in its hierarchical treatment. Rather than generate contours from left to right, as if without projection or memory, global highs and lows are established according to a few paradigmatic shapes and the remaining syllables in the speech melody are filled in at successive levels of lesser stress. Figure 27.14 shows the result, combining the contour analysis of Figure 27.13 with the metrical/durational analysis of Figure 27.10, but now with these methods applied to the entire poem. Contained within this seemingly transparent musical notation are the structures of phonological stress, the prosodic hierarchy, the metrical grid, duration, and pitch height. The success of the derivation can be judged informally by its naturalness as a reading.

A usual prosodic analysis would have stopped before this point. From a musical perspective, there is yet another step to take, an analysis of the hierarchical patterns of recurrence of sounds. Traditional poetic analysis treats verbal recurrences such as rhyme, alliteration, and assonance as primitive sequential patterns: *aabb, abab,* and so forth. Music theory, in contrast, has a highly developed approach to recurrence in the form of prolongational structure.

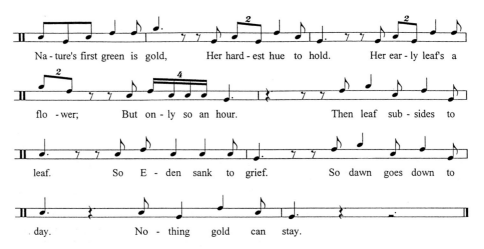

Figure 27.14 Metre and durations (from Figure 27.10) combined with a contour analysis of the entire poem.

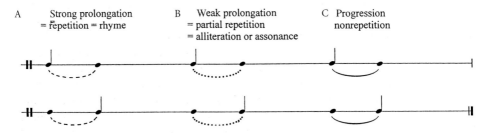

Figure 27.15 Repertory of prolongational connections.

Figure 27.15 gives three kinds of prolongational connection: (1) strong prolongation or repetition, represented by a dashed slur; (2) weak prolongation or partial repetition, represented by a dotted slur; and (3) progression or nonrepetition, represented by a solid slur. In each case the superordinate element can precede or succeed the elaborating element.

Musical prolongational connections are derived through a combination of time-span segmentation and tonal pitch stability.[2,14] Poetry incorporates the former through the prosodic hierarchy but lacks any counterpart to the tonal system. The better musical analogy, then, is to atonal music, for which event salience largely replaces event stability.[14] That is, when hearing atonal surfaces, and given the absence of acoustic or idiom-specific criteria to select stable from unstable events within hierarchical time spans, the listener tends to organize embellishing events in relation to events that have greater surface prominence within the framework of the time-span hierarchy. In phonological terms, relative surface prominence is equivalent to relative stress. Hence prosodic prolongation can be viewed as a kind of atonal prolongation, in which the elements being prolonged are not pitch structures but degrees of timbral similarity mediated by stress within the prosodic hierarchy. (This approach extends beyond my earlier treatment, in which synthesized vowels are

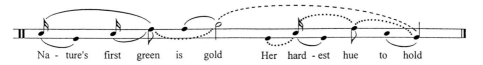

Figure 27.16 Prolongational structure for the first couplet. The contours are retained from Figure 27.14.

related prolongationally by similarity but without the incorporation of nested patterns of stress.[15]) The three prolongational categories continue intact: the repetition of rhyme equals strong prolongation; the weaker repetition of alliteration or assonance equals weak prolongation; and syllabic nonrepetition equals progression.

The syllables connected in the prolongational analysis of the first couplet follow the parsing of the prosodic hierarchy in Figure 27.2 and the hierarchical contour in Figure 27.13d. Each connection forms a progression, weak prolongation, or strong prolongation, according to the degree of repetition of sound. Figure 27.16 illustrates, retaining the structural notation of Figure 27.13d. In the first line, 'ture's' attaches as a progression from 'Na-', 'first' to 'green', and 'is' to 'gold'. At the next level, 'Na-' attaches to 'green' because both have three *x*s. Then 'green' attaches to 'gold', as a weak prolongation because of the alliteration between 'green' and 'gold'. The second line creates a similar pattern, but with more internal alliteration. Finally, at the level of the couplet, the two syllables with four *x*s, 'gold' and 'hold', form a rhyming strong prolongation. Note that it is timbral similarity rather than pitch that is connected prolongationally, for 'gold' is in the highest pitch category while 'hold' is in the lowest. The resulting graph shows not isolated instances of alliteration and rhyme, as in traditional prosodic analysis, but the richer relationship of partial repetitions nested within superordinate rhymes—'green' is to 'gold' as 'hue' is to 'hold'. Progressions between dissimilar syllables occur as relatively local connections. This approach can be extended to the poem as a whole.

This account of prosodic prolongational structure has skipped some derivational stages involving technicalities of the theory of musical reduction. The main point is that we can indeed transplant most of the mechanisms of the musical theory to the poetic realm.

Connections

Let us step back from the derivation of the Frost analysis and assume that the music-analytic methods outlined here have validity for modelling the sonic organization of poetry in general. To what extent do these methods extend to the analysis of ordinary speech? Briefly, ordinary speech possesses phonological stress, the prosodic hierarchy, and contour, so the application of these components should continue intact. The phonological stresses of ordinary speech, however, are irregular enough to inhibit the inference of a metrical grid. Similarly, ordinary speech lacks significant patterns of syllabic repetition, so that the sense of a timbral prolongational structure is weakened. These attenuated perceptions are reflected in the model by weakened metrical and prolongational derivations.

A complementary approach to the study of the relationship between music and poetry would be to develop a rigorous theory of textsetting.[16] That listeners have strong intuitions about whether a poetic line is well- or ill-set to music is in itself an indication of the parallels between the two media. Generally, the stronger the correlation between the common formal structures of poetry and music, the more idiomatic the textsetting. That is, a textsetting tends to match up the stresses, metrical positions, durations, phrasings, contours, and formal patterns of a poem and its musical realization. The idiom-specific traditions of *Sprechstimme* in early 20th-century German musical expressionism and of hip hop in current American popular music show how far music and language can merge along these dimensions.

The overall thrust of the Frost analysis is that the mental representation of the sounds of metrical, rhymed poetry and of music, whether texted or not, share a good deal more organization than has usually been supposed. Perhaps this commonality has not been adequately recognized because in certain basic respects the two media are unlike: poetry has words and phrases with propositional meaning; music has a hierarchical, multidimensional pitch space.[14,17] The analysis of the Frost reflects these differences by omitting references both to the poem's imagery or meaning and to musical concepts such as specific pitches and intervals, scales, harmony, key, voice leading, counterpoint, or tonal tension and relaxation.

It seems reasonable to suppose that well-founded theoretical parallels and distinctions have counterparts in brain structure and function. Appropriate theory can thus guide and interpret neurological findings. We may inquire, then, to what extent the commonalities and differences discussed here are instantiated in brain structure and function. The present analysis predicts, as one would expect, that there is not a single music area and a single language area, but that musical and linguistic functions are spread out in different structural and functional components. It further predicts that those brain modules that process rhythm, contour, and timbral relationships are the same in music and language, while those that process purely pitch structures and purely linguistic structures occupy different parts of the brain. Figure 27.17 illustrates.

Current neuropsychological evidence offers some support for this view. Studies of patients with brain lesions that affect musical and linguistic processing indicate that musical and phonological contours are processed in the same area but that musical pitch intervals are processed in different structures, with an apparent one-way channel from contour processing to intervallic pitch processing.[18–20] If so, individuals with deficits that inhibit their ability to process musical or linguistic contour are also unable to process specific pitch relations. This makes intuitive sense, for if a listener cannot tell up from down, how could he or she distinguish between a minor third and a perfect fourth? However, individuals unable to process musical pitch might still be able to process contour. People who are musically tone-deaf do not speak in a monotone. (In this connection, tone languages such as Chinese depend not on fixed pitch categories and intervals but on relative pitch height and contour.[21] Thus, a person could remain competent in speaking a tone language despite an inability to distinguish musical pitch relationships.)

Neuropsychological evidence also suggests a bifurcation in musical processing between pitch and rhythm. There is partial justification for this from music theory, in which grouping and metre are distinct components from both tonal reduction and tonal pitch space.[2,14] Support for this division comes not only from neuropsychology but from experiments in music cognition.[22] In the details, however, the story is bound to be more complex. From a

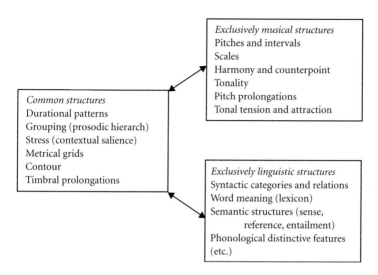

Exclusively musical structures
Pitches and intervals
Scales
Harmony and counterpoint
Tonality
Pitch prolongations
Tonal tension and attraction

Common structures
Durational patterns
Grouping (prosodic hierarch)
Stress (contextual salience)
Metrical grids
Contour
Timbral prolongations

Exclusively linguistic structures
Syntactic categories and relations
Word meaning (lexicon)
Semantic structures (sense,
        reference, entailment)
Phonological distinctive features
(etc.)

Figure 27.17 Hypothesized brain organization of musical and linguistic structures.

music-theoretic perspective, pitch is one of the inputs to the derivation of grouping and metre. For example, a tonal cadence signals a grouping boundary, and harmonic rhythm is a strong determinant of metre. Similarly, the derivation of pitch reduction depends on the position of pitches and chords within nested time spans based on grouping and metre. Yet tonal space itself—the system (or systems) of pitches, intervals, scales, chords, tonal regions, tonal attractions, degrees of sensory and cognitive consonance, and degrees of mutual proximity and stability—remains, at a theoretical level, independent of duration, grouping, and metre. Figure 27.17 projects this overall picture: except for contour and timbral prolongations, all of the items listed under 'common structures' belong to the domain of rhythm, which music and poetry share, and most of the items listed under 'exclusively musical structures' belong to tonal space.

Note that the category 'exclusively linguistic structures' in Figure 27.17 includes not just syntactic and semantic features but some phonological aspects as well, such as distinctive features.[8] Moreover, the perceptual organization of speech may not fully submit to a general, Gestalt-based auditory account.[23] These qualifications nevertheless do not undermine the convergence between theoretical and empirical treatments for the domains listed under 'common structures.'

Presumably these exclusive and common structures are a consequence of human evolution. In this view, the roots of music and language are the same, in the form of premusical and prelinguistic communicative and expressive auditory gestures involving shapes of duration, stress, contour, timbre, and grouping.[24] We still communicate with infants and higher mammals in this manner. These elementary shapes appear to lie at the basis of expressive utterance in language and of musical expression (an idea that goes back at least to Rousseau[25]). With evolution came specialization: music and language diverged in their most characteristic features, pitch organization in music and word and sentence meaning in language. Poetry straddles this evolutionary divergence by projecting, through the addition to ordinary speech of metrical and timbral patterning, its common heritage with music.

References

1. **Winn, J.** (1981) *Unsuspected Eloquence: A History of the Relations between Poetry and Music.* New Haven: Yale University Press.

2. **Lerdahl, F.** and **R. Jackendoff** (1983) *A Generative Theory of Tonal Music.* Cambridge, MA: MIT Press.

3. **Lerdahl, F.** and **J. Halle** (1991) Some lines of poetry viewed as music. In J. Sundberg, L. Nord, and R. Carlson (eds) *Music Language, Speech, and Brain.* Wenner-Gren International Symposium Series. Longon: Macmillian.

4. **Lerdahl, F.** and **X. Chabot** (1991) A theory of poetry as music and its exploration through a computer aid to composition. *Proc. Intl Computer Music Conf.*

5. **Hayes, B.** Personal communication.

6. **Hayes, B.** (1989) The prosodic hierarchy in poetry. In P. Kiparsky and G. Youmans (eds) *Phonetics and Phonology: Rhythm and Meter.* New York: Academic.

7. **Liberman, M.** and **A. Prince** (1977) On stress and linguistic rhythm. *Linguistic Inquiry* 8, 249–36.

8. **Chomsky, N.** and **M. Halle** (1968) *The Sound Pattern of English,* second printing. Cambridge, MA: MIT Press.

9. **Oehrle, R. T.** (1989) Temporal structures in verse design. In P. Kiparsky and G. Youmans (eds) *Phonetics and Phonology: Rhythm and Meter.* New York: Academic.

10. **Becker, J.** and **A. Becker** (1979) A grammar of the musical genre *Srepegan. J. Music Theory* 23, 1–44.

11. **Handel, S.** (1989) *Listening.* Cambridge, MA: MIT Press.

12. **Pierrehumbert, J.** (1980) *The Phonology and Phonetics of English Intonation.* MIT Ph.D. Dissertation.

13. **Ladd, D. R.** (1996) *Intonational Phonology.* Cambridge, UK: Cambridge University Press

14. **Lerdahl, F.** (2001) *Tonal Pitch Space.* New York: Oxford University Press.

15. **Lerdahl, F.** (1987) Timbral hierarchies. *Contemporary Music Rev.* 1, 135–60.

16. **Halle, J.** and **F. Lerdahl** (1994) A generative textsetting model. *Curr. Musicol.* 55, 3–26.

17. **Krumhansl, C. L.** (1990) *Cognitive Foundations of Musical Pitch.* New York: Oxford University Press.

18. **Peretz, I.** (1993) Auditory agnosia: a functional analysis. In S. McAdams and E. Bigand (eds) *Thinking in Sound: The Cognitive Psychology of Human Audition.* Oxford: Oxford University Press.

19. **Peretz, I.** (2001) Le cerveau musical. In J. J. Nattiez (ed.) *Enciclopedia Einaudi della musica.*

20. **Patel, A. D.** and **I. Peretz** (1997) Is music autonomous from language? A neuropsychological appraisal. In I. Deliége and J. Sloboda (eds) *Perception and Cognition of Music.* Hove, UK: Psychology Press.

21. **Yung, B.** (1991) The relationship of text and tune in Chinese opera. In J. Sundberg, L. Nord, and R. Carlson (eds) *Music, Language, Speech, and Brain.* Wenner-Gren International Symposium Series. London: Macmillan.

22. **Palmer, C.** and **C. L. Krumhansl** (1987) Independent temporal and pitch structures in determination of musical phrase. *J. Exp. Psychol. Hum. Percept. Perform.* 13, 116–26.

23. **Remez, R. E., P. E. Rubin, S. M. Berns,** *et al.* (1994) On the perceptual organization of speech. *Psychol. Rev.* 101, 129–56.

24. **Brown, S.** (2001) The 'Musilanguage' model of music, In N. L. Wallin, B. Merker, and S. Brown (eds) *The Origins of Music.* Cambridge, MA: MIT Press.

25. **Rousseau, J.-J.** (1960) Essai sur l'origine des langues. In J. H. Moran and A. Gode (trans.) *On the Origin of Language.* Chicago: University of Chicago Press.

CHAPTER 28

DOES EXPOSURE TO MUSIC HAVE BENEFICIAL SIDE EFFECTS?

E. GLENN SCHELLENBERG

Abstract

Reports that exposure to music causes benefits in nonmusical domains have received widespread attention in the mainstream media. Such reports have also influenced public policy. The so-called 'Mozart effect' actually refers to two relatively distinct phenomena. One concerns short-term improvements in spatial abilities that are said to occur after listening to music composed by Mozart. The other refers to the possibility that formal training in music yields nonmusical benefits. A review of the relevant findings indicates that the short-term effect is small and unreliable. Moreover, when it is evident, it can be explained by between-condition differences in listeners' arousal level or mood. By contrast, the effect of music lessons on nonmusical aspects of cognitive development is still an open question. Several studies have reported positive associations between formal music lessons and abilities in nonmusical (e.g. linguistic, mathematical, and spatial) domains. Nonetheless, compelling evidence for a causal link remains elusive.

Music and nonmusical abilities

The present report evaluates claims that exposure to music produces benefits in nonmusical domains. These claims began to influence public policy as soon as they came to public notice.[1] For example, Zell Miller, the former Governor of Georgia, budgeted for the distribution of classical music recordings to each infant born in state. Moreover, Florida mandates daily doses of classical music in state-run preschools.

Researchers (e.g. Ref. 2) and journalists (e.g. Refs 3–6) have generated confusion by failing to clarify the distinction between the short-term consequences of music listening and the long-term consequences of formal training in music. Indeed, results from both types of studies have been merged to yield the dictum, 'music makes you smarter'. But passive listening to music, a ubiquitous activity, bears little resemblance to formal training, which involves lessons and systematic practice (see also Ref. 7). Thus, separate evaluation of the short-term benefits of musical exposure and the long-term side effects of music lessons could help to clarify the issues.

Examination of the effects of previous experience on learning and behaviour has a rich tradition in the history of psychology. 'The *transfer* of training from old to new situations is part and parcel of most, if not all, learning. In this sense the study of transfer is coextensive with the investigation of learning'[8] (p. 1019, emphasis added). In addition, hundreds of psychological examinations of *priming* have investigated how prior exposure to a stimulus affects subsequent processing of the same stimulus or a closely related stimulus.[9,10] If exposure to music causes welcome side effects, we would expect such effects to arise from transfer or priming. Moreover, some researchers who argue for the nonmusical benefits of exposure posit a specific neuropsychological basis for such benefits.[2,11–13] Presumably, this hypothesized cortical process would be compatible with other cortical processes that are demonstrably relevant to music.

Transfer and priming

Transfer and priming occur in positive and negative forms. Positive transfer occurs when previous experience in problem solving makes it easier to solve a new problem,[8,14] typically by accelerating learning. As such, positive transfer describes successful generalization of a process or strategy. One example involves reasoning with analogies.[15] Previous exposure to analogies (e.g. *Lawyer* is to *client* as *doctor* is to ????; the correct answer is *patient*) can lead to greater success at finding the missing piece in new analogies. Similar research is available on metaphor and the transfer of skills.[14] A common theme across transfer effects is *similarity*;[14,16] positive transfer is more likely to occur when there are more similarities between the old and new problems.

Negative transfer is the opposite of its positive counterpart; previous experience interferes with solving a new problem.[8] Negative transfer, which is often called *interference*, can occur proactively or retroactively. Proactive interference is evident when previous learning makes subsequent learning relatively difficult. For example, a new problem is approached with an old mental set that is inefficient or inappropriate for the new context. By contrast, retroactive interference refers to difficulty accessing mental representations because of intervening experience between initial encoding and retrieval.

Roughly speaking, priming can be considered the 'short term' or 'low level' relative of transfer. Anderson[17] defines priming as 'an enhancement of the processing of a stimulus as a function of prior exposure' (p. 459). In a classic experiment,[18] participants were asked to identify words presented briefly in the visual modality. Performance was superior for words that were seen prior to the word-identification test. The 'low level' nature of this sort of priming is evident in greater priming effects following open-ended instructions (e.g. study the word) compared to compulsory semantic processing (e.g. generate an antonym), the latter condition involving 'deeper' levels of processing.[19] It is clear that priming does not require conscious awareness, as reflected in the priming effects observed in amnesics.[20]

Negative priming refers to situations in which the processing of a 'target' stimulus is *inhibited* by prior exposure.[21] For example, when participants are presented with two words (a 'target' and a 'distractor') and required to name only one (the target), performance on subsequent trials is relatively slow when the target word was previously a distractor. Most priming studies examine *repetition* priming, or subsequent processing of an identical stimulus.[10] Nonetheless, cross-modal and cross-language priming effects are also observable. For people who are bilingual in Spanish–English, auditory presentation of a partial sentence in Spanish (the priming stimulus) can facilitate visual recognition of a target English word, provided that the target was implied by the sentential prime.[22] There are higher level, *associative*[17] or *semantic*[9] priming effects, in which word processing (e.g. 'butter') is facilitated by previous presentation of an associated word (e.g. 'bread').[23]

This brief review of transfer and priming provides a context for evaluating specific claims about exposure to music. These claims posit remarkable positive side effects of exposure to certain types of music, side effects that, in principle, are closely related to transfer and priming. My intention is to situate claims that *music makes you smarter* in the context of cognitive psychology, which will permit a review and evaluation of such claims with reference to well established cognitive phenomena. A secondary goal is to situate the neuronal mechanism advanced as the basis of associations between music and nonmusical abilities in the domain of cognitive neuropsychology.

The Mozart effect

The current debate about musical exposure and its side effects was inspired, in part, by Rauscher *et al.*[24] who reported that brief exposure (10 min) to a Mozart sonata generates short term increases in spatial-reasoning abilities (the *Mozart effect*). Each participant in their study was tested in three conditions. Participants in one condition listened to a Mozart sonata before completing three tests of spatial abilities. Participants in the other two conditions listened to a relaxation tape or sat in silence before completing the tests. Performance on the first spatial test (but not the next two) was superior in the 'Mozart' condition. This finding attracted considerable attention because it appeared in a highly prestigious journal, *Nature*, and because the investigators translated their finding into an IQ-score improvement of approximately eight points (i.e. half a standard deviation). Indeed, the popular conclusion that 'music makes you smarter' followed directly from this IQ translation.

Closer examination of the method of Rauscher *et al.*[24] raises questions about the validity of their findings. The choice of comparison conditions is particularly problematic. Sitting in silence or listening to a relaxation tape for 10 min is less arousing or interesting compared to listening to Mozart. Moreover, mood-states are known to influence performance on problem-solving tasks, with superior performance associated with positive affect.[25–27] Thus, the effect could have arisen from differences in arousal or mood rather than from exposure to Mozart.

Because the Mozart effect is at odds with the literature on priming and transfer, alternative explanations of the source of the effect (i.e. the arousal/mood hypothesis) seem all the more credible. Improved spatial skills following exposure to a Mozart sonata do not represent an instance of repetition priming (i.e. the priming stimulus was not repeated). Nor are they an instance of associative priming. How is passive listening to a musical stimulus 'associated' with performance on a visually presented test of spatial skills? Evidence for associative priming typically involves pairs of words with an obvious semantic association (nurse–doctor, bread–butter). How, then, could an auditory (musical) stimulus prime performance on a task with no obvious link to music? Transfer as an explanatory framework also raises more questions than it answers. Transfer typically involves applying a learned skill or strategy to a new context. But what is learned by listening passively to a piece of music? Something about the music, no doubt, but it is difficult to rationalize how the transfer of such knowledge could yield improved performance on a spatial task.

In short, the Mozart effect is a radical claim about cognitive processes that is difficult to reconcile with known principles and findings in cognitive psychology. It comes as no surprise, then, that attempted replications have produced mixed results (for reviews see Refs 11, 28–30). Although many published studies have failed to replicate the effect, a meta-analysis that included some unpublished studies concluded that the effect was moderate but robust.[29] Because the Mozart effect studies have been reviewed elsewhere, the present report focuses on the issues raised by selected studies.

Consider the replication reported by Rauscher *et al.*,[13] who pretested their participants with a Paper-Folding-and-Cutting (PF&C) test (one of the spatial tests used in the original study). Participants were then divided into three groups of equivalent abilities. One group heard Mozart during three subsequent test sessions. A second group sat in silence during the three sessions. A third group heard a minimalist piece by Philip Glass during the first session, an audio-taped story in the second session, and a repetitive piece of dance music in the third session. After each session, the PF&C test was administered again. Although the Mozart group showed a significantly larger improvement in performance than did the other two groups after the first session, there was no difference between the Mozart and comparison groups after the next two sessions. The advantage of Mozart over silence and Glass conditions in the first test session did not extend or clarify the original finding. Participants may find repetitive, minimalist music as boring or unarousing as silence. The null findings in the second and third sessions also raise doubts about the reliability of the effect.

Rauscher[11,31] suggests that the numerous replication failures can be explained primarily by differences in the spatial tasks that have been used as outcome measures. She claims that the effect can be obtained with 'spatial-temporal' tasks (e.g. the PF&C task and other tasks involving mental transformation of visual images), but not with 'spatial-recognition' tasks. This distinction is based on the idea that perceiving and remembering music involves identifying changes and systematic transformations in musical patterns (e.g. motives) that occur over time. Thus, 'transfer' from music listening to the spatial domain should be limited to tasks involving mental manipulation of visual images, which also takes time. Indeed, the time required is linearly related to the amount of manipulation.[32] This distinction is curious in light of the original findings,[24] which indicated that the effect was identical across spatial tasks, temporal or otherwise. In a subsequent reanalysis of the original data,[11] however, the advantage of the Mozart effect proved to be significant on only one of the three spatial tests that were administered, the 'temporal' PF&C task, but not on the two nontemporal tests. Nonetheless, mean scores were highest in the Mozart condition across tests, and the design precluded tests of the two-way interaction between the listening conditions and the spatial tests. In other words, despite their conclusion and interpretation, the data did not support Rauscher's hypothesis (i.e. that the influence of Mozart's music on spatial abilities depends on the temporal nature of the tasks). Moreover, the temporal/nontemporal distinction cannot explain why several attempts to replicate the original findings failed to do so, even though the outcome measure was a task that met Rauscher's criteria for spatial-temporal status.[33–35] Finally, the distinction does not address the problem that the effect, when evident, may be a consequence of differences in arousal or mood.

In *all* cases in which the Mozart effect has been evident, comparison conditions involved repetitive music, sitting in silence, or listening to relaxation tapes. As noted, these comparison conditions might seem boring to participants (compared to listening to music), promoting relatively low levels of cognitive arousal or negative mood states. As a first attempt to address this possibility, Nantais and Schellenberg[36] replicated and extended the original findings. In their first experiment, each participant was tested on the PF&C task twice, once after listening to 10 min of music and once after sitting in silence for 10 min. For some participants, the music was the same Mozart piece used by Rauscher and her colleagues. For others, a piece by Schubert (from the same compact disk as the Mozart piece, performed by the same pianists) was used instead. This experiment was also the first to use a computer-controlled procedure administered to participants individually. Indeed, the potential impact of group dynamics on the results of earlier studies is unknown.[13,24,33,35,37] (Imagine a classroom of undergraduates being required to sit in silence for 10 min!)

As shown in Figure 28.1 (upper left panel), performance on the PF&C test was better after listening to Mozart than after sitting in silence. In other words, the Mozart effect was

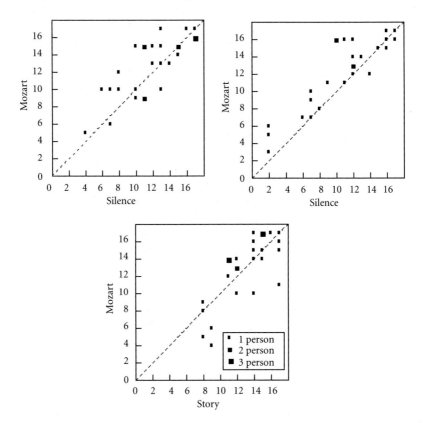

Figure 28.1 Scores on the paper-folding-and-cutting task for participants tested by Nantais and Schellenberg.[36] Each participant was tested twice. The upper left panel illustrates scores after listening to Mozart or sitting in silence. A piece by Schubert was used instead of Mozart for other participants (upper right panel). A third group was tested after listening to either Mozart or a narrated story (lower panel). The line on the diagonal represents equivalent performance across conditions.

replicated. Nonetheless, an identical effect was evident when the Mozart composition was substituted with the piece by Schubert (Figure 28.1, upper right panel). One would predict such a 'Schubert effect' if the comparison condition (silence) was depressing levels of performance. For both groups, performance also improved from the first to the second testing session, revealing a simple practice effect. In a second experiment, a Mozart condition was contrasted with a comparison condition that involved listening to a narrated short story (potentially as engaging as listening to music) instead of sitting in silence. The Mozart effect disappeared (Figure 28.1, lower panel), as one would predict if the experimental (Mozart) and comparison (story) conditions were equally engaging, and if the source of the Mozart effect stemmed from differences in arousal or mood. Perhaps even more important was the finding that performance interacted with listeners' preferences. Those who preferred Mozart over the story performed better on the PF&C test after listening to Mozart. Those who preferred the story performed better after listening to the story (Figure 28.2). These findings provide support for the suggestion that short-term effects of music on tests of spatial abilities stem from differences in arousal or mood rather than from listening to Mozart. Although the figure implies that participants who preferred Mozart performed better regardless of condition, the main effect of preference was marginal ($p = 0.09$).

Further support for the 'arousal or mood' hypothesis comes from a meta-analysis of 20 Mozart-silence comparisons.[28] Successful replications of the Mozart effect were attributed to cognitive arousal, which is predominantly a right-hemisphere function,[38–40] as are tests of complex spatial abilities.[40,41] This view helps to explain why the Mozart effect tends to be slightly larger when the control condition consists of relaxation instructions, which are designed to reduce arousal, instead of sitting in silence.[28]

Another way to interpret the Mozart effect is provided by a new theory based on a large body of findings on the association between mood and cognition.[42] The theory proposes that positive mood states increase circulating levels of the neurotransmitter dopamine.

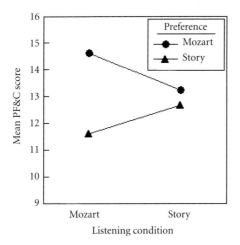

Figure 28.2 Paper-folding-and-cutting (PF&C) scores from Nantais and Schellenberg's[36] participants as a function of testing condition (Mozart or story) and preference (Mozart or story).

During periods of positive affect, dopamine is released from the ventral tegmental area, which has projections to the prefrontal cortex. A variety of cognitive tasks that show improvement when positive affect is induced[26] may be influenced by the effects of dopamine on prefrontal function. It is possible, then, that the Mozart effect is another way in which positive affect influences performance in a problem-solving task. In short, although the seemingly mysterious Mozart effect may indeed have a neuropsychological explanation, listening to music is just one of many ways to induce arousal or positive affect.

The meta-analysis presented by Chabris[28] and the results of Nantais and Schellenberg[36] are consistent with the idea that differences in arousal or mood are the actual source of the Mozart effect, but neither report tested this hypothesis directly. Thompson, Schellenberg, and Husain[43] attempted such a test using the PF&C task as their outcome measure. Each of their participants was tested once in a music condition and once in a silence condition (as in, Ref. 36, Experiment 1). Arousal and mood were measured after listening to the music using the Profile of Mood States[44] and a subjective rating scale. Participants were also asked to rate how much they enjoyed the music. For some participants, the music condition consisted of the same Mozart piece used in the original Mozart-effect study; for others, a piece by Albinoni was used instead. Albinoni's 'Adagio' was selected because it is considered to be a stereotypical example of slow, sad-sounding music.[45] By contrast, the Mozart sonata is pleasant and happy sounding. Hence, the prediction was that increases in performance on the PF&C task would be evident for music compared to silence in the Mozart group but not in the Albinoni group.

This prediction was upheld by the data. As shown in Figure 28.3, the Mozart group showed a robust improvement in PF&C scores after listening to Mozart compared to sitting in silence. By contrast, the Albinoni group performed more-or-less identically in the music and silence conditions. More importantly, the advantage of the music over the

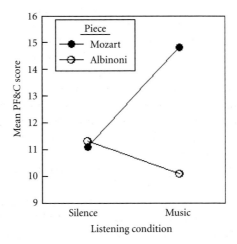

Figure 28.3 Scores on the paper-folding-and-cutting (PF&C) task for participants tested by Thompson *et al.*[43] Each participant was tested twice, once after listening to music and once after sitting in silence. For some participants, the musical piece was the Mozart sonata used by Rauscher *et al.*[24] For others, it was Albinoni's Adagio.

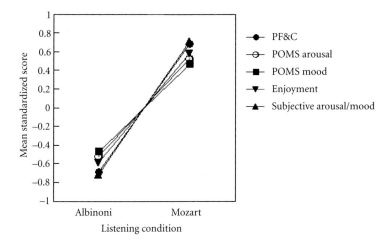

Figure 28.4 Standardized scores for Thompson *et al.*'s[43] participants after listening to a piece composed by Mozart or a piece composed by Albinoni. The variables include the paper-folding-and-cutting (PF&C) task, two subscales from the Profile of Mood States that measured arousal and mood, enjoyment ratings, and a subjective measure of arousal and mood.

silence condition in the Mozart group disappeared when the arousal, mood, or enjoyment variables were held constant. As shown in Figure 28.4, differences between the Mozart and Albinoni conditions on the post-test measures of arousal, mood, and enjoyment were virtually identical to between-condition differences in performance on the PF&C task. In short, the results were completely consistent with the notion that the Mozart effect is an epiphenomenon of arousal or mood.

The theoretical framework that Rauscher and her colleagues use to explain the Mozart effect is called the 'Trion model'.[46,47] The model states that specific cortical firing patterns are present over large areas of the cortex when one performs, composes, or listens to music. Because these patterns are considered to be spatial-temporal in nature, they are said to be highly similar to patterns evident during spatial-temporal reasoning. Both processes involve perceiving and thinking about rule-governed transformations that occur over time. The model describes more than a simple associative or connectionist network, in which one group of neurons is connected to another group. Rather, it posits actual similarities in cortical firing patterns for (1) passive listening to music and (2) actively participating in a task requiring spatial-temporal reasoning.

If we examine the neuropsychological research on music processing, however, the basic tenets of the Trion model seem implausible. The research of Peretz and her colleagues is particularly relevant. Peretz has shown that much of music perception and cognition is relatively modular, and, moreover, that individual aspects of music cognition are relatively modularized and independent of other aspects.[48] For example, melody and rhythm are processed independently and in different parts of the brain,[49–51] lyrics are processed independently of tunes[52] and perceiving musical emotion is independent of memory for music.[53,54] Most importantly, Peretz has studied brain-damaged patients with amusia and none has exhibited accompanying deficits in spatial abilities. For example, one of her amusic patients could not discriminate tones that differed by gross differences in pitch yet she continued to drive safely around Montréal. In short, there is substantial evidence for modularity of music processing and for independence of various aspects of music. Such evidence is inconsistent with the notion that cortical activity is similar across a variety of musical activities (performing, composing, and listening), and that such patterns of activation are identical during spatial-temporal reasoning.

Long-term side-effects of music lessons

Although the short-term Mozart effect appears to be independent of Mozart in particular and of music in general, it is still possible that positive, relatively long-term cognitive side effects result from taking music lessons. Indeed, the two issues may be orthogonal. To anticipate the conclusion, the relevant findings reviewed below are consistent with the idea of an association between musical training and nonmusical benefits (see also Ref. 7), but they fall far short of being conclusive.

Musical abilities and nonmusical abilities   Several studies have examined whether musical *ability* (rather than musical *training*) is correlated with other kinds of abilities. Positive associations imply that improving one's musical ability through formal lessons would be accompanied by nonmusical benefits. In correlational designs, however, it is always impossible to make firm conclusions about the direction of causation when associations are discovered. It is also impossible to rule out the possibility that the association stems from a third, unidentified variable.

Gromko and Poorman[55] examined children between the ages of 4 and 13 who were enrolled in a private school. Their goal was to determine whether musical aptitude is related to children's ability to use symbols. In an initial testing session, children completed the tonal subtest of Gordon's[56,57] musical aptitude measures. During a second session, children were tested on two tasks, one that required them to match short melodies with graphic representations and another that required them to draw graphic representations of the contour of short melodies. Performance on all three measures improved with age, and each measure was significantly correlated with the other two. These findings confirm that children's musical aptitude is predictive of their ability to interpret and produce symbolic representations of music. Because each of the outcomes was associated with age, however, it is impossible to determine whether the associations would still be in evidence if differences in age were held constant (i.e. the authors did not report partial correlations).

In an examination of performance on musical and spatial tasks that required analogical reasoning, children from 6 to 12 years of age were tested on their ability to transfer a given relation between one pair of stimuli to a novel pair.[58] As the age of the children increased, performance on both tasks improved. Moreover, age-related improvements were virtually identical across tasks. As with the study by Gromko and Poorman,[55] however, the association between the music and spatial tasks could be a consequence of the fact that older children performed better on both tasks.

Lamb and Gregory[59] studied the association between reading and musical abilities in a sample of 5-year-old children. Reading abilities and phonemic awareness were positively associated with pitch-discrimination abilities but not with the ability to discriminate timbres. These associations remained in evidence when differences in age and nonverbal intelligence were held constant. Virtually identical associations between reading abilities and musical abilities (with differences in age and IQ held constant) were reported for a sample of 9-year-old children.[60] Although these findings do not address the issue of causation, they provide evidence of an association between reading and musical abilities that is independent of age or general intelligence.

Douglas and Willatts[61] tested a sample of 8-year-olds to examine whether literacy and musical ability are associated. Pairs of tones were presented in a pitch-discrimination task that required children to identify whether the second tone was higher, lower, or the same as the first. A rhythm-discrimination test required children to respond 'same' or 'different' to pairs of sequences played on a wood block. Literacy was measured with tests of reading and spelling. All measures showed significant pairwise correlations. When differences in receptive vocabulary were held constant, however, reading and spelling measures were associated with rhythm-discrimination abilities but not with pitch-discrimination abilities. Whereas these findings suggest that rhythm-discrimination abilities are better than pitch-discrimination abilities at predicting literacy, the results of Lamb and Gregory[59] imply that pitch-discrimination abilities are a better predictor than timbre-discrimination abilities.

Finally, Lynn, Wilson, and Gault[63] examined the association between musical aptitude and general intelligence (Spearman's g) in groups of children 10 years of age. Children were administered rhythm- and pitch-discrimination tasks as well as tests of general intelligence. Each of the music measures was positively associated with each of the measures of intelligence. These results suggest that musical aptitude is a function of general intelligence. Alternatively, musical aptitude may be a valid estimate of g. Although the association between musical *aptitude* and intelligence is provocative, it remains to be seen whether music *lessons* actually promote improvements in cognitive abilities.

Music lessons and nonmusical abilities: correlational and quasiexperimental studies   Other researchers have tested the possibility that music lessons are associated with nonmusical abilities. Again, because we can never be sure that those with and without musical training are identical on other potentially relevant dimensions (e.g. socioeconomic status and overall IQ), unequivocal determinations of causation are impossible.

A classic example of a relevant quasiexperiment is Chan, Ho, and Cheung's[62] study of female college students in Hong Kong (mean age of 20 years). The authors compared the verbal and visual memory abilities of women with no musical training to those of women who had taken 6 years of music lessons before the age of 12. Although the groups did not differ on the visual-memory task, the musically trained group outperformed the untrained group on the verbal-memory task. Unfortunately, despite the authors' claim that the groups were matched according to years of education (with alpha = 0.01), closer inspection of the findings revealed that the musically trained group had significantly more education (with alpha set to a standard 0.05 value). In other words, it is impossible to determine whether the verbal advantage stemmed from music lessons rather than from additional years of education. Indeed, we would predict better verbal skills to accompany higher levels of education.

Hassler, Birbaumer, and Feil[64] examined verbal fluency and visual-spatial abilities in children 9–14 years of age, some of whom were taking music lessons. The children were classified into one of three groups: (1) musically talented and capable of composing or improvising, (2) musically talented but not capable of composing or improvising, or (3) nonmusicians. The groups did not differ on a test of spatial relations, but significant differences were found on tests of verbal fluency and visualization abilities, with the musically talented children outperforming the nonmusicians. At a follow-up test two years later, significant differences were found for each of the three outcome variables.[65] Nonetheless, students in the composing/improvising group had more music lessons than the other musically talented group, yet no differences between these groups on the outcome measures were evident. As such, this study provides equivocal support for the idea that music lessons are accompanied by advantages in nonmusical domains.

Two studies compared the nonmusical abilities of children enrolled in a Kodály music program with those of a comparison group who were not taking music lessons.[66,67] The Kodály program is known for intensive training and placing great emphasis on singing and the development of sequential skills. The program also incorporates clapping, the use of hand signs, and simple musical notation. Hurwitz and his colleagues examined the sequencing and spatial skills of a group of 7-year-olds. Children in the Kodály group had taken music lessons for approximately 7 months, with 40-minute lessons 5 days per week. The sequencing task involved tapping mechanical keys in a regular manner, or in time with a metronome after the metronome was turned off or its rate had been changed. Children were also given tests of spatial abilities, plus a Stroop-like test of interference. The Kodály group outperformed the comparison children on the Stroop test and on some of the spatial tests. In a separate examination of children who had completed 1 year of Kodály instruction, the Kodály group performed better than a comparison group on a reading test even though the two groups had performed identically a year earlier. A subsequent study of 4- and 5-year-olds' understanding of prenumber concepts showed a benefit of Kodály training only for 5-year-old girls.[67] These results suggest that training in music may lead to nonmusical improvements, yet it is impossible to ascertain whether nonmusical aspects of Kodály training or preexisting differences between groups may have influenced the results.

Schellenberg[68] used a correlational approach to examine whether music lessons are predictive of intellectual development in a group of 147 children ranging in age from 6 to 11 years. The outcome measure was a standard IQ test (Wechsler Intelligence Scale for Children—Third Edition). His approach is noteworthy because he also measured three variables that are likely to be confounded with music lessons: socioeconomic status (measured as family income), parental education (which would be correlated with parental IQ), and time spent in nonmusical extra-curricular activities. Of the four variables he measured, music lessons had the strongest association with IQ ($r = 0.38$, $p < 0.0001$). The data are illustrated in Figure 28.5. Moreover, when the other three potentially confounding variables were held constant, the partial association between music lessons and IQ remained significant. Although these findings are consistent with the proposal that music lessons confer nonmusical benefits, it is impossible to rule out two alternative explanations: (1) children with higher IQs may be more likely to take music lessons, and (2) an as-yet-unidentified variable could be influencing IQ *and* the likelihood of taking music lessons.

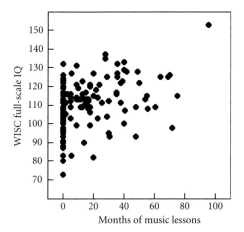

Figure 28.5   IQ scores from children tested by Schellenberg[68] as a function of months of music lessons.

Music lessons and nonmusical abilities: experimental studies   The next group of studies had more-or-less random assignment of participants to experimental conditions. Thus, provided that comparison conditions were selected appropriately, we should be able to determine whether music lessons actually 'cause' nonmusical cognitive advantages. As with most of the short-term (Mozart effect) studies, however, none of the studies in this group used comparison conditions that preclude the possibility of alternative explanations for the findings.

For example, 6-year-old children who were taught music for 7 months by means of the Kodály method showed improvements in mathematical and reading abilities that surpassed those of children without such training.[69] The researchers' goal was to examine possible by-products of a 'test arts' (Kodály) program that was implemented in some first-grade classes but not in others. They examined two first-grade classes in each of two schools that were designated as 'test arts' classrooms, and another two from both schools that were 'standard arts' classrooms. If we assume that the classrooms were assigned to the two arts programs at random, we can consider the design to approximate a 'true' experiment. The reported advantage for the test-arts classes is remarkable when we consider that in the previous year, children in the test-arts classes were actually *behind* the standard-arts children in terms of the proportion who had reached the national average grade level. Although these results are promising, children in the standard-arts classrooms did not participate in activities focusing on 'sequenced skill development' as did children in the test-arts (Kodály) classrooms. Again, this confounding makes it impossible to attribute the remarkable recovery and achievements of the test-arts classrooms to training in music per se, rather than to other nonmusical aspects of the Kodály program.

In another study, 4-year-old children who received individual 10-min piano lessons once or twice a week for 6–8 months performed better on a test of spatial skills than children assigned to comparison conditions.[12] Nonetheless, other aspects of the design question the reliability of the effect. For example, some of the children had 33 per cent more lessons than other children, yet this additional training in music had no effect on performance. Moreover, the primary comparison condition involved playing with commercial software programs on a computer. Although a computer instructor provided one-on-one instruction about how to use the computer and open the programs, the software (not the instructor) was designed to teach the children basic skills in reading and arithmetic. As such, superior levels of performance in the piano group could be the consequence of additional instruction from an adult.

Standley and Hughes[70] found that children in prekindergarten classes (4–5 years of age) who took 15 music lessons over a period of 2 months showed enhanced prereading and writing skills compared to other children. Children in the comparison condition were exposed to the regular prekindergarten curriculum but had no additional lessons of any kind. Again, it is impossible to determine whether the observed numerical and verbal benefits arose specifically from music instruction or from pedagogical differences that were independent of musical training. The investigators noted that 'it was also apparent from the children's reaction that the music activities provided pleasure and excitement about academic participation, possibly generating long range motivation for reading and writing' (p. 83). Nonmusical activities that generate similar levels of pleasure and excitement could generate similar increases in motivation.

Gromko and Poorman's[55,71] study of 3- and 4-year-old children enrolled in a private Montessori school is similar to Standley and Hughes'[70] study described above. Children in the music group were provided with weekly group music lessons in addition to the regular curriculum, but the comparison group received no additional lessons of any sort. As such, the modest gains in nonverbal IQ witnessed for the music group relative to the comparison group can be attributed simply to additional educational instruction from an adult.

Three recent experimental studies suffer from similar methodological problems. Each compared young children enrolled in music-education programs with children in 'control' groups who had no comparable extraschool activities.[72–74] One study provided 3 years of piano lessons free of charge to children in the fourth to sixth grade.[73] These 'piano' children performed better than children in a control group on a comprehensive test of cognitive abilities after the first and second years, but the difference disappeared after the third year. Between-group differences during the first 2 years stemmed solely from differences in spatial abilities. In another study, kindergartners were provided with group keyboard lessons for 8 months.[74] The keyboard children showed greater improvement than a control group on tests of spatial abilities, but there was no difference between groups on a test of recognition. A third study examined the influence of a 30-week structured music curriculum on cognitive development.[72] Treatment and control groups of 6-year-olds were administered six subtests from the Stanford-Binet Intelligence Test before and after the curriculum. The treatment group showed relatively larger gains on a single subtest that measured capacity of short-term memory (Bead Memory).

Another recent study examined possible side-effects of group keyboard lessons that were provided free of charge to children 6–8 years of age.[75] A control group had computer lessons with a commercial software program designed to improve English-language skills. Both groups were also given lessons intended to enhance spatial abilities by playing with a software program designed by the researchers. Unfortunately, the main outcome variable consisted of scores on a testing version of the same spatial software, which has unknown reliability and validity. Moreover, aggregate scores on the outcome tests did not differ between groups. The investigators reported a significant advantage for the keyboard group on a subtest of mathematical fractions and proportions, and they concluded that improved musical and spatial skills lead to improved mathematical abilities. These results would be more convincing if they had been obtained with standardized tests, and if the piano group had performed better overall, or at least on subtests for which clear predictions were made a priori.

In an initial attempt to rectify some of the shortcomings of earlier experiments, Thompson, Schellenberg, and Husain[76] tested whether music lessons influence children's ability to interpret the emotions expressed by nonlinguistic cues (i.e. *prosody*) in speech. Six-year-olds were assigned randomly to a year of music lessons, a year of drama lessons, or no lessons. After the lessons were completed, the children were tested on their ability to label the emotion (happy, sad, fearful, or angry) conveyed by semantically neutral sentences spoken in English (e.g. *the chair is made of wood*) or in Tagalog, and by tone sequences that mimicked the prosody of the sentences. The children with music lessons performed better than the no-lessons children on these tasks. In fact, their performance was equivalent to children who took drama lessons, which focused specifically on using prosody to convey emotions. A separate test of adult participants suggested that such effects are long-lasting. Specifically, adults who started music lessons during childhood performed better on prosody-decoding tasks than did adults with no musical training.

The studies just reviewed provide consistent *suggestive* evidence that music lessons have positive nonmusical side effects. Nonetheless, specifics of the reported associations vary widely from study to study. If we suspend our disbelief, however, and assume that music education affects abilities in other areas, how could we account for this influence?

A number of neurological studies describe ways in which music lessons affect cortical development. Compared to nonmusicians, accomplished players of string instruments show increased representation in the cerebral cortex for the fingers of their left hand,[77] which implies that musical training can alter patterns of cortical organization. Indeed, cortical representations are especially large for those who begin music lessons at an early age when the brain is relatively plastic. Although the size of the corpus callosum is larger in musicians than in nonmusicians, this effect is particularly notable in musicians who began taking lessons before the age of seven.[78] Relatively large brain asymmetries are also evident among musicians who have absolute (perfect) pitch,[79] and this relatively rare ability to name and produce pitches in isolation is evident predominantly among musicians who begin lessons in early childhood.[80] Moreover, the representation of piano tones in the auditory cortex differs in musicians than in nonmusicians,[81] although genetic factors or simple exposure to music could also play a role.[82] Finally, specific cortical areas in the right hemisphere are activated when reading a musical score but not when reading one's primary or secondary language.[83]

Consequences of an enriched environment on other species (e.g. rats and mice) include denser patterns of dendritic branching and a greater number of hippocampal neurons.[84,85] If music education represents an enrichment of a child's environment, such enrichment could promote neurological development, which could, in turn, influence abilities in other domains. Music, however, is simply one of many ways to enrich a child's environment. Moreover, music education is a complex process that involves many different dimensions.

We know that schooling improves a wide variety of cognitive skills and that this association is not simply a by-product of maturation.[86-89] For young children in particular, schooling is more effective in smaller classes.[90-92] Reviews of intervention programs for children who are at risk of academic failure suggest that extended one-on-one contact with a supportive adult is a common feature of successful interventions.[93,94] Thus, music lessons, which are typically taught individually or in small groups, may confer nonmusical benefits for children by providing close and extended contact with an adult other than a parent or teacher. If this is the case, then similar side effects should be evident with other types of lessons that provide similar levels of contact (e.g. chess, drawing).

Music lessons may be unique, however, because of their focus on a particular combination of factors, such as hours of individual practice, learning to read music, attention and concentration, timing, ear training, sight reading, constructive feedback from the instructor, and exposure to music.[95] Thus, positive transfer effects to nonmusical domains, such as language, mathematics, or spatial reasoning, could be similarly unique for individuals who take music lessons. On the other hand, music lessons are likely to improve many *general* skills, such as the ability to attend to rapidly changing temporal information, skills relevant to auditory stream segregation, the ability to detect temporal groups, sensitivity to signals of closure and other gestalt cues of form, emotional sensitivity and expressiveness, and fine motor skills. These general skills should be particularly likely to transfer to a variety of nonmusical domains.

As someone who took music lessons from the age of five and practised regularly for the next 11 years, I feel changed—probably for the better—in ways that seem specific to my involvement with music. It remains to be seen, however, whether this personal observation will withstand the test of rigorous experimental investigation.

Acknowledgements

Preparation of this article was supported by a grant from the International Foundation for Music Research. Bill Thompson and Sandra Trehub provided helpful comments on an earlier draft.

References

1. **Kolata, G.** (8 August 1999). Muddling fact and fiction and policy. *New York Times* WK5.
2. **Shaw, G. L.** (2000) *Keeping Mozart in Mind.* San Diego: Academic Press.
3. **Calamai, P.** (26 August 1999) Mozart theory creates discord in the scientific community. *Toronto Star* A28.
4. **Ingram, J.** (11 May 1997) More proof music lifts young IQs. *The Toronto Star* F8.
5. **Martin, S.** (October, 1994) Music lessons enhance spatial reasoning skills. *APA Monitor* 5.
6. **Motchuk, A.** (15 March 1997) Can Mozart make maths add up? *New Scientist* 17.

7. **Hetland, L.** (2000) Learning to make music enhances spatial reasoning. *J. Aesthetic Education* 34(3/4), 179–238.

8. **Postman, L.** (1971) Transfer, interference and forgetting. In J. W. Kling and L. A. Riggs (eds) *Woodworth and Schlosberg's Experimental Psychology*, 3rd edn. New York: Holt, Rinehart and Winston, pp. 1019–32.

9. **Neely, J. H.** (1991) Semantic priming effects in visual word recognition: a selective review of current findings and theories. In D. Besner and G. W. Humphreys (eds) *Basic Processes in Reading: Visual Word Recognition* Hillsdale, NJ: Erlbaum, pp. 264–336.

10. **Tulving, E. and D. L. Schachter** (1990) Priming and human memory systems. *Science* 247, 301–6.

11. **Rauscher, F. H. and G. L. Shaw** (1998) Key components of the Mozart effect. *Perceptual and Motor Skills* 86, 835–41.

12. **Rauscher, F. H., G. L. Shaw, L. J. Levine, E. L. Wright, W. R. Dennis,** and **R. L. Newcomb** (1997) Music training causes long-term enhancement of preschool children's spatial-temporal reasoning. *Neurol. Res.* 19, 2–8.

13. **Rauscher, F. H., G. L. Shaw,** and **K. N. Ky** (1995) Listening to Mozart enhances spatial-temporal reasoning: towards a neurophysiological basis. *Neurosci. Lett.* 185, 44–7.

14. **Robins, A.** (1996) Transfer in cognition. *Connection Science*, 8, 185–203.

15. **Gick, M. L. and K. J. Holyoak,** (1983) Schema induction and analogical transfer. *Cognitive Psychol.* 15, 1–38.

16. **Gentner, D., M. J. Ratterman,** and **K. D. Forbus** (1993) The roles of similarity in transfer: separating retrievability from inferential soundness. *Cognitive Psychol.* 25, 524–75.

17. **Anderson, J. R.** (1995) *Cognitive Psychology and its Implications*, 4th edn. New York: Freeman.

18. **Jacoby, L. L.** (1983) Perceptual enhancement: persistent effects of experience. *J. Exp. Psychol.: Learning, Memory, Cognit.* 9, 21–38.

19. **Craik, F. I. M. and R. S. Lockhart** (1972) Levels of processing: a framework for memory research. *J. Verbal Learning Verbal Behav.* 11, 671–84.

20. **Graf, P., L. R. Squire,** and **G. Mandler** (1984) The information that amnesic patients do not forget. *J. Exp. Psychol.: Learning, Memory, Cognit.* 10, 164–78.

21. **May, C. P., M. J. Kane,** and **L. Hasher** (1995) Determinants of negative priming. *Psychological Bulletin* 118, 35–54.

22. **Hernandez, A. E., E. A. Bates,** and **L. X. Avila** (1996) Processing across the language boundary: a cross-modal priming study of Spanish-English bilinguals. *J. Exp. Psychol.: Learning, Memory, Cognit.* 22, 846–64.

23. **Meyer, D. E. and R. W. Schvaneveldt** (1971) Facilitation in recognizing pairs of words: evidence of a dependence between retrieval operations. *J. Exp. Psychol.* 90, 227–34.

24. **Rauscher, F. H., G. L. Shaw,** and **K. N. Ky** (1993) Music and spatial task performance. *Nature* 365, 611.

25. **Benedict, R. H. B., M. Dobraski,** and **M. Z. Goldstein** (1999) A preliminary study of the association between changes in mood and cognition in a mixed geriatric psychiatry sample. *J. Gerontology* 54B, 94–9.

26. **Isen, A. M.** (1999) Positive affect. In T. Dalgleish and M. Power (eds) *The Handbook of Cognition and Emotion*. New York: Wiley, pp. 521–39.

27. **O'Hanlon, J. F.** (1981) Boredom: practical consequences and a theory. *Acta Psychologica* 49, 53–82.

28. Chabris, C. F. (1999) Prelude or requiem for the 'Mozart effect'? *Nature* 400, 826–7.

29. Hetland, L. (2000) Listening to music enhances spatial-temporal reasoning: evidence for the "Mozart effect". *J. Aesthetic Education* 34(3/4), 105–48.

30. Jenkins, J. S. (2001) The Mozart effect. *J. Royal Society of Medicine* 94, 170–2.

31. Rauscher, F. H. (1999) Prelude or requiem for the 'Mozart effect'? *Nature* 400, 827–28.

32. Shepard, R. and J. Metzler (1971) Mental rotation of three-dimensional objects. *Science* 171, 701–3.

33. Steele, K. M., K. E. Bass, and M. D. Crook (1999) The mystery of the Mozart effect: failure to replicate. *Psychol. Sci.* 10, 366–9.

34. Steele, K. M., K. M. Brown, and J. A. Stoecker (1999) Failure to confirm the Rauscher and Shaw description of recovery of the Mozart effect. *Perceptual and Motor Skills* 88, 843–8.

35. Steele, K. M., S. Dalla Bella, I. Peretz, T. Dunlop, L. A. Dawe, G. K. Humphrey, R. A. Shannon, K. L. Kirby, Jr, and C. G. Olmstead (1999) Prelude or requiem for the 'Mozart effect'? *Nature* 400, 827.

36. Nantais, K. M. and E. G. Schellenberg (1999) The Mozart effect: an artifact of preference. *Psychol. Sci.* 10, 370–3.

37. Steele, K. M., T. N. Ball, and R. Runk (1997) Listening to Mozart does not enhance backwards digit span performance. *Perceptual and Motor Skills* 84, 1179–84.

38. Heller, W. and J. B. Nitschke (1997) Regional brain activity in emotion: a framework for understanding cognition in depression. *Cognit. Emotion* 11, 637–61.

39. Robertson, I. H., J. B. Mattingley, C. Rorden, and J. Driver (1998) Phasic alerting of neglect patients overcomes their spatial deficit in visual awareness. *Nature* 395, 169–72.

40. Tucker, D. M., A. Hartry-Speiser, L. McDougal, P. Luu and D. deGrandpre (1999) Mood and spatial memory: emotion and right hemisphere contribution to spatial cognition. *Biol. Psychol.* 50, 103–25.

41. Ditunno, P. L. and V. A. Mann (1990) Right hemisphere specialization for mental rotation in normals and brain damaged subjects. *Cortex* 26, 177–88.

42. Ashby, F. G., A. M. Isen, and A. U. Turken (1999) A neuropsychological theory of positive affect and its influence on cognition. *Psychol. Rev.* 106, 529–50.

43. Thompson, W. F., E. G. Schellenberg and G. Husain (2001) Arousal, mood, and the Mozart effect. *Psychol. Sci.* 12, 248–51.

44. McNair, D. M., M. Lorr, and L. F. Droppleman (1992) *The Profile of Mood States*, 3rd ed. San Diego: Educational and Industrial Testing Service.

45. Krumhansl, C. L. (1997) An exploratory study of musical emotions and psychophysiology. *Canadian J. Exp. Psychol.* 51, 336–52.

46. Leng, X. and G. L. Shaw (1991) Toward a neural theory of higher brain function using music as a window. *Concepts in Neurosci.* 2, 229–58.

47. Leng, X., G. L. Shaw, and E. L. Wright (1990) Coding of musical structure and the trion model of the cortex. *Music Percept.* 8, 49–62

48. Peretz, I. (2001) Music perception and recognition. In B. Rapp (ed.) *The Handbook of Cognitive Neuropsycho.* Hove, UK: Psychology Press, pp. 521–40.

49. Peretz, I. (1996) Can we lose memories for music? A case of music agnosia in a nonmusician. *J. Cognitive Neurosci.* 8, 481–96.

50. Peretz, I. and R. Kolinsky (1993) Boundaries of separability between melody and rhythm in music discrimination: a neuropsychological perspective. *Quarterly J. Exp. Psychol.* 46A, 301–25.

51. Peretz, I. and J. Morais (1989) Music and modularity. *Contemporary Music Rev.* 4, 277–91.

52. **Besson, M., F. Faïta, I. Peretz, A.-M. Bonnel,** and **J. Requin** (1998) Singing in the brain: independence of lyrics and tunes. *Psychol. Sci.* 9, 494–8.

53. **Peretz, I.** and **L. Gagnon** (1999) Dissociation between recognition and emotional judgements for melodies. *Neurocase* 5, 21–30.

54. **Peretz, I., L. Gagnon,** and **B. Bouchard** (1998) Music and emotion: perceptual determinants, immediacy, and isolation after brain damage. *Cognit.* 68, 111–41.

55. **Gromko, J. E.** and **A. S. Poorman** (1998) Developmental trends and relationships in children's aural perception and symbol use. *J. Res. Music Education* 46, 16–23.

56. **Gordon, E.** (1979) *Primary Measures of Music Audiation.* Chicago: G. I. A. Publications.

57. **Gordon, E.** (1982) *Intermediate Measures of Music Audiation.* Chicago: G. I. A. Publications.

58. **Nelson, D. J.** and **A. L. Barresi** (1989) Children's age-related intellectual strategies for dealing with musical and spatial analogical tasks. *J. Res. Music Education* 37, 93–103.

59. **Lamb, S. J.** and **A. H. Gregory** (1993) The relationship between music and reading in beginning readers. *Educational Psychol.* 13, 19–27.

60. **Barwick, J., E. Valentine, R. West,** and **J. Wilding** (1989) Relations between reading and musical abilities. *British J. Educational Psychol.* 59, 253–7.

61. **Douglas, S.** and **P. Willatts** (1994) The relationship between musical ability and literacy skills. *J. Res. Reading* 17, 99–107.

62. **Chan, A. S., Y. C. Ho,** and **M. C. Cheung** (1998) Music training improves verbal memory. *Nature* 396, 128.

63. **Lynn, R., R. G. Wilson,** and **A. Gault** (1989) Simple musical tests as measures of Spearman's *g. Personality and Individual Differences* 10, 25–8.

64. **Hassler, M., N. Birbaumer,** and **A. Feil** (1985) Musical talent and visual-spatial ability: a longitudinal study. *Psychol. Music* 13, 99–113.

65. **Hassler, M., N. Birbaumer,** and **A. Feil** (1987) Musical talent and visual-spatial ability: onset of puberty. *Psychol. Music* 15, 141–51.

66. **Hurwitz, I., P. H. Wolff, B. D. Bortnick,** and **K. Kokas** (1975) Nonmusical effects of the Kodály music curriculum in primary grade children. *J. Learning Disabilities* 8, 167–74.

67. **Neufeld, K. A.** (1986) Understanding of selected pre-number concepts: relationships to a formal music program. *Alberta J. Educational Res.* 32, 134–9.

68. **Schellenberg, E. G.** (2003) *Music lessons and IQ.* Paper presented at the biennial meeting of the Society for Research in Child Development, Tampa, FL.

69. **Gardiner, M. F., A. Fox, F. Knowles,** and **D. Jeffrey** (1996) Learning improved by arts training. *Nature* 381, 284.

70. **Standley, J. M.** and **J. E. Hughes** (1997) Evaluation of an early intervention music curriculum for enhancing prereading/writing skills. *Music Therapy Perspectives* 15, 79–85.

71. **Gromko, J. E.** and **A. S. Poorman** (1998) The effect of music training on preschoolers' spatial-temporal task performance. *J. Res. Music Education* 46, 173–81.

72. **Bilhartz, T. D., R. A. Bruhn,** and **J. E. Olson** (2000) The effect of early music training on child cognitive development. *J. Applied Dev. Psychol.* 20, 615–36.

73. **Costa-Giomi, E.** (1999) The effects of three years of piano instruction on children's cognitive development. *J. Res. Music Education* 47, 198–212.

74. **Rauscher, F. H.** and **M. A. Zupan** (2000) Classroom keyboard instruction improves kindergarten children's spatial-temporal performance: a field experiment. *Early Childhood Research Quarterly* 15, 215–28.

75. Graziano, A. B., M. Peterson, and G. L. Shaw (1999) Enhanced learning of proportional math through music training and spatial-temporal reasoning. *Neurol. Res.* 21, 139–52.

76. Thompson, W. F., E. G. Schellenberg, and G. Husain (2002) *Decoding speech prosody: Do music lessons help?* Manuscript under review.

77. Elbert, T., C. Pantev, C. Wienbruch, B. Rockstroh, and E. Taub (1995) Increased cortical representation of the fingers of the left hand in string players. *Science* 270, 305–7.

78. Schlaug, G., L. Jäncke, Y. Huang, J. F. Staiger, and H. Steinmetz (1995) Increased corpus callosum size in musicians. *Neuropsychologia* 33, 1047–55.

79. Schlaug, G., L. Jäncke, Y. Huang, and H. Steinmetz (1995) In vivo evidence of structural brain asymmetry in musicians. *Science*, 267, 699–700.

80. Takeuchi, A. H. and S. H. Hulse (1993) Absolute pitch. *Psychol. Bull.* 113, 345–61.

81. Pantev, C., R. Oostenveld, A. Engelien, B. Ross, L. E. Roberts, and M. Hoke (1998) Increased auditory cortical representation in musicians. *Nature* 392, 811–3.

82. Monaghan, P., N. B. Metcalfe, and G. D. Ruxton (1998) Does practice shape the brain? *Nature* 394, 434.

83. Nakada, T., Y. Fujii, K. Suzuki, and I. Kwee (1998) 'Musical brain' as revealed by highfield (3 tesla) functional MRI. *Neuroreport* 9, 3853–6.

84. Greenough, W. T. and F. R. Volkmar (1973) Pattern of dendritic branching in occipital cortex of rats reared in complex environments. *Exp. Neurol.* 40, 491–504.

85. Kemperman, G., H. G. Kuhn, and F. H. Gage (1997) More hippocampal neurons in adult mice living in an enriched environment. *Nature* 386, 493–5.

86. Ceci, S. J. (1991) How much does schooling influence general intelligence and its cognitive components? A reassessment of the evidence. *Dev. Psychol.* 27, 703–22.

87. Ceci, S. J. and W. M. Williams (1997) Schooling, intelligence, and income. *American Psychologist* 52, 1051–8.

88. Morrison, F. J., E. M. Griffith, and D. M. Alberts (1997) Nature-nurture in the classroom: entrance age, school readiness, and learning in children. *Dev. Psychol.* 33, 254–62.

89. Morrison, F. J., L. Smith, and M. Dow-Ehrensberger (1995) Education and cognitive development: a natural experiment. *Dev. Psychol.* 31, 789–99.

90. Blatchford, P. and P. Mortimore (1994) The issue of class size for young children in schools: what can we learn from research? *Oxford Rev. Education* 20, 411–28.

91. Ehrenberg, R. G., D. J. Brewer, A. Gamoran, and J. D. Willms (2001) Class size and student achievement. *Psychol. Sci. Public Interest* 2, 1–30.

92. Mosteller, F. (1995) The Tennessee study of class size in the early school grades. *Future of Children* 5, 113–27.

93. Barnett, W. S. (1995) Long-term effects of early childhood programs on cognitive and school outcomes. *Future of Children* 5, 25–50.

94. Lazar, I. and R. Darlington (1982) Lasting effects of early education: a report from the consortium for longitudinal studies. *Monographs of the Society for Research in Child Development* 47(2–3), Serial No. 195.

95. Lamont, A. (1998) Responses to Katie Overy's paper: respondent 3. *Psychol. Music* 26, 201–4.

INDEX